The Contact a Family Directory

The essential guide to medical conditions, disabilities and support

2008 edition

Editor: Natalie Ridgway and Sasha Henriques MSc

Researcher: Sasha Henriques MSc

Foreword by Professor Sir Al Aynsley-Green
Children's Commissioner for Engl

GH00702422

cͻntact a family
for families with disabled children

Contact a Family Helpline 0808 808 3555

Published by:
Contact a Family,
209-211 City Road
London EC1V 1JN
United Kingdom

Tel: 020 7608 8700
Fax: 020 7608 8701
Tel: 0808 808 3555 Helpline
Tel: 0808 808 3556 Textphone

e-mail: info@cafamily.org.uk
Web: http://www.cafamily.org.uk

Registered Charity Number 284912
Charity registered in Scotland No. SC039169
Limited Company Number 1633333
VAT Reg No. GB 749 3846 82

Typeset and designed by Natalie Ridgway and Dean Casswell, Contact a Family
Printed by Hobbs the Printers, Hampshire

CONTENTS

New entries/articles for this 2008 edition are denoted with a ■
Entries that have been substantially revised or rewritten are denoted with a ◆

The Contact a Family Directory 2008

Contact a Family Helpline 0808 808 3555

Contact a Family Helpline 0808 808 3555

Contact a Family Helpline 0808 808 3555

FOREWORD

As President of Contact a Family, one of my main areas of interest is disabled children. In my former role of National Clinical Director for Children, I made over three hundred and fifty visits to children's services across the length and breadth of the country. While there is excellent work being done in many areas, one of the major problems I have seen is the lack of understanding of children's needs and children's services in the minds of people who matter. They don't always understand why the needs of children are different from those of adults. In some areas, children are seen as an 'add on' and the services provided for them are not part of the mainstream. Another difficulty is the poor understanding between health, social care and education.

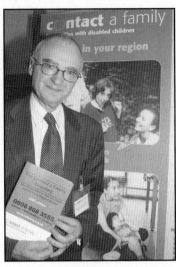

That is why I am delighted that disabled children have been included as one of four local priority groups for service improvement in the NHS in England, through the operating framework announced in December 2007. This is the first time that disabled children have been a priority group for the NHS. This announcement coincided with confirmation that disabled children were also a priority for the Department for Children, Schools and Families in the Children's Plan.

This year, the roll out of extra support for families through the 'Aiming High for Disabled Children' programme will begin from April onwards. Later in 2008, information prescriptions will be given to all adults and children in England with a long-term condition or social care need, in consultation with a health or social care professional. These prescriptions will guide parents to relevant and reliable sources of information to allow them to feel more in control and better able to manage their child's condition. I know how important it is that when a child is diagnosed with a disability, long-term or rare condition, families have access to good quality information. That is why I am delighted to write the foreword to the 2008 Directory, which remains a key of source of help and information for families and those working with them.

Finally, I'd like to say how honoured I am to be President of Contact a Family. I am proud to work with the staff, and I will do my best to help achieve even greater success for children and their families in the future.

Professor Sir Al Aynsley-Green
President, Contact a Family

ACKNOWLEDGMENTS

The Contact a Family Directory is a vital resource for everyone working in the field of child health. We are committed to producing a publication of the highest possible quality, reliability and accuracy. This year we have added a further nine new entries.

There are numerous contributors to the success of The Contact a Family Directory that we must acknowledge. Our first thanks must go to the increasing number of patient and family support organisations who are now featured in The Contact a Family Directory.

We also thank the specialist medical professionals who continue to provide support, guidance and information for individual entries. This includes Professor Michael Patton, Professor of Medical Genetics, St George's Hospital, London and Dr Ed Wraith, Consultant Paediatrician, Royal Manchester Children's Hospital, who have been involved with The Contact a Family Directory from the beginning, along with the other members of Contact a Family's Medical Advisory Panel. We acknowledge individual contributors by listing their names as part of the relevant entry.

Special thanks also go to the Children and Families Directorate within the Department for Children, Schools and Families who support the work of Contact a Family in many ways and who fund the work of our Information Officer who has responsibility for researching The Contact a Family Directory.

Both versions of The Contact a Family Directory continue to thrive - the yearly paper edition and the monthly online version at **www.cafamily.org.uk**. The website has 1.7 million visits per year and is an essential tool for parents and professionals searching for health information on the web. We also have a complimentary website **www.makingcontact.org** which allows families to link in a safe environment.

During 2008, we intend to launch a variety of new features for the online version including links to other reliable sources of information for each condition and message boards for subscribers.

Finally I would like to thank my colleagues Mark Robertson, Sasha Henriques, Louise Derbyshire and Natalie Ridgway who work so hard every year to produce The Contact a Family Directory.

Rosey Foster
Chair
Contact a Family

ABOUT CONTACT A FAMILY

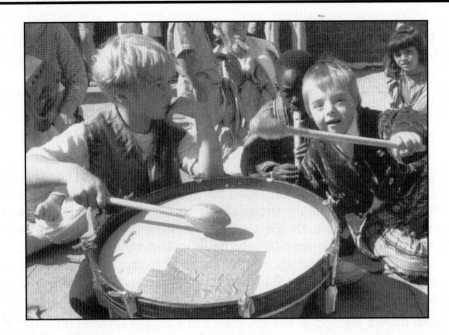

Contact a Family provides advice, information and support to families with disabled children across the UK. This includes children with specific and rare disorders, children who develop acute and long-term health conditions and children with special educational needs.

We give development advice and support to UK-wide groups concerned with specific conditions and rare disorders, many but not all of which are listed in *The Contact a Family Directory*. We also hold details of new support groups in the process of formation.

We provide information, development advice and support to local parent groups and individual parents, anywhere in the UK. This service is provided by experienced staff working from our UK office, national offices, regional offices and local community projects. Contact details for all our offices are given below.

We also run a Family Support Service in different parts of the United Kingdom which enables us to offer one to one support to families caring for a disabled child. For details of where these staff are based please refer to our website or call our helpline.

Between 2004 and 2007 Contact a Family, supported by the Big Lottery, entered into an three year partnership with the Royal College of Paediatrics and Child Health (RCPCH). From this work the UK wide Parents and

Paediatricians Together Project was developed. This project helped paediatricians ensure that parents of disabled children got access to the information and support they need by putting them in touch with Contact a Family. Secondly, it started to create new frameworks for co-operation between parents and paediatricians which helped influence paediatric and child health services across the UK.

Although the Big Lottery part of the project ended in 2007 the project still operates in London funded by the City Bridge Trust. However strands of the work continue in other parts of the UK. Please contact our individual country offices for further details.

We also raise awareness of the issues facing families with disabled children to both central and local government and other policy making bodies.

Our helpline provides a comprehensive advice and information service to parents. Our helpline is staffed by a team of experienced Parent Advisers who provide advice and information on many aspects of the day to day issues that affect families such as welfare benefits; employment rights; immigration advice; sources of grants and charitable funding; services available and how to access them along with details of national and local support groups. This information is supported by a range of factsheets on subjects which include benefits, education rights, community care, holidays, siblings, and living without a diagnosis.

As well as providing information on specific conditions and rare disorders, the Parent Advisers will link families by putting them in touch with UK support groups for specific conditions and local support groups for families of children with any disability or specific health condition. Where no support network exists, particularly in the case of very rare syndromes, the Parent Advisers will try and link families on a one-to-one basis. This service is also available via the Internet from our family linking website **http://www.makingcontact.org**

Contact a Family works in close co-operation with other statutory and voluntary organisations with an interest in disabled children and their families.

Further details of Contact a Family's work are available on our website **http://www.cafamily.org.uk**

If you would like to become involved with Contact a Family or support our work please contact us.

UK office

Contact a Family, 209-211 City Road, London EC1V 1JN
Tel: 0808 808 3555 Helpline (10am-4pm, Mon-Fri and 5.30-7.30pm, Monday)
Textphone: 0808 808 3556   Tel: 020 7608 8700   Fax: 020 7608 8701
e-mail: info@cafamily.org.uk

Contact a Family Helpline 0808 808 3555

Northern Ireland office

Contact a Family Northern Ireland, Bridge Community Centre, 50 Railway Street,
Lisburn BT28 1XP
Tel: 028 9262 7552   e-mail: nireland.office@cafamily.org.uk

Scotland office

Contact a Family Scotland, Craigmillar Social Enterprise and Arts Centre, 11/9 Harewood
Road, Edinburgh EH16 4NT
Tel: 0131 659 2930   e-mail: scotland.office@cafamily.org.uk

Wales office

Contact a Family Cymru, 33-35 Cathedral Road, Cardiff CF11 9HB   Tel: 029 2039 6624
Fax: 029 2039 6625   e-mail: wales.office@cafamily.org.uk

Regional offices

Contact a Family North East England Region
The Dene Centre, Castle Farm Road, Newcastle upon Tyne NE3 1PH
Tel/Fax: 0191 213 6300   e-mail: northeast.office@cafamily.org.uk

Contact a Family North West England Region
6th Floor, St. James House, Pendleton Way, Salford M6 5FW
Tel: 0161 743 0700   Fax: 0161 743 0711   e-mail: northwest.office@cafamily.org.uk

Contact a Family West Midlands Region
Prospect Hall, 12 College Walk, Selly Oak, Birmingham B29 6LE
Tel: 0121 415 4624   Fax: 0121 415 4922   e-mail: westmids.office@cafamily.org.uk

Project offices

Ealing Contact a Family
First Floor, St. Andrew's Church Centre, Mount Park Road, London W5 2RS
Tel: 020 8810 8151   e-mail: ealing.office@cafamily.org.uk

Lewisham Contact a Family
1 Forman House, Frendsbury Road, Brockley, London SE4 2LB
Tel: 020 7635 6333 Fax: 020 7732 8494   e-mail: lewisham.office@cafamily.org.uk

Southall Contact a Family
St. Georges Community Centre, 8-12 Lancaster Road, Southall UB1 1NW
Tel: 020 8571 6381   e-mail: southall.office@cafamily.org.uk

Southwark Contact a Family
54 Camberwell Road, London SE5 0EN
Tel: 020 7277 4436   Fax: 020 7703 6449   e-mail: southwark.office@cafamily.org.uk

Sutton and Merton Contact a Family
Hill House Community Centre, Bishopsford Road, Morden SM4 6BL
Tel: 020 8640 5525   e-mail: sutton.office@cafamily.org.uk

Wandsworth Contact a Family
1 Siward Road, London SW17 0LA   Tel: 020 8947 5260
Fax: 020 8947 9506   e-mail: wandsworth.office@cafamily.org.uk

HOW TO USE THE
CONTACT A FAMILY DIRECTORY

Introduction

Learning that an individual or a child has a disability is always a traumatic experience however sensitively the initial communication is handled. *The Contact a Family Directory* is a positive response to difficulties encountered by individuals, parents and professionals alike when they seek reliable and up-to-date information.

In Contact a Family's experience, individuals, parents and professional workers frequently need to know about specific conditions and rare disorders and the related support organisations. Through the publication of *The Contact a Family Directory,* Contact a Family is addressing this need.

Contact a Family maintains a database of a substantial number of specific conditions and rare disorders in addition to those listed in *The Contact a Family Directory*. **Therefore if individuals, parents or professionals wish to enquire about a particular condition for which there is no entry in *The Contact a Family Directory* it is worth contacting our freephone Helpline, Tel: 0808 808 3555 Text: 0808 808 3556 e-mail: helpline@cafamily.org.uk** For all other enquirers, call Contact a Family's UK office, Tel: 020 7608 8700 and you will be directed to the relevant Information Officer.

Alphabetical entries

As *The Contact a Family Directory* is published annually, Contact a Family is able to up-date existing entries and to introduce new ones. All entries for specific conditions and rare disorders are in alphabetical order. **However, many conditions and syndromes are known by alternative names and readers are therefore advised to consult the Index if a particular term or name cannot be located.**

Each entry contains a short medical description of the condition together with details of inheritance patterns and prenatal diagnosis. This information is followed by details of the related support networks: their activities, publications, and what they offer to families. It should be noted that some groups are very small and are run by individuals or parents who offer one-to-one linking and mutual support between families. Some of the listed Contact Groups prefer to be reached in the first instance through Contact a Family. If users of *The Contact a Family Directory* have difficulty in contacting a support group, please telephone Contact a Family, Tel: 020 7608 8700.

Index

The Index identifies all the specific conditions and rare disorders covered by *The Contact a Family Directory*. Synonyms and alternative names for these conditions will be found in the Index, cross-referenced to the appropriate entry in the alphabetical section of *The Contact a Family Directory*. The Index features the alphabetical entries of specific conditions and rare disorders in bold type.

Medical terms

Many medical terms are explained within the medical text of an entry. Otherwise, readers are advised to consult a standard medical dictionary such as Mosebys Medical, Nursing and Allied Health Dictionary. The online dictionary of the US National Institutes of Health can also be used, Web: http://www.nlm.nih.gov/medlineplus/mplusdictionary.html

Keep up to date

Your copy of *The Contact a Family Directory* will become a less useful resource over a period of time, as medical understandings of conditions often changes and new support groups are established every year. We therefore strongly advise all purchasers to destroy this copy in April 2009 and obtain the next edition.

Contact a Family will seek to ensure that *The Contact a Family Directory* remains accurate and useful. We will be grateful to receive any information or comments from readers to help us improve *The Contact a Family Directory*.

BACKGROUND INFORMATION

The Contact a Family Directory includes entries for:

- disorders which are life limiting to, or life threatening in, childhood or adolescence;
- chronic disorders affecting children and adults;
- disorders with paediatric and adult forms;
- adult onset disorders.

The information shown in current entries also covers adults with the disorders.

Contact a Family is committed to the provision of high quality, authoritative descriptive material about a large range of disabilities and medical conditions, some of which are very rare.

The medical texts provided in *The Contact a Family Directory* are written for non-specialist, multi-disciplinary professionals involved with families and individuals. They are also designed to provide accessible information for families and individuals, for information purposes only.

There are thought to be about eight thousand inherited disorders and thousands of non-inherited medical conditions.

When *The Contact a Family Directory* was first published in 1991, Contact a Family chose to cover those disorders which have established UK support organisations. Although priority is given to carrying entries where there is an established support organisation for the specific disorder, *The Contact a Family Directory* Editorial Board has decided to commence including entries for disorders where Contact a Family has received a substantial number of enquiries but where there is no support organisation. All these entries aim to cross refer to more general entries where support and information are available for individual features of the disorder.

All medical texts appearing in *The Contact a Family Directory* have been written by, or approved by, the leading medical experts on the disorder with details of the authorship and date of last update shown at the end of each entry.

Contact a Family and the Editorial Board of *The Contact a Family Directory* reserve the right to remove details of support organisations that do not meet requirements of effective response to enquirers. In these cases, the medical text is retained for information purposes. Contact a Family has a Medical Advisory Panel which also advises on *The Contact a Family Directory*:

Contact a Family Helpline 0808 808 3555

Genetics Professor Michael Patton, Professor of Medical Genetics, St George's Hospital Medical School, London, UK.

Metabolic Disorders Dr J E (Ed) Wraith, Consultant Paediatrician, Willink Biochemical Unit, Royal Manchester Children's Hospital, Manchester, UK.

Ophthalmic Conditions Miss Isabelle Russell-Eggitt, Consultant Ophthalmic Surgeon, Great Ormond Street Hospital, London, UK.

Behavioural Phenotypes Professor Jeremy Turk, Professor of Developmental Psychiatry and Consultant Child & Adolescent Psychiatrist, Department of Clinical Developmental Sciences, St. George's Hospital Medical School, London, UK.

Endocrine Disorders Dr Richard Stanhope, Consultant Paediatric Endocrinologist, Institute of Child Health/Great Ormond Street Hospital, London, UK.

Neurological Disorders Professor Brian Neville, Professor of Childhood Epilepsy, Institute of Child Health/Great Ormond Street Hospital, London, UK.

Cardiac Disorders Dr Robert Yates, Consultant Fetal and Paediatric Cardiologist, Great Ormond Street Hospital, London, UK.

Dermatology Professor John Harper, Consultant in Paediatric Dermatology, Great Ormond Street Hospital, London, UK.

Haematology and Oncology Professor Finbarr Cotter, Professor of Experimental Haematology, St Bartholomew's Hospital, London, UK.

Gastroenterology Professor Peter Milla, Professor of Paediatric Gastroenterology & Nutrition, Great Ormond Street Hospital, London, UK.

Immunisation and Community Paediatrics Dr D Elliman, Consultant in Community Child Health, Islington Primary Care Trust, London, UK and Great Ormond Street Hospital, London, UK, Immunisation Co-ordinator, Islington Primary Care Trust and Chair, Sub-Committee on Child Health, National Screening Committee.

Orthopaedic Conditions Mr Daniel Porter, Senior Lecturer & Hon. Consultant in Orthopaedic Surgery, University of Edinburgh, Edinburgh, UK.

Immunisation and Community Paediatrics Dr Helen Bedford, Institute of Child Health, London, UK.

Respiratory Medicine Professor A Bush, Professor of Paediatric Respirology, Royal Brompton Hospital, London, UK.

Development Disorders Professor A Le Couteur, Professor of Child and Adolescent Psychiatry, Newcastle University, Newcastle upon Tyne, UK.

Rheumatology Professor T Southwood, Professor of Paediatric Rheumatology, University of Birmingham, Birmingham, UK.

MEDICAL INFORMATION ON THE INTERNET: SEEKING QUALITY

This article is designed to provide advice on the identification of reliable medical information on the Internet. Families of children with any disability or additional need and professionals working with them can also call the Contact a Family Helpline on 0808 808 3555 for further help and explanation.

It is not difficult to find information on subjects such as medical conditions/ disorders, treatments, drug and other therapies and research on the Internet. Indeed, people have been known to have bought drug and other treatments through the Internet without seeking a diagnosis from a doctor. In one well known case an Internet surfer suffered acute kidney failure after drinking oil of wormwood obtained online. *Weisbord SD, Soule JB, and Kimmel PL, Poison on line: acute renal failure caused by oil of wormwood purchased through the internet. New England Journal of Medicine, 1997. 337: 825.*

Identifying descriptions of conditions and disorders whose writers are named, and their qualifications given, needs some knowledge.

Consumers – parents, carers and professionals – using the Internet to find medical information, need to evaluate what they find before deciding what information is useful for them and their advisers. The date when information was written, the author together with details of their qualification to write on the subject, and the source of the material such as a university, hospital or government deprtment are three of the important items to look for. There are important reasons to know these details – material can be out of date having been superseded by newer knowledge and treatments; unless the material is dated a decision on what information is useful and relevant to discuss with medical advisers cannot be made. If validating information is not given, the consumer will be unable to differentiate between types of information such as that provided by a medical expert, personal information written by an individual based on their own experience which might not be typical or 'insight' material from a number of people on a support group website. With the provision of proper validation, all material has its own importance and relevance for different needs.

Contact a Family medical texts carry endorsements in the following form *Medical text written June 1996 by Professor P Beighton, Department of Human Genetics, University of Cape Town, Cape Town, South Africa. Last updated April 2004 by Professor H A Bird, Professor of Pharmacological Rheumatology, Leeds General Infirmary, Leeds, UK.*

Contact a Family and the Information Management Research Institute (IMRI), School of Informatics, Northumbria University, Newcastle upon Tyne, UK, have produced advice to consumers looking for medical information on the Internet and for support groups who are planning or revamping websites. The guidelines produced by our 'Judge: Websites for health' Project can be found at Web: http://www.judgehealth.org.uk and they are designed to address concerns that some of this information is inaccurate, misleading or even dangerous. Support group websites are important sources of health information. It is vital that these websites are well designed and contain good quality information, with indications of currency, authorship and provenance as well as balance.

Contact a Family also subscribes to the guidelines of *Health on the Net*. These guidelines for quality health sites can be found on the HON site, Web: http://www.hon.ch which also gives a quality mark for sites following the guidelines. The Contact a Family site carries the Health on the Net quality mark.

In your search for information, you may come across 'my story' sites. These are Internet sites developed by individuals or families who have a specific disorder. Some of these sites are of a high standard with excellent links to verifiable hospital and university sites. However, even if they indicate that the medical information has been checked by a medical expert, this may be specific to that individual or family member and not be typical. These sites often give the name of a medical expert and you can then get in touch to check on the general nature of the disorder.

There are also a number of e-mail groups on the internet; many are available through http://uk.groups.yahoo.com or you can register with our confidential e-mail service http://www.makingcontact.org

You are likely to be in touch with people who are genuine, but remember, some may have extreme views and some may not be genuine. It should also be remembered that the way a medical condition affects an individual can vary enormously in severity. Each description offered by an affected individual will be personal and may not be reflected in the same way in others diagnosed with the same condition. Individuals may recommend treatments that may not suit every individual.

A leaflet entitled 'Finding Medical Information on the Internet' has been produced by Contact a Family and approved by the Royal College of Paediatrics and Child Health. Copies can be obtained from Contact a Family's Helpline, Tel: 0808 808 3555 or e-mail: helpline@cafamily.org.uk

Contact a Family Helpline 0808 808 3555

Search suggestions
Search engines
Web: http://www.google.co.uk
Web: http://uk.yahoo.com
Web: http://www.freesearch.co.uk

Metasearchers
Web: http://www.ask.co.uk
Web: http://www.dogpile.co.uk

Health sources
There is an ever growing range of excellent websites on the Internet giving detailed information about specific conditions and rare disorders. The websites below all conform to quality criteria. It is important to present information in a style that is easily accessible to people with visual and other difficulties but it is especially important with medical information that the website providers adhere to the basic validations of accuracy, currency and relevancy. Some of this information is provided on the page and some can be found in a separate page describing the purpose and authorship of the information on the website. However, dating of information should be found on the page even if the authorship is found elsewhere.

Genetic information
Where a disorder is inheritable, the acknowledged first source of information is the **Online Inheritance in Man (OMIM)**. This is the online version of the Atlas of Mendelian Inheritance in Man, edited by Professor Victor McCusick of Johns Hopkins Hospital, Baltimore. It is made available on the Internet, as are the information resources of the National Institutes of Health and MEDLINE, by the US government. The OMIM home page, Web: http://www.ncbi.nlm.nih.gov/omim contains helpful information about using the resource. A little time spent looking at the links shown in the left hand bar will be useful.

It should be remembered that this is a huge resource and contains information on many sub-types of syndromes and care should be taken to check that the entries found cover the correct forms of the disorders.

There are two main areas of interest. Firstly, the detailed history of the disorder from when it was first identified until the present. This text has copious references to MEDLINE (qv), mostly to abstracts but sometimes to full texts of articles.

The other very important section is the Clinical Synopsis. This provides a list of features of the condition by body system. It is most important to remember that not all individuals will display all the features mentioned and the degree of severity will vary greatly. General information about medical disorders will, of necessity, cover the most severe scenario. Identification of the degree of severity of a disorder in an individual should be discussed with a medical adviser.

PubMed Web:http://www.ncbi.nlm.nih.gov/pubmed is a service of the National Library of Medicine which provides access to over 11 million **MEDLINE** citations back to the mid-1960's and additional life science journals. Again, this service is provided on the Internet by the US Government. This searchable database is a first port of call to identify published research in the world's learned journals. As articles cover human and animal subjects, foreign language articles and 40 years of information, you will often wish to refine your search narrowly. Under the main search window, select Limits and fill in the range of information you need using the check boxes; also make use of the very informative Help|FAQ option in the side bar.

Further online resources

Web: http://www.cafamily.org.uk *Look out for new features in our online version of the Directory, from summer 2008. This will include direct links to other reliable sources of information on conditions.*

Web: http://intute.ac.uk *A UK universities and partners database of web resources for education and research.*

Web: http://www.nlm.nih.gov/medlineplus/encyclopedia.html *Extensive medical encyclopaedia made available by US National Library of Medicine.*

Web: http://ninds.nih.gov/disorders *Excellent information on a range of neurological disorders provided by the US National Institutes of Health with further links to research.*

Web: http://www.nih.gov/icd *Gives links to all the US National Institutes of Health; many of them have very extensive searchable databases.*

Web: http://www.rarediseases.org/search/rdbsearch.html *The site of NORD - National Organization for Rare Disorders which gives access to abstracts of its information on a huge range of disorders as well as the networks that support the disorder. This is an American site but is very useful where there is no equivalent UK support network.*

Web: http://www.dh.gov.uk *Gives access to the index of all governmental organisations such as the Department of Health; information and full texts of DoH publications, Health of the Nation targets, helplines etc.*

Web: http://www.library.nhs.uk *UK National Library for Health has a wide range of information and is able to search across multiple health resources including The Cochrane Library, BMJPG Clinical Evidence, NHS Direct and specialist libraries including Cancer, Child Health and Respiratory diseases.*

Web: http://www.liv.ac.uk/cfgd *The Cochrane Collaboration Cystic Fibrosis & Genetic Disorders Group.*

Web: http://www.nhsdirect.nhs.uk *The online arm of the UK National Health Service.*

Web: http://bpsu.inopsu.com *The British Paediatric Surveillance Unit site detailing its work in surveillance of rare disorders in children and giving links to published information.*

Web: http://www.emedicine.com/search.html *Very good site for information on a wide range of disorders. Fully authored and dated on page with references and e-mail links to writers and editors.*

Web: http://www.ich.ucl.ac.uk *Link to the UK's foremost children's hospital. Contains extensive archive of paediatric resources and the latest in care and research developments.*

Web: http://www.ukgtn.nhs.uk *List of available NHS genetic testing services accessed via GPs*

Web: http://www.orpha.net *A database providing information on rare diseases orphan drugs.*

Web: http://www.yourchildshealth.nhs.uk *An introduction to child health topics.*

Web: http://www.nhs.uk *NHS Choices, a site providing information on conditions, treatments, local services and healthy living*

Contact a Family Helpline 0808 808 3555

AN INTRODUCTION TO BEHAVIOURAL PHENOTYPES

The term 'behavioural phenotype' refers to those aspects of an individual's development and behaviour which can be attributed to the presence of a specific genetic or other biological anomaly. It covers vulnerability to psychiatric and psychological disturbance as well as cognitive (intellectual) abilities. The concept is not a new one. However it has only recently been widely accepted because of the earlier emphasis on social determinants of psychological state and behaviour. The emphasis is on a predisposition towards certain behavioural tendencies. Not all individuals with the same genetic anomaly will show a particular behaviour, and not all those that do will show it to the same degree. Such behaviours are important in that they may give a clue to the presence of an underlying genetic cause for the individual's developmental and behavioural difficulties. They may also indicate what combinations of interventions are likely to be most effective.

Acknowledgement of a biological basis to certain behavioural traits does not reduce the importance of psychological and social factors, which can have an added effect on the biologically caused tendencies. It is also important to note that psychological, educational and social interventions are often highly effective. Nonetheless, accepting that such problems are primarily caused by genetic, as opposed to family or other social, factors can be an enormous relief for parents who may be feeling guilty; believing they have created their son's or daughter's difficulties. Such a diagnosis is important for a number of other reasons as well:

- The individuals' and families' basic human rights to know of underlying causes of developmental and behavioural difficulties which may affect the ability to lead a full and satisfying life without assistance;
- The potential to receive information on likely developmental progress and challenges (including behavioural ones) the individual is likely to experience;
- Facilitation of the grief process relating to having a disability, or having a family member who has a disability or genetic disorder;
- Assistance in focussing on the future and developing suitable plans;
- Awareness of the need for familial genetic counselling;
- Potential to relate to appropriate support groups.

The first use of such a concept was by Langdon Down in his original description of individuals with Down syndrome (see entry). He described a characteristic profile of personality traits. These included strong powers of imitation, a lively sense of humour and the ridiculous, obstinacy and amiability.

His proposal has received substantial criticism over the years, not least because of the wide variability in personality profiles witnessed in people who have Down syndrome, just as in the general population. But recent research has supported the notion that there is a greater similarity personality and temperament-wise between people with Down syndrome than would be expected by chance. It has also confirmed the increased risk amongst people with Down syndrome of developing Alzheimer's presenile dementia and depression - two common causes of 'challenging behaviour' in people with learning disabilities (see entry). Conversely, young people with Down syndrome show relatively low rates of the two major neurodevelopmental disorders of childhood, namely Autism Spectrum disorders and Attention Deficit-Hyperactivity Disorder (see entries). Note that people with Down syndrome can and do get both these conditions. On such occasions they are often overlooked with subsequent failure to institute a suitable learning programme. The issue is one of 'diagnostic overshadowing' where all the individual's problems tend to be attributed to their having Down syndrome (or learning disability) rather than other diagnoses being considered.

The first modern use of the term behavioural phenotype was in relation to young people with the X-linked condition Lesch-Nyhan syndrome. This rare problem is transmitted on the X chromosome, hence all known sufferers are males. Individuals with Lesch-Nyhan syndrome often seem normal at birth but later develop marked limb movement difficulties as well as severe self-mutilation including knuckle gnawing and lip biting. This compulsive-like behaviour is a major cause of ill health and personal distress for the individuals concerned and their carers yet remains extremely resistant to psychological and medical treatments.

Much research has confirmed that the frequency, duration and intensity of self-injurious behaviour is closely linked to personal experiences, how one has been treated by others, and how one's surroundings are structured and organised. However the likelihood of self-injury and its nature or type appear to be driven substantially by the underlying genetic cause of the learning disability. There are many examples of this in addition to the above. Individuals with Cornelia de Lange syndrome (see entry) are prone to lip biting. People with Prader-Willi syndrome (see entry) overeat voraciously unless helped to resist the overwhelming urges. They are thus at high risk of serious obesity with all its associated health problems including diabetes mellitus (see entry). Those with Fragile X syndrome (see entry) often bite their hands (usually at the base of the thumb) in response to anxiety or excitement. Individuals with Smith-Magenis syndrome (see entry), caused by a micro-deletion on the short arm of chromosome 17, frequently head-bang and pick and pull at their finger and toenails. They have also been reported as being at increased risk of inserting objects into their bodily orifices. Individuals with the rare condition

Hypomelanosis of Ito (see entry) often display self-injury in the form of wrist and knuckle biting. However, self-injury may be explicable largely in terms of the individual's social and environmental circumstances. For example, people with another rare condition, Aicardi syndrome (see entry), do head bang a lot, but probably no more than expected for their general levels of developmental ability and social circumstances.

When considering behavioural phenotypes, it is useful to separate psychological processes, which may be involved, into several categories:
- Profile of intellectual strengths and needs;
- Speech and language skills;
- Concentration skills, impulse control and freedom from distractibility;
- Social functioning;
- Self-injurious tendencies;
- Other psychological difficulties such as obsessive-compulsive tendencies, anxieties, mood disorders and aggression;
- Interaction with physical features which affect behaviour, for example enlarged tongue affecting language in people with Down syndrome, joint laxity predisposing to clumsiness in people with Fragile X syndrome.

Intellectual strengths and needs

Some genetic conditions have a specific effect on the likely level of intelligence. They may even cause a particular pattern of strengths and needs. Usually an underlying specific genetic cause for a person's learning disability is not discovered despite intensive investigation. The most common known genetic cause of learning disability is Down syndrome which has a prevalence of approximately 1 in 650 individuals. Most people with Down syndrome have an extra chromosome 21 which has occurred as a new mutation rather than having been inherited. There is a rare cause of Down syndrome known as a translocation where a fragment of one chromosome has become detached, and stuck on to another one. This form is inherited. People with Down syndrome have very variable intellectual abilities - usually in the mild to moderate learning disability range. Their social functioning is typically higher than their cognitive (intellectual) abilities. The most common inherited cause of learning disability is Fragile X syndrome, which occurs in 1 in 4,000 to 6,000 individuals. People with Fragile X syndrome experience very variable intellectual abilities but these are usually in the mild to moderate learning disability range. They often have strengths with language skills yet particularly special needs with numeracy and visuo-spatial abilities. In addition, their rate of intellectual growth may slow down towards adolescence because of particular difficulties with dealing with sequences of information ('sequential information processing'). The genetics of Fragile X syndrome is extremely complicated. A few boys and men may have quite a substantial genetic abnormality yet appear relatively unaffected. Conversely as many as a third of so-called female carriers experience developmental and behavioural difficulties. These may be extreme for example severe learning difficulties and autism. Conversely they may be very subtle, showing themselves as specific difficulties with mathematics, or problems in organising information in one's mind and planning ahead. Children with velocardiofacial (VCF) syndrome, caused by a microdeletion on the long arm of chromosome 22, also typically attain higher verbal than performance IQ scores, as do girls and women with Turner syndrome (see entry), who have just the one X chromosome. In contrast, individuals with Klinefelter syndrome (see entry), who have three sex chromosomes (one Y and two X's) have problems more with language and other verbal tasks. Most individuals with Williams syndrome (see entry) (idiopathic hypercalcaemia) have learning disability and need special schooling. They too have particular difficulties with visuo-spatial and motor skills yet have strikingly good expressive language even though their comprehension lags somewhat behind.

Speech and language skills

Speech and language abilities and styles can be surprisingly affected by having a particular genetic syndrome. People with Fragile X syndrome often have a jocular style to their conversation with up and down ('litanic') swings of pitch and many perseverations (going on and on about the same thing) and repetitions (saying the same word or phrase repeatedly). They also show language features suggestive of Autism Spectrum disorders such as echolalia (repetition of phrases) even in the presence of a friendly and socially aware personality. Williams syndrome characteristically produces superficially grammatically correct, complex and fluent language which may lead to overestimation of general intellectual ability. In some conditions, such as Angelman syndrome (see entry) (caused by problems on chromosome 15), verbal communication is usually absent. In others such as velocardiofacial syndrome, there is early onset receptive and expressive language impairment.

Attentional skills and overactivity

The association of high activity levels with inattentiveness, restlessness, fidgetiness, impulsive tendencies and marked distractibility is well recognised. Such features are common in people who have learning disability and often reflect their general developmental level. Occasionally they may be indicative of a specific developmental delay as in Attention Deficit-Hyperactivity Disorder. Many genetic conditions seem to predispose to such problems - to the extent that it is tempting to speculate on a general non-specific genetic predisposition. However, some genetic syndromes have been shown to have a particular association with these problems. These include Fragile X syndrome, Tuberous Sclerosis (see entry), Williams syndrome, Cornelia de Lange syndrome, Sotos syndrome (see entry), Sanfilippo syndrome (see entry, Mucopolysaccharide diseases and associated diseases), Marfan syndrome (see entry), Smith-Magenis syndrome and Turner syndrome. In some instances the problem is more one of inattentiveness rather than overactivity, as in Turner's syndrome. Gross motor overactivity may be the major concern as in Smith-Magenis syndrome and Tuberous Sclerosis. There is sometimes evidence for at least some of the above behavioural difficulties to be far more severe than expected for the individuals' ages and general levels of developmental ability. For example, boys with Fragile X syndrome are usually more inattentive, restless and fidgety than their learning disabled peers, even though their activity levels may be similar. Furthermore, boys with Fragile X syndrome do not seem to automatically grow out of these problems, unlike many individuals without genetic anomalies or learning difficulties. Overactivity, poor concentration and distractibility are also common in Williams syndrome, and attentional deficits and hyperactivity have been reported as common in Sotos syndrome and velocardiofacial syndrome. Restlessness, hyperactivity and inattentiveness may develop after three or four years of life, as in Sanfilippo syndrome.

Social functioning

The ability and drive to relate to other people, to have some idea of their needs and how they are feeling, and to be able to let others know one's own thoughts and feelings are crucial developmental skills. The combination of multiple qualitative impairments in social functioning with language difficulties, poor imagination skills and marked obsessional tendencies is consistent with a diagnosis of autistic spectrum disorder. These conditions are known to be associated with learning disability. Over two thirds of people with autism have learning disabilities as well. As above, the presence of autistic features in people with so many different genetic anomalies suggests a general vulnerability. Again however, certain genetic syndromes do seem to have a particular association, and even sometimes a strikingly characteristic profile of autistic-like features. People with Fragile X syndrome often display shyness and social anxiety, an aversion to direct eye contact, delayed imaginary (make-believe) play, echolalia and repetitive speech and self-injury in the form of hand biting as well as some repetitive activities, in particular hand flapping. There is an increased rate of autism in Fragile X syndrome, but the profile of 'autistic-like' features is often seen even in those without autism. There is also good evidence that Autism Spectrum disorders are unusually common in tuberous sclerosis and that they can not be explained by the presence of epilepsy or the associated learning disability. Conversely autism may be surprisingly rare as in Down syndrome. Over-sociability may be a problem as in Williams syndrome. Individuals may be very chatty with a particularly well-developed social use of language. They are often outgoing, socially disinhibited and excessively affectionate yet still frequently have great problems making friends with others of similar age. Social impairments are frequent in girls with Turner's syndrome where it has been proposed that the risk of autistic disorders is dependent on which parent you have inherited your single X chromosome from.

Other psychological difficulties

Common childhood difficulties may be associated with particular genetic conditions. For example people with Down syndrome and Prader-Willi syndrome are prone to breathing difficulties while sleeping ('sleep apnoea'). This may contribute to excessive daytime drowsiness. People with Smith-Magenis syndrome and Sotos syndrome are also prone to severe sleep difficulties. In addition, people with Sotos syndrome are vulnerable to frequent severe tantrums, as are those with XYY syndrome who also show an increased rate of conduct disorders. Some behaviours may be quite unusual such as the paroxysmal (sudden excessive) laughter in Angelman's syndrome, 'self-hugging' ('spasmodic upper body squeeze') in Smith-Magenis syndrome and the midline hand wringing and hyperventilation (overbreathing) in Rett syndrome (see entry).

Other biological causes of behavioural difficulties

It is not only genetic problems that can create patterns of behavioural difficulty. Infections, particularly before birth or early in life can have an influence. For example, congenital rubella (German measles) is a well-established cause of autism as well as severe learning difficulties and visual and hearing problems. Obsessive-compulsive disorder may result from infection with the streptococcus bacterium (paediatric autoimmune neurodevelopmental disorder associated with streptococcus (PANDAS)). Fetal Alcohol Spectrum disorder (see entry) is a very common cause of diminished intellectual ability, expressive and receptive language problems, irritability, hyperactivity and difficulty perceiving social cues. Hydrocephalus (see entry) ('water on the brain') can be associated with problems sequencing information and impulse control.

Contact a Family Helpline 0808 808 3555

Helping people who have a genetically determined behavioural phenotype and their families

Knowledge and awareness of behavioural phenotypes is not just of use diagnostically. It is also critical in the early development of a suitable support package covering medical, psychological, educational and social aspects. For example, people with Prader-Willi syndrome need help from an early age to acquire healthy eating habits and routines. The family should be fully informed and aware of the condition and its consequences and should where appropriate have received genetic counselling. They should have had attention paid to the suitability of their living environment and whether they are receiving all appropriate benefits. They should be offered the opportunity to link with appropriate support groups. The individual concerned should receive a thorough educational evaluation incorporating knowledge of the genetic condition along with the person's unique profile of developmental strengths and needs. Careful consideration is required regarding educational placement and curriculum, including essential therapeutic components such as speech and language work. Help should be available for associated challenging behaviours, familial difficulties coping and the needs of siblings. Early intervention packages such as Portage should be in place. Occasionally the judicious use of medication in addition to the above may be helpful for specific behavioural problems.

Medical text written October 2000 by Professor J Turk. **Last reviewed July 2004 by Professor J Turk, Professor of Developmental Psychiatry and Consultant Child & Adolescent Psychiatrist, Department of Clinical Developmental Sciences, St. George's Hospital Medical School, London, UK.**

REFERENCES
GRAHAM, P.J., TURK, J. & VERHULST, F. (1999) Child Psychiatry: A Developmental Approach. (Pp. 84-109 'Intelligence & Learning Disorders') Oxford: Oxford University Press.
O'BRIEN, G. & YULE, W. (1995) Behavioural Phenotypes. London: MacKeith Press.
O'BRIEN G. (2002) B1ehavioural Phenotypes in Clinical Practice. London: MacKeith Press.
TURK, J. & SALES, J. (1996) Behavioural Phenotypes and their Relevance to Child Mental Health Professionals. Child Psychology & Psychiatry Review, 1, 4-11.

PROCEDURES AND MANAGEMENT

In the course of the management of many of the disorders described in the Contact a Family Directory of Specific Conditions, Rare Disorders and UK Family Support Groups, various procedures and management programmes are used. For some of these there are organisations which can provide further information.

A range of useful addresses can be found in the Helpful Organisations entry.

Contact a Family publishes a factsheet "*Aids, Equipment and Adaptations*" which gives extensive information about a wide range of services and suppliers useful for families of disabled children and adults. Access to the full range of Contact a Family factsheets, Guides for Parents, Reports, Newsletters and the Group Action pack can be found at Web: http://www.cafamily.org.uk/publications.html Access and subscription for Contact a Family's eNewsletters can be found at Web: http://www.cafamily.org.uk/whatsnew.html

Artificial feeding

Many individuals and families have to use artificial nutrition therapy (enteral or parenteral). Parenteral Nutrition is nutrition delivered directly into a main vein near to the heart. Enteral Nutrition refers to nutrition delivered via tubes into the digestive system. Tubes can be inserted down the nose into the stomach (Naso-gastric feeding) or directly into the stomach (Gastrostomy) or small bowel (Jejunostomy): this is also called a Percutaneous Endoscopic Jejunostomy (PEJ).

Association of young people with ME
Web: http://www.ayme.org.uk/article.php?sid=10&id=164
Very good information on tube feeding.

PINNT, PO Box 3126, Christchurch BH23 2XS e-mail: PINNT@dial.pipex.com
Web: http://www.pinnt.com
PINNT (Patients on Parenteral or Enteral Feeding) covers enteral feeding - nasogastric; gastrostomy and jejunostomy - feeding and with parenteral nutrition (intravenous feeding). PINNT and Half PINNT, the paediatric arm of PINNT, provide help and information when a decision on any of these types of feeding is made.

The British Association for Parenteral and Enteral Nutrition
Web: http://www.bapen.org.uk
Provides information and articles for professionals.

Bone Marrow Transplantation Units
Great Ormond Street Hospital, London WC1N 3JH   Tel: 020 7813 7862 PALS service
Web: http://www.ich.ucl.ac.uk
The Bone Marrow Transplant Unit at Great Ormond Street Hospital (GOSH) treats children with Blood, Immunodeficiency, Metabolic disorders and Juvenile Idiopathic Arthritis. GOSH has one of the largest BMT centres in the world for treating children with immunodeficiencies.

Contact a Family Helpline 0808 808 3555

Bristol Royal Hospital for Children, Paul O'Gorman Building, Upper Maudlin Street, Bristol BS2 8BJ   Tel: 0117 342 8461
Web: http://www.ubht.nhs.uk/your-hospitals/bristol-royal-hospital-for-children.html
The Bristol Royal Hospital for Children has the largest paediatric Bone Marrow Transplantation Unit in the UK and takes international referrals. The conditions treated include blood disorders, solid tumour and genetic metabolic disorders.

Newcastle General Hospital, Westgate Road, Newcastle upon Tyne NE4 6BE
Tel: 0191 256 3460   Web: http://www.bubblefoundation.org.uk
The Bone Marrow Transplant Unit at Newcastle General Hospital treats babies and children with immunodeficiency disorders, solid tumours and Juvenile Idiopathic Arthritis.

Challenging behaviour
Many children with a range of disorders display challenging behaviour.

Challenging Behaviour Foundation, The Old Courthouse, New Road Avenue, Chatham ME4 6BE Tel: 01634 838739   Fax: 01634 828588   e-mail: info@thecbf.org.uk
Web: http://www.thecbf.org.uk
The Challenging Behaviour Foundation produces free information leaflets on various aspects of challenging behaviour such as physical interventions, equipment and safety, self injurious behaviour and a booklist for parents. An information pack is available on request (4 x 1st class stamps appreciated towards costs). For individual information sheets, please send SAE or visit the CBF website.

Cochlear Implants
Where people cannot benefit from conventional hearing aids, cochlear implants may be helpful in picking up incoming sounds and sending electrical pulses directly to the auditory nerves. However, such electronic devices cannot completely restore normal hearing.

CICS Group, PO Box 28843, London SW13 0WY   e-mail: info@cicsgroup.org.uk
Web: http://www.cicsgroup.org.uk
The CICS Group provides support before, during or after a child's cochlear implant and offers practical help with everyday problems.

Colostomy
A colostomy is a surgically created opening into the colon through the abdomen. The purpose of a colostomy which may be temporary or permanent, is to allow stools to bypass a damaged or diseased part of the colon.

Colostomy Association, PO Box 8017, Reading RG6 9DF   Tel: 0800 587 6744 Helpline Tel: 0118 986 7597   Fax: 0118 956 9095   e-mail: cass@colosomyassociation.org.uk
Web: http://www.colostomyassociation.org.uk

Ileostomy
Inflammatory bowel diseases such as Crohn's disease and ulcerative colitis (see entry) can sometimes cause such damage to the patient's large intestine (colon) that it may be necessary for the surgeon to remove it entirely. With a Brooke ileostomy, the lower end of the small intestine (ileum) is brought out through the abdominal wall and the body's waste matter is collected in an externally attached bag. Alternatively, the patient who has ulcerative colitis may be able to choose to have an internal pouch, which involves the construction of a reservoir from a section of ileum. Someone who has a pouch does not need an external bag. People who have Crohn's disease cannot usually have an internal pouch.

ia (the Ileostomy and Internal Pouch Support Group), Peverill House, 1 - 5 Mill Road, Ballyclare BT39 9DR   Tel: 0800 0184 724 Helpline   Fax: 028 9332 4606
e-mail: info@iasupport.org   Web: http://www.the-ia.org.uk
ia provides a visiting service and also supports individuals, including parents of children and young people, by e-mail and by telephone.

Incontinence
Where there are structural, developmental or psychological difficulties, incontinence may arise.

Enuresis Resource & Information Centre, 34 Old School House, Britannia Road, Kingswood Bristol BS15 8DB   Tel: 0117 960 3060   Fax: 0117 960 0401
e-mail: info@eric.org.uk   Web: http://www.eric.org.uk

Incontact, SATRA Innovation Park, Rockingham Road, Kettering, NN16 9JH
Tel: 01536 533255 e-mail: info@incontact.org   Web: http://www.incontact.org
Provides support and information to people with bladder and bowel problems and their carers.

Limb abnormalities, acquired and congenital limb absence
STEPS (for contact details see Lower Limb Abnormalities)
Steps covers lower limb abnormalities and has extensive information about all issues, including prosthetics, facing families of children with a lower limb abnormality.

Reach (for contact details see Upper Limb Abnormalities)
Reach covers upper limb abnormalities and provides insurance cover for the 'good arm' of children over 2 years of age (UK only) as an automatic benefit of membership and has a wide range of information available.

Limbless Association, Queen Mary's Hospital, Roehampton Lane,
London SW15 5PN   Tel: 020 8788 1777   Fax: 020 8788 3444
e-mail: enquiries@limbless-association.org   Web: http://www.limbless-association.org
The Limbless Association provides information, advice and support for people of all ages who are without one or more limbs. It has a nationwide network of volunteer visitors (within the UK) who are all amputees themselves, offering support and encouragement to prospective amputees, carers and those already trying to come to terms with limb loss or deficiency.

Pain management
Action for Sick Children, Web: http://www.actionforsickchildren.org/parents.html
Good information on injections and pain. Also covers other subjects allied to children going into hospital.

Paediatric Pain Profile (PPP), Web: http://www.ppprofile.org.uk
The Paediatric Pain Profile is a pain assessment tool for children with severe and complex disbility. Pages on their website describe the development and testing of the tool. The PPP can be downloaded from their website. For further information please contact Anne Hunt
e-mail: ahunt@uclan.ac.uk Tel: 01772 895 148

Pain Concern, PO Box 13256, Haddington EH41 3YD   Tel: 01620 822572 (Mon-Fri, 9am-5pm; Fri, 6.30pm-7.30pm)   e-mail: info@painconcern.org.uk
Web: http://www.painconcern.org.uk
Provides information and support for pain sufferers and those who care for them. A selection of factsheets and leaflets is available. The listening-ear helpline provides an opportunity to talk to another pain sufferer.

Contact a Family Helpline 0808 808 3555

The Pain Relief Foundation, Clinical Sciences Centre, University Hospital Aintree, Lower Lane, Liverpool L9 7AL   Tel: 0151 529 5820   Fax: 0151 529 5821
e-mail: secretary@painrelieffoundation.org.uk   Web: http://www.painrelieffoundation.org.uk
Information on chronic pain conditions. Send an A4 50p SAE plus £1.

British Pain Society, Third Floor, Churchill House, 35 Red Lion Square, London WC1R 4SG   Tel: 020 7269 7840   Fax: 020 7831 0859
e-mail: info@britishpainsociety.org   Web: http://www.britishpainsociety.org
Information booklet. Send an A4 SAE. A list of pain management clinics is also available.

Restricted growth and over growth

Restricted Growth Association (for contact details see Restricted Growth)
The Association has welfare and counselling services together with a regional contact network. It gives information about clothing, employment, mobility and home aids.

Child Growth Association (for contact details see Restricted Growth)
The Association supports and advises families of children and adults with restricted and over growth disorders. It has very good growth charts available.

Tracheostomy

A tracheostomy is performed where there is a temporary or permanent obstruction in the airway. An artificial opening is made in the trachea (windpipe) into which a tube is inserted. It is through this tube that the child or adult breathes. It is necessary to keep the airway clear by sucking out the secretions which form.

ACT (for contact details see Tracheostomy)
Offers support and encouragement to families and contact with others where possible.

Transplants

NHS Blood and Transplants, Oak House, Reeds Crescent, Watford WD24 4QN
Tel: 01923 486 800   Fax: 01923 486801   Web: http://www.nhsbt.nhs.uk
*NHS Blood and Transplant (NHSBT) was established as a Special Health Authority in October 2005. Its remit is to provide a reliable, efficient supply of blood, organs, information and associated services through its three branches: **UK Transplant**, Web: http://www.uktransplant.org.uk; **National Blood Service**, Web: http://www.blood.co.uk; and **Bio Products Laboratory**, Web: http://www.bpl.co.uk*

Urostomy and other urinary diversions

When the function of the bladder is affected by nerve damage or specific disorders such as Abdominal Exstrophies, Bladder Exstrophy, Spina Bifida, Hirschsprung's Disease, Cancer or Multiple Sclerosis (see entries) surgery can divert the urinary flow to an alternative site of output by means of an urostomy or other form of Urinary Diversion.

Urostomy Association, 18 Foxglove Avenue, Uttoxeter ST14 8UN   Tel: 01889 563 191
Fax: 01889 568 222   e-mail: info.ua@classmail.co.uk
Web: http://www.uagbi.org
The Urostomy Association has Young Persons Advisors (Male and Female).

Ventilation

Breathe On, Knight Cottage, Sackmore Lane, Marnhull DT10 1PN
Tel. 01258 820951 (answer phone)   e-mail. victoria@breatheon.org.uk
Web: http://www.breatheon.org.uk
Supports the families of children on long term ventilation.

Visible difference

There are a number of causes of face and body differences in children and adults for which there are a number of organisations that can provide information, advice and help. These causes include trauma and birth defects/syndromes.

Let's Face It (for contact details see Facial Difference)
Let's Face It has built up an extensive resource of information for people for whom automobile accidents, burns, cancer or birth defects/syndrome have caused a facial difference. The organisation aims to offer friendship on a one to one basis, provide information about prosthetics and other aids and raise awareness of facial difference and issues facing individuals to the medical, nursing and allied health professions.

Changing Faces (for contact details see Facial Difference)
Changing Faces provides information, support and advice to anyone with a disfigurement and their family. It has information and advice for employers to encourage equal opportunities in the workplace and for schools to promote awareness. It offers advice for healthcare professionals in developing new models of healthcare and build coping strategies and self-confidence for patients.

British Red Cross, 44 Moorfields, London EC2Y 9AL   Tel: 0844 871 11 11
Fax: 020 7562 2000   e-mail: information@redcross.org.uk
Web: http://www.redcross.org.uk
The British Red Cross aims to rebuild confidence by teaching the application of cover creams to disguise disfiguring skin conditions such as scarring, rosacea, vitiligo, tattoos, leg veins and other dermatological conditions. Services are provided through local branches, details available from UK office. The service only deals with prescribable camouflage products and a letter of recommendation goes to the service user's GP after consultation with a British Red Cross volunteer practitioner.

British Association of Skin Camouflage, PO Box 202, South Park Road, Macclesfield SK11 6FP   Tel: 01625 871129   e-mail: basc9@hotmail.com
Web: http://www.skin-camouflage.net
The British Association of Skin Camouflage promotes, support or further the remedial techniques of camouflage for the relief of those who need to be restored to confidence in a normal appearance and thereby to help improve their quality of life.

Cancerbackup (for contact details see Cancer)
Cancerbackup has extensive information on its website about Hair Loss and Wigs and Prosthesis & equipment needed by individuals and families of children as a consequence of Cancer.
Children and young people can access the Captain Chemo Website at
Web: http://www.royalmarsden.org/captchemo Further information is also available from local hospital based Children's Cancer and Leukaemia Group centres at 22 locations in the UK
Web: http://www.cclg.org.uk/public/about_us/introduction/centres.html
A lot of the information may be useful even if the cause is not cancer related.

Other sources of information

Institute of Child Health,
Web: http://www.ich.ucl.ac.uk/factsheets
A wide range of factsheets providing information relating to disorders, procedures and hospitalisation.

ANTENATAL, NEONATAL AND CHILDHOOD SCREENING: A SUMMARY FOR PROFESSIONALS

What is screening?

Although screening programmes have now been in place for many years in the UK and other countries around the world, there is still confusion as to what they can and cannot achieve. A screening test for a disorder is one offered to a large group of people who have no symptoms of the disorder. They are usually selected on the basis of their age or sex or the fact that they are pregnant. The screening test will pick out the people who are at highest risk of having the disorder in question. It cannot usually divide for certain those who have the disorder from those who don't have it. For most tests, some people with a positive result will turn out not to have the disorder ('false positive') and some with a negative result will subsequently be shown to have the disorder ('false negative'). Those people who have a positive result on the screening test are usually offered a further test ('diagnostic test'), which will pick out much more accurately those who have the disorder.

The term 'screening programme' includes the screening test, the diagnostic test and any treatment or action that follows on from these. To be of value, the quality of life of the person being screened, or their family, should be improved as a result of some change that results from the screening programme. This could be the early treatment of a disease so its adverse effects are minimised, or it may be allowing a pregnant woman to choose whether she wishes to continue with a pregnancy when the unborn baby has a serious disease. This latter is referred to as 'informed choice' and the success of such a programme cannot be judged by how many babies with a disease are terminated. It must be evaluated on the basis of the proportion of women who feel that they have received enough information and support to allow them to proceed in the way that is best for them. The benefits of the programme should outweigh any hazards, of which there are always some, such as anxiety generated.

Because screening, apart from the neonatal bloodspot programme, was somewhat haphazard, the National Screening Committee (NSC) was set up in 1996 to advise the UK Health Ministers on screening policy. In its first report, the NSC defined a screening test as:

'The systematic application of a test or enquiry, to identify individuals at sufficient risk to benefit from further investigation or direct preventive action, amongst persons who have not sought medical attention on account of symptoms of that disorder.'

The NSC is responsible for providing advice on those screening programmes which are to be implemented, those which are to be discontinued and those which are to be amended. Individual screening programmes are assessed against a set of criteria covering the condition, the test, the treatment options and effectiveness and acceptability of the screening programme. Assessment in this way is intended to ensure that more good than harm is achieved at a reasonable cost.

Appropriate information must be offered at every stage of the screening programme and where an abnormal test result occurs, counselling should be available.

The NSC has a subgroup known as the Fetal, Maternal and Child Health Coordinating Group. It is responsible for looking at issues in pregnancy and childhood.

Antenatal screening

Antenatal screening is undertaken for a number of conditions in the mother and unborn baby. For conditions in the mother, for example anaemia and raised blood pressure, treatment is available during the antenatal period to improve her health and indirectly that of the baby. For conditions in the baby, the screening test may enable a mother to make an informed choice about continuation of the pregnancy or allow treatment to improve the baby's health to be started as soon as possible.

1. Screening for maternal disease

Screening for maternal disease involves monitoring pregnancies to try to select those where, even though the pregnant woman appears well, she has a condition such as anaemia, HIV infection, syphilis or high blood pressure which could be harmful to the unborn baby. Once the condition has been discovered, treatment can be started to lessen the effect of the disease on the unborn baby. Immunity to rubella is checked, so that any non-immune mothers can be vaccinated after delivery. If a mother is found to be infected with hepatitis B, then her baby can be immunised soon after birth to prevent him/her becoming infected.

2. Screening for abnormalities of the unborn baby

Screening for fetal abnormality is offered to pregnant women as part of routine maternity care. Screening falls into two main groups – those that make use of ultrasound examination and those that rely on a blood test.

Ultrasound examination has the potential to show a number of structural abnormalities of the unborn baby. Abnormalities of the heart, spine, face and brain can be picked up as can neural tube defects (see entry, Spina Bifida). Early detection allows a mother to make an informed choice about the continuation of her pregnancy and, in some cases, treatment can be planned to take place soon after the baby is delivered.

Blood tests and/or ultrasound scans may indicate that the unborn baby has a high risk of being affected by Down syndrome (see entry). If this is the case then a further 'diagnostic' test – either chorionic villus sampling or amniocentesis (see section on Pre-Natal Diagnostic Techniques in Patterns of Inheritance) depending on how far the pregnancy has progressed - may confirm the presence or absence of the condition in the unborn baby. A blood test on the mother may also show that the unborn baby might have a disorder of its blood such as sickle cell disorder (see entry), thalassaemia (see entry), or haemolytic disease (Hemolytic disease - US) of the newborn (a form of severe anaemia in the baby arising because it has a different blood group from its mother). In this case, however, further tests would need to be performed to confirm this.

The results of antenatal blood tests are only capable of providing an *estimate* of the risk of a fetal abnormality and cannot definitely confirm the presence or absence of a specific condition during pregnancy. As such, screening test results are reported as a probability or risk of an affected pregnancy. These are described as:

- screen positive results - where the pregnancy is identified as having a high chance of a fetal abnormality;
- screen negative results - where the pregnancy is identified as having a low chance of a fetal abnormality.

However, there are a number of limitations of screening:

- Firstly, the tests currently available are capable of detecting a *limited* number of fetal abnormalities only. Many fetal abnormalities are not identified by the tests currently offered to women during pregnancy. This means that every woman has a small chance of having a pregnancy affected by a fetal abnormality even if they have had all the screening tests. For example, the screening tests cannot pick up whether a child will have autism or psychiatric problems;

- Secondly, the results of screening tests are not one hundred per cent accurate. The reason for this, as previously indicated, is that screening tests cannot completely distinguish those pregnancies affected with particular fetal abnormalities from those which are not. Therefore:
  - For some pregnancies shown to have a high chance of fetal abnormality (positive screen), the unborn baby will not have the condition screened for. These are called *'false positive results.'* In fact, for certain conditions, the majority of women found to be in the high risk group have a normal diagnostic test and go on to have healthy babies;
  - Conversely, for some pregnancies shown to have a low chance of fetal abnormality (negative screen), the baby will be affected by the condition. The number or proportion of these so-called *'false negative results'* varies with the type of screening test. A negative screen result does not mean that an affected pregnancy has been completely excluded.

  In fact, the accuracy of many screening tests depends on knowing how far advanced a pregnancy is at the time the test is performed. This is why all women have an ultrasound examination early in pregnancy;

- Thirdly, while screening tests incur no physical harm to the mother, some diagnostic tests carry a small risk of miscarriage. Following a positive screen result, therefore, women who decide to undergo diagnostic testing, such as chorionic villus sampling, amniocentesis or blood sampling from the fetus, may lose the unborn baby as a result of the procedure. This is one reason why invasive diagnostic procedures are not offered to every pregnant mother as a screening test to check for the presence of a fetal abnormality;

- Fourthly, screening cannot give complete reassurance to women and may generate anxiety.

Antenatal counselling
Informed decision-making

The National Screening Committee (NSC) has proposed that the key objective of screening programmes is to enable people to make informed choices. Individuals have a limited time during pregnancy in which to make decisions about screening and diagnostic testing. Typically, the decisions they face include:

- Whether or not to be screened;
- Which conditions to be screened for;
- Which test(s) to have.

Contact a Family Helpline 0808 808 3555

Women whose pregnancies are found to be at risk (that is a positive screen result) would need to consider:
- Whether or not to undergo prenatal diagnostic testing;
- Which test(s) to have;
- If the baby is found to be affected whether or not to continue with the pregnancy.

Antenatal screening and diagnostic tests differ significantly from tests employed in most branches of medicine. The majority of diagnostic tests in medicine are intended to guide management so that treatment may be implemented to alleviate or cure a medical condition. However, for the majority of fetal conditions which may be detected by antenatal screening, there may be no treatment currently available. In these cases the only options available for the parents are either to continue with the pregnancy and to use the test result to 'prepare themselves' for the birth of an affected child, or to accept the option of undergoing a termination of pregnancy. The very existence of screening tests will therefore mean that many parents will face the decision of whether or not to continue with their pregnancy. As there is likely to be a continuing rapid growth in genetic science, leading to the introduction of new screening tests, it is possible that many more couples will be faced with difficult dilemmas arising from screening and diagnostic testing concerning termination for fetal disease or abnormality.

Information needs
The provision of up-to-date information and high quality counselling and support enables women and couples to make the choices which they consider best. In this regard, The Royal College of Obstetricians and Gynaecologists recommend that:
- Women and their partners should feel free to exercise the options of their choice;
- Screening and diagnostic tests must only be undertaken with the knowledge and consent of the individual woman;
- For all aspects of antenatal screening, women and their partners must be given verbal information supported by suitable written or audiotape/ audio-visual, if required;
- For all aspects of antenatal screening, women and their partners should be aware of the risks and benefits associated with each test;
- It is suggested that there should be a policy on how, and when, women and their partners are given results. Results of specific tests such as those for fetal abnormality or HIV should be given in person;
- Individuals should be informed of all the results of any tests undertaken.

- Women should be fully supported and be offered access to specialist advice and support if required. This may include counselling or specialist advice for genetic disorders, HIV or haemoglobinopathy, etc. It should also include referral to self-help groups including ARC - Antenatal Results and Choices (see entry, Fetal Abnormality);
- Women should be satisfied with the service offered. Adherence to these policies can be audited.

Antenatal support

In order to minimise the emotional distress often associated with screening programmes, individuals may be offered accurate and sensitive counselling at various stages including:

- Prior to screening, during which individuals are given the opportunity to make an informed choice about whether or not to have particular tests;
- After screening, during which individuals are given the results of investigations and presented with the options for future action. At this time, support is offered to individuals in decision-making;
- Post-decision making, during which information from subsequent investigations is given, support is offered concerning the decision about whether or not to continue with an affected pregnancy and the implications for the future are discussed;
- Prior to a subsequent pregnancy, in which parents are helped to make decisions about antenatal diagnostic tests and cope with the huge burden of anxiety which often accompanies subsequent pregnancies (even if all goes well).

Quality assurance and monitoring

Quality assurance and monitoring are essential components of any screening programme and it is one of the NSC's responsibilities to set national standards. Currently, service provision across the four UK countries is fragmented leading to variation in policy and practice in antenatal screening. To illustrate this, different screening tests are offered in different regions, some at the same stage of pregnancy and some at different stages. Some screening tests indicate the risk of fetal abnormality at term whilst others express this risk at the time of screening. Variation in screening policies has resulted in the provision of screening on an inequitable basis and an overall line of responsibility would help to reduce such inequality.

Looking to the future, resources made available through the NHS plan have allowed the setting up of an Antenatal Screening Programme Development Project. This consists of a small national team with regional co-ordinators.

By improving the overall quality and co-ordination of antenatal screening programmes, it is hoped that women will be offered better information and support to enable them to make the choices they consider best.

Neonatal screening and childhood screening

1. Neonatal screening

Neonatal screening is offered so that the presence of a congenital disorder in the newborn may be identified as soon as possible after birth and treatment offered. Neonatal screening aims to ameliorate disabling conditions that impair a child's quality of life. The timeliness of screening ensures that appropriate treatment may begin and lead to the maximum possible reduction of the adverse effects of the condition.

Screening takes a number of forms in the neonatal period:

- A very small quantity of blood is taken from the baby's heel between the fifth and eighth day after birth. Currently all babies are tested for phenylketonuria, congenital hypothyroidism (see entry, Thyroid Disorders) cystic fibrosis and sickle cell disorders. A pilot of screening for MCADD (Medium chain acyl-coA dehydrogenase deficiency), another inborn error of metabolism (see entry, Metabolic diseases), been completed and screening will be introduced nationally by spring 2009;
- All babies have a routine physical examination after birth. A general examination ensures that there are no visible malformations and more specifically, the eyes are examined for conditions such as cataracts (see entry), the heart for heart defects (see entry), the hips for developmental dyspasia (see entry, Congenital Dislocation and Developmental Dysplasia of the Hip) and the testes for cryptorchidism;
- All babies have their hearing tested in the first four to five weeks of life.

2. Childhood screening after the neonatal period

- All babies have a physical examination at 6-8 weeks. This takes the same form as that in the neonatal period;
- It is recommended that all children have their vision assessed between four and five years old by someone specially trained to do so. This will take some time to institute;
- All children should have their height, weight and hearing screened at school entry.

Quality assurance and monitoring

There is variation in practice and policy in neonatal and childhood screening. There is currently a structure of child health screening co-ordinators in England who work closely with the antenatal co-ordinators.

Conclusion

Screening has significant differences from clinical practice as the health service is targeting apparently healthy people and offering to help individuals to make better informed choices about their health. However, as the NSC has pointed out, there are risks involved in screening and it is important, therefore, that individuals have realistic expectations of what a screening programme can deliver. Although screening may have the potential to save lives or improve quality of life through the early diagnosis of serious conditions, it is not a foolproof process. As such, whilst screening may reduce the risk of developing a condition or its complications, it cannot offer a guarantee of protection. The NSC has indicated that in any screening programme, there is an irreducible minimum of false positive results (people wrongly reported as having the condition) and false negative results (people wrongly reported as not having the condition). The NSC is increasingly presenting screening as risk reduction because of this. The NSC believe that what is required is overall direction, a written policy, specified funding and line responsibility, at the same time, preserving local commitment. It will be interesting to see the extent to which service providers will encourage public awareness of screening in the future.

Glossary

Screening test This is a test which is designed to identify those individuals who are at a high enough risk of having a particular disorder to warrant the offer of a diagnostic test. A screening test may be a procedure, such as a blood test, or it may be the asking of a question, such as 'How old are you?'

Screening programme This includes screening, diagnosis and the management of a condition.

Positive result (on a screening test) This is a result which indicates that an individual is at high risk of a condition.

Negative result (on a screening test) This is a result which indicates that an individual is at low risk of a condition.

False positive result A positive result is indicated where the condition is not present.

False negative result A negative result is indicated where the condition is present.

Sensitivity of a screening test This refers to the ability of the test to accurately detect those who have a condition. A highly sensitive test has a sensitivity approaching 100 per cent. The consequence of a test which lacks sensitivity is that individuals are informed that they do not have a condition when in fact they do (false negative).

Specificity of a screening test The ability of the test to accurately identify those who do not have the condition. A highly specific test has a specificity approaching 100 per cent. The consequence of a test which lacks specificity is that an individual is informed that they have a condition when in fact they do not (false positive).

Positive predictive value The proportion of people with a positive test result who have the condition.

Further information on the NSC and the screening programmes is available at Web: http://www.library.nhs.uk/screening

Additional reading

Collins, J. and Dezateux C. (2001) *The UK National Newborn Screening Programme Centre: Working towards quality in partnership.* Great Ormond Street Hospital for Children NHS Trust

Elliman, D.A.C., Dezateux, C., Bedford, H.E. *Newborn and childhood screening programmes: criteria, evidence, and current policy.* Arch Dis Child 2002;87:6-9.

Health Departments of the United Kingdom (1998) *First Report of the UK National Screening Committee* http://www.nsc.nhs.uk/pdfs/nsc_firstreport.pdf

Health Departments of the United Kingdom (2000) *Second Report of the UK National Screening Committee* http://www.nsc.nhs.uk/pdfs/secondreport.pdf

Royal College of Obstetricians & Gynaecologists (1995) *Report of the Audit Committee's Working Group on Communication Standards*, Royal College of Obstetricians & Gynaecologists, London.

Royal College of Obstetricians and Gynaecologists http://www.rcog.org.uk has a range of useful information in its *Guidelines* section.

Medical text written November 2002 by Contact a Family. Approved November 2002 by Dr David Elliman. **Last updated November 2007 by Dr David Elliman, Consultant in Community Child Health, Islington Primary Care Trust, London, UK and Great Ormond Street Hospital, London, UK and member of the National Screening Committee and Dr Helen Bedford, Senior Lecturer in Children's Health, Institute of Child Health, London, UK and past member of the Sub-Committee on Child Health, National Screening Committee.**

PATTERNS OF INHERITANCE

Introduction

Genetics is the branch of biology concerned with heredity and individual characteristics. Specific conditions and rare syndromes may have a genetic basis. Where this is the case there will be a variety of causes. For example the causes may include a **single abnormal gene**, a **chromosomal abnormality** or a **genetic predisposition allied to other factors**.

This section includes a glossary of genetic terms used throughout *The Contact a Family Directory* and it is written for the non-specialist. We shall concentrate mainly upon two forms of inheritance: the single abnormal gene and chromosomal abnormalities. Illustrations are used to explain certain patterns of inheritance.

The human body is made up of billions of cells. At the centre of each cell is a special compartment called the nucleus which stores threads of DNA (Deoxyribonucleic Acid) arranged in chromosomes. The chromosomes are in their turn composed of fifty thousand to one hundred thousand genes which contain the genetic blue print determining each individual's characteristics.

The ovum and sperm each carry twenty-three chromosomes and on fertilisation the chromosomes combine to give a total of twenty-three pairs, forty-six chromosomes in total. One pair of chromosomes determines the sex of the individual: males have an X and Y chromosome, while females have two X chromosomes.

Inheritance will depend upon the arrangement of the genes and the status mode of the gene, that is, autosomal dominant, autosomal recessive or X-linked recessive. (These terms are defined in the Genetics glossary).

1. Single abnormal gene

A mutant (abnormal) gene is one where a gene may be considered as a variant of a 'normal' gene. This change may occur spontaneously by chance and have no significance for the individual concerned. In other cases, the gene which mutates (changes its character) may give rise to specific inherited disorders where there is no previous family history. Such a gene, in specific circumstances determined by status, can cause a specific disorder. Inheritance may be autosomal dominant, autosomal recessive or X-linked recessive.

More research has shown that in many conditions there may be different spelling mistakes or mutations in the gene which can cause the disease. For example, in cystic fibrosis over two hundred different mutations can occur in the gene, but they mostly produce the same disease pattern.

Contact a Family Helpline 0808 808 3555

Autosomal dominant inheritance

Autosomal means that males or females are equally affected. In dominant inheritance the chance of passing on the disorder is fifty per cent for each pregnancy. If the gene is inherited it will result in an affected individual. Examples of such conditions are Huntington's Chorea or Tuberous Sclerosis. In some cases **penetrance** may not be complete in some individuals, resulting in a mild form of the condition. Sometimes the condition with autosomal dominant inheritance may arise due to a mutation in egg or sperm, and in such cases there would be no preceding history. This is illustrated in the diagram below.

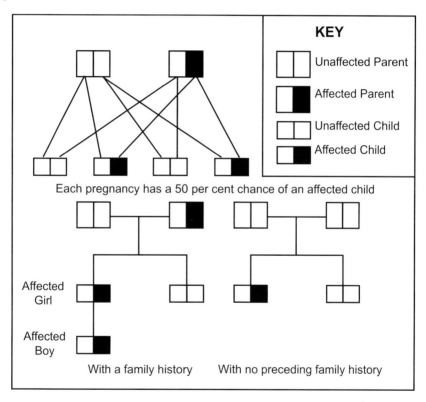

Autosomal recessive inheritance

In this form of inheritance the affected gene is recessive: two of the same gene mutations are required for the child to be affected by the disorder. In such cases the parents are unwitting carriers of the gene. The risk of an affected child being born will be twenty-five per cent for each pregnancy. Examples of such conditions are Friedreich's Ataxia, Cystic Fibrosis or Phenylketonuria.

Unless the parents are related, the chances of marrying a carrier of the same recessive gene is low, though the incidence of the existence of recessive genes in the population varies with conditions. Genetic counselling can help to predict the occurrence for individual families.

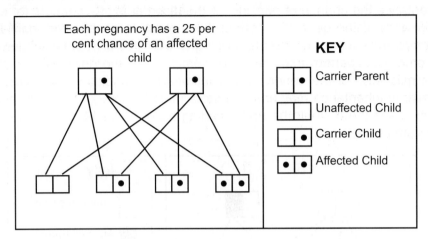

X-linked recessive inheritance

This is a recessive form of inheritance where the mother carries the affected gene on the X chromosome. This means that girls are carriers and that usually only boys are affected by the disorder. Examples of such disorders are Duchenne Muscular Dystrophy, Haemophilia (Hemophilia - US) or Hunter disease (a mucopolysaccharide disease.)

Affected men will not pass the condition on to their sons but all their daughters will be carriers. This is because a man passes his Y chromosome on to his sons and his X chromosome to his daughters.

In some rare situations, female carriers may show mild features of an X-linked disorder, for example in Fragile X syndrome.

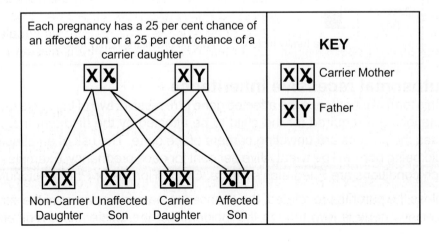

X-linked dominant inheritance

There are few examples of this type of inheritance, one such is Coffin-Lowry syndrome. In this form males and females are both affected. An affected female will have a fifty per cent chance of passing the disorder on to both her sons and her daughters. An affected male will pass the condition on to all his daughters, but not to his sons.

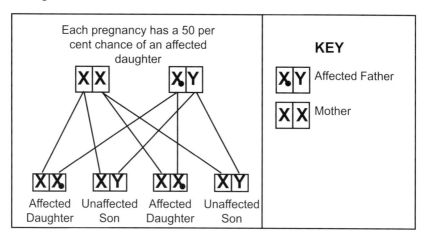

Each pregnancy has a 50 per cent chance of an affected daughter

KEY

X Y Affected Father

X X Mother

X X Affected Daughter X Y Unaffected Son X X Affected Daughter X Y Unaffected Son

Mitochondrial inheritance

The genetic material (DNA) is largely located in the nucleus of the cell, but in the surrounding cytoplasm of the cell there are small bodies called mitochondria which are responsible for energy production and also carry their own genes and DNA. These genes can also be passed on during reproduction. However, the pattern of inheritance is not always predictable since there is a chance element in determining the amount of cytoplasm and hence the amount of mitochondrial DNA that is passed on. Mitochondrial DNA is passed on through the egg but not by the sperm as it is only the nucleus of the sperm that enters the egg during fertilisation. Hence the pattern we see with mitochondrial inheritance is transmission through an affected female to a variable number of male and female offspring, but no transmission from an affected male.

Imprinted genes

In most cases it will not matter whether the gene or chromosome defect is inherited from the mother or father – the effect on the child will be the same. However there are some genes and chromosome regions in which there will be a different effect depending on which parent the abnormality has come from. For example, a deletion of chromosome 15 from the father in the sperm will cause Prader-Willi syndrome (see entry) whereas the same deletion of chromosome 15 from the mother in the egg will cause a different condition called Angelman syndrome (see entry). With these imprinted genes it is necessary to have both the maternal and paternal contribution in early embryonic development in the womb. It is likely that the need for a contribution from both parents has arisen in evolutionary terms with sexual reproduction and has been recognised as a barrier to certain forms of cloning.

2. Chromosomal abnormalities

A chromosome is a rod like structure present in the nucleus of all body cells, with the exception of the red blood cells, and which stores genetic information in the form of genes. The chromosome is like the wrapping round the genes. Normally human beings have twenty-three pairs of chromosomes, forty-six in total. The ova and sperm carry one of each pair, twenty-three chromosomes each. On fertilisation the chromosomes combine to give a total of forty-six. One pair of chromosomes in each individual is designated XX or XY. Normally a female has an XX pair and a male an XY pair.

A chromosomal abnormality occurs when there is a defect in a chromosome or in the arrangement of the genetic material on the chromosome. Chromosomal abnormalities give rise to specific physical features, but it should be stressed that there may be wide variations in the severity of the symptoms in individuals with the same chromosome abnormality.

Additional material may be attached to a chromosome; absence of a whole or part of a chromosome may occur, and defective formation of the chromosome may also occur. Increases and decreases in chromosomal material interfere with normal body function and development. Chromosomal abnormalities give rise to specific physical features.

There are two main types of chromosomal abnormality which may occur during meiosis and fertilisation. These are known as numerical aberrations and structural aberrations.

Numerical aberrations

Where these occur there is a failure in chromosome division resulting in cells with an extra chromosome (twenty-four chromosomes) or a deficiency (twenty-two chromosomes). Such abnormal gametes can result in anomalies such as Down syndrome (forty-seven chromosomes) or Turner syndrome (forty-five chromosomes). The following are examples of numerical aberrations; **triploidy, trisomy, monosomy** and **mosaicism**.

Structural aberrations

Where these occur there is a rearrangement in the location of, or a loss of, genetic material. These include: **deletions, duplications, inversions, ring formations and translocations (balanced, unbalanced and robertsonian.)**

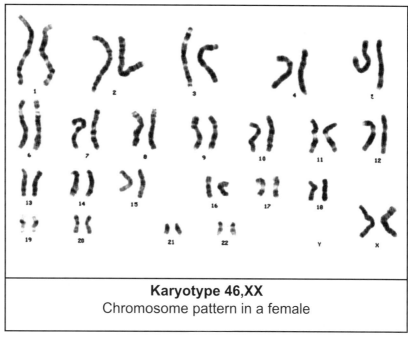

Karyotype 46,XX
Chromosome pattern in a female

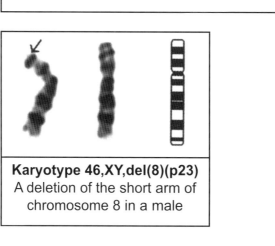

Karyotype 46,XY,del(8)(p23)
A deletion of the short arm of
chromosome 8 in a male

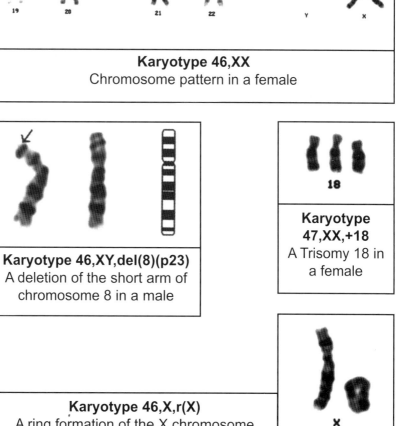

18

**Karyotype
47,XX,+18**
A Trisomy 18 in
a female

Karyotype 46,X,r(X)
A ring formation of the X chromosome

X

When cultured under specific conditions fragile sites may be located on the X chromosome. This gives rise to Fragile X syndrome where boys are worse affected but one third of affected girls also have some degree of learning difficulty.

Descriptions of particular chromosomal formations are often written in a shortened form. This type of contraction indicates the total number of chromosomes, the sex of the individual and the abnormal chromosome number. For example a girl with Cri du Chat syndrome would be shortened to 46,XX,5p- that is, the affected child has forty-six chromosomes, is a female (XX) and has a deletion of the short arm of chromosome 5. If this was in the form of a ring it would be 46,XX,r(5). A trisomy could be written as 47,XY, + 21, a male with Down syndrome.

Gene mapping is the area of genetic research that identifies at which chromosome site the gene is located. This is the first stage in trying to identify specific disease genes.

Gene markers are variations in the DNA or genetic material which lie close to the site of a disease gene and may be used for 'tracking' the disease through a family to provide prenatal or presymptomatic diagnosis.

Gene tracking is the process through which Gene Markers are followed through a family by genetic testing. When a specific marker is inherited with the disease in a significant number of individuals, then it may be used to assist in prenatal tests.

Fluorescent In Situ Hybridisation (FISH) is a new and promising technique for using fluorescent labelled gene markers in chromosome analysis. It allows the recognition of small deletions and rearrangement which would previously have been undetected. It may also provide a rapid method of detecting chromosome abnormalities.

3. Genetic pre-disposition allied to other factors

Such conditions combine a pre-disposition to develop a disease with other factors which may also contribute. There may be an undefined familial history of the condition. Where two affected children are born there may be an increased risk of recurrence. An example of a condition which falls into this category is Cleft Lip and Palate (see entry).

4. Genetic counselling

This is available at regional genetic centres throughout the country. Genetic counselling can quantify risks for particular parents in their individual circumstances. It can also provide support and advice for families who already have an affected child and wish to enlarge their family. A list of regional genetics centres is included on page 60.

Prenatal diagnostic techniques

There are a number of techniques which are used to diagnose prenatal defects in fetuses whose mothers are at risk of having a baby with an abnormality. Risks may include a family history of an anomaly, or that the parents have already had one child with, for exmaple, a heart defect. On the other hand prenatal testing may be performed on the grounds of the age of the mother. Common techniques are:

Amniocentesis

A sample of amniotic fluid (the 'waters') is taken through the abdominal wall. The sample of fluid is then analysed and certain biochemical, chromosomal or neural tube defects can be identified. Results may take three to four weeks. Amniocentesis can identify: metabolic diseases where the affected enzyme has been previously identified; chromosome defects; and neural tube defects (such as Spina Bifida, see entry).

Chorionic villus sampling

After fertilisation of the ovum by the sperm, the fertilised body forms a cell mass. The inner cells of this mass form the fetus, while the outer cells form the placenta. These outer cells become embedded in the wall of uterus (womb) forming placental material with the same origin as the fetus. These chorion cells can be tested to indicate fetal abnormality.

A catheter is introduced through the vagina or abdominal wall and using ultrasound scanning is guided to the chorionic villi. This test can be performed at ten to twelve weeks and chromosome results are available within two weeks. Hence results of abnormalities are obtained earlier than by amniocentesis.

The test can identify: metabolic defects where the affected enzyme has been isolated; chromosomal defects; and certain single gene defects where the specific gene has previously been identified. In these latter groups, results may be available in one or two days.

Fetoscopy

In this technique the mother and the fetus are both heavily sedated and an endoscope is fed through the abdominal wall into the uterus. A needle is then inserted through the tube. This method allows samples of fetal blood, liver or skin to be taken.

The advantages of fetoscopy are that the fetus can be seen and tissue and blood sampled. Additionally therapy such as blood transfusion may be given. Fetoscopy has largely been superseded by early prenatal diagnosis and ultrasound. It is available only in a few specialist centres.

Ultrasound scanning

A widely used technique involving the use of ultrasonic waves (sound waves of a high frequency which cannot be heard by the human ear) to scan the fetus and measure it. The fetus can be seen on the screen enabling skeletal and other abnormalities to be identified. Fetal measurements taken at the scan can be compared with average 'normal' fetal age measurements to identify anomalies.

Scans are normally performed between sixteen to twenty weeks. Conditions which may be identified include Spina Bifida, Hydrocephaly and Microcephaly (see entries). In some conditions like Tuberous Sclerosis, where heart tumours may contribute to the diagnosis, an additional scan may be performed at twenty to twenty-two weeks. The technique is widely used and has no specific risks for mother or fetus.

Medical text written 1991 by Professor Michael Patton. Last updated October 2004 by Professor Michael Patton. **Last reviewed August 2005 by Professor Michael Patton, Professor of Medical Genetics, St George's Hospital Medical School, London, UK.**

DICTIONARIES AND GLOSSARIES

Medical terms are usually formed of a number of parts which include a root, a prefix and/or a suffix. Knowledge of how terms are built up help in the understanding of medical terminology. For example, **hyper-** means excessive or increased and **hypo-** means deficient or decreased thus **hypertension** is higher than normal blood pressure and **hypotension** is lower than normal blood pressure.

Web: http://www.malattiemetaboliche.it/articoli/prefixs_suffixs.pdf (0.5Mb) *Extensive training resource of medical terms, prefixs & suffixs.*

General medical dictionaries

Web: http://www.childrenfirst.nhs.uk/kids/hospital/dictionary *Clear descriptions of range of medical terms for children and parents.*

Web: http://www.nelh.nhs.uk/directories.asp *Detailed explanation of medical terms available at the UK National electronic Library for Health (NeLH).*

Web: http://www.nlm.nih.gov/medlineplus/mplusdictionary.html *Short explanation of medical terms from the US government MedlinePlus.*

Genetic glossaries and information

Web: http://www.genome.gov/glossary.cfm *US National Institute of Health (NIH) Glossary of Genetic Terms.*

Web: http://www.gig.org.uk/education.htm *Genetic glossary and explanation of inheritance modes.*

Glossary of medical terms used

ABNORMAL A variation from the normal. In the case of genes an abnormal gene may result in a specific disorder.

ACQUIRED A condition or disease originating after birth. An acquired condition is not hereditary.

ACUTE A sudden onset of symptoms or disease which may be severe and/or brief in duration.

AUTOSOMAL Something which pertains to the autosome which is any chromosome other than the X and Y (set chromosomes). In practice it means that the abnormal gene can affect males or females equally.

AUTOSOMAL DOMINANT Where an individual possesses an altered gene that individual will demonstrate characteristics of the disorder. The condition will be transmitted to children with a 50 per cent chance of an affected child for each pregnancy.

AUTOSOMAL RECESSIVE Where an individual carries an altered gene this will not affect the individual him or herself. However, when two carriers of the same altered gene have children there is a 25 per cent chance of an affected child for each pregnancy.

BALANCED TRANSLOCATION Occurs when two chromosomes break and exchange places leaving the same amount of genetic material. An individual with a balanced translocation will be unaffected, but children may be affected in a variety of ways.

CARRIER An individual who carries the abnormal gene for a specific condition without symptoms (also referred to as heterozygote).

CATHETER A tube used either for withdrawing fluid from a body cavity or for introducing fluid to a body cavity.

CELL The basic structural unit of all living organisms. It is surrounded by a membrane and contains a nucleus which carries genetic material.

CHORIONIC VILLUS SAMPLING A method of collecting the chorion cells from the pregnant mother. Chorion cells are situated on the wall of the uterus (womb). They have the same origin as the fetal cells and can, therefore, be analysed to detect certain fetal abnormalities in the fetus.

CHROMATID The two halves into which a chromosome is longitudinally divided at mitosis and meiosis.

CHROMOSOME A rod like structure present in the nucleus of all body cells (with the exception of the red blood cells) which stores genetic information. Normally, humans have 23 pairs, the unfertilised ova and each sperm carrying a set of 23 chromosomes. On fertilisation the chromosomes combine to give a total of 46 (23 pairs).

CHRONIC Long-term or prolonged disease or condition which can persist or progress over a long period of time.

CONGENITAL A condition which is present at birth, although it can be recognised prenatally, at birth or many years later. A Congenital disorder can be genetic or acquired at any time during fetal development.

DELETION The absence of genetic material on a chromosome.

DIZYGOTIC Two cells having been fertilised resulting in twins.

DNA Deoxyribonucleic acid is the 'building block' for all genetic material.

DUPLICATION Occurs where a chromosome or part of a chromosome is duplicated. This may happen during cell division prior to fertilisation.

ENZYME A protein substance which is essential to the correct functioning of biochemical reactions which break down food into essential chemicals required by the body and/or break down toxic by-products in our bodies.

FAMILIAL Characteristic of some or all members of a family.

FETOSCOPY Method of prenatal diagnosis where the inside of womb and the developing fetus can be examined visually and sampling can be performed using a fetoscope.

FRAGILE SITE A site on a chromosome where genetic material may be prone to break. In Fragile X syndrome there is a fragile site on the female X chromosome.

GENETIC COUNSELLING Information and support provided by a specialist doctor, usually a geneticist, to parents who have known conditions in their families or who are concerned about the future possibility of genetically transmitted conditions.

IDIOPATHIC A disease or syndrome that is of unknown cause.

IMPRINTING Refers to the phenomenon whereby the effect of inheriting a gene is different depending on whether the inheritance was from the mother or father e.g. Prader Willi syndrome and Angelman syndrome.

INVERSION Occurs where a chromosome breaks in two and becomes reattached after turning round 180°. Providing no chromosome material is lost, this abnormality should have no effect on the individual. However, that individual may carry the risk of producing eggs or sperm with the incorrect amount of chromosome material.

HOMOZYGOTE A homozygote has a double dose of an altered gene as in an affected individual with an autosomal recessive disorder.

MEIOSIS The process of cell division which results in a cell where the 23 pairs of chromosomes split into two, each with 23 chromosomes. These cells are the female ova (eggs) and the male sperm.

MITOCHONDRIA Refers to the small bodies which are responsible for energy production and also carry their own genes and DNA.

MITOSIS Division of all cells except the reproductive cells with chromosome numbers and genetic make-up identical to that of the parent cell.

MONOSOMY The total loss of one of a pair of chromosomes. This occurs, for example, in Turner syndrome where one X chromosome is lost leaving a total of 45 chromosomes.

MOSAICISM Where a genetic or chromosomal abnormality does not occur in all body cells. The proportion of normal to abnormal cells will determine the severity of the disorder.

MUTANT A gene which has undergone change from the normal gene. This mutation may be an established one or a new sporadic mutation.

NEURAL TUBE DEFECT Occurs when there is a defective development of the spinal cord and the brain. Conditions such as Spina Bifida and Anencephaly (absent brain) are examples of such developmental defects.

NUCLEUS Portion in the centre of each cell which contains the chromosomes with their genetic material.

OVUM Female egg: reproductive cell carrying 23 chromosomes.

PENETRANCE The degree to which an individual who carries a dominant gene may show symptoms of the disorder.

PLACENTA A complex structure occurring in pregnancy. It is attached to the wall of the womb and connected to the fetus by the umbilical cord. The fetus receives its nourishment through the placenta and the vessels of the umbilical cord.

PREDISPOSITION (GENETIC) That the individual concerned is intrinsically more prone to develop a particular disorder.

RING FORMATION Occurs where the ends of a chromosome bend over and fuse together with a loss of genetic material.

ROBERTSONIAN TRANSLOCATION Occurs when translocations of chromosomes involve end to end fusion with the loss of the short arms. The balanced carrier has 45 chromosomes and is normal, any children may be affected in number of ways.

SPERM (abbreviation of spermatozoon) The male reproductive cell carrying 23 chromosomes

STATUS MODE (PATTERN OF INHERITANCE) Describes how the gene is inherited: for example, autosomal dominant, autosomal recessive or X-linked.

TRANSLOCATION Occurs where there is a rearrangement in which a piece of one chromosome is transferred to another with a different number.

TRIPLOIDY The presence of a full extra set of chromosomes. This abnormality is invariably lethal and would lead to a miscarriage or stillbirth.

TRISOMY The addition of a complete extra chromosome to a pair.

TWINS May be genetically identical (monozygous) when they arise from a single fertilised egg or non-identical (dizygous) when they arise from two separate eggs.

X-LINKED RECESSIVE The form of inheritance where the abnormal gene is carried on the X chromosome. It is a form of inheritance where girls are usually carriers and boys are affected. This is because the male Y chromosome does not carry the compensatory normal gene.

"We walked out of the hospital feeling stunned and alone. We had to wait two weeks to speak to the consultant. Those two weeks seemed an eternity, so we went straight to the internet to find more information, and completely terrified ourselves. You are then left to deal with a child with a rare disorder."
Parent.

REGIONAL GENETICS CENTRES

North Thames
Mothercare Unit of Clinical Genetics & Fetal Medicine
Institute of Child Health, 30 Guilford Street, London WC1N 1EH   Tel: 020 7905 2647

Kennedy Galton Centre for Clinical Genetics, Level 8V, Northwick Park Hospital, Harrow HA1 3UJ   Tel: 020 8869 2795

North West
Chester Regional Clinical Genetics Service
Moston Lodge, Countess of Chester Hospital, Liverpool Road, Chester CH2 1UL
Tel: 01244 364754

Mersey Regional Clinical Genetics Service
Royal Liverpool Children's Hospital, Eaton Road, West Derby, Liverpool L12 2AP
Tel: 0151 252 5238

Manchester Regional Genetics Service
Department of Medical Genetics, St Mary's Hospital, Hathersage Road, Manchester
M13 0JH   Tel: 0161 276 6506   Fax: 0161 276 6145

Manchester Paediatric Genetics Unit
Royal Manchester Children's Hospital, Hospital Road, Pendlebury, Manchester M27 4HA
Tel: 0161 727 2335   Fax: 0161 727 2328

Northern
Northern Genetics Service
International Centre for Life, Central Parkway, Newcastle upon Tyne NE1 3BZ
Tel: 0191 241 8600   Fax: 0191 241 8799

Yorkshire Regional Genetics Service
Ashley Wing, St James's University Hospital, Beckett Street, Leeds LS9 7TF
Tel: 0113 206 5555   Fax: 0113 246 7090

Northern Ireland
Regional Genetics Centre, Department of Medical Genetics, Floor A
Belfast City Hospital Trust, 97 Lisburn Road, Belfast BT9 7AB
Tel: 028 9026 3874   Fax: 028 9023 6911

Oxford and Anglia
East Anglian Medical Genetics Service
Addenbrooke's NHS Trust, Box 134, Hills Road, Cambridge CB2 2QQ
Tel: 01223 216446   Fax: 01223 217054

Oxford Regional Genetics Service
Department of Clinical Genetics, The Churchill, John Radcliffe NHS Trust, Old Road,
Headington, Oxford OX3 7LJ   Tel: 01865 226026

Scotland
North of Scotland Regional Genetics Service
Department of Medical Genetics, Medical School, Foresterhill, Aberdeen AB9 2ZD
Tel: 01224 552120   Fax: 01224 559390

Contact a Family Helpline 0808 808 3555

East Scotland Human Genetics Laboratories
Department of Pathology, Ninewells Hospital and Medical School, Dundee DD1 9SY
Tel: 01382 632035   Fax: 01382 640966

South East Scotland Clinical Genetics Service
Department of Clinical Genetics, Molecular Medicine Centre, Western General Hospital,
Crewe Road South, Edinburgh EH4 2XU   Tel: 0131 651 1012   Fax: 0131 651 1013

West of Scotland Regional Genetics Service
Ferguson-Smith Centre for Clinical Genetics, Yorkhill, Glasgow G3 8SJ
Tel: 0141 201 0808   Fax: 0141 201 0261

South Thames
South Thames (East) Regional Genetics Centre
Clinical Genetics Department, 7th Floor, New Guy's House, Guy's Hospital, London
SE1 9RT   Tel: 020 7188 1364   Fax: 020 7188 1369

South West Thames Regional Genetics Services
St Georges Hospital Medical School, Cranmer Terrace, London SW17 0RE
Tel: 020 8725 0574   Fax: 020 8725 3444

South West
Regional Cytogenetics Services
Southmead Hospital, Bristol BS10 5NB   Tel: 0117 959 5570

Clinical Genetics Department
Royal Hospital for Sick Children, St Michaels Hill, Bristol BS5 5BJ   Tel: 0117 928 5652

Clinical Genetics Department
Royal Devon & Exeter Hospital (Heavitree), Gladstone Road, Exeter EX1 2ED
Tel: 01392 405726   Fax: 01392 405739

Wessex Clinical Genetics Service
Level G, Princess Anne Hospital, Coxford Road, Southampton SO16 5YA
Tel: 023 8079 6166   Fax: 023 8079 4346

Trent
Department of Clinical Genetics
Leicester Royal Infirmary, Leicester LE1 5WW   Tel: 0116 258 5736   Fax: 0116 258 6057

Nottingham Department of Clinical Genetics
City Hospital, Hucknall Road, Nottingham NG5 1PB   Tel: 0115 962 7728
Fax: 0115 962 8042

North Trent Department of Clinical Genetics
Sheffield Children's Hospital, Sheffield S10 2TH   Tel: 0114 271 7025   Fax: 0114 273 7467

Wales
Institute of Medical Genetics
University Hospital of Wales, Heath Park, Cardiff CF14 4XW   Tel: 029 2074 4028

West Midlands
West Midlands Regional Clinical Genetics Service
Clinical Genetics Unit, Birmingham Women's Hospital, Edgbaston, Birmingham B15 2TG
Tel: 0121 627 2630   Fax: 0121 627 2618

Contact a Family Helpline 0808 808 3555

CHILDREN'S HOSPITALS

The details below are for children's hospitals; for general hospitals with children's wards, families should ask for the main information point, for the increasing number of Patient Advice and Liaison Services (PALS) offices, or should check individual hospital websites, links to which are available at Web: http://www.nhs.uk/root/localnhsservices/orgs/hospitals

Aberdeen
Royal Aberdeen Children's Hospital, Westburn Road, Aberdeen AB25 2ZG
Tel: 0845 456 6000   e-mail: carol.cameron@arh.grampian.scot.nhs.uk
e-mail: i.pucci3@nhs.net   Web: http://www.nhsgrampian.org
For information about services at the hospital, families should contact the Community Children's Nurses. There is accommodation for all families at the hospital and a range of specialist nurses. Specialist community nurses work to ensure that children can be treated at home if at all possible. There is also a range of secondary and tertiary services provided to the children of Orkney and Shetland, with some links to Highland and Tayside.

Brighton
Royal Alexandra Children's Hospital, Eastern Road, Brighton BN2 3JN
Tel: 01273 696 955 Web: http://www.bsuh.nhs.uk
Families can contact the Lead Nurse (Paediatrics), for general information about the hospital's services. There is a Ronald McDonald House providing free 'home away from home' accommodation for families of children having in-patient treatment. Please contact the House Manager, to check for availability of rooms, Tel: 01273 328145 ext.2226.

Belfast
Royal Belfast Hospital for Sick Children, 180 Falls Road, Belfast BT12 6BE
Tel: 028 9063 3139 (General office)
Web: http://www.royalhospitals.org/ourservices/paediatric.html
Families information needs can be obtained by contacting the hospital's general office. The hospital has a Citizen's Advice Bureau office open Mon-Thur (details of opening hours through the General Office). There is a Sargent Cancer Care for Children House which provides accommodation for families of children having cancer treatment. There is also range of other accommodation available at the hospital for families.

Birmingham
Birmingham Children's Hospital, Steelhouse Lane, Birmingham B4 6NH
Tel: 0121 333 9999   Tel: 0121 333 8403 (PALS service)
Tel: 0121 333 8505 (Child and Family Information Centre)
Tel 0121 333 8016 (Interpreting Services Team)
e-mail: child.infoctr@bch.nhs.uk   Web: http://www.bch.org.uk
The "Welcome to Birmingham Children's Hospital" booklet gives families general information about the hospital's services and facilities. For more information about the hospital, families can contact the Child and Family Information Centre. The Information Centre provides a free and confidential information service. They have information about childhood illness, disabilities, local and national support groups and general health promotion. Internet access is also available. The hospital also has an interpreting services team. There is a parent Accommodation Centre in the hospital for parents of long stay patients. Nearby accommodation is also provided by Edward's Trust, Tel: 0121 237 5656 Web: http://www.edwardstrust.org.uk

The Contact a Family Directory 2008

Bristol
Bristol Royal Hospital for Sick Children, Paul O'Gorman Building, Upper Maudlin Street, Bristol BS2 8BJ   Tel: 0117 342 8461   e-mail: bchinfo@ubht.swest.nhs.uk
Web: http://www.ubht.nhs.uk/bch
The hospital has a very good information booklet that can be downloaded from the website. Details of the specialties of the hospital and of the facilities of all the wards are also available. The hospital has a Family Information Room which provides written, verbal or electronic information to support parents and patients before, during and after treatment.

Cardiff
The Children's Hospital for Wales, University Hospital of Wales, Heath Park, Cardiff CF14 4XW   Tel: 029 2074 7747
Web: http://www.cardiffandvale.wales.nhs.uk
The Children's Hospital for Wales is based at the University Hospital of Wales. Accomodation for families of children receiving treatment can be arranged. Information about the location of the hospital and facilities at the hospital are on the main Cardiff and Vale NHS Trust website.

Edinburgh
Royal Hospital for Sick Children, 9 Sciennes Road, Edinburgh EH9 1LF
Tel: 0131 536 0070 (Family Support Services)   e-mail: kate.mitchell@luht.scot.nhs.uk
Pre-admission information is available to families through the Family Support staff who provide physical and emotional support to families with a child in hospital. Directions and maps can also be obtained here. There are three parent units run by the service providing facilities for both residential and non-residential families. Accommodation is provided on a priority basis. CLIC villa is available to families of haematology/oncology patients. The Special Needs Information Point (SNIP) provides emotional support and information on a wide range of issues including medical conditions and benefits. A text phone is available for parents and young people with a hearing impediment. To contact SNIP, Tel: 0131 536 0583 e-mail: snip@btinternet.com

Glasgow
Royal Hospital for Sick Children, Family Support & Information Service, Women's & Children's Directorate, Dalnair Street, Glasgow G3 8SJ
Tel: 0141 201 0707 (Family Information Centre)   e-mail: family.information@yorkhill.scot.nhs.uk
Web: http://www.show.scot.nhs.uk/yorkhill
The Family Support & Information Centre offers emotional, practical support & information for families who have a child in hospital. The centre offers a drop in facility for support & information. There is a quiet area and also an area for information leaflets please feel free to contact if you require further information.

Liverpool
Royal Liverpool Children's NHS Trust, Alder Hey, Eaton Road, Liverpool L12 2AP
Tel: 0151 252 5161 (PALS)   Tel: 0151 228 4811 ext. 3809 (Child and Family Information Centre)
Web: http://www.alderhey.org.uk
On the parents and carers pages of the Trust website there is a copy of "Welcome to Alder Hey" booklet that contains a host of useful information including maps and directions to the hospital as well as accommodation arrangements. The Trust has a Patient Advice and Liaison Service (PALS) service which provides information and advice on Trust services, and a host of health and care information to enquirers. The Parents and Carers Council and Children's and Young People Council are well established in the Trust and continue to work with staff to make "Alder Hey an even better place".

Contact a Family Helpline 0808 808 3555

London

Evelina Children's Hospital, St Thomas' Hospital, Lambeth Palace Road, London SE1 7EH
Tel: 020 7188 7188   e-mail: kic@gstt.nhs.uk   Web: http://www.guysandstthomas.nhs.uk
The Evelina Children's Hospital is based at St Thomas' Hospital in London. It has an extensive website with information detailing the hospital's location, facilities and hospital school. There are pull-out beds in the hospital where a parent can stay. For information about Ronald McDonald House accommodation for families of children receiving treatment at the hospital, ask the nurse in charge and for Gassiot House accommodation call the accommodation office on Tel: 020 7188 0276 (Mon-Fri; 9am-5pm). Accommodation is allocated on a priority basis.

Great Ormond Street Hospital, London WC1N 3JH   Tel: 020 7405 9200
Tel: 020 7813 8151 Family Services Department   Tel: 020 7829 7862 PALS
e-mail: pals@gosh.nhs.uk   Web: http://www.gosh.nhs.uk/pals
There are downloadable fact sheets and a large amount of useful information on the website which give details of both the hospital and the Institute of Child Health. Web: http://www.ich.ucl.ac.uk (For 'adults'). Web: http://www.childrenfirst.nhs.uk (With separate sections for 'tots', 'kids' and 'teens'). The hospital is able to provide on-site and off-site accommodation for over 1,000 parents of children having in-patient care. Accommodation is guaranteed for two parents with children in ITU (intensive care unit) and guaranteed for one parent with children in other wards. There are downloadable factsheets and a large amount of useful information on the website which give details of both the hospital and the Institute of Child Health. The PALS department is able to provide information about any matter relating to treatment at the hospital.

Manchester

Royal Manchester Children's Hospital, Hospital Road, Pendlebury, Manchester M27 4HA
Tel: 0161 727 2903 (PALS service)

Booth Hall Children's Hospital, Charlestown Road, Blackley, Manchester M9 7AA
Tel: 0161 220 5555 (PALS service)   Fax: 0161 220 5557
Web: http://www.cmmc.nhs.uk/hospitals/childrens
The hospitals have Family Counsellors and a Family Care Team. Advice, information and support is available for patients and families when a child is in hospital. Both hospitals have a PALS services. There is a very good parent information leaflet on the hospitals' joint website.

Sheffield

Sheffield Children's Hospital, Western Bank, Sheffield SO10 2TH
Tel: 0114 271 7594 PALS service   Fax: 0114 276 6073
e-mail: linda.towers@sheffch-tr.trent.nhs.uk
Web: http://www.sheffield.nhs.uk/hospitals/childrens.html
Information about services at the hospital, and to help resolve concerns, can be obtained from the PALS service. There is accommodation for parents and a very informative web site.

CHILDREN'S HOSPICES

For comprehensive information, contact:
The Association of Children's Hospices
First Floor, Canningford House, 38 Victoria Street, Bristol BS1 6BY   Tel: 0117 989 7820
Fax: 0117 929 1999 Web: http://www.childhospice.org.uk

A hospice pack is available from:
ACT - Association for Children with life-threatening conditions and Their families
Orchard House, Orchard Lane, Bristol BS1 5DT   Tel: 0117 922 1556   Fax: 0117 930 4707
e-mail: info@act.org.uk Web: http://www.act.org.uk

For information on Hospices for adults, contact:
Hospices Information
Help the Hospices, Hospice House, 34-44 Britannia Street, London WC1X 9JG
Tel: 0870 903 3903 Web: http://www.hospiceinformation.info

The following individual Hospices provide a wide variety of services, advice and information relevant to children with life-threatening conditions and their carers. Contact a Family's Helpline 0808 808 3555 is able to provide further information.

Acorns Children's Hospice Birmingham
103 Oak Tree Lane, Selly Oak, Birmingham B29 6HZ   Tel: 0121 248 4850
Web: http://www.acorns.org.uk

Acorns Children's Hospice Walsall
Walstead Road, Walsall WS5 4LZ   Tel: 01922 422500   Web: http://www.acorns.org.uk

Acorns Children's Hospice Worcester
350 Bath Road, Worcester WR5 3EZ   Tel: 01905 767676   Web: http://www.acorns.org.uk

Brian House
Low Moor Road, Bispham, Blackpool FY2 0BG   Tel: 01253 358 881
Web: http://www.brianhouse.inthefylde.org.uk

Butterwick Children's Hospice
Middlefield Road, Stockton-on-Tees TS19 8XN   Tel: 01642 607748
Web: http://www.butterwick.org.uk

Chase Children's Hospice Service
Christopher's, Old Portsmouth Road, Guildford GU3 1L P   Tel: 01483 230960
Web: http://www.chasecare.org.uk

Chestnut Tree House
Dover Lane, Poling, Arundel BN18 9PX   Tel: 0845 450 5820
Web: http://www.chestnut-tree-house.org.uk

Children's Hospice South West
Little Bridge House, Redlands Road, Fremington, Barnstaple EX31 2PZ
Tel: 01271 325270 Web: http://www.chsw.co.uk

Children's Trust
Tadworth Court, Tadworth KT20 5RU   Tel: 01737 365000
Web: http://www.thechildrenstrust.org.uk

Contact a Family Helpline 0808 808 3555

Claire House Children's Hospice
Clatterbridge Road, Bebbington, Wirral CH63 4JD   Tel: 0151 343 0883
Web: http://www.claire-house.org.uk

Demelza House Hospice Care for Children
Rook Lane, Bobbing, Sittingbourne ME9 8DZ   Tel: 01795 845200
Web: http://www.demelzahouse.org

Demelza-James Hospice at Home
Red Lion House, Magham Down, Hailsham BN27 1PN   Tel: 01323 446460

Derian House Children's Hospice
Chancery Road, Astley Village, Chorley PR7 1DH   Tel: 01257 271271
Web: http://www.derianhouse.co.uk

Donna Louise Trust
Treetops, 1 Grace Road, Trentham, Stoke on Trent ST4 8FN   Tel: 01782 654440
Web: http://www.donnalouisetrust.org

Douglas House
Magdalen Road, Oxford OX4 1RZ   Tel: 01865 794749
Web: http://www.helenanddouglas.org.uk

East Anglia's Children's Hospices (Ipswich)
6 Walker Close, Ipswich IP3 8LY   Tel: 01473 714194   Web: http://www.each.org.uk

East Anglia's Children's Hospices (Milton)
Milton, Cambridge CB4 6AB   Tel: 01223 860306   Web: http://www.each.org.uk

East Anglia's Children's Hospices (Quidenham)
Quidenham, Norwich NR16 2PH   Tel: 01953 888603   Web: http://www.each.org.uk

Eden Valley Children's Hospice (day care only)
Durdar Road, Carlisle CA2 4SD   Tel: 01228 810 801   Web: http://www.edenvalleyhospice.org.uk

Francis House
390 Parrs Wood Road, Didsbury, Manchester M20 5NA   Tel: 0161 434 4118
Web: http://www.francishouse.org.uk

Haven House Foundation
The White House, Mallinson Park, Woodford Green IG8 9LB   Tel: 020 8505 9944
Web: http://www.havenhouse.org.uk

Helen House
37 Leopold Street, Oxford OX4 1QT   Tel: 01865 728251
Web: http://www.helenanddouglas.org.uk

Hope House
Nant Lane, Morda, Oswestry SY10 9BX   Tel: 01691 671999
Web: http://www.hopehouse.org.uk

Horizon House
18 O'Neill Road, Newtownabbey BT36 6WB   Tel: 028 9077 7635
Web: http://www.nihospicecare.com

Iain Rennie Hospice at Home
52a Western Road, Tring HP23 4BB   Tel: 01442 890222   Web: http://www.irhh.org

Jessie May Trust
35 Old School House, Kingswood Foundation Estate, Britannia Road, Kingswood
Bristol BS15 8DB   Tel: 01179 582172   Web: http://www.jessiemaytrust.org.uk

Keech Cottage Children's Hospice
Great Barminham Lane, Luton LU3 3NT   Tel: 01582 492339   Web: http://www.pasque.org

Little Havens Children's Hospice
Daws Heath Road, Thundersley, Essex SS7 2LH
Tel: 01702 552200   Web: http://www.littlehavens.org.uk

Martin House
Grove Road, Clifford, Boston Spa, Wetherby LS23 6TX   Tel: 01937 845045
Web: http://www.martinhouse.org.uk

Naomi House
Stockbridge Road, Sutton Scotney, Winchester SO21 3JE   Tel: 01962 760060
Web: http://www.naomihouse.org.uk

Rachel House
Avenue Road, Kinross KY13 8FX   Tel: 01577 865777   Web: http://www.chas.org.uk

Rainbow Trust (South)
Rainbow House, 47 Eastwick Drive, Great Bookham, Leatherhead KT23 3PU
Tel: 01372 453309 Web: http://www.rainbowtrust.org.uk

Rainbow Trust (North)
Rainbow Fearnstone, Allendale Road, Lowgate, Hexham NE46 2NL   Tel: 01434 602961
Web: http://www.rainbowtrust.org.uk

Rainbows - The East Midlands Children's Hospice
Lark Rise, Hazel Road, Loughborough LE11 2HS   Tel: 01509 638 000
Web: http://rainbows.eazytiger.net

Richard House Children's Hospice
Richard House Drive, London E16 3RG   Tel: 020 7511 0222
Web: http://www.richardhouse.org.uk

Robin House
Boturich, Balloch, Alexandria G83 8LX   Tel: 01389 722055   Web: http://www.chas.org.uk

St Andrew's Children's Hospice
Peaks Lane, Grimsby DN32 9RP   Tel: 01472 350908
Web: http://www.standrewshospice.com

St Oswald's Children's Hospice
Regent Avenue, Gosforth, Newcastle-upon-Tyne NE3 1EE   Tel: 0191 285 0063
Web: http://www.st-oswalds.org

Shooting Stars Children's Hospice
The Avenue, Hampton TW12 3RA   Tel: 020 8481 8180   Web: http://www.shootingstar.org.uk

Ty Gobaith
Tremorfa Lane, Groesnydd, Conwy LL32 8SS   Tel: 01492 651900
Web: http://www.hopehouse.org.uk

Ty Hafan - Children's Hospice in Wales
Hays Road, Sully CF64 5XX
Tel: 01446 739993   Web: http://www.tyhafan.org

Zöe's Place Life Health Centre
Yew Tree Lane, West Derby, Liverpool L12 9HH   Tel: 0151 228 0353
Web: http://www.zoes-place.org.uk
Zöe's Place accepts babies up to the age of three years.

Contact a Family Helpline 0808 808 3555

HELPFUL ORGANISATIONS

The organisations listed below provide a wide variety of services, advice and information relevant to children with disabilities and their carers. The Contact a Family Helpline 0808 808 3555 is able to provide further information.

Aids and equipment

Disabled Drivers Association
Ashwellthorpe, Norwich NR16 1EX   Tel: 0870 770 3333   Fax: 01508 488173
e-mail: ddahq@aol.com   Web: http://www.dda.org.uk
Provides information and practical help on mobility issues for disabled people.

Disabled Living Foundation
380-384 Harrow Road, London W9 2HU   Tel: 0845 130 9177 Helpline
Tel: 020 7289 6111   e-mail: advice@dlf.org.uk   Web: http://www.dlf.org.uk
Comprehensive information service on aids/equipment for people with disabilities.

MedicAlert
1 Bridge Wharf, 156 Caledonian Road, London N1 9UU   Tel: 0800 581420 Helpline
Tel: 020 7833 3034   Fax: 020 7278 0647   e-mail: info@medicalert.co.uk
Web: http://www.medicalert.org.uk
The Emergency Identification System for people with hidden medical conditions.

Bereavement

Bereavement Service Department
Great Ormond Street Hospital, London WC1N 3JH   Tel: 0800 282986 Helpline (7-10pm; & Mon- Fri, 10am-1pm; & Wed 1-4pm)   Tel: 020 7813 8551   Fax: 020 7813 8516
Web: http://www.childdeathhelpline.org.uk

Child Bereavement Trust
Aston House, High Street, West Wycombe, High Wycombe HP14 3AG
Tel: 0845 357 1000 Information & support service line   Tel: 01494 446648
Fax: 01494 440057   e-mail: enquiries@childbereavement.org.uk
Web: http://www.childbereavement.org.uk

Compassionate Friends
53 North Street, Bedminster, Bristol BS3 1EN   Tel: 08451 23 23 04 Helpline
Tel: 0117 953 9639   e-mail: info@tcf.org.uk   Web: http://tcf.org.uk
Support for bereaved parents.

Cruse Bereavement Care
126 Sheen Road, Richmond TW9 1UR   Tel: 0870 167 1677 Helpline   Tel: 020 8332 7227
Fax: 020 8940 7638   e-mail: info@crusebereavementcare.org.uk
Web: http://www.crusebereavementcare.org.uk
Web: http://www.rd4u.org.uk (Young Person's web site)
Bereavement help and information.

The Alder Centre
Alder Hey Children's Hospital, Eaton Road, Liverpool L12 2AP   Tel: 0800 282986 Helpline (7-10pm; & Mon- Fri, 10am-1pm; & Wed 1-4pm)   Tel: 0151 252 5391   Fax: 0151 252 5513
Web: http://www.childdeathhelpline.org.uk
A partnership between professionals and trained volunteers, virtually all of whom are bereaved parents, who offer befriending and emotional support to others who have suffered a similar experience.

Carers

Carers UK
20-25 Glasshouse Yard, London EC1A 4JT   Tel: 0808 808 7777 Carers Line (Wed & Thur, 10am-12noon & 2pm-4pm)   Tel: 020 7490 8818   Fax: 020 7490 8824
e-mail: info@ukcarers.org   Web: http://www.carersonline.org.uk
Advice, information and campaigning for carers.

Carers Scotland
91 Mitchell Street, Glasgow G1 3LN   Tel: 0141 221 9141   e-mail: info@carerscotland.org
Web: http://www.carerscotland.org

Carers Wales
River House, Ynsbridge Court, Gwaelod-y-Garth, Cardiff CF15 9SS
Tel: 0292 081 1370   e-mail: info@carerswales.org.uk   Web: http://www.carerswales.org

Crossroads Care
10 Regent Place, Rugby CV21 2PN   Tel: 0845 450 0350   Fax: 01788 565 498
e-mail: communications@crossroads.org.uk   Web: http://www.crossroads.org.uk
Co-ordinates schemes for care of disabled people in their own homes.

Crossroads Scotland
24 George Square, Glasgow G2 1EG   Tel: 0141 226 3793   Fax: 0141 221 7130
e-mail: info@crossroads-scotland.co.uk   Web: http://www.crossroads-scotland.co.uk
Care Attendant Schemes providing short breaks for carers across Scotland.

Princess Royal Trust for Carers
142 Minories, London EC3N 1LB   Tel: 020 7480 7788   Fax: 020 7481 4729
e-mail: info@carers.org   Web: http://www.carers.org
Provides access to support, advice and services through its network of carers' centres.

Funding

Family Fund
Unit 4, Alpha Court, Monks Cross Drive, Huntington, York YO32 9WN
Tel: 0845 130 4542   Text: 01904 658085   Fax: 01904 652 625
e-mail: info@familyfund.org.uk   Web: http://www.familyfund.org.uk
A national charity offering financial assistance and information to families caring for a child/ children with special needs and disabilities under the age of 16 years.

React
St Luke's House, 270 Sandycombe Road, Kew, Richmond TW9 3NP   Tel: 020 8940 2575
Fax: 020 8940 2050   e-mail: react@reactcharity.org   Web: http://www.reactcharity.org
Grants for the special aids/equipment needs of children with life-threatening conditions.

General support organisations

Barnardo's
Tanners Lane, Barkingside, Ilford IG6 1QG   Tel: 020 8550 8822   Fax: 020 8551 6870
e-mail: dorothy.howes@barnardos.org.uk   Web: http://www.barnardos.org.uk
Barnardo's helps the most vulnerable children and young people transform their lives and fulfil their potential.

Contact a Family Helpline 0808 808 3555

BDF Newlife
BDF Centre, Hemlock Business Park, Hemlock Way, Cannock WS11 7GF
Tel: 08700 70 70 20   Nurse Helpline   Tel: 01543 468888   Fax: 01543 468999
e-mail: info@bdfnewlife.co.uk   Web: http://www.bdfcharity.co.uk
Provides support service for families, funds medical research, creates awareness and encourages prevention of birth defects.

SSAFA
19 Queen Elizabeth Street, London SE1 2LP   Tel: 0845 1300 975
e-mail: info@ssafa.org.uk   Web: http://www.ssafa.org.uk
National charity helping serving and ex- Service men, women and their families, including widows and widowers in need.

The Cedar Foundation
Malcolm Sinclair House, 31 Ulsterville Avenue, Belfast BT9 7AS   Tel: 028 9066 6188
Fax: 028 9068 2400   email: info@cedar-foundation.org
Web: http://www.cedar-foundation.org
Northern Ireland charity supporting people with disabilities to be fully included in their communities.

Government
Directgov
Web: http://www.direct.gov.uk/carers - Information for carers
Web: http://www.direct.gov.uk/disability - Information for disabled people
Directgov provides a single point of online access to government carers and disability services and information - including financial support, rights, independent living and much more.

ParentsCentre
Web: http://www.parentscentre.gov.uk - helping you to help your child.
Information and support for parents on how to help with your child's learning, including advice on choosing a school and finding childcare.

Short Term Breaks
Provision of short term breaks varies widely. Information can be obtained from local social services and voluntary organisations such as **Barnardos**,
Web: http://www.barnardos.org.uk and **NCH**, Web: http://www.nch.org.uk
Contact a Family national and regional offices have details of information services and providers in their area.

Umbrella organisations
ACT - Association for Children with life-threatening or terminal conditions and Their families
Orchard House, Orchard Lane, Bristol BS1 5DT   Tel: 0845 108 2201 Helpline
Tel: 0117 922 1556   Fax: 0117 930 4707   e-mail: info@act.org.uk
Web: http://www.act.org.uk
Campaigns for children's palliative care services, promotes models of good care and provides information for families and professional workers. Also runs Web: http://www.act4families.org.uk giving the latest developments in palliative care and an opportunity for families to exchange information and give feedback on the issues they face.

Brain and Spine Foundation
7 Winchester House, Cranmer Road, Kennington Park, London SW9 6EJ
Tel: 0808 808 1000 (Helpline)   Tel: 020 7793 5900 (Admin)   Fax: 020 7793 5939
e-mail: helpline@brainandspine.org.uk   Web: http://www.brainandspine.org.uk
Provides an information service for patients, carers and health professionals; an education
programme for GPs and medical undergraduates; and workbooks for schools and colleges
as well as supporting a wide range of neuroscience research projects. Provides information
and support for children and young people through Headstrong
Web: http://www.headstrongkids.org.uk

Council for Disabled Children
8 Wakely Street, London EC1V 7QE   Tel: 020 7843 1900   Fax: 020 7843 6313
e-mail: cdc@ncb.org.uk   Web: http://www.ncb.org.uk/cdc
Promotes collaborative work between different organisations providing services and
support for children and young people with disabilities and special educational needs.

Genetic Interest Group
Unit 4D, Leroy House, 436 Essex Road, London N1 3QP   Tel: 020 7704 3141
Fax: 020 7359 1447   e-mail: mail@gig.org.uk   Web: http://www.gig.org.uk
Forum of voluntary organisations concerned with policy for genetic disorders.

Long-Term Medical Conditions Alliance
202 Hatton Square, 16 Baldwins Gardens, London EC1N 7RJ   Tel: 020 7813 3637
Fax: 020 7813 3640   e-mail: info@lmca.org.uk
Web: http://www.lmca.org.uk
The umbrella body for national voluntary organisations working to meet the needs of
people with long-term health conditions.

National Parent Partnership Network (NPPN)
Council for Disabled Children, 8 Wakley Street, London EC1V 7QE   Tel: 020 7843 6058
e-mail: drussell@ncb.org.uk   Web: http://www.parentpartnership.org.uk
Supports the work of the parent partnership services which provide information and advice
to parents, particularly during statutory assessment and the issuing of a statement.

Patients Forum
Riverbank House, 1 Putney Bridge Approach, London SW6 3JD   Tel: 020 7736 7903
Fax: 020 7736 7932   e-mail: info@thepatientsforum.org.uk
Web: http://www.thepatientsforum.org.uk
A network of national and regional organisations representing the healthcare interests of
patients, their families and carers.

Transplant Support Network
Springfield Mills, Oakworth Road, Keighley BD21 1SL   Tel: 0800 027 4490 Helpline
e-mail: info@tsnet.demon.co.uk   Web: http://www.transplantsupportnetwork.org.uk
The Network provides support and information for all those who have had a transplant.

OVERSEAS ORGANISATIONS FOR SPECIFIC CONDITIONS AND RARE DISORDERS

Australia
Association of Genetic Support of Australasia (AGSA)
Web: http://www.agsa-geneticsupport.org.au

Canada
Canadian Organization for Rare Disorders   Web: http://www.cord.ca

Europe
European Organization for Rare Disorders   Web: http://www.eurordis.org

France
Alliance Maladies Rares   Web: http://www.alliance-maladies-rares.org

Germany
Bundesarbeitsgemeinschaft Hilfe für Behinderte e.V.   Web: http://www.bagh.de

Denmark
KMS   Web: http://www.kms-danmark.dk

Netherlands
Vereniging Samenwerkende Ouder- en Patiëntenorganisaties
Web: http://www.vsop.nl

New Zealand
Parent to Parent New Zealand   Web: http://www.parent2parent.org.nz

Norway
Senter for Sjeldne Funksjonshemningler   Web: http://www.frambu.no

USA
Birth Defect Research for Children   Web: http://www.birthdefects.org

National Organization for Rare Disorders (NORD)   Web: http://www.rarediseases.org

MUMS National Parent-to-Parent Network   Web: http://www.netnet.net/mums

Self-help clearinghouses
Web: http://www.mentalhelp.net/selfhelp/selfhelp.php?id=859_
Self-help clearinghouses can provide information on local support groups, including groups not affiliated with any national self-help organisation. In addition, many of the clearinghouses provide consultation to help individuals develop needed new groups. Some provide training workshops, distribute 'how to' materials, and publish directories and newsletters.

CONTACT A FAMILY PUBLICATIONS

Contact a Family produces a range of guides covering issues affecting families, regardless of their children's disability or condition. Individual copies are available free of charge, multiple copies from £1. The full publications list and order from is available from Contact a Family, 209-211 City Road, London EC1V 1JN. The guides include:

- **A guide to claiming Disability Living Allowance for children** helps parents and professionals through the claiming process with information on how to appeal if unsuccessful.
- **About families with disabled children** is a guide for students and professional workers which highlights some of the issues that are part of a parent's daily experience of caring for a disabled child; it also details key legislation.
- **Aids, equipment and adaptations** gives information on where to obtain special equipment and how to adapt your home.
- **A parents' guide to direct payments in England and Wales** and **A parents' guide to direct payments in Scotland** explains how to go about getting direct payments and how they work in practice.
- **Benefits, tax credits and other financial assistance** explains the range of benefits, tax credits and financial support that families may be entitled to, as well as details of other organisations that may provide financial assistance.
- **Dealing with debt - Scotland, Dealing with debt - England and Wales** and **Dealing with debt - Northern Ireland** provide pointers for families in debt. Research shows that families looking after a child with a disability are particularly likely to face debt problems. It is estimated that, on average, bringing up a child with a disability costs three times what it costs to bring up another child.
- **Disabled children's services in England and Wales** and **A guide to assessments and services in Scotland** look at social services/social work assessments and the rights of families to get the support they need.
- **Education Maintenance Allowance** looks at how to get a weekly payment for your son or daughter if they stay on at school, college or training after compulsory schooling.
- **Fathers** gives some practical information to fathers of children with disabilities as well as sharing the experiences of other dads.
- **Finding and paying for childcare** advises on access to quality childcare which can be an issue for any family, but may be particularly important - and often more difficult - if you are looking after a disabled child.
- **Grandparents** attempts to identify some of the feelings and needs

grandparents may experience as well as highlighting ideas for those grandparents who are unsure how best to support parents/carers of a child with a disability.

- **Help with council tax bills** includes information about the different schemes that exist for reducing a council tax bill.
- **Holidays, play and leisure** provides details of organisations that have regular up-to-date information about holidays for people with disabilities, sources of finance, and details of specialist holiday providers.
- **Money when your child reaches 16** explains what happens to benefits and tax credits when a child turns 16, and whether they should start claiming in their own right.
- **Preparing for adult life and transition England and Wales** and **Preparing for adult life and transition in Scotland** identify the main areas that parents and young people need to think about. It explains the Transition Plan, the essential starting point in planning for the future.
- **Relationships and caring for a disabled child** uses comments and views from parents themselves, along with some practical information about services and entitlements, to act as a guide for all parents of disabled children struggling with relationship issues
- **Siblings** brings together the experiences of brothers and sisters of children with disabilities and provides ideas for parents on dealing with the wide range of emotions and issues that can arise.
- **Special educational needs - England**, **Special educational needs - Wales** and **Additional support for learning - Scotland** provide a brief introduction to the processes involved in getting extra help at school and other education settings for a child with special educational needs.
- **The NHS and caring for a disabled child** explains what your rights are within the NHS and what services you should expect to receive.
- **The tax credits guide** includes a 'ready reckoner' to help assess tax credit entitlement.
- **Understanding your child's behaviour** looks at particular aspects of behaviour such as intellectual strengths and needs, speech and language, concentration skills and impulse control, interpersonal functioning and tendency to self-harm.
- **Working** is aimed at parents of disabled children who are thinking about returning to work or are currently in employment. It includes information about the support available to make that transition back into employment and your rights when in work.

We also publish **When your child has additional needs**, a guide for parents and **Concerned about your child** which explains the help available and encourages parents to talk to their doctor or health visitor should they have concerns about their child's development.

IMMUNISATION

Immunisation is the use of a vaccine to protect against disease. When a vaccine is given, the body's immune system is stimulated to produce memory cells and substances called antibodies which protect against future infections. Vaccines contain either:

- the live germ (bacteria or virus) which has been toned down (attenuated) so that usually it does not cause the disease or, if so, it is usually in a mild form; or
- the killed germ; or
- part(s) of the germ or things the germ produces.

Vaccines also contain small quantities of other substances to enable them to work properly.

The Routine Childhood Immunisation Schedule in UK (from September 2006)

Vaccine	Recommended age of administration
Diphtheria, tetanus, pertussis (DTP), Inactivated polio vaccine (IPV) and Haemophilus influenzae type b (Hib) – DTP/IPV/Hib, a single injection	8 weeks.
Pneumococcal conjugate vaccine (PCV)	8 weeks.
DTP/IPV/Hib and Meningococcal C vaccine (Men C)	12 weeks.
DTP/IPV/Hib, PCV and Men C	16 weeks.
Hib/Men C booster	12 months.
Measles, mumps & rubella (MMR) and PCV	13 months.
MMR - 2nd dose	Any time after 1st dose as long as at least three months have elapsed, or one month if after 18 months old. Usually given with pre-school booster below.
DTP/IPV	Three years four months.
Td/IPV	At, or before, time of leaving school. From 2008, Human Papilloma Virus (HPV) vaccine will be given to girls in year 8 at school. There will also be a catch-up campaign for older children in the school years beginning autumn 2009 and autumn 2010.

BCG used to be offered to all children in secondary school, but as the pattern of disease has changed, this is no longer the case. Instead, the vaccine is offered to all babies and children who are thought to be at higher risk of catching the disease. In some areas, this will mean that all babies are offered the vaccine.

It is normal for parents to have concerns and questions about immunisation. There are very few reasons for withholding immunisation. They are usually temporary and include:

- if the child is unwell or has a fever on the day of immunisation, in which case the vaccination should be postponed;
- if the child is taking any medicines that affect the immune system, including steroids or has a disease that affects the immune system;
- if the child has an unstable neurological condition.

Side-effects of immunisation include swelling or redness around the site of the injection, temperature or irritability.

Parents of children with special needs may have concerns relating to immunisation and their child's specific condition. Children who have certain specific conditions may be more at risk from childhood diseases and therefore immunisation is encouraged. Where the condition affects the immune system (e.g. Primary Immunodeficiencies, see entry) vaccination may not work very well and, in some cases, live vaccines may be dangerous. In such circumstances, vaccination should always be discussed with the child's paediatrician. It is always helpful for parents to discuss any concerns they may have regarding immunisations with their health visitor or general practitioner or with the paediatrician involved in the care and management of their child.

Medical text written June 2000 by Dr David Elliman and Dr Helen Bedford. **Last updated October 2007 by Dr David Elliman, Consultant in Community Child Health, Islington Primary Care Trust, London, UK and Great Ormond Street Hospital, London, UK, Immunisation Co-ordinator, Islington Primary Care Trust and Dr Helen Bedford, Senior Lecturer, Centre for Paediatric Epidemiology and Biostatistics, Institute of Child Health, London, UK.**

Further information on this and the Immunisation Programme can also be obtained from:

Immunisation Programme
Department of Health, Room 602A, Skipton House, 80 London Road, London SE1 6LH
Fax: 020 7972 5758   Web: http://www.immunisation.org.uk
Group details last confirmed August 2006.

The Health Promotion Agency for Northern Ireland
18 Ormeau Avenue, Belfast BT2 8HS   Tel: 028 9031 1611
Web: http://www.healthpromotionagency.org.uk/Work/Parentschild/immunisation/menu.htm
Group details last confirmed August 2006.

Health Education Board Scotland
Woodburn House, Canaan Lane, Edinburgh EH10 4SG   Tel: 0131 536 5500
Text: 0131 536 5503   Web: http://www.hebs.scot.nhs.uk
Group details last confirmed August 2006.

Other organisations providing parents with alternative views:

Justice Awareness and Basic Support (JABS)
1 Gawsworth Road, Golborne, Warrington WA3 3RF   Tel: 01942 713565
Fax: 01942 201323   e-mail: jabs@jabs.org.uk   Web: http://www.jabs.org.uk
Offers support to parents who believe their children have a health problem following immunisation.
Group details last confirmed August 2006.

The Informed Parent
PO Box 4481, Worthing BN11 2WH   Tel/Fax: 01903 212969
Web: http://www.informedparent.co.uk
Provides an alternative view of immunisation to the official stance and supports parents regardless of decisions made.
Group details last confirmed August 2006.

All service providers are now expected to involve parents in developing services for disabled children. Contact a Family can help with its two new practical consultation guides, one for parents and one for professionals, published in partnership with the Council for Disabled Children and available from Contact a Family.

22q11 DELETION SYNDROMES

22q11 Deletions: DiGeorge syndrome (DGS); velo-cardio-facial syndrome (VCFS); Shprintzen syndrome; CATCH 22

Background

The chromosome 22q11 deletion is found in a wide variety of apparently unrelated conditions. The deletion was first recognized in 1981 in Di George syndrome, affecting the heart, calcium and resistance to infection and occasionally the palate. Velo-cardio-facial syndrome (VCFS) with disorders in structure and function of the palate, heart defect and a facial appearance with features similar to each other, also known as Shprintzen syndrome, was considered a quite separate condition until the genetic basis was found to be the same as Di George in 1988. In Japan it was called conotruncal anomaly face syndrome. It has also been called CATCH 22, after some of the most important medical features (C=cleft palate, A=appearance, T=thymus/ immunology deficiency, C=calcium salt low, H=heart defect), but this name is not favoured when describing people.

The effects can be seen as a range of severity from mild to moderate in VCFS, to more severe in Di George syndrome.

What are the symptoms?

The main features found in the 22q11 deletion are numerous and affect every body system but the severity varies from person to person with two people from the same family not necessarily showing the same features to the same extent. These features include:

Heart problems (see entry, Heart Defects) which affect about seventy-five per cent of people with 22q11 deletion. The most common heart problems are: tetralogy of Fallot (a combination of four heart defects), interrupted aortic arch (failure of development of a section of the main artery supplying the body), ventricular septal defect (hole in the ventricle of the heart which allows blood to flow where it should not) and right aortic arch (instead of the usual left side).

Learning disabilities (see entry, Learning Difficulties) affect about sixty-five per cent people with 22q11 deletion and include: slow development of speech and language; poor concentration; and an inability to reach age appropriate milestones. The child may have difficulty at school with arithmetic, comprehension and problem solving, but may be particularly good at learning by rote and reading. The learning difficulties may be associated with a smaller than usual head size or rarely, by craniosynostosis (where the bones in the skull close before they should). ADHD - Attention Deficit Hyperactivity Disorder (see entry) is more common than usual, making learning difficult, and may not respond to the usually recommended medicines. Early intervention can help reduce the problems.

Cleft palate (see entry, Cleft Lip and/or Palate) and velopharyngeal insufficiency are found in around sixty per cent of people with 22q11 deletion. The palate (or roof of the mouth) closes off the nose from the back of the mouth during speech and can contribute to a delay in speech and language. Regurgitation through the nose during swallowing can also occur, although it is not very common. This effect on speech and swallowing is called velopharyngeal insufficiency (VPI). Problems that might occur include a cleft palate (where there is a hole in the palate) or a submucous cleft (where the roof of the mouth may look fine, but the muscles are not in the right position). Another problem which may be present is weakness and in-coordination of the muscles in the roof of the mouth. VPI also occurs in some patients because the adenoids are poorly developed or the base of the skull is shortened. VPI results in an excessively nasal sounding voice, and makes consonant sounds more difficult.

Speech problems (see entry, Speech and Language Impairment) are common with clefts or VPI but may also result from developmental delay, learning difficulties, or hearing difficulties which are caused by problems with the Eustachian tubes (which drain fluid from the ear). This can cause glue ear, middle ear infections which are made worse or more frequent than usual due to the immune deficiency, developmental delay or learning difficulties.

Feeding difficulties are common in infancy and early childhood because of the combination of cleft palate and/or VPI, and regurgitation of stomach contents into the gullet and mouth (gastro-oesophageal reflux). There may also be problems with chewing and swallowing solids (dysphagia) which may benefit from specialist help.

People with 22q11 deletion tend to have similar facial features including almond shaped eyes, elongated facial features often with flat cheek bones, a long, 'strong' nose with a relatively broad and prominent nasal bridge, small nostrils, and small jaw. The ears may be small, prominent, and folded over at the top. The fingers are thin, and tapering at the ends with small underdeveloped nails. These features become easier to identify as the child grows older.

As some degree of thymus or T-cell malfunction is frequent, children often have infections due to impaired immunity but it is unusual for it to fail completely, and any immune problems often improve with age.

The parathyroid glands in the neck may be underactive which causes low levels of calcium in the blood, called hypocalcaemia, and this may cause convulsions. These are unusual after infancy, even if the hypocalcaemia persists. Hypothyroidism (underactive thyroid) (see entry, Thyroid Disorders) and growth hormone deficiency (see entry) occurs occasionally. As individuals with 22q11 are generally among the smallest ten per cent, their growth should be monitored. Any slowing of growth may need to be checked in case of nutritional and hormone deficiencies.

Emotional responses may be immature so some children may have difficulty in making relationships with children of their own age, or sometimes they may avoid eye contact. Extremes of rapid mood swings or behaviour varying from quiet inactivity to hyperactivity, and unexpected temper outbursts may cause serious management difficulties. After childhood, depression and other psychiatric conditions, including schizophrenia (see entry), have been found to be somewhat commoner than in the general population.

Kidney problems (see entry, Kidney disease) are found in thirty-five per cent of people with 22q11 deletion. It is quite common for a kidney to be absent, or for one kidney to be smaller than the other although its condition generally doesn't get worse. However, even if a child does not seem to have a kidney problem, an ultrasound examination should be made to confirm this.

Bone and muscle problems are more common in people with 22q11 deletion than usual. Problems that can occur include: scoliosis (curvature of the spine) (see entry), Sprengel's shoulder (where the shoulder blade is in a higher position than normal), talipes (club foot) (see entry, Lower Limb Abnormalities) and rheumatoid arthritis (see entry, Arthritis (Juvenile Idiopathic)).

Muscle tone is often reduced. A lack of muscle bulk is common, so the children appear to have a small build. Joints that can be extended more than usual (hypermobility) may result in complaints of leg pains on walking and exercise. Hernias occur due to muscle weakness. Constipation is more common as the gut muscles don't work so well. Testicles may not descend at the normal age.

Eye abnormalities include coloboma (deficiency in a local spot of the eyeball's layers) (see entry), some developmental differences from usual and small cataracts (see entry) which are unlikely to need intervention.

Rarely, a laryngeal web may cause breathing difficulties from birth.

Inheritance patterns and prenatal diagnosis
Inheritance patterns

In 22q11 Deletion syndromes, each chromosome has a long (q) and short (p) arm. In this syndrome a tiny part is missing (deleted) from the long arm (q) of one of the two chromosomes 22's at position 11 on that chromosome. In very few individuals it is not possible to show this chromosome deletion even though they undoubtedly have the condition.

In many affected children the deletion has started in the particular egg or sperm which went to form them, just by chance when the chromosomes were being copied to pass on, but in a small number (ten per cent) one parent has it and has passed it on. The deletion is shown by the FISH (fluorescence in-situ hybridisation) test, when instead of both chromosome 22's 'lighting up' with a special fluorescent DNA tag only one does. If a parent carries the 22q11 deletion, the inheritance mode is autosomal dominant. When neither parent shows the deletion there is still a one to two per cent risk of another affected child as it may only be carried in the germinal cells of the parents' ovaries or testes.

22q11 deletion occurs in around 1 in 4,000 of the population. The very variable ways it affects individuals can result in a lengthy time to obtain a diagnosis.

Prenatal diagnosis

Amniocentesis or Chorionic villus sampling will detect the chromosome 22 deletion. Ultrasound scans can detect most heart defects.

Medical text written August 2003 by Dr A Habel, Consultant Paediatrician, Great Ormond Street Hospital, London, UK.

Further online resources

Medical texts in *The Contact a Family Directory* are designed to give a short, clear description of specific conditions and rare disorders. More extensive information on this condition can be found on a range of reliable, validated websites. Further information on these resources can be found in our **Medical Information on the Internet** article on page 21.

Support

Max Appeal

Lansdowne House, 15 Meriden Avenue, Stourbridge DY8 4QN
Tel: 0800 389 1049 Freephone Helpline   Tel: 01384 821227
e-mail: info@maxappeal.org.uk   Web: http://www.maxappeal.org.uk
The Appeal is a National Registered Charity No. 1088432, established in 1999. It provides support for all forms of 22q11 deletions including DiGeorge syndrome, Velo-Cardio-Facial syndrome, Shprintzen syndrome and the 22q11 form of Opitz G/BBB syndrome. It offers contact with other families and has regional groups. It is developing international and research links. It publishes a quarterly newsletter and has a wide range of information available, details on request. The Appeal has over 470 members.
Group details last updated May 2007.

AARSKOG SYNDROME

Aarskog syndrome: Aarskog-Scott syndrome

Background

Aarskog syndrome is a rare inherited condition described in 1970 by Dr D Aarskog and Dr C I Scott in 1971. It is a development disorder characterised by short stature with facial, genital and skeletal anomalies. The condition affects mainly males, although females may have milder features. Aarskog syndrome is associated with a wide range of features and not all features of the syndrome will be found in each individual; it affects individuals differently.

It has been estimated that the syndrome affects about 1 in 1,000,000 births but mildly affected individuals may not have been identified so the incidence may be considerably higher. Aarskog syndrome is caused by mutations in the FGDY1 gene found on the X chromosome.

What are the symptoms?

Aarskog syndrome is associated with:

- a characteristic facial appearance which may include a rounded face;
- a 'widow's peak' hairline;
- hypertelorism and ptosis (wide set eyes with 'drooping eyelids');
- palpebral fissures (large downward slanted eyes);
- a shawl scrotum (the pouch containing the testes enclosing the base of the penis);
- possible undescended testes and inguinal hernias;
- short stature that may not be obvious until the child is between one to three years old;
- some tissue webbing between fingers, joint hypermobility, abnormal shortness of fingers and toes and a single crease across the palm of the hands;
- hyperflexible joints.

Other features can include:

- late dentition (eruption of teeth) with more frequent caries (tooth decay) and some missing second teeth and cleft lip/palate;
- mild learning disability in about ten per cent of individuals with Aarskog syndrome. Dyspraxia, Dyslexia and ADHD can also be present. Social skills are not affected in Aarskog syndrome although boys may lack confidence;
- later puberty for some boys than their peers. Some males may show reduced fertility;

- occasional anomalies of the cervical vertebrae (bones of the spine in the neck area), cervical spine hypermobility and spina bifida. Pectus excavatum (depressed chest) has been noted.

How is it diagnosed?

Diagnosis is based on the recognition of the distinctive pattern of craniofacial anomalies, disproportionate short stature, characteristic urogenital anomalies and shortening of the distal extremities (hands and feet). X-rays can reveal other distinctive abnormalities.

How is it treated?

Aarskog syndrome cannot be cured but there may be surgical procedures and physiotherapy available for specific features of the syndrome. Where growth is very restricted, growth hormone treatment has proved effective for some individuals.

Inheritance patterns and prenatal diagnosis

Inheritance patterns

Aarskog syndrome is inherited as an X-linked recessive condition.

Prenatal diagnosis

Prenatal testing may occasionally be available in cases where a family member has a known mutation but it is not usually possible.

Medical text written September 2004 by Contact a Family. Approved September 2004 by Dr M Porteous, Consultant Clinical Geneticist and Reader in Clinical Genetics, Western General Hospital, Edinburgh, UK.

Further online resources

Medical texts in *The Contact a Family Directory* are designed to give a short, clear description of specific conditions and rare disorders. More extensive information on this condition can be found on a range of reliable, validated websites. Further information on these resources can be found in our **Medical Information on the Internet** article on page 21.

Support

There is no effective support group for Aarskog syndrome. Families can use Contact a Family's Freephone Helpline for advice, information and, where possible, links to other families. Contact a Family's web-based linking service Making Contact.org can be accessed at http://www.makingcontact.org

ABDOMINAL EXSTROPHIES

Gastroschisis: Exomphalos

Background

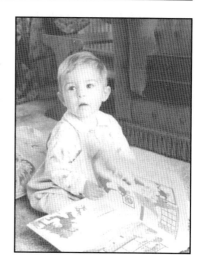

Exomphalos, otherwise known as omphalocoele or omphalocele, is a condition where the umbilicus is abnormally large. In its most severe variant, the umbilicus measures more than 10cm in diameter and the abdominal organs protrude into the base of the umbilical cord. Associated abnormalities, particularly involving the heart, are common.

Gastroschisis is a condition where the intestine protrudes from the abdomen through a hole in the abdomen wall beside the umbilicus.

What are the causes?

Gastroschisis is associated with young maternal age, mothers under twenty being twelve times more likely to have infants with Gastroschisis. It is usually not associated with other abnormalities. (The Aetiology of Gastroschisis; Curry J et al British Journal of Obstetrics and Gynaecology 107: 1339-1346; Nov 2000).

How is it treated?

Many affected infants will have had the abnormality detected during pregnancy. Early surgery is usually required and the majority of infants survive.

Inheritance patterns and prenatal diagnosis

Inheritance patterns

None known

Prenatal diagnosis

Diagnosis can be effected by ultrasound scan.

Medical text written May 1994 by Mr N E Dudley, Consultant Surgeon, John Radcliffe Hospital, Oxford, UK. **Last updated November 2006 by Mr J Curry, Consultant Paediatric Surgeon, Great Ormond Street Hospital, London, UK.**

Further online resources

Medical texts in *The Contact a Family Directory* are designed to give a short, clear description of specific conditions and rare disorders. More extensive information on this condition can be found on a range of reliable, validated websites. Further information on these resources can be found in our **Medical Information on the Internet** article on page 21.

Support

GEEPS (Gastroschisis, Exomphalos, Exstrophies Parents Support)
e-mail: geeps@btinternet.com   Web: http://www.geeps.co.uk
GEEPS is a parent support group, established in 1991. It currently offers support for the families of affected children by e-mail and through the website.
Group details last confirmed February 2008.

In December 2006, the Disability Equality Duty came into force. All public authorities must look at ways to ensure disabled people are treated equally.

ABDOMINAL MIGRAINE

Background

Abdominal migraine is an idiopathic disorder seen mainly in children. The symptoms are of recurrent episodes of midline abdominal pain with attacks lasting one to seventy-two hours and complete normality between episodes.

What are the symptoms?

The episodes of pain are of moderate to severe intensity and is felt in the midline of the abdomen, usually around the umbilicus, or poorly localised. The attacks of pain are usually accompanied by anorexia and nausea and about half of the patients will vomit with at least some attacks. Marked pallor is commonly noted during the attacks although some patients may appear flushed. The pain is severe enough to interfere with normal daily activities and many children describe their mood during the attack as one of intense misery. The attacks are self limiting and resolve spontaneously and patients are completely well and symptom free between attacks.

The onset of attacks of abdominal pain may be at any time of day but occurs most frequently first thing in the morning on waking. Associated symptoms include photophobia (sensitivity to light), phonophobia (sensitivity to sound) and dizziness in many children.

The symptoms of abdominal migraine normally appear in childhood before puberty, reaching a peak at the age of twelve years and thereafter falling rapidly. In most patients the symptoms of abdominal migraine will resolve with age but in one third of patients the symptoms will persist until the teenage years. Most patients will develop migraine headaches. Very occasionally the onset of symptoms may be during the teenage years or in adults.

How is it diagnosed?

Recurrent abdominal pain is a common problem in children although most do not have abdominal migraine. The diagnosis should only be used where the specific features of the condition are present.

How is it treated?

Acute attacks of abdominal migraine are usually treated by rest and the condition frequently resolves with sleep. Patients should be allowed to lie down undisturbed in a quiet and dark room. Simple analgesic drugs may be helpful in relieving attacks.

There is good evidence from a controlled clinical study that Pizotifen may reduce the frequency and intensity of attacks when given regularly as a prophylactic agent. It has been suggested that Propranolol may also be effective but no controlled clinical trials have been carried out.

Inheritance patterns and prenatal diagnosis
Inheritance patterns
A family history of migraine is frequently seen in abdominal migraine and as with other forms of migraine, the condition appears more commonly to be inherited from the mother.
Prenatal diagnosis
None.

Medical text written October 2002 by Dr D N K Symon. **Last updated June 2007 by Dr D.N.K. Symon Consultant Paediatrician, University Hospital of Hartlepool, Hartlepool, UK.**

Support
There is no support group specifically for Abdominal Migraine but support and information can be obtained from the Migraine Action Association or the Migraine Trust (see entry, Migraine). Families can also use Contact a Family's Freephone Helpline for advice and information on any aspect of caring for their child.

ACHONDROPLASIA

Background

Achondroplasia is a rare genetic condition affecting bone growth. It is one of the most common causes of restricted growth with disproportionate short stature.

Achondroplasia literally means 'no cartilage growth', but in reality it refers to reduced bone formation at the 'growth plate' (a section of cartilage at either end of the bone, responsible for growth). This results in shortened limbs. The tissues around the limbs are not affected and continue to grow leading to bulky arms and legs. Growth charts designed specifically for children with Achondroplasia can be used to monitor growth. Achondroplasia is mainly a physical condition with affected people generally having a normal range of intelligence.

Many practical difficulties can be overcome with a little imagination and there is no reason why someone with Achondroplasia should not participate fully in society. It is important that the person themselves is able to find their own limits and boundaries and that these are not imposed by society.

What are the symptoms?

People with Achondroplasia have a range of characteristics including:

- A near normal trunk length with shorter arms and legs;
- A large head with prominent forehead and flattened bridge of the nose;
- An increased curvature of the lower spine (lumbar lordosis);
- Bowing of the lower legs;
- Possible crowded teeth;
- Short, broad feet and hands with separation between middle and ring fingers (the 'trident' hand);
- Flexible joints.

Babies with Achondroplasia may develop motor skills and mobility more slowly than normal because of the combination of a heavier head and shorter arms and legs, but ultimately development should be within the expected normal range.

How is it diagnosed?

Some of the medical complications that can be associated with Achondroplasia include:

- Glue ear/hearing impairment;
- Speech impairment;
- Breathing problems in young children;
- Sleep apnoea (severe snoring leading to respiratory problems) in adults, especially if weight is not controlled;
- Hydrocephalus;
- Spinal stenosis leading to compression of nerves to the limbs resulting

in pain and/or numbness;
- Back problems;
- Joint problems due to leg bowing.

How is it treated?

Many of the problems associated with Achondroplasia can be detected and reduced through regular health surveillance checks by a paediatrician and through lifestyle changes such as a good diet and regular exercise (following consultation with a physician).

People with Achondroplasia have a normal life expectancy.

Inheritance patterns and prenatal diagnosis

Inheritance patterns

Most people with Achondroplasia are born to average size parents. Achondroplasia is due to a change in the gene that codes for Fibroblast Growth Factor Receptor 3. (FGFR3). In almost all cases the single base change is exactly the same. The prevalence of Achondroplasia is 1 in 25,000 children.

Average size parents of a child with Achondroplasia have a very small chance of having another child with the condition.

For parents with Achondroplasia the inheritance pattern is autosomal dominant.

Prenatal diagnosis

Ultra sound scans may detect disproportionately short limbs at around twenty-five weeks of pregnancy. For couples where one or both has the condition, a chorionic villus sampling test is available at twelve weeks of pregnancy.

Medical text written March 2002 by Dr M Wright, Consultant Clinical Geneticist, Institute of Medical Genetics, International Centre for Life, Newcastle upon Tyne, UK based on information written by Dr W Christian. **Last updated August 2006 by Dr W Christian, Paediatric Specialist Registrar, Bristol Royal Hospital for Children, Bristol, UK.**

Support

As Achondroplasia is a restricted growth condition, information and advice for adults and the families of children is available from the Restricted Growth Association (see entry, Restricted Growth).

ACNE

Acne: Acne Vulgaris

Background

Acne is a chronic inflammatory condition affecting the pilo sebaceous unit. This is the canal through which the hair grows and into which the associated oil gland pumps oil. Pilo sebaceous units are found over the entire body apart from the palms and soles. The anatomical site at which acne develops is dependent on the activity of the oil gland. In most people it tends to be the face but in some people acne also affects the back, chest, upper arms and even the buttocks and upper legs.

What are the causes?

Acne is caused by an abnormal response of the skin to generally normal levels of the male hormone testosterone. Both men and women produce testosterone and this hormone controls the oil production in the skin. In acne the oil glands become hypersensitive to testosterone leading to increased oil production, a partial blockage in the pore that allows oil to drain on to the surface of the skin. Eventually this leads to pooling of oil within the hair shaft, inflammation, infection and the development of red and then pussy spots.

Acne is a self limiting condition but it is impossible to predict how long it will last. Seventy percent of people will resolve within four or five years but other patients may suffer from acne for decades before it eventually resolves. During the time that it is active acne can cause significant scarring of the skin and can also have a profound effect on the psychological well being of the sufferer.

How is it treated?

Acne is a very treatable disease and the aims of treatment are to prevent both physical and psychological scarring. Acne should never be ignored - it is no good waiting to grow out of it as it may be very persistent and can cause a major impact on quality of life. The earlier it is treated the better the end result. Considerable advances have been made over the last decade in the treatment of acne including the development of a variety of light therapies and the new development of laser therapy for acne. Acne scarring is also becoming more treatable with a number of new techniques coming on line.

Medical text written May 1994 by Dr T Chu. **Last updated June 2006 by Dr T Chu, Consultant Dermatologist, Hammersmith Hospital, London, UK.**

Further online resources

Medical texts in *The Contact a Family Directory* are designed to give a short, clear description of specific conditions and rare disorders. More extensive information on this condition can be found on a range of reliable, validated websites. Further information on these resources can be found in our **Medical Information on the Internet** article on page 21.

Support

Acne Support Group

PO Box 9, Newquay, TR9 6WG   Tel: 0870 870 2263

e-mail: alison.dudley@btopenworld.com   Web: http://www.stopspots.org

The Group is a National Registered Charity No.1026654, established in 1992. The Group also supports those with Rosacea. It offers support to those affected and their families. It publishes a biannual newsletter and has a wide range of information available, details on request. Please send SAE. The Group has over 7,000 enquiries a year.

Group details last confirmed June 2006.

A donation of £1,000 would fund the production costs of one of our guides for an entire year. A donation form is on page 1088.

ACOUSTIC NEUROMA

Acoustic Neuroma: Vestibular Schwannoma

Background

An Acoustic Neuroma is a non-cancerous, usually slow growing, tumour of the VIII cranial nerve. Acoustic neuromas are one of the most common brain tumours affecting approximately 1 in 100,000 persons a year. The tumour is usually located at the base of the brain where the nerve leaves the skull and enters the bony structure of the inner ear.

What are the symptoms?

As Acoustic Neuromas grow very slowly, symptoms are likely to arise after the age of thirty. The more common features are hearing loss (see entry, Deafness), tinnitus (see entry) and imbalance; less commonly headaches on awakening or on movement, vertigo, pain, numbness of the face or some vision difficulties are reported.

How is it diagnosed?

While a physical examination may identify some signs such as unilateral facial drooping, drooling or unsteadiness on walking, an acoustic neuroma is more likely to be diagnosed on a neurological assessment, taking the individual's history and performing other tests such as MRI (magnetic resonance imaging) and hearing tests. The latter may also include tests of balance (electronystagmography and calorics) and a brainstem auditory evoked response (BAER).

How is it treated?

Removal of small acoustic neuromas aims to prevent facial paralysis but larger neuromas pressing on facial nerves can be removed but may result in some paralysis. Very large tumours compressing the brainstem can lead to hydrocephalus (build up of fluid in the brain), and a life threatening rise in intracranial pressure. In this case surgery aims to relieve the hydrocephalus and the increased intracranial pressure. Radiosurgery is also used in appropriate cases. In some very small tumours there are minimal or no symptoms; in these cases regular MRI scans may be the only checks that need to be made.

Inheritance patterns and prenatal diagnosis

Inheritance patterns

There is a known association of acoustic neuroma with Neurofibromatosis type 2 (NF2), an autosomal dominantly inherited disorder with complete penetrance. In NF2 there is a defect in a tumour suppressor gene on chromosome 22.

Prenatal diagnosis
Not as yet.

Medical text written July 2002 by Contact a Family. Approved July 2002 by Dr R Davies, Consultant Audiological Physician, National Hospital for Neurology and Neurosurgery, London, UK.

Further online resources

Medical texts in *The Contact a Family Directory* are designed to give a short, clear description of specific conditions and rare disorders. More extensive information on this condition can be found on a range of reliable, validated websites. Further information on these resources can be found in our **Medical Information on the Internet** article on page 21.

Support

British Acoustic Neuroma Association (BANA)
Oak House, Ransom Wood Business Park, Southwell Road West, Mansfield NG21 0HJ
Tel: 0800 652 3143   Tel: 01623 632143   Fax: 01632 635313
e-mail: admin@bana-uk.com   Web: http://www.bana-uk.com
*The Association is a National Registered Charity No. 1024443, established in 1992.
It works to support affected individuals and to promote and support research into the
disorder. It also supports research into procedures assisting the rehabilitation of individuals
and has a network of local groups. It publishes a quarterly magazine 'Headline News' and
has information available, details on request. The Association has over 1,100 members.*
Group details last updated February 2008.

ACQUIRED APLASTIC ANAEMIA

Acquired Aplastic Anaemia: aAA; Acquired Aplastic Anemia (US)

Background

Acquired Aplastic Anaemia (aAA) affects around 2 in 1,000,000 children every year. Affected children develop low blood counts due to failure of production by the bone marrow.

What are the causes?

Although aAA can be triggered by viral infections, drugs or exposure to toxic substances in most cases there is no evidence of a specific cause. The disorder may be due either to a defect in early blood forming cells (stem cells) or to an attack by the body's own immune system, especially T lymphocytes.

How is it treated?

aAA rarely improves spontaneously and treatment by a bone marrow transplant or immune suppressive drugs is required. Both these treatments are now highly effective so that most children respond well. The commonly used drugs for immune suppression are anti-lymphocyte globulin (ALG) and cyclosporin (CSA). With both forms of treatment supportive care including intermittent blood and platelet transfusion and antibiotics are usually necessary until the bone marrow recovers.

Inheritance patterns and prenatal diagnosis

Inheritance patterns

None.

Prenatal diagnosis

None.

Medical text written July 1997 by Dr D Webb. **Last reviewed October 2003 by Dr D Webb, Consultant Paediatric Haematologist/Oncologist, Great Ormond Street Hospital, London, UK.**

Support

AA Support Group Co-ordinator

Aplastic Anaemia Trust, 16 Sidney Road, Borstal, Rochester ME1 3HF

Tel: 0870 487 0099   e-mail: support@theaat.org.uk

Web: http://www.theaat.org.uk

The Trust is a National Registered Charity No. 1107539. Originally established in 1985 as the Marrow Environment Project, it joined with the Aplastic Anaemia Support Group in 2000 to form the Aplastic Anaemia Trust. The Trust offers support and information to families affected by Aplastic Anaemia. It produces a quarterly newsletter, holds national meetings and encourages contact between families. The Trust is in contact with over 450 families.

Group details last updated October 2007.

ACUTE DISSEMINATED ENCEPHALOMYELITIS (ADEM)

Acute Disseminated Encephalomyelitis: ADEM

Background

Acute Disseminated Encephalomyelitis (ADEM) accounts for up to one third of all known cases of encephalitis. This illness was first described two hundred and fifty years ago by the distinguished English physician, Clifton, who noted that it occurred occasionally in patients who had smallpox. The white matter of the brain is predominantly affected and under the microscope it can be seen that there is invasion around small veins by white blood cells from the blood. Where these cells accumulate, myelin is destroyed. The illness has been poorly understood and a variety of terminologies used to describe it, these include post infectious, parainfectious or post vaccinial.

What are the symptoms?

The clinical presentation of ADEM, despite different causes, is similar. The illness usually begins with non specific symptoms such as fever, headache, stiff neck, vomiting and anorexia. These are rapidly followed by depression of consciousness in which the patient may become confused, stuporous, delirious and occasionally entering into coma. During this early period neurological examination usually shows focal neurological signs such as bilateral optic neuritis, ataxia of the limbs, clumsiness in walking, paralysis down one side and seizures may occur. The duration of these symptoms is variable, some cases lasting a few weeks to a month, and other fatal cases having a rapid progressive course over a number of days. The clinical sign that correlates most closely with the prognosis is the level of consciousness. The illness usually has monophasic course, that is once it is over, further attacks rarely develop. Recently long term studies of patients with ADEM have shown that a small number develop multiple sclerosis later on.

What are the causes?

This illness usually follows in the wake of exanthema (rapidly erupting rash) or after other viral infections or immunisations. There is usually a latent period of days to two to three weeks.

The cerebrospinal fluid (CSF) is frequently abnormal showing an increase in white cells and protein. The electroencephalogram (EEG) is abnormal in most cases showing diffuse slowing. Magnetic resonance imaging (MRI) typically shows multiple areas of abnormality in the white matter of the brain.

How is it diagnosed?

The differential diagnoses of ADEM include acute meningitis, acute viral encephalitis and acute multiple sclerosis. Differentiation of these diseases is not easy, certainly in the early stages. In viral encephalitis the CSF is often abnormal and a rise in specific viral antibody may occur. To distinguish ADEM from multiple sclerosis in the initial phases may be more difficult. Magnetic resonance imaging and CSF examination may help.

The brain at post mortem may appear entirely normal or may show the signs of congestion. Histologically the basic lesions consist of infiltrations of mononuclear cells from the blood which occur around small veins in the white matter. Demyelination occurs and is limited to the area of the perivenous cellular cuff. These are different from the lesions found in multiple sclerosis.

There is general agreement that a causative organism cannot be isolated from the central nervous system of patients with ADEM. The association of the disease with an antecedent infection or immunisation suggests an immunological process and detailed laboratory studies involving measurement of anti-brain antibodies and of cellular immune responses to specific myelin antigens have shown that these patients have indeed mounted an allergic response against their own brain constituents.

How is it treated?

The ideal form of treatment is immunomodulation to be instituted without delay once the diagnosis is made. High doses of steroids can often lead to a very rapid resolution of symptoms with an excellent prognosis. Overall the prognosis is good where the diagnosis is made early and the appropriate therapy instituted without delay.

Inheritance patterns and prenatal diagnosis

Inheritance patterns

Not applicable.

Prenatal diagnosis

Not applicable.

Medical text last updated October 2000 by Professor C Hawkins. **Last reviewed October 2005 by Professor C Hawkins, Professor of Clinical Neurology, Keele University and Consultant Neurologist to the Regional Neuroscience Centre, Stoke-on-Trent, UK.**

Further online resources

Medical texts in *The Contact a Family Directory* are designed to give a short, clear description of specific conditions and rare disorders. More extensive information on this condition can be found on a range of reliable, validated websites. Further information on these resources can be found in our **Medical Information on the Internet** article on page 21.

Support

Acute Disseminated Encephalomyelitis (ADEM) is a form of Encephalitis. Details of the Encephalitis Support Group appear under the separate entry, Encephalitis.

ADAMS-OLIVER SYNDROME

Adams Oliver syndrome: Absence Defect of Limbs, Scalp and Scull; Congenital Scalp Defects with Distal Limb Reduction Anomalies

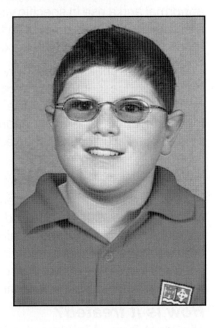

Background

Adams Oliver syndrome is a rare disorder identified in 1945 by Dr F H Adams and Dr C P Oliver, characterised by congenital scalp and skull defects.

What are the symptoms?

The syndrome is characterised by congenital scalp and skull defects. These defects can range from mild, with some skin and hair defect, through to severe when there may be defects of the underlying bone.

Rarely, bleeding occurs from dilated veins that are sometimes associated with severe scalp defects. Other features that may occur include eye anomalies, accessory nipples, cutis marmorata telangiectatica congenita (a rare condition seen at or soon after birth, mainly affecting the blood vessels of the skin creating a mottled or marbled pattern on the skin), haemangiomas (see entry, Vascula Birthmarks), skin tags and woolly hair.

Intellectual development is generally within normal limits, even in individuals with large cranial bone defects, although learning disabilities have been reported.

Limb defects, ranging from small fingers and toes through to severe involvement of long bones, can also occur. In very severe cases, the lower limb can be absent below mid-calf. However, it is common for people with the affected gene to have minimal scalp or limb abnormality.

What are the causes?

Although the underlying mechanism of the disease is not known it has been suggested that it could result from an early embryonic vascular abnormality.

How is it treated?

Although bald ulcerated areas of the skull usually heal on their own, occasionally plastic surgery is needed.

While surgery may be indicated for some of the skull defects, treatment is otherwise symptomatic. Management focuses on ameliorating the effects of any skull or limb defects.

Inheritance patterns and prenatal diagnosis

Inheritance patterns

Autosomal dominant. Genetic counselling is recommended for families affected by this condition.

Prenatal diagnosis

No specific test is available. A detailed eighteen week ultrasound scan may detect the more severe limb and cranial defects.

Medical text written December 1993 by Dr D Ravine, Senior Registrar, Institute of Medical Genetics, University Hospital of Wales, Cardiff, UK. **Last updated February 2003 by Contact a Family. Approved February 2003 by Mr D E Porter, Senior Lecturer & Hon. Consultant in Orthopaedic Surgery, University of Edinburgh, Edinburgh, UK.**

Further online resources

Medical texts in *The Contact a Family Directory* are designed to give a short, clear description of specific conditions and rare disorders. More extensive information on this condition can be found on a range of reliable, validated websites. Further information on these resources can be found in our **Medical Information on the Internet** article on page 21.

Support

Adams-Oliver Syndrome Support Group

14 College View, Connah's Quay, Deeside CH5 4BY   e-mail: sandy.ivins@btinternet.com
The Group is a contact group, established in 1993. It offers moral support through shared experiences. The Group is in touch with over 50 families in the UK, Canada, Europe, South America and the Middle East.
Group details last confirmed June 2007.

ADDISON DISEASE

Background

Addison disease, first described in 1849 by Dr T Addison, is a rare condition which is due to the destruction of the adrenal cortex leading to a deficiency or absence of cortisol and other adrenal hormones. The symptoms are due to the failure of the production of cortical hormones, which are responsible for the rate at which sugar is made available to the tissues of the body, and the amount of salt lost from the body.

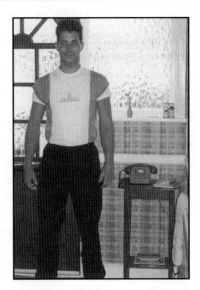

What are the symptoms?

The symptoms of chronic adrenal failure have a very gradual onset, so that the condition is difficult to appreciate. Lack of energy, malaise, or giddiness when standing up, are almost always present. There is usually an increase in skin pigmentation. Often, the development of an intercurrent illness decompensates the condition which suddenly deteriorates into circulatory collapse, hypoglycaemia and, if untreated, death.

What are the causes?

The deficiency may have a number of causes, such as auto-immunity, tuberculosis, or it may be spontaneous.

How is it treated?

The condition, once diagnosed, can be successfully treated with replacement hormones. Extra steroid hormones will be necessary to cover periods of intercurrent illnesses and surgical stress.

Inheritance patterns and prenatal diagnosis

Inheritance patterns

The condition may occasionally be genetic: for example, there is an X-linked form of the disease which is related to adrenoleukodystrophy.

Prenatal diagnosis

None

Medical text written November 1991 by Contact a Family. Approved by Professor Michael Patton, Professor of Medical Genetics, St George's Hospital Medical School, London, UK and Dr J E Wraith, Consultant Paediatrician, Royal Manchester Children's Hospital, Manchester, UK. **Last updated September 2005 by Dr R Stanhope, Consultant Paediatric Endocrinologist, Great Ormond Street Hospital, London, UK.**

Contact a Family Helpline 0808 808 3555

Further online resources

Medical texts in *The Contact a Family Directory* are designed to give a short, clear description of specific conditions and rare disorders. More extensive information on this condition can be found on a range of reliable, validated websites. Further information on these resources can be found in our **Medical Information on the Internet** article on page 21.

Support

Addison's Disease Self Help Group

21 George Road, Guildford GU1 4NP   e-mail: info@addisons.org.uk
Web: http://www.addisons.org.uk
The Group is a National Registered Charity No. 1106791 started in 1984. It offers contact with others with same condition. It publishes a bi-monthly newsletter and has information available, details on request. Please send SAE for information. The Group represents 14 affected children and 800 adults.
Group details last updated May 2007.

The Contact a Family Helpline provides information on a range of issues including benefits, special educational needs, and adapting your home. Call the helpline for more information.

ADRENOLEUKODYSTROPHY

Adrenoleukodystrophy: Schilder's disease; Sudanophilic Leukodystrophy

Background

Adrenoleukodystrophy (ALD) is a life threatening genetic disorder which only occurs in males and affects the adrenal gland and white matter of the nervous system. It is caused by the accumulation of long chain fatty acids in the cells and tissues of an affected child. ALD was first recognised in 1923 and since then several hundred cases have been reported from many countries.

What are the symptoms?

There are several forms of ALD. In the severe (childhood cerebral) form, boys usually develop normally until they reach between the ages of four to ten years of age when behavioural changes, such as loss of memory and emotional instability, may be experienced in varying degrees. There may also be difficulty with vision, hearing and motor function. Adrenal function may also be impaired (Addison disease) leading to nausea, vomiting, and changes in skin colour. Addison disease is commonly associated with gonadotrophin deficiency and may present with failure to enter puberty. There is continuous progressive deterioration of the nervous system. The rate of deterioration varies in each individual child.

A milder form of this illness, called adrenomyeloneuropathy (AMN) also occurs in males during late adolescence, or early adult life. It is usually characterised by adrenal impairment, immature sex organ development and varying degrees of difficulty with walking and motor function.

Symptoms of ALD are occasionally seen in female carriers. The vast majority have mild symptoms. Very rarely cerebral ALD has been described.

How is it treated?

The only form of treatment that has been shown to be effective in early cerebral ALD is bone marrow transplantation, but it is ineffective in advanced disease. Lorenzo's oil has been widely used but its effectiveness remains unknown.

Inheritance patterns and prenatal diagnosis

Inheritance patterns

X-Linked recessive

Prenatal diagnosis

Amniocentesis is available to carrier women only.

Medical text written May 1994 by Dr R Schwarz, Consultant Paediatrician, Central Middlesex Hospital, London UK. **Last updated April 2004 by Dr A Velodi, Consultant Paediatrician and Honorary Senior Lecturer, Metabolic Unit, Great Ormond Street Hospital, London, UK.**

Further online resources

Medical texts in *The Contact a Family Directory* are designed to give a short, clear description of specific conditions and rare disorders. More extensive information on this condition can be found on a range of reliable, validated websites. Further information on these resources can be found in our **Medical Information on the Internet** article on page 21.

Support

ALD Family Support Trust

4 Morley House, 320 Regent Street, London W1B 3BB   Tel/Fax: 020 7631 3336
e-mail: info@aldfst.org.uk   Web: http://www.aldfst.org.uk
The Trust is a National Registered Charity No. 1024690, established in 1993. It offers support by telephone and letter and links families where possible. It has information available, details on request. The Trust has 200 family members with around 270 affected children.
Group details last updated September 2006.

ALD Life

PO BOX 43642, London SE22 0XR   Tel: 020 8473 7493   e-mail: info@aldlife.org
Web: http://www.aldlife.org
ALD Life is a National Registered Charity No.1106008, established in 2001. It offers support, practical advice and networking opportunities both nationally and internationally. It funds research and provides grants to families and individuals for bereavement, support during bone marrow transplant and specialised equipment not available elsewhere. There is a quarterly newsletter and linking wherever possible. The group is in touch with 150 families, approximately 70 of them in the UK. ALD Life have also now opened a charity shop in Penge, London SE20 to further their fundraising.
Group details last updated July 2007.

AGENESIS OF THE CORPUS CALLOSUM

Background

Agenesis of the Corpus Callosum (ACC) is a rare neurological condition. The Corpus Callosum is a bridge of white matter joining the two cerebral hemispheres of the brain. It forms during the course of brain development. The frequency with which it fails to form is normally not known as its total or partial absence can only be demonstrated with brain imaging procedures and these will usually only be performed if individuals have neurological abnormalities. Hence there may well be many asymptomatic individuals with partial or complete callosal agenesis.

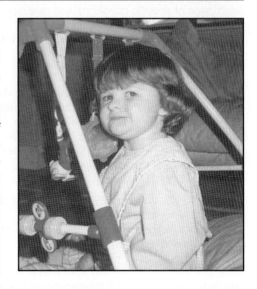

What are the symptoms?

The clinical manifestations are best described under two headings: syndromic and non-syndromic.

Non-syndromic are more common and affected patients usually present with a large head, seizures and developmental delay. Hypertelorism (widely spaced eyes) occurs in many also. Seizure control may be difficult to achieve. Although the head can be very large ventricular shunting procedures for hydrocephalus are not indicated or helpful.

Many neurological syndromes also include agenesis of the corpus callosum. All of these have additional brain malformations and affected individuals are usually severely disabled often with dysmorphic characteristics and global developmental delay. Often associated with other midline cerebral and cranial abnormalities such as septo-optic dysplasia (see entry), it is sometimes associated with pituitary dysplasia. Because of this fits are sometimes due to hypoglycaemia (growth hormone and cortisol deficiency) as well as due to structural brain abnormality.

What are the causes?

Callosal agenesis may be and often is associated with other developmental brain anomalies and it is often these, rather than the callosal agenesis itself, which is the cause of subsequent neurological disability.

Inheritance patterns and prenatal diagnosis

Inheritance patterns

In the non-syndromic form of callosal agenesis genetic transmission is rare although there are a few autosomal recessive, X-linked and dominant cases on record. Genetic advice to affected individuals and their families can be helpful therefore. More frequently the non-syndromic form of callosal agenesis is an anomaly of brain development that is post conceptually determined, sometimes in association with chromosomal abnormalities.

In the syndromic form of callosal agenesis referral for precise neurological diagnosis is required. The majority of these syndromes do occur sporadically but these are occasional kindreds reported with familial incidence. Again dominant, X-linked and recessive disorders have been described whilst the Aicardi syndrome (see entry) is thought to result from an X-linked dominant mutation.

Prenatal diagnosis

Agenesis of the Corpus Callosum is undetectable through routine prenatal tests. ACC may be detected with a scan at eighteen weeks.

Medical text written November 1998 by Dr L Rosenbloom. Last updated December 2001 by Dr L Rosenbloom. **Last reviewed May 2005 by Dr L Rosenbloom, Consultant Paediatric Neurologist, Alder Hey Children's Hospital, Liverpool, UK.**

Further online resources

Medical texts in *The Contact a Family Directory* are designed to give a short, clear description of specific conditions and rare disorders. More extensive information on this condition can be found on a range of reliable, validated websites. Further information on these resources can be found in our **Medical Information on the Internet** article on page 21.

Support

Corpal

20 Tollbar, Rushden, Northampton NN10 6DP   Tel: 01933 386817

e-mail: accCorpal@yahoo.co.uk

CORPAL is a National Registered Charity No. 1086019, re-established in 1997. It offers support by telephone and letter and links families where possible. It publishes an occasional newsletter and has information available, details on request. Please send SAE. The organisation is in touch with over 270 families.

Group details last confirmed September 2007.

AICARDI SYNDROME

Background

Aicardi syndrome is a very rare neurological condition due to a congenital abnormality of brain development. The characteristic features consist of under development or absence of the development (agenesis) of a brain structure known as the corpus callosum, a form of epilepsy (infantile spasms) and an abnormality to the structure and appearance of the retina of the eyes.

It is an example of one of the syndromic causes of Agenesis of the Corpus Callosum. In Aicardi syndrome, in addition to the structural abnormality of the corpus callosum (see entry), other structures within the brain can also be abnormal. This can result in a variety of types of brain cyst and/or abnormal structure within areas of both grey or white matter of the brain.

What are the symptoms?

Learning Disability (see entry) is a constant feature and varies from moderate to the more commonly seen severe picture.

The associated epilepsy (see entry) classically takes the form of 'infantile spasms' or is 'spasm-like.' Other types of epileptic fit may be seen. The epilepsy usually occurs by two months of age, it is often difficult and remains difficult to control. Investigating it with electroencephalogram studies may reveal a pattern characteristic of these spasms (hypsarrhythmia). This form of epilepsy is sometimes referred to as West syndrome (see entry). As such, Aicardi syndrome can be considered to be a 'symptomatic' cause of West syndrome.

The abnormalities at the back of the eye, evident only on internal examination with an ophthalmoscope, are to the structure of the choroid and retina. They appear as distinctive multiple, round 'footprint shaped' yellow-white lesions. The level of vision depends upon the extent of these retinal lesions and the severity of any associated learning disability.

The condition is associated with a host of other variable manifestations. These can include abnormalities of the bony structure of the spine, spinal curvature (see entry, Scoliosis), cleft lip and palate (see entry).

The spectrum of disability within Aicardi syndrome is wide. Its severity is to some extent determined by the extent of the underlying brain abnormality.

The majority of recognised cases are severely affected with persisting epilepsy. Life expectancy can be severely limited. There are some children with a milder structural brain abnormality who, although suffering visual handicap and learning difficulties, may have some understanding of language, some independent mobility and be responsive to their environment.

Aicardi syndrome is not the same as, and has no link to, a separate neurological condition referred to as Aicardi-Goutiers syndrome.

Psychological and behavioural characteristics

The information below has been drawn up by Dr Orlee Udwin of the Society for the Study of Behavioural Phenotypes.

Nearly all children with Aicardi syndrome have severe learning difficulties. Most have no expressive language and remain totally dependent on adults for their self care. However, there are a few girls who have some understanding of language, can walk with support or independently and are fairly responsive to the environment. Self-injurious behaviours and aggression towards people and objects have been reported in some studies and may be involuntary. Disturbed sleep (possibly due to fitting) and waking in the night are also common problems.

Inheritance and prenatal diagnosis

Inheritance patterns

The condition only occurs in girls. This is explained genetically by it being an X-linked dominant condition with lethality in males. Reoccurrence within a family appears to be extremely uncommon.

Prenatal diagnosis

Although structural brain abnormalities may sometimes be evident on antenatal ultrasound scan, this is not the case in the majority of cases of Aicardi syndrome. There is no prenatal diagnosis available.

Medical text written February 2000 by Dr K R E Pohl, Consultant Paediatric Neurologist, Guy's Hospital, London, UK. Psychological and behavioural characteristics written by Dr Orlee Udwin of the Society for the Study of Behavioural Phenotypes. **Last reviewed August 2005 by Dr L Rosenbloom, Consultant Paediatric Neurologist, Alder Hey Children's Hospital, Liverpool, UK.**

Further online resources

Medical texts in *The Contact a Family Directory* are designed to give a short, clear description of specific conditions and rare disorders. More extensive information on this condition can be found on a range of reliable, validated websites. Further information on these resources can be found in our **Medical Information on the Internet** article on page 21.

Support

Support for Aicardi syndrome is available from CORPAL (see entry, Agenesis of the Corpus Callosum)

AICARDI-GOUTIÈRES SYNDROME

Aicardi-Goutières syndrome: AGS; Pseudo-TORCH syndrome; microcephaly-intracranial calcification syndrome (MICS); Cree encephalitis

Background

In 1984, Jean Aicardi and Françoise Goutières, two French paediatric neurologists, described an early onset genetic brain disorder mimicking the features of viral infections affecting a child in the womb. Clinical indicators of the disease include:

- Calcification (the accumulation of calcium) in the brain, seen on a CT scan;
- Changes in the white matter (whitish nerve tissue) of the brain and spinal cord brain best seen on an MRI scan;
- Raised levels of white cells, interferon-alpha and pterins (proteins produced by the body to fight viral infection) in the cerebrospinal fluid following a lumbar puncture;
- Distinctive 'chilblain-like' lesions on the hands and feet which are usually worse in the cold.

Four different genes (see table) have been identified that, when damaged by a mutation, can cause AGS. Only one gene is involved in any one family.

Gene	Chromosome Position	Other names	Percentage of families with mutations
AGS1	3	TREX1/DNaseIII	35%
AGS2	13	RNASEH2B/FLJ11712	45%
AGS3	11	RNASEH2C/AYP1	15%
AGS4	19	RNASEH2A	<5%

What are the symptoms?

Broadly speaking there are two types of presentation in AGS. Some babies, especially those with AGS1 mutations, experience problems at or very soon after birth. Features include feeding difficulties, abnormal neurological signs, low platelets (blood cells involved in clotting) and liver abnormalities. In contrast, other children, often those with AGS2 mutations, develop normally for the first few weeks or months of life. They then experience the sudden onset of a period of intense irritability, cry a lot for hours at a time, sleep poorly and develop fevers without infection. During this period there is a loss of skills. After a few months the disease process seems to 'stop'. Many individuals with AGS are still stable in their late teens and early twenties. Typical neurological features of AGS include learning problems, stiffness of the limbs with poor trunk and head control and impairment in muscle tone (dystonia) of the limbs. Although the neurological problems seen in AGS are often severe, a small number of children, usually those with AGS2 mutations, show good communication skills.

What are the causes?

At the moment we do not know how changes in TREX1 and the RNASEH2 complex cause AGS. These genes make chemicals called nucleases which break down DNA and RNA. During the normal life-cycle of our cells, nucleases clean up naturally produced waste DNA and RNA. A failure of this process can induce the body to mount an immune reaction against its own DNA and RNA. A similar immune reaction is seen in response to viral DNA and RNA following an infection. This would explain why the clinical features of AGS and viral infection overlap and why we see high levels of the anti-viral agent interferon-alpha in children with AGS.

Inheritance patterns and prenatal diagnosis

Inheritance patterns

Aicardi-Goutières syndrome is an autosomal recessive genetic disorder. This means that for a couple with one affected child there is a 1 in 4 risk of having a further affected child in any future pregnancy.

Prenatal diagnosis

The availability of genetic testing allows us to confirm the diagnosis of AGS in most, but not all, families. This is important in view of the associated 1 in 4 risk of recurrence. For some couples, if both mutations can be identified in their child it may be possible to offer testing during a subsequent pregnancy.

Medical text written March 2007 by Dr Yanick Crow, Senior Lecturer and Honorary Consultant, Department of Clinical Genetics, Ashley Wing, St James's University Hospital, Leeds, UK.

Further online resources

Medical texts in *The Contact a Family Directory* are designed to give a short, clear description of specific conditions and rare disorders. More extensive information on this condition can be found on a range of reliable, validated websites. Further information on these resources can be found in our **Medical Information on the Internet** article on page 21.

Support

While there is no specific support group for families of children in the UK for this condition, information is available from Climb (see entry, Metabolic diseases) and support is available from a group of families under the umbrella of Climb.

ALBINISM

Albinism: Hypopigmentation; Oculo-cutaneous albinism; Ocular albinism

Background

Albinism is a group of genetic disorders in which the affected individual has reduced or absent pigmentation. It is thought that about 1 in 20,000 people are affected with albinism. All ethnic groups and both genders appear to be affected by albinism which presents in the neonatal period.

What are the symptoms?

People with albinism may have:

- Reduced visual acuity (the ability to see detail at close and long distance) see entry, Vision Disorders in Childhood;
- Nystagmus;
- Photophobia (abnormal sensitivity to light);
- Strabismus (inability of one eye to attain vision with the other; squint).

There are two main types of albinism:

Ocular albinism (OA) predominantly affects the eyes with affected individuals often having only slightly lighter skin and hair colour than other family members and it usually leads to nystagmus (see entry). Many individuals may have been given a diagnosis of 'idiopathic nystagmus'.

Oculo-cutaneous albinism (OCA) affects the eyes and skin to a very variable extent. Features include:

- Reduced pigmentation of the iris and retina of the eye;
- Lighter than usual hair and skin. Typically, individuals may have no pigmentation and have skin that does not tan and snow-white hair. However some individuals have brown hair and can tan.

There are rare variants of OCA:

- Hermansky-Pudlak syndrome which presents with easy bruising and affected individuals may have lung, bowel and bleeding features;
- Chediak-Higashi syndrome which there is an increased susceptibility to infection and bleeding.

What are the causes?

Albinism is caused when there is a fault in the production of melanin (any of the range of black, dark brown, reddish brown, or yellow pigments).

How is it diagnosed?

Diagnosis can be made by the observation of the characteristic features of the disorders. An ophthalmologist will be involved in identifying the ocular features and abnormalities of the visual system via a Visually Evoked Potential

(VEP) test which shows a detailed record of electrical activity in the visual pathways to the brain. Genetic tests are not yet available except rarely on a research basis.

How is it treated?

Treatment for albinism is symptomatic and aims to ameliorate the problems caused by the disorder. High sun protection factor (SPF) sunscreen, sun glasses and clothing to protect the skin can all be helpful.

A range of telescopic and microscopic optical devices can provide great improvement in acuity by spreading the features of the object being viewed over a larger area of the abnormal macula (the central part of the retina).

Inheritance patterns and prenatal diagnosis

Inheritance patterns

Ocular albinism is X-linked. Oculo-cutaneous albinism is autosomal recessive. Genetic counselling should be sought.

Prenatal diagnosis

Not currently available.

Medical text written August 2006 by Contact a Family. Approved August 2006 by Miss Isabelle Russell-Eggitt FRCS FRCOphth, Consultant Ophthalmic Surgeon, Great Ormond Street Hospital, London, UK.

Support

Albinism Fellowship (UK & Ireland)

PO Box 77, Burnley BB11 5GN   Tel: 01282 771900 Helpline (Answer phone)
e-mail: info@albinism.org.uk   Web: http://www.albinism.org.uk
The Fellowship is a Scottish Registered Charity No. SC009443, established in 1979. The Fellowship provides advice and support for people with an interest in albinism and a range of appropriate services that provide information, raise awareness, challenge misrepresentation, improve self-esteem and give opportunities to meet other people affected by the condition. The Fellowship is a voluntary self-help, sociable and positive organisation that aims to provide information and support for people with an appropriate interest in the condition. Their vision is that all people with albinism have the opportunity to realise their full potential.
Group details last updated February 2008.

ALBRIGHT HEREDITARY OSTEODYSTROPHY

Background

Albright Hereditary Osteodystrophy (AHO) is a genetic condition characterised by a wide range of features. These include short stature in adulthood, a tendency for obesity and brachydactyly (shortening of the bones in the hands and feet). Other features may include a rounded face, wide neck and small subcutaneous ossifications (hard lumps under the skin). Some individuals with AHO have delayed learning skills. The range and severity of symptoms varies from one person to another. The height and weight of individuals with AHO can be normal, particularly in childhood.

There are two types of AHO. These are 'AHO with Pseudo Hypoparathyroidism' (PHP) and 'AHO with Pseudo Pseudo Hypoparathyroidism' (PPHP). Both types have the same cause and both types can occur within the same family.

What are the symptoms?

AHO with Pseudo Hypoparathyroidism (PHP)

In addition to the characteristics described above, in PHP the body is unable to respond to various hormones. One such hormone is the parathyroid hormone (PTH). This is important as it maintains levels of calcium and phosphate in the blood. In PHP, parathyroid hormone is produced in normal amounts by the parathyroid gland and released into the blood. However, the body is 'resistant' to its effects and this causes various symptoms. Individuals have low calcium levels (hypocalcemia), high phosphate levels (hyperphosphatemia) and elevated parathyroid hormone in the blood. Signs of hypocalcemia include tingling in the fingers, muscle cramps, possible seizures (fits) and cataracts. Hypocalcemia typically begins in childhood. Another hormone which the body is unable to respond to in PHP is the thyroid stimulating hormone (TSH) which makes the thyroid gland produce thyroid hormone. The effects of lack of thyroid hormone are a tendency to weight gain, dry skin and hair, lack of energy and to feel the cold.

AHO with Pseudo Pseudo Hypoparathyroidism (PPHP)

Individuals with AHO with Pseudo Pseudo Hypoparathyroidism (PPHP) do not have low levels of calcium but do have the range of the physical features described above.

How is it treated?

Fortunately, the low calcium levels as experienced with this condition can be treated with vitamin D, and low thyroid can be treated with thyroxine.

Contact a Family Helpline 0808 808 3555

Inheritance patterns and prenatal diagnosis

Inheritance patterns

AHO is inherited as an autosomal dominant trait. Changes in a gene on chromosome 20 are associated with the features of this condition.

Prenatal diagnosis

AHO may be tested for using chorionic villus sampling (CVS) or amniocentesis during pregnancy, but only if the specific genetic change causing AHO in the family has been found. Genetic counselling may be helpful for individuals and families affected by this condition.

Medical text written October 2003 by Contact a Family. Approved October 2003 by Dr L Wilson, Consultant in Clinical Genetics, Institute of Child Health, London, UK.

Support

A support group for Albright Hereditary Osteodystrophy is being formed. Families can use Contact a Family's Freephone Helpline for advice, information and, where possible, links to other families. Contact a Family's web-based linking service Making Contact.org can be accessed at http://www.makingcontact.org

ALEXANDER DISEASE

Background

Alexander disease is a rare genetic, degenerative disorder of the nervous system with effects on the mid brain and cerebellum; in the most common infantile form of the disease, the frontal white matter is involved. It is one of a group of genetic disorders called the leukodystrophies. The term leukodystrophy comes from the Greek words, 'leuko' meaning white and referring to the 'white matter' of the nervous system and 'dystrophy' meaning imperfect growth or development. In Alexander disease, the growth of the white matter of the brain, or myelin sheath, is affected. The brain stem may be particularly involved; in rare adult forms of the condition resulting in unusual signs such as flapping movement of the palate (palatal myoclonus), limb paralysis and clumsy movements. Cerebellar disease also occurs.

What are the symptoms?

The onset of Alexander disease may occur at any time during infancy or adulthood. For many individuals onset is between birth and two years, with the average being six months. This infantile form of the disease affects boys and girls and leads to delayed development and dementia. The condition is characterised by an enlarged brain and head (megalencephaly), progressive spasticity (stiffness of the arms and/or legs), cerebellar ataxia (see entry) and dementia. Infants fail to thrive, show delayed mental and physical development, and have seizures. Hydrocephalus (see entry) may occur. Sadly, the outlook is generally poor and children rarely survive past the age of five to six years.

What are the causes?

The disease is due principally to mutations in a gene for glial fibrillary acidic protein (GFAP) that maps to chromosome 17q21; all mutations to date have been heterozygous. Mutations suspected in another gene, NADH-ubiquinone flavoprotein-1, have not been detected in the majority of Alexander disease patients.

How is it diagnosed?

An exact diagnosis of Alexander disease may not be possible without post mortem examination of brain or nerve tissues. Brain biopsy or autopsy specimens show a characteristic appearance on microscopy of the brain tissue. Degeneration of supporting cells (astrocytes) leads to long eosinophilic (red staining) masses known as Rosenthal fibres that are usually found in relation to blood vessels. For some, therefore, a diagnosis of this disease is not possible within the child's lifetime. Genotype analysis at the GFAP locus is now possible and may allow confident diagnosis in a majority of cases if the disease is suspected.

In addition to the infantile form of Alexander disease, very rare juvenile and adult forms have also been described. These forms occur less frequently and have a longer course of progression. Onset of the juvenile form of Alexander disease occurs between seven to fourteen years of age and sadly, death usually occurs within ten years after the onset of symptoms. It is, however, not certain whether the disorders described in older children and adults are the same disorder and should be described as Alexander disease.

There is also a condition attributed to, or resembling Alexander disease called Parkinsonism-dementia complex of Guam. This neurodegenerative disease is characterised by amyotrophy (failure of development, or wasting, of muscles), parkinsonian features including rigidity, bradykinesia (slowed ability to start and continue movements) and resting tremor and dementia.

How is it treated?

Thankfully, advances in gene therapy for neurodegenerative disease do offer the hope that more definitive treatment for Alexander disease will become available as part of international research efforts to treat leukodystrophies.

Inheritance patterns and prenatal diagnosis

Inheritance patterns

Some cases of Alexander disease are sporadic (or non-familial.) However, there are a number of families with more than one affected child. In these cases of Alexander disease the inheritance pattern is unclear and has yet to be subject to molecular analysis of the GFAP gene. Recently heterozygous mutations in a gene encoding GFAP have been strongly associated with Alexander disease, which is presumed to be transmitted as an autosomal dominant trait, although uncharacterised rare mechanisms may operate (mosaicism).

Prenatal diagnosis

It is now recommended for subsequent pregnancies in which mutations in GFAP can be sought.

Medical text written November 2000 by the Alzheimer's Society. Approved November 2000 by Professor T M Cox. **Last updated January 2008 by Professor T M Cox, Professor of Medicine, University of Cambridge, Cambridge, UK.**

Further online resources

Medical texts in *The Contact a Family Directory* are designed to give a short, clear description of specific conditions and rare disorders. More extensive information on this condition can be found on a range of reliable, validated websites. Further information on these resources can be found in our **Medical Information on the Internet** article on page 21.

Support

As Alexander disease is a metabolic disease, support and advice are available from Climb, (see entry, Metabolic diseases). Climb supports the families of children and young people with metabolic diseases; there is currently no designated UK support group for adults with this metabolic disease. Support for dementia can be obtained from the Alzheimer's Society (see entry, Alzheimer's disease).

During 2008 there will be increased short breaks in 21 pilot areas of England because of a government programme called 'Aiming High for Disabled Children'. For more information about the programme ring the helpline.

ALKAPTONURIA

Background

Alkaptonuria is a rare metabolic disorder which was first described in 1902 by Sir Archibald Garrod. The three major features are arthritis, bluish-black pigmentation in connective tissue and urine that turns black when exposed to air. Individuals are affected differently by the range and severity of features. Alkaptonuria is found in all populations, however, it is especially frequent in individuals of Czech or Dominican descent. The condition affects males and females equally. Individuals are not usually aware of Alkaptonuria until their thirties and forties when symptoms become apparent. Children and young adults are usually asymptomatic.

What are the symptoms?

Alkaptonuria may discolour the outer ears, nose and whites of the eyes with bluish-black pigment. Vision is not affected. The teeth and nails may also be a bluish-black colour. A dusky discolouration on the skin of the hands may be apparent. Pigment appears when individuals perspire, causing discolouration of clothing.

Homogentisic acid (HGA) accumulated in the urine causes this to turn black. Darkening may not occur for several hours after urinating and many individuals never observe any abnormal colour in their urine.

In later life, Alkaptonuria may affect the heart, kidney and prostate. The condition does not cause developmental delay or cognitive impairment and lifespan of affected individuals is generally not reduced.

What are the causes?

Alkaptonuria is caused by the deficiency of an enzyme known as homogentisic acid oxidase (HGAO). Normally, this enzyme performs a crucial step in a metabolic pathway by converting a chemical, homogentisic acid (HGA), into another form to meet the body's needs. As normal amounts of the HGAO enzyme are missing, HGA is not broken down and accumulates in the body. Some is eliminated in the urine, and the rest is deposited in body tissues where it is harmful. The result is a blue-black discolouration of connective tissue including bone, cartilage and skin (otherwise known as ochronosis).

The build-up of HGA leads to premature progressive degeneration in the joints. Chronic joint pain is one of the first symptoms of Alkaptonuria. Arthritis of the spine, knees and hips causes symptoms of stiffness, pain, swelling and limited motion. Males tend to have an earlier onset of arthritic symptoms with a greater degree of severity than females. Deposits of pigment may cause cartilage to become brittle and eventually to fragment.

How is it treated?

Some of the symptoms of Alkaptonuria may be controlled with treatment.

Inheritance patterns and prenatal diagnosis

Inheritance patterns

Alkaptonuria is inherited as an autosomal recessive trait. Changes in the HGD gene on chromosome 3 are associated with the features of Alkaptonuria. This condition was one of the first 'inborn errors of metabolism' and one of the first conditions for which recessive inheritance was proposed.

Prenatal diagnosis

This may be possible and further information, including genetic counselling, should be sought from your doctor.

Medical text written September 2003 by Contact a Family. Approved September 2003 by Dr L Ranganath, Consultant Physician in Clinical Chemistry, Liverpool University Medical School, Liverpool, UK.

Further online resources

Medical texts in *The Contact a Family Directory* are designed to give a short, clear description of specific conditions and rare disorders. More extensive information on this condition can be found on a range of reliable, validated websites. Further information on these resources can be found in our **Medical Information on the Internet** article on page 21.

Support

Alkaptonuria Society

12 High Beeches, Childwall, Liverpool L16 3GA   Tel: 0151 737 1862

e-mail: manager@alkaptonuria.info

Web: http://www.alkaptonuria.info

The Society provides support and information by phone and through the website. It has an online discussion board which is used by people from around the world.

Group details last confirmed May 2007.

ALLERGIES

Background

Allergy is an altered immune response to a substance which is eaten, inhaled or injected and which is harmless in most people. Substances (allergens) as diverse as pollen, penicillin and bee venom produce reactions which vary in severity from a mild rash or itching/sneezing to bronchial asthma and, occasionally severe, life-threatening anaphylactic shock (see entry, Anaphylaxis).

What are the symptoms?

Food allergy characteristically presents with multiple symptoms (lip swelling, tightness in the throat, rhinitis, abdominal pain, nettlerash and/or asthma and, rarely, life-threatening anaphylaxis). Rhinitis presents with itch/sneezing, watery nasal discharge and associated eye symptoms during the pollen season. Allergic asthma presents with cough, sensation of tightness in the chest, wheeze and breathlessness.

There is a history of immediate symptoms on exposure to these allergens and sensitivity may be confirmed either by skin prick testing with the relevant allergen and/or a blood test which measures the level of allergy-related IgE antibodies in the blood to the relevant allergen. However, these tests must always be interpreted in the context of a patient's symptoms on exposure to the relevant allergen, otherwise false-positive tests will occur. Occasionally, there is no particular time relation between exposure and symptoms so diagnosis may be difficult. Also, spontaneous remission may occur.

What are the causes?

In principle any substance can cause an allergy. Common ingested allergens include peanut, fish, eggs and milk. Injected substances include drugs (antibiotics) and insect venom (wasp stings). Inhaled allergens which may cause rhinitis and asthma (see entry) include house dust mite, pollens and animal danders. Common skin sensitisers include latex and house dust mite. Occupational allergy includes asthma, rhinitis or dermatitis which occurs following exposure to a particular substance in the work place.

Diseases which may be caused or aggravated by allergy include:
- Asthma;
- Hayfever/rhinitis;
- Conjunctivitis;
- Acute urticaria (nettlerash, hives) - Chronic urticaria, however, is frequently not due to an allergy;
- Food allergy;
- Drug allergy;

- Venom allergy;
- Anaphylaxis.

How is it diagnosed?

Diagnosis of allergies is usually straightforward although it may sometimes be difficult and time consuming. In general, there is a period of exposure prior to development of symptoms during which sensitisation occurs. Only a proportion of sensitised (atopic) people go on to develop symptoms (allergies) following re-exposure to the allergen. For example, egg and milk allergy commonly occur in infancy when exposure to these foods is most common. Allergic asthma occurs later in childhood following exposure to inhalant allergens including house dust mites and animal danders, whereas hayfever peaks in adolescence/early adulthood following repeated exposure to seasonal pollens, the 'Allergy March.'

Inheritance patterns and prenatal diagnosis

Inheritance patterns

Allergy is commonly, although not always, associated with a family history of allergic disorders. The likelihood of allergy is greater if one or both parents have an allergy.

Prenatal diagnosis

None, although a family history in both parents is very commonly associated with allergic manifestations in offspring.

Medical text written November 1991 by Contact a Family. Approved November 1991 by Dr J Brostoff, Consultant Immunologist, Middlesex Hospital, London UK. Last updated July 2002 by Professor S R Durham. **Last reviewed May 2006 by Professor S R Durham, Professor of Allergy & Respiratory Medicine, Imperial College, London, UK.**

Further online resources

Medical texts in *The Contact a Family Directory* are designed to give a short, clear description of specific conditions and rare disorders. More extensive information on this condition can be found on a range of reliable, validated websites. Further information on these resources can be found in our **Medical Information on the Internet** article on page 21.

Support

Allergy UK

3 White Oak Square, London Road, Swanley BR8 7AG   Tel: 01322 619898
Fax: 01322 663480   e-mail: info@allergyuk.org   Web: http://www.allergyuk.org
Allergy UK is a National Registered Charity No. 1104845, established in 1991. It offers: information, advice and support to people with allergies; details of NHS allergy clinics and allergy specialists; and translated cards for people who are travelling abroad identifying the carrier as having a serious allergy and providing emergency information. Activities include raising awareness among doctors, nurses, pharmacists, health visitors and dieticians by way of advanced training to diploma and degree level. It has a wide range of information available, details on request. Allergy UK receives over 40,000 enquiries a year. They also run Web: http://www.blossomcampaign.org which offers advice and information for parents and children regarding social exclusion of children due to allergies.
Group details last updated August 2007.

Contact a Family Helpline 0808 808 3555

Action against Allergy

PO Box 278, Twickenham TW1 4QQ   Tel: 020 8892 2711
e-mail: AAA@actionagainstallergy.freeserve.co.uk
Web: http://www.actionagainstallergy.co.uk
The organisation is National Registered Charity No. 276637. It offers: access to a telephone support network and co-ordination of an Allergy information centre and library. A specialist referral service provides contact details for NHS and private allergy specialists. It publishes a newsletter three times a year and has a wide range of information available, details on request. The organisation has approximately 2,000 members.
Group details last confirmed January 2007.

Latex Allergy Support Group

PO Box 27, Filey YO14 9YH   Mob: 07071 225838 (Mon-Fri, 7pm - 10pm)
e-mail: latexallergyfree@hotmail.com
Web: http://www.lasg.co.uk
The Group is a National Registered Charity No. 1104845, established in 1996. It supports affected individuals and their families and raises awareness amongst the public, healthcare workers, schools and other at risk groups. It publishes a quarterly newsletter, 'Bouncing Back' and has information available, details on request.
Group details last confirmed September 2007.

"It was so frustrating not being able to talk to another mother whose child had the same condition so we could share things, the way you do if your child gets measles. Through Contact a Family, I was able to speak to a mother who also had a child with a rare disorder and within a few hours had found a group of people who could really understand what we were going through." Parent.

ALOPECIA

Background

Hair is produced by structures in the skin known as hair follicles. Normally, a hair on the scalp will grow for a number of years. Eventually the hair stops growing and is shed two or three months later. A new hair then grows in its place.

The term alopecia is used to describe hair loss. There are several different types and causes of alopecia.

Male Balding
Male Balding: Male pattern hair loss; Androgenetic alopecia

Male balding is the most common type of alopecia. Half of the male population has some degree of balding by the age of fifty and only about 1 in 5 men over the age of seventy keeps a full head of hair. It usually starts as gradual hair thinning on the crown and recession of the hairline. This process may continue to complete loss of hair over the front and top of the scalp leaving a horseshoe pattern of hair remaining around the sides and back of the head.

Female Pattern Hair Loss
Female Pattern Hair Loss: Female androgenetic alopecia

Female pattern hair loss is a common form of hair thinning in women. The changes in hair growth are similar to those in male balding but the pattern of hair loss is usually different and it is very rare for it to progress to true balding.

Alopecia Areata
Alopecia Areata (AA) is thought to be an autoimmune disorder. In an autoimmune disorder the body's own defence system attacks the body; in the case of AA, it attacks the hair follicles. AA can start at any age, including during childhood, and affects males and females of all ethnic groups.

What are the symptoms?
Male Balding
During male balding there is a gradual shortening of the growth period of the hair, so hairs will not grow as long, and a delay in the replacement of the hair after the old hair falls out. Eventually the hair follicles shrink, a process called miniaturisation, so that the hair becomes finer as well as shorter. Finally when the follicle gets too small, no hair grows.

Female Pattern Hair Loss
Female pattern hair loss can start at any age from early teens onward. The hair becomes gradually thinner, making it easier to see the scalp. Thinning

usually affects the front and top of the scalp but it can be all over the scalp. In most women the frontal hairline does not recede, unlike male balding.

Alopecia Areata

The main feature of AA is the development of one or more bald patches on the scalp about the size of a large coin.

Individuals with AA may also experience any of the following:

- The development of further patches;
- Bald patches on body hair, beard, eyebrows and eyelashes;
- Pitted or ridged nails;
- Rarely, Alopecia Totalis, the loss of all scalp hair;
- Rarely, Alopecia Universalis, the loss of all hair on the body.

In most people the hair grows back but in some cases new patches of hair loss develop before hair grows back on old areas. Sometimes bald patches overlap and merge into larger areas. Almost all people who have a bout of AA will get it again, though episodes of hair loss may be many years apart.

What are the causes?

Male Balding

Male balding is caused by hormone reactions and a genetic predisposition. Most balding men, though not all, have a family history of balding. The balding tendency can probably be inherited from either father or mother but at present we have only a limited understanding of the genes that are responsible.

Female Pattern Hair Loss

As in men, there can be a genetic predisposition to hair thinning that runs in families. Some women with female pattern hair loss have increased levels of male-type hormones in their bloodstream but most do not and the cause of the hair loss is not yet known.

Alopecia Areata

The exact mechanism in AA has not been identified but it is thought that it can be triggered in a number of ways that include environmental factors, infection, viruses, sunlight or the stress of events such as bereavement or accidents. Genetic predisposition is also thought to play a part as up to twenty per cent of people with AA have a close relative similarly affected. People with AA are slightly more likely than the general population to develop other autoimmune disorders such as Thyroid disease (see entry), Vitiligo (see entry) or Diabetes (see entry).

Other causes of alopecia include:

- Chemotherapy or radiotherapy for cancer;
- Under active thyroid gland (see entry, Thyroid disorders);
- Childbirth. Some women experience excessive hair shedding two to three months after childbirth. This is temporary and recovers fully after

a few months in almost all women;

- Increased hair shedding may also occur following various illnesses, especially those associated with a high temperature or rapid weight loss;
- Fungal infections of the skin (mainly in children);
- Some medical drugs;
- Genetic diseases. Hair loss or thinning is a feature of many genetic abnormalities, such as ectodermal dysplasias, although all of these conditions are rare.

How is it diagnosed?

The diagnosis of male balding is made on the overall appearance and pattern of hair loss. Any other types of loss such as in patches, all over loss of hair or rapid progression of hair loss are likely to result from other causes.

How is it treated?

Male Balding

For many men, male balding is not a serious problem (though most would prefer to keep their hair!) However, some men are bothered by hair loss and are keen to do something about it. The treatment options include:

- Hair styling, such as clean shaving the head, hair weaving or hair pieces;
- Minoxidil lotion. This will help to slow down or stop hair loss and may produce some new hair growth. It works best when used in early balding – it will not regrow hair on a bald scalp. Treatment must be continued to maintain the benefits. Minoxidil lotion can be bought from pharmacies and is not available on the NHS;
- Finasteride tablets. Finasteride interferes with the effect of male hormones on hair follicles and halts or slows the balding process in over eighty per cent of men. About two thirds of men taking finasteride experience some regrowth of hair. Like minoxidil lotion, finasteride works best in the early stages of balding and the benefits will be lost within a few months if treatment is stopped. This type of drug is not available on the NHS;
- Surgical intervention to transplant hair from the back of the head to the crown of the head or, more radically, flap-surgery in which an area of scalp is transplanted from one area of the head to another.

Female Pattern Hair Loss

For women, the cosmetic appearance of their hair is generally more important to their self-esteem than in men, and women are more likely to want treatment. The treatment options include:

- Hair cosmetics, hair styling – a good hairdresser can be helpful;
- Minoxidil lotion. About two thirds of women will get some increase in

hair growth with minoxidil lotion. This takes six to twelve months to achieve and treatment has to be continued to maintain the response;

- Drugs that block the action of male-type hormones can help in some women but they are not licensed for treating hair loss. Finasteride is not approved for use in women;
- Hair transplantation can help in selected cases.

Alopecia Areata

There are several different treatments for AA but none is very effective and none cures the disease. In people who are minimally affected, the hair is likely to regrow on its own and no treatment is needed. In others, treatments such as topical (locally applied) creams, solutions rubbed into the scalp and steroid injections/creams can be used but these have a limited success. For women with extensive AA a wig or hairpiece is often the best option. Wigs tend to be less suitable for men.

Emotional and psychosocial stress can be caused to individuals and the support organisations can be very helpful.

Additional information

A NHS leaflet, *HC11 – Help with health costs*, giving information about prescription of wigs is available at Web:
http://www.dh.gov.uk/assetRoot/04/07/80/85/04078085.pdf or can be ordered from Department of Health, PO Box 777, London SE1 6XH
Tel: 08701 555455 Fax: 01623 724524.

Inheritance patterns and prenatal diagnosis

Inheritance patterns

No specific pattern has been identified but AA is likely to appear in more than one member of an affected family.

Prenatal diagnosis

Not applicable

Medical text written July 2005 by Contact a Family and Dr A Messenger, Consultant Dermatologist, Royal Hallamshire Hospital, Sheffield, UK.

Further online resources

Medical texts in *The Contact a Family Directory* are designed to give a short, clear description of specific conditions and rare disorders. More extensive information on this condition can be found on a range of reliable, validated websites. Further information on these resources can be found in our **Medical Information on the Internet** article on page 21.

Support

Hairline International – the Alopecia Patients' Society

Lyons Court, 1668 High Street, Knowle, Solihull B93 0LY   Tel: 01564 785 980

e-mail: elizst@aol.com Web: http://www.hairlineinternational.com

The Society is a patient support network, established in 1989. It provides information and support to people who have differing kinds of hair loss including early, total and radical hair loss. Full details of the Society are available (SAE A4 envelope). Hairline International responds to over 2,000 enquiries a year.

Group details last updated July 2005.

Alopecia UK

5 Titchwell Road, London SW18 3LW   Tel: 020 8333 1661

e-mail: info@alopeciaonline.org.uk   Web: http://www.alopeciaonline.org.uk

Alopecia UK provides information, advice and support for people with experience of alopecia areata, totalis and universalis and their families. It is primarily, but not exclusively, website-based. The website receives over 25,000 visits per month and, in addition to information, offers a discussion forum, as well as membership with regular updates, and local support groups.

Group details last confirmed March 2007.

ALPHA THALASSAEMIA – MENTAL RETARDATION ON THE X-CHROMOSOME

Alpha Thalassaemia (Alpha Thalassemia – US) – Mental Retardation on the X-Chromosome: Alpha Thalassaemia Mental Retardation syndrome; Mental Retardation on the X-Chromosome; ATR-X

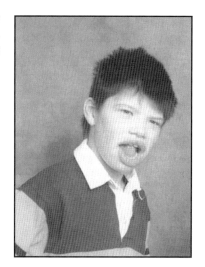

Background
ATR-X syndrome is an inheritable condition which affects boys. The effects of the condition include learning difficulties, a characteristic facial appearance and mild anaemia. The anaemia results from a mild form of thalassaemia similar to, but quite distinct from, ß Thalassaemia (see entry, Thalassaemia Major) which is common in the Mediterranean and South-East Asia and is not associated with learning difficulties.

World-wide, over one hundred and fifty affected families have been identified with this condition. The underlying gene was identified in 1995.

What are the symptoms?
Affected boys have severe learning difficulties and milestones are delayed. Speech is usually not achieved. Affected boys tend to suffer frequent colds and recurring chest infections. Most of the boys have genital abnormalities, most frequently undescended testes. Feeding problems and regurgitation are commonly present. Sleep disturbance and mouthing may occur in some children.

How is it diagnosed?
The red blood cells of someone affected by ATR-X syndrome have a tell-tale appearance under the microscope which allows the diagnosis of ATR-X to be confirmed by a simple blood test.

Inheritance patterns and prenatal diagnosis
Inheritance patterns
X-Linked. It is often possible to identify female carriers of the ATR-X syndrome by family studies.

Prenatal diagnosis

This may be possible in some families where there is already one affected family member. Advice from the Regional Genetics Centre may be sought prior to pregnancy.

Medical text written February 1993 by Dr D Higgs and Dr R Gibbons, MRC Molecular Haematology Unit, Institute of Molecular Medicine, John Radcliffe Hospital, Oxford UK.
Last updated June 2007 by Dr R Gibbons, MRC Molecular Haematology Unit, Institute of Molecular Medicine, John Radcliffe Hospital, Oxford, UK.

Further online resources

Medical texts in *The Contact a Family Directory* are designed to give a short, clear description of specific conditions and rare disorders. More extensive information on this condition can be found on a range of reliable, validated websites. Further information on these resources can be found in our **Medical Information on the Internet** article on page 21.

Support

ATR-X Support Group
82 The Crescent, Northwich CW9 8AD   Tel: 01606 44943
e-mail: davidwalker825@btinternet.com
The group was established in 1991 and is in contact with Professor Douglas Higgs and Dr Richard Gibbons, the leading authorities on the condition. It offers support for families of affected children and linking of families where possible. The Group maintains a national register of families. It publishes a newsletter and is in touch with the families of 70 affected children and adults in the UK and overseas.
Group details last updated February 2007.

Contact a Family Helpline 0808 808 3555

ALSTRÖM SYNDROME

Background

Alström syndrome is a very rare, hereditary genetic disorder first described by C.H. Alström in Sweden in 1959. There are over two hundred cases known worldwide.

What are the symptoms?

The first sign usually noticed in affected children is an involuntary rapid movement of the eye (nystagmus) and light sensitivity which begins in infancy and eventually leads to retinopathy (a degeneration of the retina, the thin, light sensitive lining at the back of the eye) and blindness.

As infants and toddlers, affected children are generally overweight. Hearing impairment usually begins before the children are ten years old. Later, in young adulthood, children develop high levels of insulin in the blood, diabetes mellitus, and slowly progressive kidney problems.

Other findings observed in some Alström syndrome patients include a darkening of areas of the skin called acanthosis nigricans, scoliosis or curvature of the spine, short stature, an underactive thyroid gland, elevation of enzymes in the liver, and dilated cardiomyopathy (a dysfunctioning of the heart muscle). Kidney failure can occur in the second to fourth decade of life. Urological problems can occur, rarely leading to the need for catheterisation or even urinary diversion.

Inheritance patterns and prenatal diagnosis

Inheritance patterns

Autosomal recessive

Prenatal diagnosis

For current information about prenatal diagnosis, contact Alström Syndrome UK.

Medical text written October 1999 by Contact a Family based on information provided by the Jackson Laboratory, Maine, USA. Approved October 1999 by Dr R Paisey. **Last updated January 2004 by Dr R Paisey, Consultant Physician, Torbay Hospital, Torquay, UK.**

Further online resources

Medical texts in *The Contact a Family Directory* are designed to give a short, clear description of specific conditions and rare disorders. More extensive information on this condition can be found on a range of reliable, validated websites. Further information on these resources can be found in our **Medical Information on the Internet** article on page 21.

Support

Alström Syndrome UK

49 Southfield Avenue, Paignton TQ3 1LH   Tel/Fax: 01803 524238 Office
e-mail: alstrom@syndromeuk.freeserve.co.uk   Web: http://www.alstrom.org.uk
The group is a National Registered Charity No. 1071196, established in 1998. It offers support to families, carers and professional workers and raises awareness of Alström syndrome in the public and medical profession. The Group fundraises for medical research and to meet individual needs, and co-ordinates an annual screening clinic alonside its annual conference. It publishes a newsletter and is in touch with 20 families. The National Specialist Commissioning Advisory Group (NSCAG) funds specialised, multi-disciplinary Alström clinics – for details contact the group as above or e-mail: kay.parkinson@alstrom.org.uk
Group details last updated January 2007.

Every Disabled Child Matters is a campaign founded by Contact a Family and other charities to get a better deal for families with disabled children. Visit www.edcm.org.uk for more information.

ALTERNATING HEMIPLEGIA

Background

Alternating hemiplegia is a condition which has transient weakness of either, or sometimes both, sides of the body. The attacks may alternate or sometimes overlap, that is the second side is affected before the first recovers. Attacks start in the first year of life and are often accompanied by unusual irregular eye movements. The attacks last from less than an hour which is unusual to sometimes several days. When the attacks are prolonged the manifestations are not apparent during sleep or for the first fifteen to twenty minutes on waking when they then return. This is a very characteristic finding and when there are bilateral attacks this may allow feeding and drinking to occur in that short clear period after waking. The episodes of hemiplegia are not epileptic in nature but epileptic seizures may co-exist and require separate anti-epileptic drug treatment.

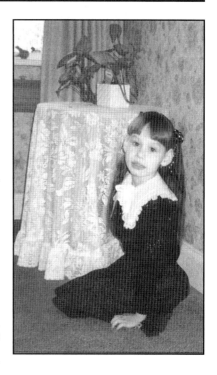

How is it caused?

The cause is not known. Affected children usually have significant learning disabilities and motor organisational problems, including unsteadiness. There is a tendency for these problems to increase with repeated episodes.

How is it treated?

Treatment is with flunarizine (a calcium channel blocker). Other drugs have not been found to be consistently helpful.

Inheritance patterns and prenatal diagnosis

Inheritance patterns

None

Prenatal diagnosis

None

Medical text written January 1994 by Dr J Wilson, Consultant Neurologist (retired – formerly of Great Ormond Street, Hospital, London, UK). Last updated June 2000 by Professor B Neville. **Last reviewed October 2004 by Professor B Neville, Professor of Childhood Epilepsy, Institute of Child Health, London, UK.**

Further online resources

Medical texts in *The Contact a Family Directory* are designed to give a short, clear description of specific conditions and rare disorders. More extensive information on this condition can be found on a range of reliable, validated websites. Further information on these resources can be found in our **Medical Information on the Internet** article on page 21.

Support

Alternating Hemiplegia Support Group

80 London Road, Datchet, Slough SL3 9LQ   Tel: 01753 546268

The Group is a self help group, established in 1993. It offers support by telephone and letter. The group is in touch with 26 families. A family meeting is held on July each year in Windsor, Berkshire.

Group details last updated September 2007.

The National Service Framework for Children in Wales was published in summer 2005

ALZHEIMER'S DISEASE

Background

Alzheimer's disease is the most common cause of dementia, responsible for just over half of the approximately seven hundred and fifty thousand people with dementia in the UK. It is a physical disease which attacks the structure of the brain.

What are the symptoms?

Typically, Alzheimer's disease begins with lapses of memory, difficulty in finding the right words for everyday objects or mood swings. Mild symptoms may be a natural effect of aging, but in Alzheimer's disease a pattern of problems emerges over six months or more.

Alzheimer's is a progressive disease and in the early stages, a person may:

- routinely forget recent events, appointments, names and faces and have difficulty in understanding what is being said;
- become confused when handling money, driving a car or using a washing machine;
- undergo personality changes, appearing to no longer care about those around them. They may become irritable, apathetic or suffer mood swings and burst into tears for no apparent reason. They may also become convinced that someone is trying to harm them.

In advanced cases people may also:

- adopt unsettling behaviour, like getting up in the middle of the night, or wandering off from their home and becoming lost;
- lose their inhibitions and sense of suitable behaviour, undressing in public or making inappropriate sexual advances.

Finally, the personality disintegrates and the person becomes totally dependent or bed-bound.

What are the causes?

Alzheimer's is a physical disease which attacks brain cells (where we store memory), brain nerves and transmitters (which carry instructions around the brain). Production of numerous chemical messengers, including acetylcholine and glutamate, are disrupted as nerve ends are attacked and cells die. The brain shrinks as gaps develop in the temporal lobe and hippo-campus, important for receiving and storing new information. The ability to remember, speak, think and make decisions is disrupted. After death, tangles and plaques made from protein fragments, dying cells and nerve ends are discovered in the brain. This confirms the diagnosis.

How is it treated?

There are now four licensed treatments available which improve the symptoms or slow down the decline in people with Alzheimer's disease. Three of these (Aricept, Exelon, Reminyl) are cholinesterase inhibitors and work on the acetylcholine chemical messenger system. The other treatment (Ebixa) works on the chemical messenger glutamate. A number of others are being developed and undergoing clinical trials. There is also accumulating evidence that a healthy lifestyle which protects the heart (regular exercise, balanced diet avoiding excessive fat or cholesterol, treatment for any high blood pressure) and involves a diet rich in antioxidants (e.g. vitamin C, vitamin E, green tea) can slightly reduce the risk of developing Alzheimer's disease.

Inheritance patterns and prenatal diagnosis

Inheritance patterns

There is no single gene for Alzheimer's disease. Genetic factors are responsible for the disease in a small number of families where the disease affects people at an early age. In the majority of these cases the disease is linked to a fault on chromosome 14. In the wider community there is a genetic component, most commonly linked to the ApoE4 gene. In these cases, genetic factors alone do not explain why some develop Alzheimer's disease, and others do not.

Prenatal diagnosis

None.

Medical text written October 2000 by the Alzheimer's Society, London, UK. **Last updated November 2004 by Professor C Ballard, Director of Research, Alzheimer's Society, London, UK.**

Further online resources

Medical texts in *The Contact a Family Directory* are designed to give a short, clear description of specific conditions and rare disorders. More extensive information on this condition can be found on a range of reliable, validated websites. Further information on these resources can be found in our **Medical Information on the Internet** article on page 21.

Support

Alzheimer's Society
Devon House, 58 St Katharine's Way, London E1W 1JX
Tel: 0845 300 0336 Helpline (Mon – Fri, 8.30am – 6.30pm)
Tel: 020 7306 0606   Fax: 020 7306 0808
e-mail: enquiries@alzheimers.org.uk   Web: http://www.alzheimers.org.uk
The Society is a National Registered Charity No 296645, established in 1979. It offers: information and advice on all forms of dementia and a network of carers groups, carers' contacts, befriending projects and telephone helplines. It publishes a monthly newsletter and has a wide range of information available, details on request. The Society has over 20,000 members.
Group details last updated November 2007.

ANAPHYLAXIS

Background

Anaphylaxis is a word coined in 1902 meaning 'without protection.' A wide variety of substances (allergens) can induce anaphylaxis. Foods and stinging insects are well known causes; however the most common cause of anaphylaxis across all age groups remains drugs. Latex rubber has also been recognised as a cause of serious allergic reactions (see entry, Allergies).

What are the symptoms?

The symptoms and signs of anaphylaxis may include one or more of: wheezing, vomiting, hives, facial swelling, abdominal pain, a feeling of impending doom, and ultimately hypotension (lowered blood pressure) with cardiorespiratory compromise. Symptoms may progress rapidly and unpredictably if treatment is not quickly administered. It is, however, reassuring that most food-induced allergic reactions are of a mild or moderate nature and do not progress to anaphylaxis.

What are the causes?

Although any food may potentially induce anaphylaxis, most food-induced reactions are due to peanut, tree nut, sesame, fin-fish, shellfish and kiwi fruit. In addition, hen's egg and cow's (or goat's) milk are important food allergens in young children which may also result in anaphylaxis. Peanuts are the most frequent cause of food induced allergic reactions. This is largely due to their allergenicity but also the fact that peanut allergy is infrequently outgrown and therefore represents a risk across all age ranges. A significant proportion of patients with peanut allergy may also be allergic to tree nuts and/or sesame allergic, and visa versa. It is therefore important that food allergic individuals are properly evaluated by an allergy specialist.

How is it diagnosed?

Diagnosis of the cause of anaphylaxis is generally easy but not always so, particularly if a meal was eaten which contained multiple food allergens or if there were possible contributing factors such as exercise or alcohol intake. Severe reactions may occur after the ingestion of small amounts of the food. Unfortunately foods are not always labelled, or food allergens are labelled with names which are not easily recognised; for example the word 'arachis' may be used to indicate peanut.

How is it treated?

All food allergic patients should be in possession of a personalised emergency plan and appropriate medications. Although mild reactions can be successfully treated with an antihistamine, intra-muscular adrenaline remains the drug of choice for moderate to severe reactions.

Inheritance patterns and prenatal diagnosis

Inheritance patterns
Often but not always a family history of allergy

Prenatal diagnosis
Not currently available but research is being carried out at the University of Southampton.

Medical text written May 2006 by Dr George Du Toit, Consultant Paediatric Allergist & Hon Senior Lecturer, Evelina Children's Hospital, Guys & St Thomas' Trust, Kings College London, UK.

Support

The Anaphylaxis Campaign
PO Box 275, Farnborough GU14 6SX   Tel: 01252 542029 Helpline   Tel: 01252 546100
Fax: 01252 377140   e-mail: info@anaphylaxis.org.uk   Web: http://www.anaphylaxis.org.uk
The Campaign is a National Registered Charity No. 1085527, established in 1994. It offers support and advice to affected people and families of affected children, and has a network of regional contact persons. Activities include operating a helpline, awareness raising and campaigning about anaphylaxis, producing a wide range of publications and educational videos, organising family fun days, meetings with expert speakers, local support groups, youth and parent workshops. It offers a membership service, which includes receipt of a newsletter three times a year, details of local events and 'product alerts' sent to warn people about inadequately labelled food relevant to their allergies. It has almost 8,000 members.
Group details last confirmed September 2007.

ANDROGEN INSENSITIVITY SYNDROME

Background

Androgen Insensitivity syndrome: Complete Androgen Insensitivity syndrome (CAIS); Partial Androgen Insensitivity syndrome (PAIS); Androgen Resistance syndrome; Testicular Feminisation syndrome; Feminising Testes syndrome; Male Pseudo-Hermaphroditism; Goldberg-Maxwell syndrome (CAIS); Morris's syndrome (CAIS); Lub's syndrome (PAIS); Reifenstein syndrome (PAIS); Gilbert-Dreyfus syndrome (PAIS)

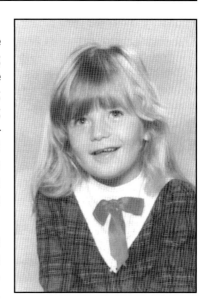

Normally, humans have twenty-three pairs of chromosomes. On fertilisation, the chromosomes combine to give a total of forty-six (twenty-three pairs). A female usually has an XX pair of sex chromosomes and a man an XY pair. The female affected by androgen insensitivity syndrome (AIS) has an XY pair of sex chromosomes.

What are the symptoms?

An affected infant has no virilisation, either during fetal life or during adult life. However, the presence of a testis does not allow the development of any internal female genitalia (no fallopian tubes, uterus or upper two-thirds of the vagina) despite having female external genitalia. The child is born an apparently normal girl. At puberty, the testes produce a large amount of the male hormone testosterone but, in the absence of its receptor, this has no effect. However, testosterone is converted to oestrogen and the girl will have normal breast development, without pubic or axillary hair, and will have no periods (there is no uterus or vagina). Because the testes are usually found in the abdomen in girls with AIS, there is a risk of them becoming cancerous.

What are the causes?

This condition is caused by a genetic defect in the androgen (male hormone) receptor, which enables the male hormone, testosterone, to have its affect.

How is it diagnosed?

AIS is not usually diagnosed at birth. The usual presentation is during childhood with a girl who has bilateral inguinal hernias, often containing the testes. Presentation may not be until the middle teenage years, when the girl enters puberty, but has no periods and also none, or minimal, pubic or axillary hair.

How is it treated?

The most important part of the management of AIS is the explanation and counselling given to the parents as to what and how to tell the child. This should involve an expert psychologist. Unlike partial androgen insensitivity (see below) the problem is compounded by not being diagnosed at birth. Certainly, full revealment of the diagnosis, including the chromosome abnormality, should be given by the time the child has become an adult.

The testes are usually removed when the diagnosis is made. Puberty should be induced at the normal age and then an accurate assessment of the vaginal size can be made. The assessment of whether to perform a vaginal dilation or a vaginoplasty (an operation to create a vagina) should be made by a gynaecologist who is expert in this field. Certainly, the girl should be counselled not to attempt intercourse until the vagina is an adequate size. There may be longer-term problems such as Osteoporosis - see entry, Osteoporosis (Juvenile).

In Partial Androgen Insensitivity, the genetic abnormality in the androgen receptor produces an incomplete block of male hormone action. In this case, the child is usually born with ambiguous genitalia and appears a poorly virilised male. The child may be brought up as either a male or a female and the management very much depends on the severity of the condition in the individual.

Inheritance and prenatal diagnosis

Inheritance patterns
X-linked recessive

Prenatal diagnosis
This is possible, through chorionic villus sampling at ten to twelve weeks and/or amniocentesis at about sixteen weeks, but seldom indicated.

Medical text written May 1997 by Dr R Stanhope. **Last reviewed October 2005 by Dr R Stanhope, Consultant Paediatric Endocrinologist, Great Ormond Street Hospital, London, UK.**

Contact a Family Helpline 0808 808 3555

Support

Androgen Insensitivity Syndrome Support Group

c/o Contact a Family, 209-211 City Road, London EC1V 1JN
Tel: 0808 808 3555 Helpline   Tel: 020 7608 8700   Fax: 020 7608 8701
e-mail: info@cafamily.org.uk   Web: http://www.aissg.org
The group is a National Registered Charity No. 1073297, established in 1992, having started informally in 1988. It offers support to families and adults affected by AIS and other XY-female conditions, with group meetings (sometimes twice) a year. It runs an online newsgroup to keep members up to date on items of interest, publishes a newsletter 'ALIAS - Learning About AIS' and has other information available, details on request. The group is in touch with several hundred affected families/individuals in the UK and has sister groups in North America and various European countries.
Group details last updated March 2007.

Contact a Family has a library and information team responding to queries from professionals and students wanting information about any aspect of working with disabled children. For more information e-mail: library@cafamily.org.uk

ANENCEPHALY

Background

Anencephaly is a condition affecting the development of the brain and often the spinal cord with a multitude of associated congenital problems. It is a condition that is non-survivable and the baby is either born dead or dies within a few hours to days of birth.

Anencephaly is what is known as an open neural tube defect in the cephalic region. This basically means that the skull and overlying scalp are absent and a severely abnormal brain structure is open to the outside. There are also significant abnormalities of the face and the neck associated with it. There are various sub-groups depending on the involvement of the neck and associated spina bifida (see entry). These abnormal deficits in the coverings of the brain are present very early in gestation, being present by the fourth week after fertilisation. The incidence varies from 1 in 1,000 to just under 7 in 1,000 in some ethnic groups. The incidences in the Western world are reducing in line with increased uptake of folic acid. Females are more prone to this than males. Twins have a higher prevalence than single births.

How is it caused?

In most cases the aetiology (cause) is unknown but there are some relations with abnormal genes.

How is it diagnosed?

Anencephaly can be detected prenatally by ultrasound sometimes as early as fourteen weeks depending on the lie of the fetus. It should be easily visible at twenty weeks on the ultrasound. Amniocentesis and measurement of the levels of alpha feta protein in the amniotic fluid can confirm the diagnosis. Alpha feta protein would be expected to be extremely high in this defect.

Inheritance patterns and prenatal diagnosis

Inheritance patterns

In most cases the aetiology (cause) is unknown but there are some relations with abnormal genes. The risk of a further pregnancy with anencephaly and spina bifida is said to be 1 in 50 if there has been one previously affected pregnancy and 1 in 5 if there have been two previously affected pregnancies. Associated abnormalities include hydro-nephrosis (excessive enlargement of the fluid collecting system for the kidneys), cleft lip and/or palate (see entry), diaphragmatic hernia (see entry), omphalocoele (abnormal abdominal wall development) and horseshoe kidneys. In addition spinal abnormalities and abnormal postures of the foot are also associated. It has been calculated that risks for a neural tube defect in relatives of affected persons are as follows: father's siblings, seven per cent; mother's sister's children, thirteen per cent;

mother's brother's children, three per cent; father's sister's children, six per cent; and father's brother's children, four per cent. Unfortunately, ninety-five per cent of these conditions occur in pregnancies in which there was nothing previously suspicious.

Prenatal diagnosis

Anencephaly can be detected prenatally by ultrasound sometimes as early as fourteen weeks depending on the lie of the fetus. It should be easily visible at twenty weeks on the ultrasound. Amniocentesis and measurement of the levels of alpha feta protein in the amniotic fluid can confirm the diagnosis. Alpha feta protein would be expected to be extremely high in this defect.

Medical text written February 2006 by Mr N Buxton, Consultant Paediatric Surgeon, Alder Hey Children's Hospital, Liverpool, UK.

Further online resources

Medical texts in *The Contact a Family Directory* are designed to give a short, clear description of specific conditions and rare disorders. More extensive information on this condition can be found on a range of reliable, validated websites. Further information on these resources can be found in our **Medical Information on the Internet** article on page 21.

Support

As Anencephaly is a neural tube disorder, information and advice is available from ASBAH, the Association for Spina Bifida and Hydrocephalus (see entry, Spina Bifida).

ANGELMAN SYNDROME

Background

Angelman syndrome is a neurodevelopmental disorder which was first described in 1965.

What are the symptoms?

The main signs and symptoms of Angelman syndrome are learning disability, jerky movements, a tendency to seizures and a happy, sociable personality. Children with Angelman syndrome usually present with delay in reaching their developmental milestones and often do not learn to sit until around one year of age. The majority of children will learn to walk but tend to have a characteristic wide-based, stiff-legged gait. General health is usually good but seizures can be a problem, particularly in childhood. Individuals with Angelman syndrome almost always have characteristic abnormalities on EEG (Electroencephalogram) testing. Many, but not all children with Angelman syndrome have a typical facial appearance with a wide, smiling mouth, deep set eyes and prominent chin. These features become more prominent as children get older. Some Angleman individuals, especially those who have chromosome 15 deletion may be fairer in complexions than the rest of their family. Adults with Angelman syndrome are much less hyperactive than younger children and have a better concentration span. They remain dependent on others, but can acquire a variety of skills to help with daily living. Medical complications in older patients include the development of joint contractures, curvature of the spine and oesophageal reflux. Seizures may also return in adulthood.

Psychological and behavioural characteristics

The information below has been updated September 2007 by Dr O Udwin, Consultant Clinical Child Psychologist, West London Mental Health NHS Trust, London UK and Dr A Kuczynski, Child Clinical Psychologist, South London & Maudsley NHS Trust, London, UK.

All individuals with Angelman syndrome have severe or profound learning disabilities. Furthermore, they have marked difficulties in their speech and language development. Early prelinguistic babbling and vocal play is often absent. Children typically acquire no more than a few words, and approximately one-third do not talk at all. Their understanding of language may be meaningfully better than their speech, and most use some nonverbal means of communication, including gestures, signs and picture boards.

Hyperactivity and 'overexcitability' is common in childhood. Many affected children find it difficult to concentrate during the day and to settle and stay asleep at night. Bedtime may provoke tantrums. The overactivity and sleep problems may decrease with age.

Children and adults are typically described as happy, sociable, and affectionate, and as enjoying physical contact. They display frequent bouts of giggling laughter and hand-clapping or flapping. Although these are often a response to what is going on around them, the humour may at times be inappropriate. Still, individuals with Angelman syndrome may be less prone to irritability and social withdrawal than others with comparable general developmental difficulties. Many of them love music and water, and are fascinated by mirrors and other reflective surfaces.

Many children with Angelman syndrome are able to learn important self-care skills, including feeding and toileting, and as they grow older they may undertake other domestic tasks, such as dusting and setting the table with assistance. However, they all require supervision in their daily lives.

Inheritance patterns and prenatal diagnosis

Inheritance patterns

Angelman syndrome may arise from a variety of genetic abnormalities, all of which involve the same part of chromosome 15 which contains the gene called UBE3A. The majority of children have a small deletion of the 15q11-13 region. Diagnostic testing for Angelman syndrome is complex. In the majority of families only one child is affected by Angelman syndrome but in 5-10% of cases brothers, sisters and extended family members may be affected. It is recommended that parents of an affected child should approach their local clinical genetics centre for genetic counselling and testing on an individual basis.

Prenatal diagnosis

Prenatal tests are available in those families where a definite genetic abnormality has been identified.

Medical text written November 1991 by Contact a Family. Approved November 1991 by Professor M Patton, Professor of Medical Genetics, St Georges Hospital Medical School, London, UK and Dr J E Wraith, Consultant Paediatrician, Royal Manchester Children's Hospital, Manchester, UK. **Last updated August 2007 by Jill Clayton-Smith, Consultant Clinical Geneticist, St Mary's Hospital, Manchester, UK. Psychological and behavioural characteristics last updated March 2004 by Dr O Udwin, Consultant Clinical Child Psychologist, West London Mental Health NHS Trust, London, UK and Dr A Kuczynski, Child Clinical Psychologist, South London & Maudsley NHS Trust, London, UK.**

Further online resources

Medical texts in *The Contact a Family Directory* are designed to give a short, clear description of specific conditions and rare disorders. More extensive information on this condition can be found on a range of reliable, validated websites. Further information on these resources can be found in our **Medical Information on the Internet** article on page 21.

A

Support

ASSERT

PO Box 13694, Musselburgh EH21 6XZ   Tel/Fax: 01268 415940

e-mail: assert@angelmanuk.org   Web: http://www.angelmanuk.org

ASSERT is a National Registered Charity No. 1021882, established in 1992. It offers support to families by telephone, e-mail and letter. Activities include: fundraising for research and group activities; participation in research studies; and raising awareness of the condition. It publishes a regular Newsletter and has information available, details on request. ASSERT holds a biennial conference and is in touch with over 450 families.

Group details last confirmed October 2007.

Contact a Family produces a guide on dealing with debt. Call the helpline for a copy.

ANIRIDIA

Aniridia: Congenital abnormality of the iris

Background

Aniridia is a rare congenital disorder of eye development. Usually part or all of the iris is absent, giving the appearance of an enlarged pupil. Sometimes the changes are more subtle with a normal pupil size and alteration of the iris appearance. There is an associated underdevelopment of the central retina (foveal hypoplasia) leading to reduced vision and nystagmus (see entry).

What are the causes?

Aniridia is caused by a defect in the PAX6 gene on chromosome 11.

How is it diagnosed?

Aniridia is usually detected soon after birth when parents notice poor vision, nystagmus and a big pupil. Genetic diagnosis is not widely available but may be possible.

How is it treated?

The condition is not curable but treatment with prescription of glasses, low vision aids and ensuring adequate help with schooling helps considerably. Complications of aniridia such as cataracts (see entry), glaucoma (see entry), corneal changes (abnormal loss of transparency and blood vessel growth) and squint can occur later in life and may reduce the vision further, but are treatable by medication or surgery.

Although many of those with aniridia will have a visual disability and are unlikely to develop enough vision to drive a car, most will have enough vision for a sighted education and cope well with the help of visual aids. It is rare to develop complete blindness.

Inheritance patterns and prenatal diagnosis

Inheritance patterns

Aniridia is caused by a defect in the PAX6 gene on chromosome 11 and is inherited in an autosomal dominant way. This can be inherited from an already affected parent (familial aniridia) or the defect can develop for the first time in an affected person (sporadic aniridia) who has no history of aniridia in the family. In those with sporadic aniridia there is no risk to their siblings but they can pass on the disease to their children. For any individual with aniridia each of their children has a 50/50 chance of being affected.

Some children with sporadic aniridia are at risk of developing Wilm's tumour of the kidney. Such children have loss of a segment (a deletion) of chromosome 11 that includes both the PAX6 gene and the neighbouring Wilm's tumour gene. Some will have the WAGR syndrome (Wilm's tumour, aniridia, genital abnormality, mental retardation). Loss of the Wilm's tumour gene can be detected by genetic testing and identifies those children who need regular testing for the tumour.

Prenatal diagnosis

This is not widely available but is possible if the particular defect of the PAX6 gene in the affected parent is known.

Medical text written October 2006 by Dr M Hingorani, Consultant Ophthalmologist, Hinchingbrooke Hospital, Huntingdon, UK.

Further online resources

Medical texts in *The Contact a Family Directory* are designed to give a short, clear description of specific conditions and rare disorders. More extensive information on this condition can be found on a range of reliable, validated websites. Further information on these resources can be found in our **Medical Information on the Internet** article on page 21.

Support

A support network for Aniridia is being developed. Families can use Contact a Family's Freephone Helpline for advice, information and, where possible, links to other families. Contact a Family's web-based linking service Making Contact.org can be accessed at http://www.makingcontact.org

ANKYLOSING SPONDYLITIS

Background

Ankylosing Spondylitis is a rheumatic disease which affects the spine. It can also affect the joints of limbs and tissues in other parts of the body. The condition is characterised by inflammation in the spinal joints followed by healing which results in additional bone growing from both sides of the joint eventually encircling it. This means that the joint is immobilised (ankylosed).

What are the symptoms?

Ankylosing spondylitis is characterised by an insidious onset usually between twenty to twenty-five years (though it can be earlier), of early morning stiffness and pain. Symptoms may improve with exercise. Pain is not always associated with the spine: it may affect the chest, buttocks or elsewhere.

What are the causes?

There is an association between a certain genetic marker (HLA B27) and the development of Ankylosing Spondylitis.

How is it treated?

Early diagnosis, treatment and special exercises can mitigate the effects of the condition.

Inheritance patterns and prenatal diagnosis

Inheritance patterns

Ankylosing spondylitis is virtually confined (in Britain) to those with the white cell blood antigen HLA B27, (seven to ten per cent of the population). However, only one fifth of those will develop the disease. The chance of children of an affected person developing the disease is between five per cent and thirty per cent.

Prenatal diagnosis

None at present.

Medical text written November 1991 by Contact a Family. Approved November 1991 by Professor M Patton, Professor of Medical Genetics, St Georges Hospital Medical School, London, UK and Dr J E Wraith, Consultant Paediatrician, Royal Manchester Children's Hospital, Manchester, UK. Last updated April 2000 by Dr A Calin (retired - formerly Consultant Rheumatologist, Royal National Hospital for Rheumatic diseases, Bath, UK. **Last reviewed October 2004 by Dr R Jacoby, Consultant Rheumatologist, Royal Devon and Exeter Hospital, Exeter, UK.**

Further online resources

Medical texts in *The Contact a Family Directory* are designed to give a short, clear description of specific conditions and rare disorders. More extensive information on this condition can be found on a range of reliable, validated websites. Further information on these resources can be found in our **Medical Information on the Internet** article on page 21.

Support

National Ankylosing Spondylitis Society (NASS)

Unit 0.2, 1 Victoria Villas, Richmond TW9 2GW   Tel: 020 8948 9117   Fax: 020 8940 7736
e-mail: admin@nass.co.uk   Web: http://www.nass.co.uk

The Society is a National Registered Charity No. 272258 and was established in 1975. It offers mutual support through a network of local branches throughout the UK providing group physiotherapy and support for people with medical/social problems. Activities include an occasional symposium. It publishes a twice yearly membership journal and has a wide range of information available, details on request. The Society has around 8,000 members.

Group details last updated April 2007.

"It was great to go somewhere where you felt relaxed, with fun things to do and meeting other families in the same position" Parent at a fun day organised by Contact a Family West Midlands.

ANOPHTHALMIA

Background

Anophthalmia is a rare developmental abnormality. It is part of a range of abnormalities in which babies are born with no eye in the eye socket (anophthalmia) or with a small eye in the eye socket (microphthalmia). Anophthalmia can affect both eyes, in which case the baby will be blind, or only one eye in which case the baby may have normal vision in the other eye.

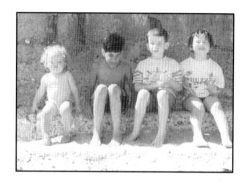

Anophthalmia or severe microphthalmia occurs in 3 to 7 in 100,000 live births. This means that in England and Wales there are only about thirty to thirty-five babies born each year with anophthalmia or severe microphthalmia. About half of these babies have other developmental problems in addition to anophthalmia.

What are the causes?

The condition is likely to occur because the delicate sequence of early developmental steps to form an eye is disrupted in some way. These signals for development in the embryo come from the genes within the developing cells. The exact mechanism is not fully understood, but a disruption of this process can occur through external factors during pregnancy or an error in the genes themselves. The occurrence of anophthalmia and microphthalmia has been related to some illnesses during pregnancy including virus infections, such as rubella (German measles) and varicella (chicken pox). It has also been linked to some drugs taken during pregnancy, including recreational drugs and thalidomide. There has been a suggestion that insecticides and fungicides used to spray crops may be related to anophthalmia, but to date there is no scientific evidence to support this. Over the last few years a few genes have been described that are important in anophthalmia or a related condition, microphthalmia. These eye development genes include SOX2, Rx, SHH (sonic hedgehog), CHX10, BCOR, and PAX6. Whilst many of these genes have only been described so far in association with a few families worldwide, SOX2 seems to be important in around ten per cent of children with anophthalmia.

How is it treated?

It is not possible to restore sight to a baby with anophthalmia affecting both eyes. However artificial eyes, usually made of acrylic and painted to look like real eyes, are used to help with the cosmetic appearance. Treatment is beneficial for these babies from a very early age. If a baby is born without an eye in the socket, the eye socket does not receive the correct signals to grow properly. This results in a small socket and it may be difficult to fit artificial eyes later to these children. Therefore it is important that babies born without an eye or with a very small eye are referred for assessment at a specialist centre as soon after the birth as possible. In this way they can be fitted with artificial eyes which will help to stimulate socket growth and will help cosmetically.

Inheritance patterns and prenatal diagnosis

Inheritance patterns

There are some families where anophthalmia and microphthalmia can be genetically inherited. However, most cases are isolated. Since anophthalmia may be genetically determined in some cases, even if there appears to be only one individual affected in the family, it is important for families to obtain accurate genetic counselling about the possible risk of any further children having a similar condition.

Prenatal diagnosis

It is possible to diagnose anophthalmia on ultrasound scan. Unfortunately the resolution of ultrasound scans at present means that it is not possible to make the diagnosis with any certainty until well into the second trimester. As anophthalmia is rare, and there is not usually more than one case within a family, the diagnosis may well not be detected until the major scan at around twenty weeks' gestation. With current knowledge, blood tests during pregnancy will not alert doctors to the possibility of anophthalmia. Amniocentesis will show up a chromosome abnormality, which occurs in a small proportion of babies with anophthalmia, usually those with several other developmental anomalies. In families where a causative gene has been identified prenatal testing may be possible.

Medical text written November 1995 by Mr A J Vivian, Consultant Ophthalmic Surgeon, West Suffolk Hospital, Bury St Edmunds, UK. **Last updated October 2004 by Miss Nicola Ragge MD FRCOphth FRCPCH, Honorary Consultant Ophthalmic Surgeon, Moorfields Eye Hospital, London, UK and Birmingham Children's Hospital, Birmingham, UK and Senior Surgical Scientist, University of Oxford, Oxford, UK.**

Further online resources

Medical texts in *The Contact a Family Directory* are designed to give a short, clear description of specific conditions and rare disorders. More extensive information on this condition can be found on a range of reliable, validated websites. Further information on these resources can be found in our **Medical Information on the Internet** article on page 21.

Support

MACS

22 Lower Park Street, Holyhead LL65 1DU   Tel: 0800 169 8088 Freephone
e-mail: enquiries@macs.org.uk   Web: http://www.macs.org.uk

M.A.C.S. (Micro & Anophthalmic Children's Society) is a National Registered Charity No.1040074, established in 1993. It offers support by telephone and letter, and linking with other families where requested. Activities include raising awareness of the condition, a network of regional family contacts, regional meetings and a family weekend/AGM. It publishes a newsletter and has information available, details on request. The organisation has over 400 UK members and over 150 overseas members.
Group details last updated July 2007.

Eyeless Trust

PO Box 1248, Slough SL2 3GH Tel: 01494 672006 (Lillian Ramsay, Social Work Consultant) Tel: 020 8852 2469 (Mari Everard, Director of Social Work)
e-mail: ANDREW.paul@eyeless.org.uk   Web: http://www.eyeless.org.uk

The Trust is a National Registered Charity No. 1028896, established in 1993. It offers counselling, support, advice and assessment of needs by qualified medical social workers. It makes grants where there is no statutory provision to cover the costs of hospital attendance, holidays for the family, children's clothing, specialised educational equipment, short breaks and respite care toiled to the needs of the family. In 2008 The Trust will be running a residential workshop for teenagers aged 16 and above to increase skills and develop independence. It has information available, details on request and is associated with a genetic research project being undertaken by Moorfields Eye Hospital. The Trust helps over 500 children with anophthalmia, many of whom have multiple disabilities.
Group details last updated November 2007.

ANXIETY DISORDERS

Background

Anxiety can be generalised often with no obvious trigger (free floating) or focused in response to a specific cause.

A **phobia** is an intense aversion which is focused on a specific object or situation. It is associated with fear of the particular stimulus, expressed as an anxiety state in particular circumstances with a specific focus when extreme. In extreme instances it is experienced by the affected individual as a panic attack.

The 'panic' attack is actually a physiological response to danger. The body prepares to 'fight or run.' To achieve this, the blood supply is diverted from one part of the body to another, the heart rate and breathing rate increase and sweating occurs. These effects produce the conscious experiences of panic and impending threat. Panic attacks are self-limiting, although phobic individuals may feel them to be life-threatening and may even believe they are experiencing a fatal event.

The focus of the attack in phobic conditions is directed to a real object or situation which becomes associated with the individual's particular fears. A phobia may reach proportions in which the individual's freedom of action is severely curtailed. In such circumstances family members are also affected.

Amongst common phobias are agoraphobia (fear of open space) and claustrophobia (fear of enclosed space), snake phobia or spider phobia.

Obsessive compulsive disorder (see entry) is a situation where the individual has to perform specific actions ('compulsions') such as washing or specific repeated thoughts ('obsessions') which may show as counting rituals. These activities in very severe cases may reach such proportions, that individuals' entire lives, and those of their families, are centred upon them.

What are the causes?

Often the cause is entirely normal and justifiable, for example an impending test, or driving a car for the first time. On other occasions the cause is less understandable, or the anxiety reaction is out of proportion. In these situations a learnt fear and avoidance response to whatever is causing the anxiety often develops (phobia).

How is it treated?

Treatment usually consists of behavioural psychotherapeutic approaches aimed at desensitizing the individual systematically to the fear inducing object or situation. Relaxation exercises are often used. 'Exposure' activities are undertaken allowing individuals to tolerate increasingly anxiety-provoking situations while practicing their ability to remain in psychological control and not panicking.

For those with obsessive compulsive disorders behavioural programmes including exposure therapy are again useful, particularly when combined with 'response prevention' strategies, encouraging sufferers to tolerate increasingly stressful situations which predispose to the obsessive-compulsive problems while remaining calm and resisting the urges. In extreme instances modern antidepressants which have strong anti-obsessional properties are prescribed.

Inheritance patterns and prenatal diagnosis

Inheritance patterns
There may be a familial tendency

Prenatal diagnosis
None

Medical text written October 2004 by Professor J Turk, Professor of Developmental Psychiatry and Consultant Child & Adolescent Psychiatrist, Department of Clinical Developmental Sciences, St. George's Hospital Medical School, London, UK.

Support

National Phobics Society

Zion Community Resource Centre, 339 Stretford Road, Hulme, Manchester M15 4ZY
Tel: 0870 122 2325   Fax: 0161 226 7727   e-mail: info@phobics-society.org.uk
e-mail: support@phobics-society.org.uk (dedicated e-mail support service)
Web: http://www.phobics-society.org.uk
The Society is a National Registered Charity No. 1113403, established in 1970. It offers one-to-one therapies such as counselling and cognitive behavioural therapy, both face to face and by telephone, clinical hypnotherapy and a nationwide network of self-help groups. It publishes a quarterly newsletter - Anxious Times - and has a wide range of information available, details on request. The Society has approximately 6,000 members and responds to over 50,000 enquiries a year.
Group details last updated August 2007.

APHASIA

Aphasia: Dysphasia

Background

Aphasia is a complex condition which can affect an individual's speech, understanding, reading or writing. It is estimated that there are around 250,000 people in the UK who have Aphasia; it can affect people of any age and occurs in men and women equally. Adults and children with aphasia may have difficulty expressing their thoughts and understanding what is being said to them through language.

What are the symptoms?

Characteristics of childhood aphasia can include, impairments of the repetition of heard sounds or words, poor attention, hyperactivity, poor eye contact, and difficulty understanding simple 'yes' or 'no' questions.

Aphasia can affect each person differently, from very mild to severe symptoms and communication difficulties which can also change from day to day or even hour to hour. They are likely to be worse when tired, unwell or under pressure.

Aphasia may make it difficult for someone to do any of the following:
- talking;
- listening;
- understanding writing;
- reading;
- using numbers.

The term Aphasia covers a wide range of language impairments and a wide range of terminology has developed over the years to describe them. The three most commonly recognised types are:
- Broca's aphasia – individuals with this type of aphasia may not be able to speak at a normal pace and often their speech is limited to short utterances of less than four words. Often referred to as 'non fluent aphasia', their ability to access words is impaired and formation of speech sounds difficult and clumsy. While they may be able to understand most speech they can be limited also in writing.;
- Wernicke's aphasia – sometimes referred to as 'fluent aphasia' an individual's ability to produce speech is not greatly affected but they may produce speech that sounds like jargon and have difficulty grasping the meanings of spoken words. As a result their spoken sentences do not flow and irrelevant words can be used. Reading and writing are often severely impaired.;
- Anomic aphasia – those who have this form of relatively less severe

aphasia are often unable to find the words for things they wish to speak about particularly significant nouns and verbs. As a result their speech often sounds empty or strange and while their grammar is unaffected, they use vague descriptions or indirectly describe meanings of words.

What are the causes?

Aphasia results from damage to the parts of the brain that control language. Damage to the brain can be caused by head injury, a brain tumour, neurological conditions, the result of stroke or a side effect of surgery on the brain. Infections of the brain such as encephalitis (see entry) can also cause this condition.

Childhood aphasia may be acquired. This happens when a child who is developing language normally suffers a head trauma or infection as described above and this disturbance disrupts their development. One form of acquired childhood aphasia is called Landau-Kleffner syndrome (see entry).

Commonly, however childhood aphasia is developmental or congenital. Children in this situation are born with a problem that arises during language development. The term developmental aphasia can be used when no evidence of neurological or other specific brain dysfunction can be found.

How is it diagnosed?

The diagnosis is based entirely on the presence of impaired development in language and related aspects of cognition and behaviour.

Speech and reading can often be unaffected but difficulty finding words is also evident in writing. Diagnosis of the condition will normally be done through a speech and language assessment. Medical examination can help determine the cause of the aphasia and assessment by a speech and language therapist can provide a basis for the best treatment.

How is it treated?

Speech and language therapy is the most common treatment offered to children with aphasia, although if there is an underlying cause this will also be treated accordingly.

Aphasia can result in significant psychosocial affects for aphasic people and for their families and they may need significant emotional and community support.

Inheritance patterns and prenatal diagnosis

Inheritance patterns

None

Prenatal diagnosis

N/A

Medical Text Written January 2008 by Contact a Family. Approved January 2008 by Professor Chris Code, Honorary Research Fellow, School of Psychology & Centre for Cognitive Neuroscience, University of Exeter, Exeter UK

Support

Aphasia information, support and advice is available from Afasic (see entry, Speech and Language Impairment)

Speakability
1 Royal Street, London, SE1 7LL
Tel: 080 8808 9572 (freephone helpline, Monday - Friday, 10am-4pm) Tel: 020 7261 9572
Fax: 020 7958 9542   Web: http://www.speakability.org.uk
Speakability is a National Registered Charity no. 295094. It supports and empowers people with aphasia to overcome the barriers they face by supporting people with aphasia and their carers through its information service, national network of Self-Help Groups and programme of activities. They are also committed to influencing individuals, organisations and statutory bodies to improve services for people living with aphasia.
Group details last updated January 2008.

"Disabled children and their brothers and sisters suffer an acute lack of the summer holiday activities that other families take for granted. Local leisure facilities, holiday playschemes and sports activities often exclude disabled children because of health and safety fears, lack of funding and inaccessible venues." Postcards from home: the experience of disabled children in the school holidays. Barnardo's. 2004.

ARBOVIRAL ENCEPHALITIDES

West Nile Encephalitis

West Nile virus is an arthropod-borne virus (i.e an arbovirus) transmitted between birds by infected mosquitos. People become infected with the virus following the bite of an infected mosquito. The virus is not transmitted from person to person. There is no evidence that a person can get the virus from handling live or dead infected birds. However, it is still recommended that bare-handed contact with dead animals is avoided.

The incubation period of a West Nile virus infection is usually five to fifteen days. Mild infections are common and include fever, headache and body aches, often with skin rash and swollen lymph glands.

Encephalitis (see entry) results when the virus invades the central nervous system destroying the brain substance with accompanying inflammation. The clinical features range from muscle weakness and paralysis; to mild confusion and behavioural changes (which may be mistaken for hysteria); and to convulsions (fits) and deep coma.

There is no specific treatment for West Nile virus. Current management consists of treating the complications of the disease such as high fever and aches, some patients are left with severe paralysis, convulsions, or raised intracranial pressure.

The simplest preventative measure is to avoid bites from the mosquitoes that carry the virus. This involves wearing long sleeves and trousers, especially during the evening when the mosquito bites and avoiding areas where stagnant water can be found – mosquito larvae need still water to develop. For further protection use an insect spray containing at least thirty per cent DEET (N,N-diethyl-3methlybenzamide) and sleep under bed-nets.

West Nile virus (genus *Flavivirus*, family *Flaviviridae*) was first identified in 1937. It was subsequently shown to have a very wide area of distribution that includes most of Africa, southern Europe, the Middle East, and even parts of the Far East. In its natural cycle, the virus is transmitted primarily between birds by mosquitoes. Classically, West Nile virus causes a non-specific febrile illness, and until recently nervous system manifestations were considered a rarity. However, in recent years the epidemiology has changed with the virus spreading to new areas and causing different disease patterns. In 1996 there was an epidemic of West Nile encephalitis in Romania, and in 1999 the virus reached the United States for the first time with an outbreak in New York. Since then it has spread across the Eastern and Central American states, and in 2002 caused its largest outbreak, with more than six thousand cases and thirty deaths reported by September 2002.

Inheritance patterns
None.
Prenatal diagnosis
None.

Japanese Encephalitis

Japanese encephalitis virus has always been recognised as a killer. Only about 1 in 300 infections results in disease, and there is a wide range of presentations from a simple febrile illness to a severe meningoencephalitis, as well as polio-like acute flaccid paralysis. There are estimated to be fifty thousand cases of Japanese encephalitis annually, with fifteen thousand deaths. The actual numbers may become clearer with the application of new simple rapid diagnostic tests. In addition to the high mortality, approximately half the survivors have severe neuropsychiatric sequelae, with their associated socioeconomic burden.

Over the last fifty years the disease has spread relentlessly across Southeast Asia, India, southern China, and the Pacific reaching Australia in 1998. Epidemics of encephalitis were described in Japan from the 1870's onwards, and Japanese encephalitis virus was first isolated from a fatal case in the 1930's. The virus causing Japanese encephalitis is a member of the Flavivirus group which derives its name from Yellow fever virus (in Latin, 'yellow' is 'flavus'). The flaviviruses are relatively new viruses, thought to derive from a common ancestor ten to twenty thousand years ago, that are rapidly evolving to fill new ecological niches. Japanese encephalitis virus is transmitted in an animal cycle between small birds by Culex mosquitoes, and pigs are important amplifying hosts. Humans become infected by Culex mosquitoes coincidentally, but are not part of the natural cycle. Recent findings in Asia raise important issues about the spread, control and pathogenesis of Japanese encephalitis. It is thought to be spread by birds, but mosquitoes blown between Pacific islands may contribute too. An expensive formalin inactivated and newer live attenuated vaccines against Japanese encephalitis are available, but not for the majority of the two point eight billion people living in affected regions. For them, the factors determining who, of all those infected with Japanese encephalitis virus, develops neurological disease may be critically important. The relative contributions of the human immune response, and viral strain differences are currently being investigated.

Inheritance patterns
None.
Prenatal diagnosis
None.

Tick-borne Encephalitis

After one to two weeks incubation the virus causes a sudden onset of fever, headache nausea and photophobia. In mild cases this resolves after a week, but in more severe cases there is a second phase of illness with meningoencephalitis or myelitis. The latter tends to cause flaccid paralysis of the upper limb and shoulder girdle. Respiratory muscle and bulbar (brainstem) involvement lead to respiratory failure and death.

Tick-borne encephalitis virus is a member of the flavivirus genus (group) that circulates in small wild animals, mostly rodents, and is transmitted between them, and to humans, by Ixodes ticks. Humans may also become infected by drinking goat's milk.

It has a wide area of distribution across Europe and the former USSR, and its seasonal incidence is reflected in one of the many pseudonyms 'Russian spring-summer encephalitis.' Genetic sequencing has allowed Western tick-borne encephalitis virus, which is endemic in Germany, Austria and much of Europe, to be distinguished from Far-Eastern tick-borne encephalitis virus which is found across the former Soviet Union.

Far Eastern tick-borne encephalitis has a higher case fatality rate, but the Western form is often associated with sequelae (after effects).

A formalin inactivated vaccine given as two doses four to six weeks apart, has been recommended for those likely to be exposed in the endemic forested areas of Europe and the former USSR. Such vaccines are now used widely in Austria.

Louping ill virus is a closely related tick-borne virus notable for being the only flavivirus found naturally in the British Isles (as well as Scandinavia). It occurs naturally among small mammals (hares, wood-lice and shrews), but is also transmitted to highland sheep which develop encephalitis. The disease is named after the leaping (or louping) demonstrated by the encephalitic sheep. Very occasionally the virus infects humans causing a meningoencephalitis, which can be severe.

Powassan virus is a distantly related tick borne flavivirus found principally among small mammals in Canada that has occasionally caused meningoencephalitis in humans.

Inheritance patterns

None.

Prenatal diagnosis

None.

Medical text written September 2002 by Dr T Solomon. **Last updated May 2007 by Dr T Solomon, Hon. Lecturer in Medical Microbiology and Tropical Medicine, University of Liverpool, Liverpool, UK.**

Further online resources

Medical texts in *The Contact a Family Directory* are designed to give a short, clear description of specific conditions and rare disorders. More extensive information on this condition can be found on a range of reliable, validated websites. Further information on these resources can be found in our **Medical Information on the Internet** article on page 21.

Support

Information and support on all forms of Encephalitis can be obtained from the Encephalitis Support Group (see entry, Encephalitis).

"The helpline was brilliant – fantastic, I can't fault it. I was getting stuck and I eventually found the people I needed to help me." Parent caller to our helpline.

ARTERIOVENOUS MALFORMATIONS

Background

An arteriovenous malformation (AVM) is a tangled web of abnormal arteries and veins connected by fistulas (abnormal corridors). AVMs are thought to be present from birth and most commonly occur in the brain. AVMs can also occur in the spine, lungs, kidney, skin and, very rarely, limbs. Because some AVMs do not result in symptoms, the exact incidence is not known. AVMs of the brain that are detected are found in about 1 in 100,000 of the general population per year. AVMs affect both sexes and all ethnic groups.

Normally, oxygenated blood is carried by arteries to body tissues through ever smaller blood vessels. The smallest blood vessels are called capillaries and form the capillary bed which is where the exchange of oxygen and nutrients for carbon dioxide and other waste products produced by the body cells (cellular wastes) takes place. Following this exchange, the blood is carried away by progressively larger blood vessels, the veins. Because AVMs lack a capillary bed, arterial blood is shunted directly from the arteries into the veins via direct communications called fistulas.

What are the causes?

The cause of AVMs is not known but it is thought that they develop as a result of a mistake in embryonic or fetal development.

Arteriovenous malformations of the brain

The main symptoms of brain AVMs include:

- Seizures/epilepsy (see entry, Epilepsy);
- Brain haemorrhage;
- Focal neurological deficits in the absence of brain haemorrhage (most often weakness or numbness);
- Ringing in the ears (known as 'pulsatile tinnitus').

Further neurological effects that largely depend on the specific position of the AVM include:

- Muscle weakness or paralysis;
- Loss of co-ordination;
- Dizziness;
- Visual disturbances;
- Problems in using or understanding language;
- Numbness, tingling, or pain;
- Memory deficits.

Vein of Galen malformation (see entry) is a rare specific form of AVM.

There are three main methods of treating AVMs of the brain:

- Embolisation, in which particles are injected to block off the blood vessels of AVMs of the brain and dura (covering of the brain);

- Stereotactic radiosurgery, in which radiation is used to treat small vascular malformations, mainly AVMs less than three centimetres across;
- Neurosurgery, in which a surgical operation is performed on the brain to disconnect an AVM of the brain or dura (covering of the brain) from the arteries that supply it and the veins that drain it.

Inheritance patterns

Rarely, AVMs may occur in the brain and lungs as a result of a condition called Hereditary Haemorrhagic Telangiectasia (see entry).

Prenatal diagnosis

The presence of an AVM may be picked up on Ultrasound scan, although this is not usually the case.

Pulmonary arteriovenous malformations

As in AVMs of the brain, a pulmonary AVM is present at birth and the capillaries essential for the full oxygenation of blood are not present. Consequently, the normal oxygenation is not carried out properly as the exchange process of oxygen and nutrients for carbon dioxide and other waste products does not occur.

The effects of pulmonary AVMs include:

- Breathing difficulties;
- Shortness of breath on physical exertion;
- Cyanosis (bluish or purplish discoloration of skin or lips as a result of poor blood oxygenation);
- Clubbing (enlargement of the tips) of the fingers;
- Audible murmur when a stethoscope is placed over the AVM;
- Warmth of the overlying skin;
- Occasionally coughing up blood.

Some people with a pulmonary AVM do not have symptoms.

Diagnosis of a pulmonary AVM is made following tests which include, chest x-rays, chest CT (computerized tomography) scan, bubble echocardiogram (scan of the heart), perfusion lung scan (x-ray examination after injection of radioactive material), pulmonary arteriogram (motion picture x-rays) or blood tests.

Treatment of pulmonary AVMs is by either surgical removal of the abnormal vessels and surrounding lung tissue or it might be possible to block the fistula with a coil when an ateriogram is carried out. If treatment is not carried out, there is a possibility of blood clots travelling from the lungs to the limbs or the brain. In the case of the latter, a stroke is a possibility.

Inheritance patterns
May be associated with conditions such as Hereditary Hemorrhagic Telangiectasia (see entry) or Juvenile polyposis with hereditary hemorrhagic telangiectasia.

Pre-natal diagnosis
This may be picked up on an ultrasound scan.

Spinal arteriovenous malformations

Spinal AVMs are very rare. They usually present to medical attention in adult life. They are a potentially treatable cause of myelopathy (any disease or disorder of the spinal cord). Myelopathies may cause any or all of the following symptoms:

- weakness of the legs;
- Disturbance of sensation over the legs, buttocks and genital areas;
- Impairment of bladder and/or bowel function.

Spinal AVMs usually involve the lower part of the spinal cord, called the thoracic cord which stretches from the neck to the small of the back.

Improvements in spinal cord imaging with Magnetic Resonance Imaging (MRI) have lead to quicker diagnosis. However, spinal AVMs are notoriously difficult to detect, and may require spinal catheter angiography (visualisation of the blood vessels after injection of a radiopaque substance) to be certain about the diagnosis.

Treatment of spinal AVMs is often difficult, and usually its objective is to limit further damage to the spinal cord, rather than alleviate the problems already caused. The two main forms of treatment are surgical excision and embolisation via a catheter in the groin. Embolisation is becoming the mainstay of treatment as technological advances in catheters and embolic glues are made.

Medical text written August 2005 by Contact a Family. Arteriovenous malformation of the brain and Spinal arteriovenous malformation information approved August 2005 by Dr R Al-Shahi, MRC Clinician Scientist and Specialist Registrar In Neurology, University of Edinburgh/ Western General Hospital, Edinburgh, UK. Pulmonary arteriovenous malformation information approved August 2005 by Dr A Jaffe, Consultant and Honorary Senior Lecturer in Respiratory Research, Great Ormond Street Hospital and Institute of Child Health, London, UK.

Further online resources

Medical texts in *The Contact a Family Directory* are designed to give a short, clear description of specific conditions and rare disorders. More extensive information on this condition can be found on a range of reliable, validated websites. Further information on these resources can be found in our **Medical Information on the Internet** article on page 21.

Support

AVM Support UK

Suite G03, Blyth CEC, Ridley Street, NE24 3AG Tel: 01670 737231

e-mail: info@avmsupport.org.uk   Web: http://www.avmsupport.org.uk

AVM Support UK was established in 2003 to offer free, patient friendly information and support to all whose lives have been affected by Arteriovenous Malformations. AVM Support UK hosts an online meeting point for people with AVMs and provides access to reliable information.

Group details last updated August 2007.

Each year, our staff organise around 150 workshops attended by over 2,500 parents.

ARTHRITIS (ADULT)

Background

There are over two hundred kinds of arthritis (some are rare, some more common), that fall into three categories: Inflammatory, Non-Inflammatory and Connective Tissue. Arthritis affects people of all ages, including children (see entry Arthritis (Juvenile Idiopathic)). In fact, some kinds of arthritis do tend to affect people in particular age groups, whilst others are more common in women than men.

Arthritis means inflammation of the joints. It is a general term that acknowledges something is wrong and is not a diagnosis in itself. Because there are so many different forms of arthritis, diagnosis can take a while and involve multiple visits to your GP or specialist (rheumatologist) and a lot of tests. Symptoms often reveal themselves gradually so it is important to tell the doctor about any new or changed symptoms. Patients should be referred to and consult a rheumatologist.

Types of Arthtitis

Some of the specific conditions are:

Osteoarthritis (OA) This is most common in hands, knees, hips, feet and spine. It usually develops gradually, over several years, and the cause is unknown. Healthy cartilage that covers the bone end in the joint is very smooth, strong and flexible. In osteoarthritis this becomes pitted, rough and brittle. Bony outgrowths (osteophytes) form at the outer edges of the joint, making it look knobbly and often there is some inflammation. The joint may become stiff and painful to move and occasionally swells. Whilst the pain itself can be very unpleasant, it does not generally make one feel unwell.

Rheumatoid Arthritis (RA) This is an inflammatory disease which mainly affects joints and tendons. This inflammation causes damage and can go on for a long time, or come and go. The body's immune system puts itself into reverse and attacks certain parts of the body instead of protecting it. This 'auto immune reaction' occurs mainly in the joints but in a 'flare-up' other organs can be affected. Tiredness and a general feeling of fatigue coupled with early morning stiffness, can last for several hours.

Secondary Arthritis This sometimes develops after an injury which damages a joint although it may not appear until many years later.

Gout This is caused by uric acid crystals in the joints. When there is too much uric acid in the tissues, it can form crystals in and around joints. If crystals enter the joint space they cause inflammation, swelling - and severe pain.

Polymyalgia Rheumatica (PMR) This is an inflammatory condition affecting the muscles in and around the shoulder and upper arm areas, buttocks and thighs. The cause of inflammation is unknown but Polymyalgia usually starts very suddenly. The main symptom is stiffness which usually restricts mobility, particularly in the early part of the day. This usually eases as the day progresses but often returns in the evenings. In contrast to rheumatoid arthritis the joints are not usually involved though occasionally there can be associated inflammation in joints such as the shoulder, hip and wrist. Frequently there is an associated loss of weight and appetite.

Ankylosing Spondylitis (AS) (see entry, Ankylosing Spondylitis).

Lupus (see entry, Lupus).

Medical text written October 2000 by Arthritis Care. Approved October 2000 by Dr D Doyle. **Last updated October 2005 by Dr D Doyle, Consultant Rheumatologist and Chairman of the Medical Advisory Panel of Arthritis Care, London, UK.**

Support
Arthritis Care
18 Stephenson Way, London NW1 2HD
Tel: 0808 800 4050 Helpline (Mon - Fri, 10am - 4pm)   Fax: 020 7380 6505
e-mail: helplines@arthritiscare.org.uk   Web: http://www.arthritiscare.org.uk
The Source - a helpline for young people with arthritis (under 26)
Tel: 0808 808 2000 (Mon - Fri, 10am - 2pm)   e-mail: thesource@arthritiscare.org.uk
Arthritis Care is a National Registered Charity No. 206563, established in 1948. It offers helpline support and advice to individuals, parents and young people. It publishes a magazine 'Arthritis News' six times a year and has a wide range of information available, details on request. Please send SAE. The organisation has 66,000 members - adults, young people and children.
Group details last confirmed March 2007.

ARTHRITIS (JUVENILE IDIOPATHIC)

Background

Arthritis means inflammation of the joint, which usually results in pain, stiffness and swelling. There are many causes of joint pain in children. However, most of these are not arthritis. There are many different forms of arthritis affecting children, some of which have specific names (listed in 'types of arthritis'.) Occasionally, it is not possible to give a particular name to a form of arthritis in a child.

Types of Arthritis

Systemic arthritis – arthritis with fever and rash, beginning in children of younger age particularly. The child may be quite unwell before arthritis becomes obvious. Other features, including swelling of the lymph glands in the neck, under the arms and

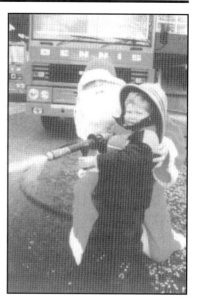

Photograph with kind permission of Belfast Telegraph

groin, may begin before diagnosis of Systemic Arthritis. Rarely, the lining of the heart or lungs may become inflamed (pericarditis or pleuritis respectively.) Some children with systemic arthritis may have problems with swollen, painful joints for many years, even into adulthood.

Polyarthritis – arthritis affecting many joints, particularly in girls. This form of arthritis may begin in the early childhood years when it affects the fingers and toes as well as larger joints. It is also associated with "silent" eye disease. In teenage girls, a different form of polyarthritis similar to adult 'rheumatoid arthritis' can be identified using blood tests for 'rheumatoid factor.' However, in most children, blood tests cannot be used to diagnose arthritis. Many patients with polyarthritis may continue to have joint problems in their adult years.

Oligoarthritis – arthritis affecting only a few joints (four or less) is the commonest form of arthritis in children. It affects young children, particularly girls, and is associated with an eye disease (chronic iridocyclitis). The eye disease can **only** be detected by 'slit lamp' examination of the eyes, which should be done every few months. Many children with oligoarthritis improve after some time, but if a few joints remain swollen, the disease is termed **persistent oligoarthritis.** If the disease worsens, and more joints become involved, it is called **extended oligoarthritis.**

Enthesitis-related arthritis – arthritis which usually begins in older boys or teenagers. It may also cause painful areas in the soles of the feet or other areas around the knees or hips where the ligaments attach to the bone. This form of arthritis is associated with a genetic factor (HLA-B27). Eventually the spine may become stiff and painful, and in adults this is known as ankylosing spondylitis (see entry).

Psoriatic arthritis – arthritis with the typical skin rash of psoriasis (see entry, Psoriatic Arthropathy). Even if the rash is absent, psoriatic arthritis can be diagnosed by other features, such as 'finger-nail pitting' or even a family history of psoriasis. Children with this form of arthritis should also be checked regularly for eye inflammation by an ophthalmologist using a slit lamp.

Inheritance patterns and prenatal diagnosis

Inheritance patterns

It is very rare to have more than one child with arthritis in one family, but there are some genetic factors passed on through the generations that may make it more likely that a child will develop arthritis. The role of the environment, e.g. bacterial or viral infections, in triggering off the disease is being questioned.

Prenatal diagnosis

None.

Medical test written February 1999 by Professor T Southwood. **Last updated January 2004 by Professor T Southwood, Professor of Paediatric Rheumatology, University of Birmingham, Birmingham, UK.**

Support

Children's Chronic Arthritis Association

Ground Floor Office, Amber Gate, City Walls Road, Worcester WR1 2AH

Tel: 01905 745595 (Mon-Fri, 10am-1pm)   Fax: 01905 745703   e-mail: info@ccaa.org.uk

Web: http://www.ccaa.org.uk

The Association is a National Registered Charity No. 1004200, established in 1988. It offers support by telephone, letter and e-mail for families of affected children and can offer area family contacts. It publishes a bi-annual newsletter and produces information booklets, details on request. Every year it organises a family educational and activity weekend. The Association has approximately 2,000 members.

Group details last confirmed August 2007.

Choices
PO Box 58, Hove BN3 5WN   Tel: 01273 430219   e-mail: info@kidswitharthritis.org
Web: http://www.kidsunlimited.info for children and teenagers with Arthritis
Web: http://www.kidswitharthritis.org
Choices is a National Registered Charity No. 1093971, established in 2001. It provides a wealth of information including a free comprehensive handbook for families of children with arthritis via the website and by phone, e-mail and letter. It is able to offer advice and work with families to ensure they receive services appropriate to their child's needs. Choices can also provide information and training for professionals working with affected families. The Choices handbook is also published in a Welsh edition. The web site for children and teenagers with arthritis is produced by children and teenagers.
Group details last confirmed October 2007.

Support is also available from Arthritis Care (see entry, Arthritis (Adult)).

"Where children have special needs and disabilities it is important that they are identified at an early stage and that identification leads directly to early intervention and support for families and children." Together from the Start - Practical guidance for professionals and disabled children (birth to third birthday) and their families DfES. 2003.

ARTHROGRYPOSIS

Arthrogryposis: Arthrogryposis Multiplex Congenita; AMC

Background

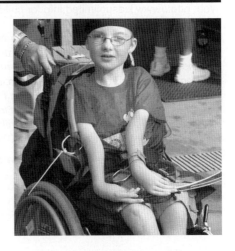

Arthrogryposis Multiplex Congenita (AMC) is not a diagnosis but a descriptive term which is used to describe a baby born with joint contractures affecting at least two different areas of the body. The joints may be fixed in a bent or straightened position. It is believed that such contractures may result from one of several processes that cause the unborn baby's limbs not to move properly at the time the joints are being formed. These processes fall into four main categories: problems with the nerve supply, the muscles, the connective or supporting tissues and external factors such as the blood supply to the baby or the shape of the womb. Approximately 1 in 5,000 babies are affected.

Arthrogryposis includes over one hundred and fifty different conditions. These include diagnoses such as Multiple Pterygium syndrome, Larsen syndrome (see entry) and Freeman Sheldon syndrome (see entry). Some are relatively mild whilst others involve problems with other organs such as the brain, nervous system or muscles.

What are the causes?

The commonest cause of AMC is amyoplasia (lack of muscle formation). This too has a recognisable pattern of joint involvement and other features. Although this condition is present at birth, it is non-progressive and it is almost certainly not inherited so that the risk of other children in the family being affected is very low.

How is it diagnosed?

Early diagnosis is important and referral to a geneticist is recommend to see if the pattern of problems can be recognised and a specific diagnosis made.

How is it treated?

The care of people with Arthrogryposis is essentially symptomatic. However early diagnosis is important so that appropriate therapy can planned. This may include early physiotherapy (including passive stretching exercises), splinting and surgery.

Inheritance patterns and prenatal diagnosis

Inheritance patterns

All types of inheritance may be implicated, including chromosomal problems. The family tree may provide clues to how the condition is inherited or passed down through the family. Even after the baby is born it may be difficult to make a specific diagnosis but it is still important that each child is assessed on an individual basis. In this way they can be given the support they need to reach their full potential at each stage of their development.

Prenatal diagnosis

If the specific genetic change that has caused the problems is known, then it may be possible to look for this in subsequent pregnancies by chorionic villus sampling (CVS) or amniocentesis. This is likely to be possible in only a very small minority of cases.

Ultrasound scanning later in the pregnancy may detect contractures or a decrease in fetal movements but it may not be possible to be sure of how severely the baby is likely to be affected.

Medical text written October 1999 by TAG (The Arthrogrypsosis Group). Approved October 1999 by Dr C Pollitt. **Last updated October 2004 by Dr C Pollitt, Specialist Registrar in Clinical Genetics, School of Biochemistry and Genetics, University of Newcastle, Newcastle upon Tyne, UK.**

Support

The Arthrogryposis Group (TAG)
Beak Cottage, Dunley, Stourport-on-Severn DY13 0TZ   Tel: 01299 825781
e-mail: taguk@aol.com   Web: http://tagonline.org.uk
The Group is a National Registered Charity No. 327508, established in 1984. It offers support, contact and information for affected children/members and their families. Activities include raising professional and public awareness of the condition; a range of family events organised by regional contacts; a national annual conference; quarterly newsletter and a wide range of information, details on request. The group represents the families of over 400 children and 300 adults who have Arthrogryposis.
Group details last updated October 2007.

ASTHMA

Background

Asthma is a complex condition that can start at any time of life. It is a condition that affects the airways - the small tubes that carry air in and out of the lungs. Children with asthma have airways that are almost always red and inflamed. These sensitive airways react badly when they have a cold or other viral infection, or when they come into contact with an asthma trigger. A trigger is anything that irritates the airways and causes the symptoms of asthma to appear.

What are the symptoms?

The usual symptoms are coughing, wheezing, breathlessness or a tight feeling in the chest. The muscle around the walls of the airways tightens so that the airway becomes narrower. The lining of the airway swells and produces a sticky mucus. As the airways narrow, it becomes difficult for the air to move in and out - this results in breathing difficulties with a wheezing or whistling noise. Some children may experience these symptoms only occasionally whilst others experience them at night, first thing in the morning or after exercise. A few may experience these symptoms all the time.

Everybody's asthma is different and one or more of a variety of triggers makes symptoms worse. These can include viral infections, exercise, cold weather and tobacco smoke. In addition, 'allergens' such as the house dust mite (a normally harmless creature that lives in beds, carpets and soft furnishings), pollen and animal fur can trigger asthma. Trying to avoid all these triggers all of the time is impossible but it is useful to encourage children with asthma to be aware of their triggers and to avoid them where possible.

Brittle Asthma

There are also a very small number of people with difficult to control asthma whose asthma is referred to as "brittle asthma". Brittle asthma is unstable and unpredictable, with frequent severe attacks. Often no consistent trigger factors can be identified. There are two types:

- **Type I**: Peak flow varies persistently day and night despite considerable medical therapy. More women than men are affected. Possible trigger factors include allergens (for example house-dust mite, pollen, cat and dog dander), life trauma or ongoing stressful situations, and symptoms related to the menstrual cycle;

- **Type II**: Attacks come on very quickly without warning and often require emergency hospital admission. Between attacks people with Type II Brittle asthma can feel well and their asthma seems well controlled. It is equally common in both men and women. Possible trigger factors include inhalation of something that causes an allergic reaction. In some people foods can be triggers for serious attacks.

What are the causes?

It is difficult to say what causes asthma and experts still do not know why it has increased. Although there are many hypotheses, asthma, like its related allergic conditions, eczema and hay fever, often runs in families and may be inherited. There are a number of other environmental factors that may contribute to someone developing asthma - many aspects of modern lifestyles, such as housing and diet might be responsible. We also know that maternal smoking during pregnancy increases the chance of a child developing asthma. Current research suggests that rather than there being one definitive cause of asthma we are more likely to find that it is a combination of genetic, environmental and lifestyle factors.

Inheritance patterns and prenatal diagnosis

Inheritance patterns

A tendency to develop asthma, eczema and hay fever may be inheritable, but environmental factors are also involved.

Prenatal diagnosis

None.

Medical text written December 2001 by Asthma UK (formerly National Asthma Campaign). Approved December 2001 by Professor Martyn Partridge. **Last updated February 2005 by Asthma UK. Approved February 2005 by Professor Martyn Partridge, MD, FRCP, Chief Medical Adviser, Asthma UK, London, UK.**

Support

Asthma UK
Summit House, 70 Wilson Street, London EC2A 2DB   Tel: 08457 01 02 03 Adviceline Tel: 08456 038 143 Supporter & Information Team   Tel: 020 7786 4900 Office Fax: 020 7256 6075 Office   e-mail: info@asthma.org.uk   Web: http://www.asthma.org.uk
The organisation is a National Registered Charity No. 802364. It offers funding for research to improve treatments and find a cure for the future, independent help and advice to everyone affected by asthma and campaigning for a better deal for people with asthma. It publishes 'Asthma News' a quarterly magazine for members. It has a wide range of information available, details on request. The organisation has approximately 20,000 members.
Group details last confirmed August 2007.

ATAXIA-TELANGIECTASIA

Background

Ataxia-Telangiectasia (A-T) is a very rare familial neurodegenerative disorder. Signs of the disorder usually become noticeable between one to four years although occasionally not until the teenage years. Affected children have problems of balance control (ataxia) and so unsteady walking is observed, as well as prominent blood vessels most commonly seen on the conjunctiva of the eyes in

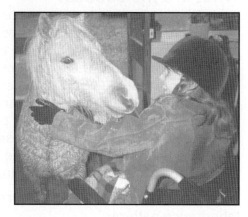

early childhood (telangiectasia). Speech problems occur but, after a period of deterioration, a stable state is reached and speech is always understandable. There is often a gradual loss of power as well as other co-ordination problems over the decades. Intelligence is normal. There is a lot of variation in how severely individuals are affected which can now be explained to some extent by recent developments in genetic understanding.

Other features of the disorder include: frequent infections due to a defect in the immune system; short stature and an increased risk of cancers.

How is it diagnosed?

The diagnostic finding is an increased sensitivity to high doses of ionising radiation. Normal x-rays pose little risk to affected individuals as radiation doses are very low. However, unnecessary x-rays should be avoided where possible.

How is it treated?

Due to the demonstration of increased levels of oxidative stress in AT cells, clinical trials are being planned with anti-oxidant therapy. Stem cell research may also lead to possible therapeutic strategies in the future.

Inheritnace patterns and prenatal diagnosis

Inheritance patterns

The mode of inheritance is autosomal recessive. In families with an affected child there would be a twenty-five per cent chance of recurrence in further pregnancies. Two genes have been found which can cause Ataxia Telangiectasia. The gene causing AT has been found. It is called ATM and is located on chromosome 11q23. Many different mutations in the ATM gene have been found. Some completely inactivate the gene causing a 'classical' picture and others may allow some function of the ATM protein and lead to a milder clinical picture. Many different mutations in the ATM gene have been found. A second gene, hMre11,has also been identified. People with hMre11 have symptoms which are less marked than A-T with a later onset of unsteadiness and jerky movements. Chromosome instability studies were also found to be less marked than in the usual cases of A-T. Both ATM and hMre11 were mapped to chromosome 11. Routine analysis for faults in this gene is not currently available on the NHS. Both genes are involved in the signalling pathway used by cells to indicate that DNA has been damaged and should be repaired.

Prenatal diagnosis

This is usually possible, but requires discussion before conception. The regional genetic centres will be able to co-ordinate this.

Medical text written November 1991 by Contact a Family. Approved November 1991 by Professor M Patton, Professor of Medical Genetics, St Georges Hospital Medical School, London, UK and Dr J E Wraith, Consultant Paediatrician, Royal Manchester Children's Hospital, Manchester, UK. **Last updated July 2005 by Dr S Ritchie, Associate Specialist in Clinical Genetics, City Hospital, Nottingham, UK.**

Further online resources

Medical texts in *The Contact a Family Directory* are designed to give a short, clear description of specific conditions and rare disorders. More extensive information on this condition can be found on a range of reliable, validated websites. Further information on these resources can be found in our **Medical Information on the Internet** article on page 21.

Support

A-T Society

IACR-Rothamsted, Harpenden AL5 2JQ   Tel: 01582 760733
Tel: 0131 667 4065 A-T Counsellor   Fax: 01582 760162   e-mail: atcharity@aol.com
Web: http://www.atsociety.org.uk
The Society is a National Registered Charity No. 1105528, established in 1989. It offers support for the newly diagnosed family, contact with other families, annual family days and youth meetings, specialist clinics at Nottingham City Hospital and Papworth Hospital and support grants for families. It publishes a twice yearly newsletter and has a wide range of information available, details on request. The society represents over 100 families and funds research into A-T.
Group details last updated June 2007.

As Ataxia-Telangiectasia is a metabolic disease, support and advice are also available from Climb (see entry, Metabolic diseases).

ATTENTION DEFICIT HYPERACTIVITY DISORDER

Attention Deficit Hyperactivity Disorder: ADHD; ADD; DAMP; Hyperkinetic Disorder

Background

Attention-Deficit/Hyperactivity Disorder (ADHD) is a common condition affecting several per cent of school age children. It is more common in boys but girls may currently be underdiagnosed. There are three subtypes: ADHD mainly inattentive, ADHD mainly hyperactive-impulsive, and ADHD combined. The first of these is sometimes referred to as ADD (Attention Deficit Disorder). When ADHD is combined with motor-perceptual problems (also referred to as Developmental Coordination Disorder or dyspraxia) some clinicians refer to DAMP (Deficits in Attention, Motor control and Perception). When problems are very severe and all the diagnostic features listed below are present the criteria for Hyperkinetic Disorder may be met. Thus, ADD, DAMP, and Hyperkinetic Disorder are all subtypes of ADHD.

Attention Deficit Hyperactivity Disorder is an impairment of either activity or attention control or both. The problem presents as a child who is always on the go, does not settle to anything, has poor concentration, poor ability to organise activities or to engage in tedious activities or tasks requiring sustained mental effort, or who cannot stay still and cannot wait for others.

What are the symptoms?

The problems are disabling, start at an early age and they are present in more than one situation, for example home and school. Sometimes affected children show underachievement at school, poor sleep, social interaction difficulties, autistic-type features (see entry, Autism Spectrum Disorders), speech-language difficulties (see entry, Speech and Language Impairement), discipline problems, temper tantrums, unpopularity, and accident-proneness. However, all these can have other causes too. IQ can be high, normal, low normal or in the learning disability range.

What are the causes?

There are several causes. Twin studies indicate a very strong genetic contribution. Environmental causes include brain damage, intolerance to certain foods, hearing impairment, toxic (including maternal alcoholism and heavy smoking) and infective agents during pregnancy. All of these may interact with psychological stress and social problems to create further behavioural and emotional difficulties. There are some specific treatments, including stimulant medication, behaviour therapy and dietary exclusion approaches in selected cases.

How is it diagnosed?

The diagnostic features are:

- **Inattentiveness** - very short attention span, over-frequent changes of activity, extreme distractibility;
- **Overactivity** - excessive movements, especially in situations expecting calm such as classroom or mealtimes;
- **Impulsiveness** - affected person will not wait their turn, acts without thinking, thoughtless rule-breaking.

Inheritance patterns and prenatal diagnosis

Inheritance patterns

There is a strong inherited contribution. DNA studies have indicated variants of some (including dopamine) genes to be more common in groups of children with ADHD. The significance in individual cases is not yet known.

Prenatal diagnosis

None

Medical text written March 2003 by Professor C Gillberg, Professor of Child and Adolescent Psychiatry, University of Göteborg, Sweden.

There are many groups and organisations providing support and information about Attention Deficit Hyperactivity Disorder including:

Support

Hyperactive Children's Support Group
71 Whyke Lane, Chichester PO19 7PD   Tel: 01243 539966
e-mail: hyperactive@hacsg.org.uk   Web: http://www.hacsg.org.uk
Provides support, information and a range of literature including 'The Journal' newsletter three times a year. Also provides training and awareness raising events.
Group details last confirmed February 2008.

CHADD (Children and Adults with Attention Deficit/Hyperactivity Disorder)
Web: http://www.chadd.org
A US national ADHD support group which provides comprehensive information, advice and support services to children, parents, adults and professional workers.

ADDA (National Attention Deficit Disorder Association)
Web: http://www.add.org
A well established US adult ADHD national association which provides comprehensive information.

A

YoungMinds

48-50 St John Street, London EC1M 4DG   Tel: 0800 018 2138 Parents' Information
Service (Mon & Fri, 10am-1pm; Tue-Thur, 1-4pm; Weds, 6-8pm) Tel: 020 7336 8445 Office
e-mail: enquiries@youngminds.org.uk   Web: http://www.youngminds.org.uk
YoungMinds is a National Registered Charity No. 1016968, established in 1989 which
is committed to improving the mental health of all children. Services include the Parents'
Information Service, a free confidential telephone helpline offering information and advice
to any adult with concerns about the mental health of a child or young person. YoungMinds
also offers consultancy, seminars and training, leaflets and booklets for young people,
parents and professionals and publishes 'YoungMinds Magazine' every two months.
Group details last updated October 2007.

adders.org

Web: http://www.adders.org
A comprehensive website covering a wide range of information on ADHD. Adders objective
is to promote awareness of ADHD and to provide information and practical help to adults
and children with the condition and their families.
Group details last confirmed August 2007.

ADDISS

2nd Floor, Premier House, 112 Station Road, Edgware HA8 7BJ   Tel: 020 8952 2800
Fax: 020 8952 2909   e-mail: info@addiss.co.uk   Web: http://www.addiss.co.uk
ADDISS is the Attention Deficit Disorder Information and Support Service for both parents
and professionals. It provides inset training for local education authorities and schools. A
large number of books and videos are for sale by mail order. ADDISS works closely with a
large number of local support groups and can refer parents to these groups.
Group details last updated January 2007.

The Mental Health Foundation

9th Floor, Sea Containers House, 20 Upper Ground, London SE1 9QB
Tel: 020 7803 1100   Fax: 020 7803 1111   e-mail: mhf@mhf.org.uk
Web: http://www.mhf.org.uk
Works to meet the needs of people with mental health problems and aims to improve
people's lives, reduce stigma surrounding mental health issues and to promote
understanding. The Foundation undertakes research and provides information (including
ADHD) for the public and social care professional workers.
Group details last confirmed February 2007.

Parentline plus

520 Highgate Studios, 53-79 Highgate Road, London NW5 1TL
Tel: 0808 800 2222 Helpline   Text: 0800 783 6783
e-mail: parentsupport@parentlineplus.org.uk   Web: http://www.parentlineplus.org.uk
Provides emotional support for parents and families concerning ADHD. Also refers to
organisations for appropriate help, advice and information about ADHD.
Group details last confirmed April 2007.

There are a number of very supportive local self help groups around the country. If you
want to contact one of these and have been unable to do so through the organisations in
this Directory please get in touch with Contact a Family.

AUDITORY PROCESSING DISORDER

Background

Auditory Processing Disorder (APD) was first noted in the USA in the mid-1960's. In 2004 it was defined by the British Society of Audiology steering group on APD as a hearing disorder resulting from problems with processing of sounds by the brain, rather than the ear and characterised by poor recognition, discrimination, separation, grouping, localisation or ordering of non-speech sounds. While people with APD may also have a problem with speech perception, those with speech perception difficulties do not necessarily have APD. Further research is being actively supported by the UK government and by hearing research charities.

Hearing starts with a complex set of actions within the outer, middle and inner ear. These actions send the sounds to the brain that interprets them so the individual can understand. This set of actions can be defined as 'listening' and carries the medical term 'auditory processing.'

If an individual's auditory processing is functioning well but there is no understanding of the sounds that are heard, the individual may have an APD. In some children with APD there may be tiny differences in the way that neurons (brain cells) are joined together, or send messages to each other. This may make it hard for sounds to be passed on to the areas of the brain that aid the understanding of language. It is possible such brain cell differences may cause APD.

What are the symptoms?

Symptoms of APD which cause difficulties to patients include:
- Understanding when listening;
- Expressing themselves clearly using speech;
- Reading;
- Understanding spoken messages and/or remembering instructions;
- Staying focussed;
- Hearing and listening in noisy places.

Many children with APD may have other language-learning difficulties such as:
- Dyslexia (see entry) – difficulties with reading and/or spelling;
- Attention Deficit Disorder (ADD) and/or Attention Deficit Hyperactivity Disorder (ADHD) (see entry) – difficulties in concentration or attention;
- Speech and Language Impairment (see entry) – difficulties in the development and/or understanding of speech and language.

How is it diagnosed?

It is thought that up to ten per cent of children may have some level of APD. There are a number of tests to diagnose APD. These will include hearing, listening and comprehension tests.

How is it treated?

There is no cure for APD but there are a number of ways to help an affected child:

- Clinic/hearing services:
  - hearing training programmes and strategies (exercises to help the child understand better when listening);
  - parental support programmes.
- In the classroom:
  - sitting near the teacher's desk to aid lip reading and other cues;
  - asking the teacher to check that the child is looking and listening when instructions are given out, especially if the teacher walks around when talking;
  - the provision by the teacher of written information to older children which might be used to consolidate verbal instructions;
  - the reduction of classroom noise (more carpeting and soft furnishings, rubber feet on table and chair legs etc);
  - the provision of listening devices to make speech clearer in noisy situations – for example, a soundfield system in the main classroom or personal fm systems.
- In the home:
  - encouraging the child to do any listening and learning exercises as prescribed;
  - checking if the child is looking and listening when necessary;
  - the reduction of background noise in the home (such as TV or radio) when trying to communicate.

Inheritance patterns and prenatal diagnosis

Inheritance patterns

There is a possibility that APD may run in families but this is as yet unknown.

Prenatal diagnosis

None.

Medical text written September 2004 by the Institute for Hearing Research. Approved September 2004 by Professor D Moore, Director, MRC Institute of Hearing Research, Nottingham, UK.

Support

APDUK

c/o Dacorum CVS, 48 High Street, Hemel Hempstead HP1 3AF
Tel: 01442 214555 (6-10pm)   e-mail: dolfrog@apduk.org
Web: http://www.apduk.org

APDUK is a largely internet-based network, established in 2002. It offers support, information and internet forums for those affected by APD, their families and interested professionals. The group aims to raise awareness and understanding of the condition, particularly among professionals, and to work to improve the diagnostic tests.
Group details last confirmed March 2007.

Contact a Family publishes research including 'Flexible Enough? Employment patterns in families with disabled children'. Contact a Family surveyed 900 parents of disabled children on the effectiveness of flexible employment rights. The findings show that there is clearly a good deal more work to be done to raise awareness of a parent's right to request flexible working arrangements.

AUTISM SPECTRUM DISORDERS
including ASPERGER SYNDROME

Background

The term Autism Spectrum Disorders (ASD) is used to describe the group of pervasive developmental disorders characterised by abnormalities in social interaction and communication and by a restricted range of repetitive behaviour and interests. These abnormalities are a pervasive feature of the disorder i.e. usually present across many settings. It is now understood that these core difficulties can manifest in individuals with varying degrees of behavioural severity, language and intellectual abilities. The presentation can be extremely variable and therefore this group of disorders is best considered as a 'spectrum'.

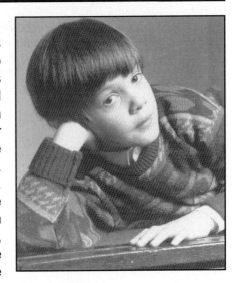

The current prevalence of ASD is around 6 to 10 in 1,000 in younger children. Boys are more commonly affected than girls. The number of children with a diagnosis of Autism/ASD appears to be increasing. This is in part explained by increased public and professional awareness and the recognition of the broader spectrum of disorder thus encompassing more children with a range of abilities.

What are the symptoms?

Affected children have difficulties in making sense of the social world and the subtleties of verbal and non verbal communication. They have difficulty understanding the feelings and emotions of other people and present with a restricted range of interests often with stereotyped repetitive behaviours. They may also experience odd responses to sensory stimuli. Approximately ten per cent of individuals with Autism may demonstrate an area of relative strengths/ability.

The spectrum includes individuals who are severely impaired with no useful speech, to those considered 'high functioning'. This latter term can be misleading in that an individual of 'high' intellectual ability may be significantly impaired in terms of social skills. Disorders that currently exist within the international classification systems such as Asperger syndrome, Infantile

Autism and Childhood Disintegrative disorder are considered to lie on the 'spectrum'.

What are the causes?

The exact cause of Autism has not yet been fully established. Research continues in a number of areas. Between six to ten per cent of children with Autism may also have a currently recognised medical condition such as Tuberous Sclerosis or Fragile X syndrome (see entries).

ASD can often be associated with other neurodevelopmental disorders (such as Learning Disability and Attention Deficit Hyperactivity disorder, see entries) and other co-morbid behavioural and mental health problems including depression, social anxiety and Obsessive Compulsive disorder (see entry). Several large scale studies have not found any evidence of the link between ASD and the MMR vaccine.

In recent years several research groups have joined to form the Autism Genome Project, one of the largest international research collaborations, to carry out further work with the aim of identifying the relatively small numbers of interacting genes that are likely to be involved.

How is it diagnosed?

There is no biological 'test' for Autism. Diagnosis is dependent on careful developmental history taking, specifically enquiring about core behaviours, and by observations and direct assessment in a variety of different settings. Diagnosis should involve a number of different professionals who have specific skills in assessing children with suspected ASD and may involve home based observations, child health/paediatric, speech and language, cognitive and occupational therapy assessment. The National Autism Plan for Children http://www.cafamily.org.uk/NAPFront.PDF recommends that each area have a locally agreed pathway for assessment and diagnosis. Following diagnosis, families will benefit from access to information about ASD specific support groups and local multi-agency services.

How is it treated?

There is no "cure" for Autism. Research findings indicate that early access to targeted behavioural and educational interventions are likely to be beneficial. However, there is no evidence for one approach being superior to another. For young children the emphasis is on ASD-specific social communication, behavioural and play (including parent-involved) interventions, and educational approaches. Early diagnosis, access to appropriate interventions, an individualised educational plan with structured support from staff with ASD expertise, alongside a family care plan is likely to help a child reach their potential. The search for dietary and pharmacological agents continues. To date there has been no large scale study to evaluate the role of gluten-

and/or casein-free diets.

ASD is a complex, life-long neurodevelopmental disability. Every individual has a unique pattern of skills and difficulties. Features may change over time although individuals are likely to continue to have difficulties throughout life. Verbal IQ has been shown to be one of the predictors of future functioning and independence. The challenge for professionals is to provide multi-agency, life-long, integrated care adapted to the changing needs of the individual and their family over time.

Inheritance patterns and prenatal diagnosis
Inheritance patterns
Genetic factors have been shown to be important with evidence from twin and family studies of an increased risk for ASD in other family members. There is a two to eight per cent risk of a subsequent sibling being affected.
Prenatal diagnosis
None

Medical text written August 2006 by Dr C Dover, Specialist Registrar in Learning Disability Psychiatry, Dr C Grayson, Consultant Paediatrician and Professor A Le Couteur, Professor of Child and Adolescent Psychiatry, Northumberland, Tyne and Wear NHS Trust, Newcastle upon Tyne, UK.

Further online resources
Medical texts in *The Contact a Family Directory* are designed to give a short, clear description of specific conditions and rare disorders. More extensive information on this condition can be found on a range of reliable, validated websites. Further information on these resources can be found in our **Medical Information on the Internet** article on page 21.

Support
The National Autistic Society
393 City Road, London EC1V 1NG   Tel: 0845 070 4004 Helpline (Mon - Fri, 10am - 4pm)
Tel: 0845 070 4003 minicom   Fax: 020 7833 9666   e-mail: autismhelpline@nas.org.uk
Web: http://www.nas.org.uk   Web: http://www.info.autism.org.uk (searchable database)
The Society is a National Registered Charity No. 269425, established in 1962. It offers information, advice and support, training courses and conferences and the promotion of research. It publishes a journal, 'Communication', four times a year and has a wide range of information available, details on request. Please send SAE. The Society represents over 17,000 members.
Group details last updated April 2007.

Scottish Society for Autism
Hilton House, Alloa Business Park, Whins Road, Alloa FK10 3SA
Tel: 0845 300 9281 Helpline   Tel: 01259 720044   Fax: 01259 720051
e-mail: autism@autism-in-scotland.org.uk   Web: http://www.autism-in-scotland.org.uk
The Society is a Scottish Charity No. SC 009068, established in 1968. It offers support, information, advice and training for parents, carers and professionals. The Society promotes and provides autism-specific education, care, support and opportunities for people of all ages with autism/Asperger syndrome in Scotland. It has a wide range of information available, with details on request and over 5,000 members, friends and supporters.
Group details last confirmed August 2007.

The International Autistic Research Organisation

49 Orchard Avenue, Croydon CRO 7NE   Tel: 020 8777 0095 (24 hours/answerphone)
Fax: 020 8776 2362   e-mail: iaro@autismresearch.wanadoo.co.uk
Web: http://www.iaro.org.uk
The Organisation is a National Registered Charity No. 802391. It provides information on autism to parents, carers or teachers. It publishes a newsletter approximately 4 times a year. The Organisation has over 400 members including those overseas.
Group details last confirmed August 2007.

Autism NI (PAPA)

PAPA Training and Resource Centre, Donard House, Knockbracken Healthcare Park,
Saintfield Road, Belfast BT8 8BH   Tel: 028 90 401729   Fax: 028 90 403467
e-mail: info@autismni.org   Web: http://www.autismni.org
Autism NI is a National Registered Charity No. XR22944, established in 1990. It has a commitment to parent support which is maintained through the activity of the network of 14 branches which also assist in active political lobbing for ASD policy and service development. Its training prospectus, newsletter and bookstore are available online as well as information on its work on early intervention and adult service support.
Group details last confirmed May 2007.

"This is the first time I've said this but I've been thinking it for years, how can you ask for help when you've got to keep your family together and be brave? And anyway who would listen, the men aren't seen to be needing support" Parent attending a Contact a Family North East event for fathers.

BANNAYAN-RILEY-RUVALCABA SYNDROME

Bannayan-Riley-Ruvalcaba syndrome: BRRS; Bannayan-Zonana syndrome; Macrocephaly, Multiple Lipomas and Haemangioma; Ruvalcaba-Myhre-Smith syndrome; Riley-Smith syndrome

Background

Bannayan-Riley-Ruvalcaba syndrome (BRRS) is a rare, congenital (present at birth) disorder. It is one of a group of syndromes called PTEN Hamartoma Tumour syndromes that also include Cowden disease and Proteus syndrome (see entry), which are associated with mutations (changes) in the PTEN gene. A number of doctors described individuals with varying symptoms that include excessive growth before and after birth, macrocephaly (large head), normal intellect or learning difficulties and hamartomas (benign tumour-like growths). This has lead to a number of differing names being given to the syndrome. It is most often called Bannayan-Riley-Ruvalcaba syndrome. The syndrome affects both males and females. It is thought that incidence of BRRS is under diagnosed due to the variable and subtle external signs of the syndrome and it is not possible to give a true picture of the likely numbers of individuals with the syndrome.

The hamartomas that are a hallmark of the syndrome are benign. Individuals with Cowden disease, which is also caused by mutations in the PTEN gene are more prone to develop other tumours and are at risk of malignancy. The risks of malignancy for individuals affected with BRRS are less clear. It has been suggested that the same regular surveillance used to screen for tumours in people with Cowden disease should be used in BRRS.

What are the symptoms?

Other features of the syndrome that have been noted include:
- Macrocephaly;
- Hypotonia (diminished muscle tone);
- Joint hypermobility;
- Delayed motor development affecting the ability to sit, stand or walk;
- Delayed speech development;
- Learning disability.

There may also be unusual skin markings including haemangiomas (tumour-like growth of small blood vessels), lipomas (benign tumour of fatty tissues), and freckling.

As in many syndromes an affected individual may not manifest all these additional features. Severity of any feature of a syndrome can vary widely.

How is it diagnosed?

Diagnosis of BRRS is made on identification of the hallmark features of the syndrome. It has been found that sixty per cent of individuals diagnosed with BRRS have a detectable mutation of the PTEN gene.

How is it treated?

BRRS cannot be cured. Treatment is symptomatic aimed at improving quality of life. Physical and speech therapy can be beneficial. Clear information about BRRS will help teachers to support children at school. From early adult life special care should be taken to monitor for the development of tumours.

Inheritance patterns and prenatal diagnosis

Inheritance patterns

Autosomal dominant.

Prenatal diagnosis

In families where the PTEN gene mutations have been diagnosed this is possible by amniocentesis at sixteen to eighteen weeks of pregnancy or by Chronic Villus Sampling (CVS) at about ten to twelve weeks.

Medical text written October 2005 by Contact a Family. **Approved October 2005 by Dr K Lachlan, Specialist Registrar in Clinical Genetics, Essex Regional Genetics Service, Southampton, UK.**

Support

Bannayan-Zonana Support Network

c/o Contact a Family, 209-211 City Road, London EC1V 1JN

Tel: 0808 808 3555 Freephone Helpline   Tel: 0808 808 3556 Text

Tel: 020 7608 8700 Admin   Fax: 020 7608 8701

The Network is a small parent support group. It provides support by letter, e-mail and telephone and has information available, details on request. The Network has access to a medical adviser and is in touch with approximately 10 families. Researchers are thought to have been in touch with 20 families in the UK.

BARDET-BIEDL SYNDROME

Bardet-Biedl syndrome: BBS; Laurence-Moon-Bardet-Biedl syndrome

Background

The syndrome is a rare inherited condition which is variable in the way in which it presents. Characteristics are: rod/cone dystrophy (atypical retinitis pigmentosa - a progressive eye condition which can lead to blindness (see entry Vision Disorders in Childhood)); obesity (usually with an early onset and resistant to treatment); polydactyly (extra fingers and/or toes); hypogenitalism (underdeveloped genitals); mild to severe learning difficulties; and kidney malformations and renal dysfunction.

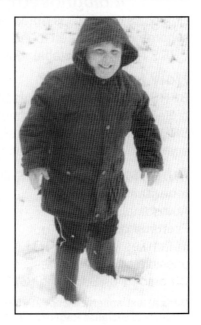

In the Middle-East and island communities such as Newfoundland, the condition is relatively common, occurring at rates of 1 in 13,500 of the population. In Europe and the UK the prevalence is much less common owing to lower consanguinity. The figure is probably between 1 in 70,000 to 100,000 of the population. Although BBS is not common it is certainly under diagnosed. As awareness of the condition increases, the number of people identified is growing every year.

How is it diagnosed?

Usually four out of six features seen in the condition are required to make the diagnosis. In addition, there are other important characteristics which need to be considered: developmental delay; speech difficulties; olfactory deficits (diminished ability to smell); diabetes mellitus; diabetes insipidus; hepatic fibrosis; and hormonal deficiencies (e.g. thyroid, testosterone).

Inheritance patterns and prenatal diagnosis

Inheritance patterns

For the majority of cases, inheritance is autosomal recessive. Although in a few cases, more than two mutations in two BBS genes may be required to manifest the condition ('triallelic inheritance'). Nine different gene defects have been shown to be responsible for the majority of cases and more are postulated. They are located on different chromosomes: BBS1 on chromosome 11 (long arm); BBS2 on chromosome 16 (long arm); BBS3 on chromosome 3 (short arm); BBS 4 on chromosome 15 (long arm); BBS5 on chromosome 2 (long arm); and most recently, BBS6 on chromosome 20 (short arm); BBS7 on chromosome 4 (long arm); BBS8 on chromosome 14 (long arm); and BBS9 on chromosome 7 (short arm). BBS1 accounts for approximately fifty per cent of cases seen in Britain and BBS2 is the second most prevalent gene.

Despite the identification of nine genes, these still only account for around forty-five per cent of all cases to date indicating that there are several more genes left to find. Nonetheless, their discovery has, in the last few years, led to an explosion in our understanding of the underlying cellular problem. It seems the problems lies in function of the cilium, a long, thin appendage that sticks out of the surface of most cells in our body and serves to sense the surrounding environment. Research is moving quickly to find out exactly what has gone wrong in the cells and the organs which they make up. This will ultimately help in the design of new diagnostic tests and perhaps therapeutic strategies. Although a sizeable proportion of families affected by BBS can now be offered gene testing in theory, simple genetic assays still need to be developed as the genes are large and looking for mutations takes time and is costly. Diagnosis is still based on clinical manifestations but molecular analysis may help confirm this in doubtful cases.

Prenatal diagnosis

A number of features can be determined on high definition ultrasound scanning of the fetus. In particular, the number of fingers and toes may be counted and specific kidney malformations seen. This, however, is not a test of exclusion of the condition. If two gene mutations can be identified in a BBS family then a molecular genetic test can be offered prenatally.

Medical text written January 1996 by Dr P L. Beales. **Last updated October 2005 by Professor P L. Beales, Professor of Medical and Molecular Genetics, Wellcome Trust Senior Research Fellow in Clinical Science, Consultant in Clinical Genetics, Molecular Medicine Unit, Institute of Child Health, London, UK.**

Further online resources

Medical texts in *The Contact a Family Directory* are designed to give a short, clear description of specific conditions and rare disorders. More extensive information on this condition can be found on a range of reliable, validated websites. Further information on these resources can be found in our **Medical Information on the Internet** article on page 21.

Support

LMBB Society

10 High Cross Road, Rogerstone, Newport NP10 9AD   Tel: 01633 718415
e-mail: chris.humphreys4@ntlworld.com   Web: http://www.lmbbs.org.uk
The Society is a National Registered Charity No. 1027384, established in 1987. It offers: support and advice to families by telephone, letter and e-mail; and contact with other families. Activities include raising awareness of the condition, an annual family conference and fundraising. It publishes a twice yearly newsletter in print and on audio cassette. It has information available, details on request. The Society represents over 200 families.
Group details last confirmed January 2007.

BARTH SYNDROME

Background

Barth syndrome is a very rare genetic disorder, which only affects males. The most serious problems in Barth syndrome are heart muscle weakness (see entry, Cardiomyopathy) and increased susceptibility to bacterial infections. This susceptibility is caused by a reduction in the number of certain white blood cells, called neutrophils. Neutrophil numbers often vary with time in this condition and patients are said to have 'cyclical neutropenia.' Other features include short stature and muscle weakness, which can lead to fatigue or delayed motor development in early childhood. Analysis of urine usually shows increased quantities of certain organic acids (3-methylglutaconic and, sometimes, 2-ethylhydracrylic).

What are the symptoms?

The features of Barth syndrome vary between different families and even within the same family, but the majority of patients develop cardiomyopathy within the first year. Typical early features are laboured breathing and poor feeding due to breathlessness ('heart failure'). Often the heart failure can be controlled by drug treatment but, in a few patients, heart transplantation may need to be considered. A few patients die suddenly, before they are diagnosed, perhaps due to a disturbance of the heart's rhythm. Other patients may die because of overwhelming infections.

What are the causes?

Barth syndrome is caused by mutations in a gene called G4.5. This gene is located on the X chromosome (Xq28). Ultimately, the genetic abnormality impairs the ability of cells to produce energy. At the cellular level, the problem is mediated by abnormalities in a protein called a tafazzin and by decreased production of a fat called cardiolipin.

How is it treated?

There is no specific treatment for Barth syndrome but many patients have a good outcome, with treatment for heart failure and appropriate use of antibiotics. The cardiomyopathy and susceptibility to infections both tend to improve as patients grow older.

Inheritance patterns and prenatal diagnosis

Inheritance patterns

Barth syndrome is inherited as an X-linked recessive trait. Because males only have one X chromosome, they only have one copy of the G4.5 gene and they run into problems if this is faulty. In contrast, females have two X chromosomes: if they have a faulty copy of G4.5, they are asymptomatic because they still have one normal copy. A carrier female can, however, pass the faulty gene on to her children: her sons have a fifty per cent chance of being affected and her daughters have a fifty per cent chance of being carriers. Detailed genetic counselling is advisable when Barth syndrome is identified in a family.

Prenatal diagnosis

Prenatal diagnosis is possible at an early stage in pregnancy in families where the mutation is known. Suitable specimens can be obtained by amniocentesis or chorionic villus sampling.

Medical text written October 2003 by Contact a Family. Approved October 2003 by Dr A Morris, Consultant Paediatrician with Special Interest In Metabolic Disease, Willink Biochemical Genetics Unit, Royal Manchester Children's Hospital, Manchester, UK.

Support

Barth Syndrome Trust

c/o Contact a Family, 209-211 City Road, London EC1V 1JN   Tel: 01794 518785
Fax: 0870 706 6360   e-mail: info@barthsyndrome.org.uk
Web: http://www.barthsyndrome.org.uk
The Trust is a National Registered Charity No. 1100835, established in 2003 to provide information and support families. It aims to raise awareness about Barth syndrome amongst health professionals and to raise funds to support research. Health professionals are welcome to contact the Trust for information. The Trust maintains strong links with world-class experts involved in treating this disorder. It also works closely with affiliated support groups around the world.
Group details last confirmed June 2007.

BATTEN DISEASE

Batten disease: Neuronal Ceroid Lipofuscinosis Type 1 (infantile); Type 2 (late infantile); Type 3 (Juvenile); NCL; Santavuori disease; Santavuori-Haltia disease (Infantile); Jansky-Bielschowsky disease (Late Infantile Type); Variant late infantile type; Vogt-Spielmeyer disease (Juvenile type); Kufs disease (Adult type)

Background

The group of diseases known as Batten disease (after the British paediatrician who first described it in 1903) or the neuronal ceroid lipofuscinoses (NCLs) are rare, genetic, progressive neurodegenerative, metabolic diseases that occur in children and adults worldwide.

What are the symptoms?

Symptoms include loss of vision, epilepsy and loss of abilities including walking, eating and talking. A number of different forms of Batten disease, including less common variants and a congenital form are known. These share similar symptoms but progress at different rates and are all genetically different. It is important to know which gene mutation causes the disease in each individual. Nine genes are known to cause Batten disease to date. The types of Batten disease are often classified by age of onset:

Infantile - onset between six months and two years, rapidly progressing with seizures, dementia, blindness and a severe loss of neurones. Death normally occurs in mid childhood.

Late Infantile - onset between two and four years, leading to seizures, blindness, loss of muscle co-ordination, mental deterioration and dementia. Death normally occurs between the ages of eight and sixteen.

Juvenile - onset between five and nine years, characterised by visual loss initially, and later seizures, loss of motor abilities and dementia. Death may occur any time from the late teens to the mid thirties.

Adult - onset normally before the age of forty, symptoms are milder than the other forms of the disease. Age of death is variable but life expectancy is shortened.

How is it treated?

Our understanding of Batten disease is improving all the time and work to develop new therapies is progressing well. However, at present there is no cure or treatment that makes a significant impact on the progressive decline in bodily functions and inevitable early death.

Inheritance patterns and prenatal diagnosis

Inheritance patterns

Autosomal recessive for all the childhood variants of NCL (neuronal ceroid lipofuscinoses), however it is thought that the very rare adult form (Kuf's disease) can be inherited in an autosomal dominant way.

Prenatal diagnosis

Prenatal diagnosis has been performed in this country within the National Health Service for infantile (gene designation CLN1), juvenile (CLN3), classical late infantile (CLN2), and variant late infantile (CLN6) NCL. It can only be done in families where there is already one affected child and the histology and genetics are known for that child. Prenatal diagnosis would be done using a chorionic villus sample which would then be split and sent for ultrastructural analysis, DNA mutation testing (infantile, late infantile and juvenile) and enzyme analysis (late infantile).

Medical text written June 1999 by Dr C Martland, Batten Disease Family Association. Approved June 1999 by Dr R Williams. **Last updated May 2004 by Dr Ruth Williams, Consultant Paediatric Neurologist, Guy's Hospital, London, UK.**

Further online resources

Medical texts in *The Contact a Family Directory* are designed to give a short, clear description of specific conditions and rare disorders. More extensive information on this condition can be found on a range of reliable, validated websites. Further information on these resources can be found in our **Medical Information on the Internet** article on page 21.

Support

Batten Disease Family Association

c/o Heather House, Heather Drive, Tadley RG26 4QR   Tel: 0115 965 4815
Web: http://www.bdfa-uk.org.uk e-mail: BDFA.info@binternet.com
THE BDFA (National Registered Charity No. 1084908) was formed in 1998 and its main aim is that no family will go through the devastating journey of Batten Disease alone. They are a supportive, informative, national networking organisation for the families, carers and professionals giving care to children and adults with Batten Disease and for promoting awareness of, and research into, the disease.
Group details last updated October 2007.

BECKER MUSCULAR DYSTROPHY

Becker Muscular Dystrophy: Becker MD

Background

Becker Muscular Dystrophy (BMD), one of the muscular dystrophies, is a rare genetic condition described in 1955 by Becker and Kiener. Like Duchenne Muscular Dystrophy (see entry), it is a muscular dystrophy associated with mutations (changes) in the dystrophin gene. An individual needs a range of proteins surrounding muscle fibres to ensure their efficient working. In BMD, a reduction of dystrophin leads to the effects seen in the condition. In Duchenne Muscular Dystrophy (DMD), there is a virtually complete absence of dystrophin while individuals with BMD have some detectable dystrophin. As a result, BMD is seen as a milder form of DMD.

As a sex-linked disorder, BMD largely affects males and its onset generally comes to medical attention in adolescence or early in adulthood but may present in childhood or middle age. It is thought to affect 1 in 30,000 males. Life expectancy may be reduced but many affected people live into their seventies or eighties.

What are the symptoms?

Features of BMD include:

- Progressive muscle weakness leading to difficulties in physical abilities such as walking or running and, later, weakness affecting the upper arms and shoulders;
- Pseudohypertrophy (enlargement without additional strength) of muscles in the calves and elsewhere;
- Cardiomyopathy (see entry). Heart disease caused by weakening of the heart muscles;
- In the later stages, respiratory muscle weakness may lead to chest infections.

There may also be learning and/or behaviour problems in some children, including difficulty in focusing attention, verbal learning and memory. Emotional difficulties may sometimes develop, perhaps as a result of the frustration or stigmatisation of living with a disability.

What are the causes?

Like Duchenne Muscular Dystrophy, it is a muscular dystrophy associated with mutations (changes) in the dystrophin gene.

Female carriers of BMD, with a mutation in the dystrophin gene on one of their two X chromosomes, are usually healthy. However, a small number of female carriers of the defective gene are manifesting carriers (females that have some of the effects of the disorder). Occasionally, a manifesting carrier may have significant muscle weakness. Manifesting carriers may also have heart problems, which appear as shortness of breath or inability to do moderate exercise. The heart problems, if untreated, can be serious.

How is it diagnosed?

Formal tests to diagnose BMD are important in order to eliminate other disorders which have similarities to BMD. A test will be made for raised levels of Creatine Kinase that are found in the blood of individuals with BMD. Further tests will be performed to confirm that the muscle weakness arises from destruction of muscle tissue rather than nerve damage. These may include genetic tests, carried out usually on a blood sample, electrical tests carried out on a muscle and/or nerve and sometimes a muscle biopsy (examination of tissue) or blood test will also be carried out.

How is it treated?

Currently there is no known cure for BMD so treatment is symptomatic aiming to control symptoms and maintain quality of life. Physiotherapy may help to maintain muscle strength and orthopaedic devices such as braces and the use of wheelchairs can improve mobility.

Inheritance patterns and prenatal diagnosis

Inheritance patterns

BMD is an X-linked condition.

Prenatal diagnosis

This is usually possible where it is known that BMD affects the family and where the particular mutation in the dystrophin gene is known. While most families have deletions or duplications of whole exons (sequence of a gene's DNA that transcribes into the structures of protein) that are relatively simple to detect, some families have point mutations (replacement of one of the basic units of DNA with another leading to a change in proteins) for which it is not so easy to offer testing. In some of these families, prenatal testing may need to rely upon linkage analysis (gene tracking) instead of mutation-detecting tests.

Medical text written August 2004 by Contact a Family. Approved August 2004 by Professor A Clark, Professor in Medical Genetics and Hon. Consultant in Medical Genetics, Institute of Medical Genetics, University of Wales College of Medicine, Cardiff, UK.

Further online resources

Medical texts in *The Contact a Family Directory* are designed to give a short, clear description of specific conditions and rare disorders. More extensive information on this condition can be found on a range of reliable, validated websites. Further information on these resources can be found in our **Medical Information on the Internet** article on page 21.

Support

As Becker Muscular Dystrophy is a Muscular Dystrophy, information, support and advice is available from the Muscular Dystrophy Campaign (see entry, Muscular Dystrophy).

BECKWITH-WIEDEMANN SYNDROME

Beckwith-Wiedemann: Exomphalos-Macroglossia-Gigantism; Neo-natal Hypoglycaemia; Visceromegaly; Hemihypertrophy

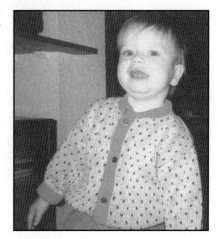

Background

Features of Beckwith-Wiedemann syndrome include:

- Macroglossia (a large tongue which may cause breathing, feeding or speech difficulties;
- Exomphalos (umbilical hernia);
- Over-growth (a high birth weight, and/or children who are bigger than their contemporaries);
- Hemihypertrophy (one side of the body grows more than the other);
- Hypoglycaemia (low blood sugar) after birth;
- Characteristic facial appearance;
- Creases or pits (indentations) of the ears.

Inheritance patterns and prenatal diagnosis

Inheritance patterns

Only a minority of cases (approximately fifteen per cent) are familial but inheritance is complex. Families should be seen by a clinical geneticist.

Prenatal diagnosis

In many cases no specific diagnosis is possible but ultrasound screening may be helpful.

Medical text written November 1993 by Dr M Elliot, Department of Clinical Genetics, Addenbrooke's Hospital, Cambridge UK. **Last updated July 2006 by Professor E R Maher, Professor of Medical Genetics, Department Medical and Molecular Genetics, University of Birmingham Medical School, Birmingham, UK.**

Support

Beckwith-Wiedemann Support Group
The Drum and Monkey, Hazelbury Bryan, Sturminster Newton DT10 2EE
Tel: 07889 211000 (mobile - day)   Tel: 01258 817573 (evenings)
e-mail: rbaker5165@aol.com   Web: http://www.bws-support.org.uk
This is a small support group started in 1988. It offers support by telephone and letter. Activities include co-operation with researchers at Birmingham University and Great Ormond Street Hospital. It publishes an occasional newsletter and has information available, details on request. The Group has nearly 200 members.
Group details last updated August 2007.

BENIGN INTRACRANIAL HYPERTENSION

Benign Intracranial Hypertension: Idiopathic Intracranial Hypertension; Pseudo Tumour Cerebri

Background

Benign Intracranial Hypertension is essentially raised intracranial pressure with papilloedema (swelling of the optic discs, which is the point where the optic nerves enter the back of the eye). It is a diagnosis arrived at when all other conditions such as brain tumours or vascular abnormalities have been excluded. In order to arrive at the diagnosis, the brain scans and measurements of the contents of the brain and spinal cord fluid should be entirely normal. The condition causes severe headaches that are not life threatening but more worryingly can cause an insidious onset of blindness that in the majority can be permanent even with treatment. It is therefore essential to detect this early and treat early to prevent the blindness occurring. It can happen in all age groups and is far more common in females but in the teenage group has an equal prevalence in males and females. The person tends to be grossly overweight. The incidence in the general population is said to be 1 to 2 in 100,000 but in overweight women in the child bearing years it is said to be 19 to 20 in 100,000. The peak incidence occurs in the third decade of life although thirty-seven per cent of cases have been reported in children. It is said to have been diagnosed in children as young as one but predominantly will be diagnosed in children in early teenage years. It is said to be a self limiting condition but there is a recurrence rate of up to forty-three per cent. The severe visual deficits involved can develop in up to 1 in 8 and these are unrelated to the previous duration of the symptoms, the degree of papilloedema, the severity of the headaches and the number of recurrences.

What are the symptoms?

The headaches are the commonest form of presentation in nearly one hundred per cent of cases. There can be dizziness, nausea, visual changes, double vision and eye pain. Papilloedema is found in all cases. Visual field defects can be detected in many. Importantly, there is normal conscious level and cognitive function despite an abnormally high intracranial pressure.

Visual loss is the most important consideration and is watched by measuring visual acuities (size of letters that can be read on a wall chart) along with visual fields. As a consequence of the visual problems being the most important, treatment is aimed at avoiding this.

What are the causes?

True Benign Intracranial Hypertension means that there is no underlying cause but the many other possible causes of similar conditions need to be excluded. There is an association with medications given for various conditions including Tetracyclin, Istotretinoin, Trimethoprim, Sametadine, Lithium, Naradoxic acid and Tamoxifen. If symptoms of Benign Intracranial Hypertension develop in the presence of these medications then they should be stopped if possible. The patient themselves can help the situation by weight loss and it is reported that simply by losing weight the symptoms can be resolved spontaneously.

How is it diagnosed?

There are said to be four diagnostic criteria: that is the CSF pressure is high; that the CSF composition is normal; that all the scanning investigations are normal; and that the signs and symptoms are solely of raised intracranial pressure (papilloedema and headache).

How is it treated?

Medical treatment involves the administration of Acetazolamide which is a drug to reduce the production of fluid inside the brain. Alternatively, Frusemide, a diuretic to reduce the amount of fluid generally, can be used. Steroids have also been tried with some success.

Surgical treatment is reserved for cases in which there has been failure of the medical approach or where there is visual loss. Serial lumbar punctures can be performed although these can be technically difficult as most patients tend to be grossly obese. Shunting can be performed and classically lumbo-peritoneal shunts (from the lumbar spine round into the abdomen) but recently these have shown to be problematic and ventriculo-peritoneal shunts are being looked at more favourably even though the ventricles (fluid cavities with the brain) are small. In cases where the vision still deteriorates despite shunting, fenestration (optic nerve sheath decompression) can be undertaken and has successfully protected the vision.

Inheritance patterns and prenatal diagnosis

Inheritance patterns

None known.

Prenatal diagnosis

Not applicable.

Medical text written February 2006 by Mr N Buxton, Consultant Paediatric Surgeon, Alder Hey Children's Hospital, Liverpool, UK.

Contact a Family Helpline 0808 808 3555

Further online resources

Medical texts in *The Contact a Family Directory* are designed to give a short, clear description of specific conditions and rare disorders. More extensive information on this condition can be found on a range of reliable, validated websites. Further information on these resources can be found in our **Medical Information on the Internet** article on page 21.

Support

Information and advice is available from ASBAH, the Association for Spina Bifida and Hydrocephalus (see entry, Spina Bifida).

"Wonderful, practical and empowering help." Parent attending a Contact a Family Wales stress management course.

BIPOLAR DISORDER

Bipolar disorder: Bipolar Affective disorder; Manic depression

Background

Bipolar Affective disorder is a mental health disorder that affects men and women equally. It usually first develops between the ages of eighteen to twenty-four. The disorder is characterised by mood swings between mania (feeling of elation or euphoria) and depression. Where the manic aspect of Bipolar Affective disorder is milder and no admission to hospital is necessary, it is called Hypomania. There are usually periods of stable mood between episodes of Bipolar Affective disorder but in the 'rapid cycling' form of the disorder there may be few or no periods of stability between episodes. Occasionally, 'mixed' episodes occur, when symptoms of mania and depression can be observed at the same time.

What are the symptoms?

Periods of mania may develop quite rapidly over a period of a few days and last for a week or longer. Aspects of mania may include a number (usually three or four) of the following:

- Unreal ideas of an individual's importance;
- Need for less sleep than normal;
- Heightened energy;
- Increased talkativeness;
- Unrealistic new activities;
- Inappropriate behaviour;
- Distracted and agitated behaviour;
- Mood change affecting personal and work life;
- Risky behaviour leading to financial difficulties;
- Possible alcohol and drug related misuse.

In Bipolar Affective disorder the depressive period lasts for at least two weeks and includes at least five of the following:

- Constant low mood for most of the day and nearly every day;
- Sleep disturbance;
- Weeping and extreme sadness;
- Tiredness and lack of energy;
- Lack of interest in most activities;
- Inability to concentrate;
- Feelings of guilt, worthlessness and suicide;
- Appetite changes;
- Problems in affection and personal relationships.

What are the causes?

The cause of Bipolar Affective disorder is not known but it is thought that genetic and environmental factors are involved. Stress factors may play a part in the further onset of the disorder in previously diagnosed individuals.

How is it diagnosed?

A diagnosis of Bipolar Affective disorder type I describes an illness with one or more manic episodes or mixed episodes. Individuals often have one or more major depressive episodes.

Bipolar Affective disorder type II is characterised by the occurrence of one or more major depressive episodes accompanied by at least one hypomanic episode.

How is it treated?

Treatment with medication is either preventative or symptomatic (treating episodes of mania and depression when they occur). Medication is usually with mood stabilising drugs such as Lithium which may also be taken in combination with other tranquilising or sedating drugs. Lithium can be taken as a long term preventative measure or a symptomatic medication.

Inheritance patterns and prenatal diagnosis

Inheritance patterns

It is thought that an individual's genetic make up might be involved as there is a higher than average change of developing the condition if other members of the family are affected.

Prenatal diagnosis

None.

Medical text written May 2005 by Contact a Family. Approved May 2005 by Professor K Ebmeier, Professor of Psychiatry, University of Edinburgh, Edinburgh, UK and Chair, Bipolar Guideline Group, Scottish Intercollegiate Guidelines Network.

Further online resources

Medical texts in *The Contact a Family Directory* are designed to give a short, clear description of specific conditions and rare disorders. More extensive information on this condition can be found on a range of reliable, validated websites. Further information on these resources can be found in our **Medical Information on the Internet** article on page 21.

Support

MDF - The Bipolar Organisation

Castle Works, 21 St. George's Road, London SE1 6ES   Tel: 08456 340 540
Fax: 020 7793 2639   e-mail: mdf@mdf.org.uk   Web: http://www.mdf.org.uk
MDF is a National Registered Charity No. 293340, established in 1983. It is a national, user-led organisation which works to enable people affected by manic depression/ bipolar disorder to take control of their lives. Services include: a network of self help groups for people with manic depression/bipolar disorder, their relatives and friends; a quarterly journal, Pendulum; publications and research papers; Self Management training programme; employment advice; travel insurance scheme; 24 hour Legal Advice Line; life assurance scheme; STEADY (the young person's self management programme); and bulletin boards and chat rooms. MDF aims to educate the public and professionals about manic depression and campaigns for greater research into methods of treatment.
Group details last confirmed February 2008.

"People who receive direct payments speak highly of them. They fundamentally alter the traditional relationship between the person using a service and the statutory services, handing back real control to the individual." Direct Payments: What are the barriers? Commission for Social Care Inspection. 2004

BLADDER EXSTROPHY

Background

The Exstrophy Epispadias complex is a spectrum of disorders ranging in severity from Epispadias through Bladder Exstrophy to Cloacal Exstrophy. All three and their variants are rare congenital abnormalities, which affect boys more frequently than girls.

What are the symptoms?

Epispadias Children with epispadias may have normal urinary control, but the majority of both boys and girls with epispadias are incontinent. In epispadias both the bladder and bladder neck (control mechanism) can be responsible. Consequently once the penis/female urethra have been corrected many children still require further surgery on the control mechanism to achieve normal control of urine.

Bladder Exstrophy The characteristic features of bladder exstrophy are: a bladder that opens directly onto the abdominal wall; abnormal genitalia; and where the bony part of the pelvis has remained open. The surgical repair is normally performed in three stages. Firstly the bladder is closed; this is undertaken soon after birth, to prevent excessive damage. To aid closure, operations on the bony pelvis may be performed. Secondly, at six to twelve months of age the epispadias repair is carried out. In boys the penis is epispadic and is corrected surgically during the second stage of the repair. In girls the clitoris is divided into two halves with the urethra running between, in addition the vagina is slightly more forward than it usually is, this is often able to be corrected at the initial repair. Finally, between three to four years of age bladder neck reconstruction is carried out, if necessary. Increasingly, the second and third stages are being combined in the first year of life. Some surgeons are now challenging this staged approach.

Cloacal Exstrophy Cloacal exstrophy is the most severe end of the epispadias-exstrophy complex , consequently the chance of normal voiding is extremely small. In addition to problems with the urine, the bowel and spine are often involved. Reconstructive surgery is usually carried out in the first few weeks of life, but these children often have long term problems gaining any urinary or faecal control. If the penis is not able to be adequately reconstructed in a boy, it may be necessary to perform bilateral gonadectomies and a feminising genitoplasty and the child be brought up as an XY female, although the child will be infertile.

How is it diagnosed?

The diagnosis is usually made at birth, or increasingly prenatally, with the exception of female epispadias that may present with urinary incontinence.

How is it treated?
Treatment in all cases is usually by surgery.

Inheritance patterns and prenatal diagnosis
Inheritance patterns
None known
Prenatal diagnosis
At present difficult but with increasing experience, prenatal diagnosis is possible.

Medical text written October 2001 by Mr D Wilcox. **Last updated January 2003 by Mr D Wilcox, Consultant Paediatric Urologist, Great Ormond Street Hospital, London, UK.**

Further online resources
Medical texts in *The Contact a Family Directory* are designed to give a short, clear description of specific conditions and rare disorders. More extensive information on this condition can be found on a range of reliable, validated websites. Further information on these resources can be found in our **Medical Information on the Internet** article on page 21.

Support
BEES Support Group
8 Burnbray Avenue, Burnage, Manchester M19 1DA   Tel: 0161 443 3174
e-mail: karen@bees-group.co.uk   Web: http://www.bees-group.co.uk
BEES (Bladder Exstrophy/Epispadias Support) is a National Registered Charity No. 1045218, established 1992. It offers support by telephone and letter, raising awareness about the condition and advice and information on incontinence. It publishes a bi-annual newsletter and has information available, details on request. Please send an SAE. Every two years BEES pays for families to attend a family weekend away at Centreparcs at various locations around the UK. This event is only offered to members. BEES is in touch with the families of 250 affected children and 100 professional workers.
Group details last updated June 2007.

BLOOM SYNDROME

Bloom syndrome: Congenital Telangiectatic Erythema

Background

Bloom syndrome was first described by Dr David Bloom in 1954. It is a rare inherited disorder with symptoms appearing in the first months of life. It affects slightly more males than females and is found in all ethnic groups but is more common in Ashkenazi Jews, with 1 in 100 being carriers of the gene responsible for development of the syndrome.

What are the symptoms?

The features found in Bloom syndrome include:

- Narrow face and redness of the skin of the face, mainly the bridge of the nose, the adjoining upper cheek areas, the lower eyelids and the lower lip. The skin problems are aggravated by sun exposure and vary in severity;
- Small size at birth and thereafter short stature. Typically, affected people only reach about 1.5m (5 feet);
- Respiratory tract and ear infections, some of which can be life-threatening;
- Normal intellect but a few cases of learning disability have been reported;
- Diabetes in about ten per cent of affected people;
- Infertility in nearly all men;
- Reduced fertility in women;
- Increased risk of malignancy. About twenty-eight per cent of individuals are thought to develop different kinds of cancer.

What are the causes?

Bloom syndrome is caused by faults in the BLM gene on Chromosome 15q26.1. When cells replicate, they have to duplicate the cell DNA code and sometimes make mistakes. These mistakes are normally checked and repaired by the body's 'house keeping' repair enzymes. The BLM gene codes for part of this repair mechanism and in Bloom syndrome it is faulty. Over time, this results in an accumulation of DNA 'faults' leading to development of the syndrome.

How is it diagnosed?

A diagnosis of Bloom syndrome can be confirmed or eliminated by a chromosome test in which the characteristic pattern of breakage or rearrangement in the chromosome is identified. Carrier status of people in the Ashkenazi Jewish population can be investigated by a blood test which can identify almost all carrier individuals.

How is it treated?

Bloom syndrome cannot be cured. However, regular monitoring can be carried out to identify any malignancies as early as possible. X-rays and other environmental exposure to compounds that cause DNA damage should be avoided if possible. Prompt treatment of infections with antibiotics is important.

Inheritance patterns and prenatal diagnosis

Inheritance patterns

Autosomal recessive.

Prenatal diagnosis

This is available to families known to be affected by the syndrome, or to be carriers, by amniocentesis or chorionic villus sampling early in the pregnancy.

Medical text written September 2006 by Contact a Family. Approved September 2006 by Professor F Cotter, Professor of Experimental Haematology, St Bartholomew's Hospital, London, UK.

Further online resources

Medical texts in *The Contact a Family Directory* are designed to give a short, clear description of specific conditions and rare disorders. More extensive information on this condition can be found on a range of reliable, validated websites. Further information on these resources can be found in our **Medical Information on the Internet** article on page 21.

Support

There is no support group for Bloom syndrome. Families can use Contact a Family's Freephone Helpline for advice, information and, where possible, links to other families. Contact a Family's web-based linking service Making Contact.org can be accessed at http://www.makingcontact.org

BRAIN INJURIES

Background

Brain injuries can be caused by injury to the head or face. Injuries to the head can cause fractures (broken bones), scalp injuries, facial injuries, eye injuries and ear injuries. Such injuries would be dealt with by the appropriate specialist doctors. Most head injuries are dealt with by doctors who have other interests than neurosurgery but who are able to deal with the common head-injured patient who does not require specialist neurosurgical service.

What are the symptoms?

Depending on the severity of the injury, there can be many possible long term problems, such as permanent memory problems, speech problems, weakness of the limbs, fits, educational developmental and emotional problems.

What are the causes?

Head injuries are caused by many things, including falls, road traffic accidents, assaults and occasionally sporting injuries. There are up to 3000 children severely brain injured each year in the UK with 40 per cent of trauma deaths being due to the head injury. Trauma causes a quarter of the deaths in children over five years of age in the UK.

How is it treated?

An injury to the brain produces changes in the patient which can be assessed to determine the severity of the injury. This enables the doctors who initially look after such a patient to determine where the patient would be best managed, either on a general ward or at a specific neurosurgical centre. Occasionally, when injuries are severe, operations are required and sometimes management on an intensive care unit is required. However, by far the majority of head injuries that most people have sustained can be managed either by simple advice from the accident and emergency department, the person being released into the care of a responsible adult, or by overnight observation in a general ward.

If long term problems result and depending on the severity, specialist care may be required in dedicated rehabilitation centres to bring about the best possible result. The effect on families can be devastating, as the injured person is often never the same as they were prior to the injury.

Inheritance patterns and prenatal diagnosis

Inheritance patterns

None.

Prenatal diagnosis

None.

Non-traumatic brain injury

Brain damage may also be caused by many non-traumatic, or non-head injury events or conditions. The more common ones include:

- meningitis and encephalitis (infections or inflammation of the brain, see entries);
- whenever there has been a lack of oxygen to the brain as occurs in:
  - near-drowning accidents;
  - cardiac arrest (heart attacks);
  - asphyxia or suffocation (e.g. inhaling smoke from fires).
- whenever there has been a lack of glucose to the brain;
- following status epilepticus (in which a tonic-clonic convulsion has lasted for more than forty-five to sixty minutes).

It is also important to understand that many of the physical, educational, emotional and behavioural problems and needs of these children and the methods of rehabilitating (which means 'putting back together again'), them are very similar to those in children who have had brain damage because of a traumatic head injury.

Medical text written October 2002 by Mr N Buxton. Last updated June 2007 by Mr N Buxton, Consultant Paediatric Neurosurgeon, Alder Hey Children's Hospital, Liverpool, UK. Non-traumatic brain injury text written October 2003 by Dr R Appleton, Consultant Paediatric Neurologist, Alder Hey Children's Hospital, Liverpool, UK.

Support

Child Brain Injury Trust
Unit 1, The Great Barn, Baynards Green, Bicester OX27 7SG
Tel: 0845 601 4939 Helpline (Mon-Wed & Fri, 10am-1pm)   e-mail: helpline@cbituk.org
Web: http://www.cbituk.org
The Trust is a National Registered Charity No. 1113326, established in 1988. It provides support, information and training on childhood acquired brain injury. It has a network of family support groups across the UK, a dedicated helpline, publications for children, training for professionals, quarterly newsletters, a small grants fund for children and events across the UK.
Group details last confirmed April 2007.

Headway
4 King Edward Court, King Edward Street, Nottingham NG1 1EW
Tel: 0808 800 2244 Helpline Tel: 0115 924 0800   Fax: 0115 958 4446
e-mail: enquiries@headway.org.uk Web: http://www.headway.org.uk
Headway, the Brain Injuries Association is a National Registered Charity No. 1025852, established in 1979. It offers information, support and services for affected individuals and their families. It also offers contact with other affected individuals and families through local groups. It publishes a quarterly newsletter and has a wide range of information available, details on request. The Association represents approximately 4,500 new cases each year as well as 100,000 individuals living with the long-term effects of head injury.
Group details last confirmed January 2007.

BRAIN TUMOURS

Background

Cells within the brain may multiply and grow into a lump or a tumour. The tumour may be localised, pressing on other parts of the brain and is described as benign. A malignant tumour may grow and invade the brain and is described as cancer (see entry). There are many different types of malignant and benign tumours in the brain, each one with different characteristics. The commonest brain tumours in children are gliomas and medulloblastomas (sometimes called PNET) although there are many others. In general these tumours do not spread to other organs outside the brain.

What are the symptoms?

Children with brain tumours can have physical problems, learning difficulties and/or speech problems as well as a deficiency of hormones produced by the pituitary gland.

How is it treated?

A large proportion of brain tumours in children are curable, but some are very aggressive and doctors are trying to improve survival by investigating new treatments in clinical trials. Children with brain tumours can have physical problems, learning difficulties and/or speech problems as well as a deficiency of hormones produced by the pituitary gland. Specialist centres have a paediatric neuro-oncology team with psychologists, physiotherapists, occupational therapists, speech therapists, play therapists, social workers, teachers and community nurses as well as doctors. They are there to help with rehabilitation and family support. Advice on growth and development is given by paediatric endocrinologists.

There are a number of specialist paediatric oncology centres each with a team of medical specialists including paediatric medical and radiation oncologists, neurosurgeons, paediatric neurologists and endocrinologists. These centres are designated as specialist centres by the Children's Cancer and Leukaemia Group (formerly the UK Children's Cancer Study Group (UKCCSG)) which oversees paediatric oncology in UK.

Inheritance patterns and prenatal diagnosis

Inheritance patterns

Brain tumours do not normally have a pattern of inheritance except where the tumour is associated with conditions such as Neurofibromatosis .

Prenatal diagnosis

None

Medical text written November 1995 by Dr M Brada, Professor of Clinical Oncology, Royal Marsden Hospital, Sutton, UK. **Last updated November 2006 by Darren Hargrave, Consultant Paediatric Oncologist, Royal Marsden Hospital, Sutton, UK.**

Support

Brain Tumour Action

25 Ann Street, Edinburgh EH4 1PL

Tel: 0131 466 3116 Befriender Line (Answerphone)

e-mail: chair@braintumouraction.org.uk   Web: http://www.braintumouraction.org.uk

Brain Tumour Action is a Scottish Charity No. SCO21490, established in 1993. It offers help and support to people living with a brain tumour and their carers. It has established a telephone befriending service and has support groups throughout the UK. Brain Tumour Action publishes a newsletter twice a year and an extensive range of information, details on request.

Group details last updated June 2007.

Brain Tumour UK

PO Box 27108, Edinburgh EH10 7WS   Tel: 0845 4500 386

e-mail: enquiries@braintumouruk.org.uk   Web: http://www.braintumouruk.org.uk

Brain Tumour UK is a National Registered Charity No. 1117538, registered in 1997 and a Company Registered in England No. 5983336. Through its website, National Helpline, local support groups and Phone Pals scheme Brain Tumour UK provides vital support and information to anyone whose life has been touched by the devastating diagnosis of a brain tumour. It also raises funds and campaigns for more research, better care and treatments. It publishes a newsletter three times a year which is sent to over 3000 contacts and hosts annual conferences for patients, families and scientists.

Group details last updated September 2007.

Samantha Dickson Brain Tumour Trust

Century House, High Street, Hartley Wintney, Hook RG27 8NY   Tel: 0845 130 9733

Fax: 0845 130 9744   e-mail: patientinfo@sdbtt.co.uk   e-mail: enquiries@sdbtt.co.uk

Web: http://www.braintumourtrust.co.uk

The Trust is a National Registered Charity No. 1060627, established in 1996. It is the largest dedicated brain tumour charity in the UK. It raises awareness and funding for brain tumour research. It also offers information and support to patients diagnosed with a brain tumour and their families. The Trust also publishes a newsletter, organises conferences. Support groups have been set up and meet regularly. Please contact the Charity for more information.

Group details last updated October 2007.

An accredited/recognised specialist centre with the correct experts is a member of the UK Children's Cancer Study Group (see entry Cancer), from where the addresses can be obtained. These addresses are also available from the Directory of Cancer Specialists published by the National Cancer Alliance (see entry Cancer).

BRITTLE BONE DISEASES – OSTEOGENESIS IMPERFECTA

Brittle Bone diseases: Osteogenesis Imperfecta (OI)

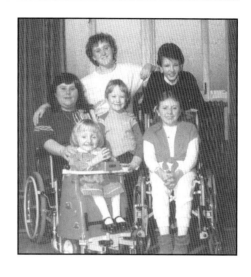

Background

Brittle bone diseases are caused by an abnormality in collagen protein that the body needs for bones as well as other structures such as skin, ligaments and teeth. The condition often leads to an increased likelihood of fractures. Abnormalities in other collagen containing tissues leads to additional problems in some patients such as lax joints, fragile teeth, blue or grey sclera (whites of eyes) and bruising. Some people with OI have short stature and some develop deafness, particularly in the teenage years or their twenties.

There are a number of types of brittle bone disease that can vary in severity from mild, in which the patient may not be correctly diagnosed and children may simply be thought to be accident prone, through to severe in which babies have multiple fractures even before birth. The frequency of fractures may increase in adolescence, following childbirth in women and during late adulthood.

How is it treated?

Fractures need to be treated but the immobilisation period should be kept to a minimum as activity allows muscles and bones to stay as strong as possible. It is important for someone with OI to have a well balanced diet with adequate calcium. There is no specific drug therapy for OI but it has been shown that a group of drugs called bisphosphonates can reduce bone loss, the number of fractures and the chronic pain experienced by these children; most children also become more mobile. Most children obtain maximum benefit from this drug over the first two years of treatment. Further research is needed to assess the benefits of treating children with brittle bone disease with this group of drugs. Some children may benefit from insertion of rods to support the bones. Regular monitoring of other functions such as hearing is required.

Inheritance patterns and prenatal diagnosis

Inheritance patterns

Type I and IV are usually autosomal dominant but new mutations often occur. There are a variety of genetic causes for type II and type III and skilled genetic counselling is necessary. There are kinds of OI which do not fit in the above categories.

Prenatal diagnosis

Severe cases may be detected by ultrasound scanning. A DNA test may be available at eight weeks for some affected families where the family has already been studied. Genetic counselling is available for affected families.

Medical text written November 2002 by Dr S F Ahmed. **Last updated March 2007 by Dr S F Ahmed, Consultant in Paediatric Endocrinology and Bone Metabolism, Royal Hospital For Sick Children, Yorkhill, Glasgow, UK.**

Further online resources

Medical texts in *The Contact a Family Directory* are designed to give a short, clear description of specific conditions and rare disorders. More extensive information on this condition can be found on a range of reliable, validated websites. Further information on these resources can be found in our **Medical Information on the Internet** article on page 21.

Support

Brittle Bone Society
Grant Paterson House, 30 Guthrie Street, Dundee DD1 5BS
Tel: 08000 282459 Freephone Helpline   Tel: 01382 204446   Fax: 01382 206771
e-mail: bbs@brittlebone.org   Web: http://www.brittlebone.org
The Society is a National Registered Charity No. 272100 (Scotland SCO10951), established in 1971. The Brittle Bone Society provides support and information to anyone affected by brittle bones (Osteogenesis Imperfecta). A newsletter is published quarterly and regional and national meetings are held throughout the year.
Group details last updated September 2007.

BRONCHO PULMONARY DYSPLASIA

Background

Bronchopulmonary Dysplasia (BPD) is a condition which occasionally occurs in premature infants who have needed respiratory support from a ventilator. It is more common the more immature the baby and is more likely to occur in babies who have required ventilation because of lung immaturity or in association with infections.

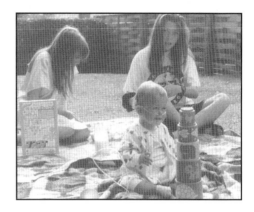

What are the symptoms?

Babies who have been affected by BPD are more prone to wheezing episodes, particularly with viral infections, during the first year of life. Some paediatricians consider it of value for babies on oxygen at home to receive protection against the respiratory syncytial virus during their first winter at home by giving them a course of injections of protective antibody.

How is it treated?

In BPD, there may be a continuing need for the baby to have some form of breathing support. This may persist for some weeks or even months with a few babies actually going home on oxygen supplementation.

Inheritance patterns and prenatal diagnosis

Inheritance patterns

No pattern has yet been identified although genes affecting the types of surfactant produced (a group of chemicals produced in the lung that facilitate lung distension and aeration and help in the fight against infections), together with genes involved in the control of inflammation in the lung, are probably important.

Prenatal diagnosis

Not applicable for this condition

Medical text written November 1991 by Contact a Family. Approved November 1991 by Professor M Patton, Professor of Medical Genetics, St Georges Hospital Medical School, London, UK and Dr J E Wraith. Consultant Paediatrician, Royal Manchester Children's Hospital, Manchester, UK. **Last updated November 2004 by Dr R Rivers, Consultant Paediatrician, Special Care Baby Unit, St Mary's Hospital, London, UK.**

Support

As BPD is a condition which affects premature infants, information, support and advice is available from BLISS (see entry, Prematurity and sick newborn).

C1 ESTERASE INHIBITOR DEFICIENCY

C1 Inhibitor Esterase Deficiency: C1 Inhibitor Deficiency; Hereditary angioedema; HAE

Background

C1 esterase inhibitor deficiency causes intermittent angioedema (swelling of face and throat) and dermal swellings. Gut oedema (swelling) may cause severe abdominal pain, which may be mistaken for acute abdominal conditions such as appendicitis. Dermal swellings are deeper and larger than urticaria ('nettle rash'). They may be painful and are not itchy.

Onset of symptoms is usually in adolescence but may occur at any age. Occasionally C1 esterase inhibitor deficiency is asymptomatic (without symptoms).

How is it diagnosed?

A diagnosis of C1 esterase inhibitor deficiency is unlikely if urticaria and itching are present. Few people affected by angioedema have C1 esterase inhibitor deficiency. Other causes of angioedema include allergies, medications (particularly ACE inhibitors such as lisinopril, often used for high blood pressure), and idiopathic (that is; no cause is identified). People who have angioedema without urticaria ('nettle rash') will normally have simple blood tests to exclude or confirm C1 esterase inhibitor deficiency (C4 complement and C1 esterase inhibitor level and function). Those who are found to have C1 esterase inhibitor deficiency would normally be referred to a specialist with an interest in this condition.

How is it treated?

The number and severity of attacks can be dramatically reduced by regular preventative medication.

If swelling occurs in the throat, the C1 esterase inhibitor deficiency is life threatening and patients should attend hospital immediately for C1 inhibitor infusion. C1 esterase inhibitor deficiency attacks can often be mistaken for anaphylaxis, but adrenaline, antihistamines and steroids are ineffective.

With appropriate treatment, people with C1 esterase inhibitor deficiency have normal life expectancy and can enjoy good health.

Inheritance patterns and prenatal diagnosis

Inheritance patterns

C1 esterase inhibitor deficiency is autosomal dominant. Non-hereditary C1 esterase inhibitor deficiency is very rare, and usually starts in middle age.

Prenatal diagnosis

Not routinely available.

Medical text written September 2001 by Dr H Longhurst. **Last updated September 2005 by Dr H Longhurst, Consultant Immunologist, St Bartholomew's Hospital, London, UK.**

Support

As C1 Esterase Inhibitor deficiency is a Primary Immune deficiency, information and advice is available from the Primary Immunodeficiency Association (see entry, Primary Immunodeficiencies).

Contact a Family produces 'When your child has additional needs' a general guide for parents with information about subjects including education, benefits, childcare and play and leisure. Call the helpline for a copy, which is also available in seven community languages and on CD.

CADASIL

CADASIL: Dementia, Hereditary Multi-infarct Type

Background

CADASIL is an acronym for Cerebral Autosomal Dominant Arteriopathy with subcortical infarcts and leucoencephalopathy.CADASIL is characterised by recurrent stroke, migraine and individuals with CADASIL can suffer from anxiety or depression.

What are the symptoms?

CADASIL is characterised by recurrent stroke (see entry) most commonly first occurring in the 30's to 50's although it is now known that the disease can be very variable and in some people may not present until their 60's. A few individuals identified with CADASIL have remained well in their 70's. The type of stroke affecting people with CADASIL are lacunar strokes (literally meaning a small lake or hole in the brain). As these strokes are small, they tend to be fairly mild and individuals often recover well. The most common type of stroke is weakness affecting one side of the body. If recurrent strokes occur, this can lead to persistent disability which is most usually arm or leg weakness, or slurring of the speech.

Migraine (see entry) is another common feature of the disease. This most commonly starts in the 20's but the onset is variable. Usually these are 'complex' migraines. This means that in addition to the headache there are short-lived neurological symptoms, most commonly, some disturbance of vision or numbness down one side of the body or speech disturbance.

Individuals with CADASIL can suffer from anxiety or depression. Depression is very frequent after any stroke and usually improves with time and treatment if necessary. However, occasionally, depression may occur before any other symptoms of CADASIL. Rarely, seizures (epilepsy) occurs as part of CADASIL. Over time, as the disease progresses, memory problems may occur and if these become severe, they are likely to occur in the 50's or 60's. An unusual feature is the onset of confusion and reduced consciousness over a period of hours or days, sometimes with fever and seizures; this often follows a migraine attack. It recovers completely over one to two weeks.

What are the causes?

It is known that CADASIL results from an abnormality in one very small part of the notch 3 gene. It is thought that the protein produced by the notch 3 gene is responsible for communication between cells within the body, although much work is still required to confirm this. As yet, it is not known why the abnormalities in the notch 3 gene in individuals with CADASIL result in the disease. Further research will be needed to understand the disease mechanism. Although this is not fully understood, it is known that patients with CADASIL suffer from progressive damage within small blood vessels. This is likely to lead to both reduced blood flow and an inability of the blood vessels to regulate blood flow. Although abnormalities in blood vessels can be found throughout the body, they appear to be most severe in the brain, and only produce problems noticed by the person with CADASIL within the brain. It is believed that the abnormalities within the brain result in reduced blood flow to certain parts of the brain.

Inheritance patterns and prenatal diagnosis

Inheritance patterns
Autosomal dominant.

Prenatal diagnosis
This may be possible for an individual member of a family with a known mutation.

Medical text written March 2003 by Contact a Family. **Last reviewed January 2008 by Professor H Markus, Professor of Neurology, St George's Hospital Medical School, London, UK.**

Support
CADASIL is a form of dementia. Information and support is available from the Alzheimer's Society (see entry Alzheimer's disease).

CHARGE SYNDROME

Background

CHARGE syndrome was initially described in 1979, the diagnostic acronym CHARGE was coined in 1982. The condition was previously known as CHARGE association but was renamed CHARGE syndrome on the identification of the gene mutation now known to be involved.

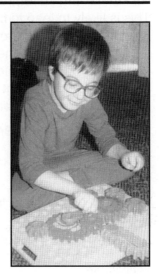

What are the causes?

About half of the individuals diagnosed with CHARGE syndrome have been found to have mutations of the CHD7 gene on Chromosome 8. As others with the syndrome have not shown this mutation, it is thought that other genes may be involved.

What are the symptoms?

The acronym CHARGE was coined to reflect the following features:

C oloboma (see entry)

H eart defects (see entry)

A tresia choanae (blockage of the nasal passages)

R estricted growth and development

G enital hypoplasia

E ar anomalies

How is it diagnosed?

Diagnosis has been historically based on fulfilling at least four out of the six diagnostic criteria in the acronym, although other features have also been variably noted.

Some of these abnormalities are more specific to CHARGE and this is now reflected in major and minor diagnostic criteria:

Major: Coloboma, Choanal Atresia, characteristic Ear Anomalies and Cranial Nerve Dysfunction.

Minor: Include the remainder of the original features plus orofacial clefting, tracheo-oesophageal fistulae (see entry) and a distinctive face.

Individuals with all four major or three major and three minor undoubtedly have CHARGE, which is now considered by many to represent a discrete syndrome.

Inheritance patterns and prenatal diagnosis
Inheritance patterns
The prevalence is estimated to be 1 in 10,000 births. Although most cases are sporadic, familial cases have been described, with a recurrence rate estimated at two to three per cent.

Prenatal diagnosis
Ultrasound scanning may detect some of the anomalies (including the ear) and genetic advice may be sought. As no consistent chromosomal abnormalities have been demonstrated, amniocentesis is not of benefit.

Medical text written December 2000 by Dr J Kirk. **Last updated August 2005 by Dr J Kirk, Consultant Endocrinologist, Birmingham Children's Hospital, Birmingham, UK.**

Further online resources
Medical texts in *The Contact a Family Directory* are designed to give a short, clear description of specific conditions and rare disorders. More extensive information on this condition can be found on a range of reliable, validated websites. Further information on these resources can be found in our **Medical Information on the Internet** article on page 21.

Support
CHARGE Family Support Group
Burnside, 50 Commercial Street, Slaithwaite, Huddersfield HD7 5JZ   Tel: 01484 844202
e-mail: cajthomas@btinternet.com   Web: http://www.widerworld.co.uk/charge
The Group is a National Registered Charity No. 1042953, established in 1987. It offers support and advice to families of affected children and linking where possible. Activities include annual Family Fun Days. It publishes a quarterly newsletter and has a wide range of information available, details on request. The Group has over 160 members.
Group details last confirmed January 2007.

CANAVAN DISEASE

Background

Canavan disease is a rare genetic, degenerative disorder of the nervous system. It is one of a group of genetic disorders called the leukodystrophies. The term leukodystrophy comes from the Greek words, 'leuko' meaning white and referring to the 'white matter' of the nervous system and 'dystrophy' meaning imperfect growth or development. In Canavan disease, there is widespread degeneration of the white matter in the brain leading to loss of sensory, motor and intellectual function.

What are the causes?

The white matter of the brain, otherwise known as myelin sheath, is a fatty covering which acts as an insulator around the nerve fibres of the brain. Myelin sheath is made up of a number of different chemicals. Canavan disease is caused by a deficiency of the normal turnover of a chemical in the brain that is required for normal white matter integrity. Canavan disease is caused by changes (or mutations) in the ASPA gene on chromosome 17. This gene is expressed in supporting cells (oligodendrocytes) involved in the formation of the myelin sheath. The disrupted formation of myelin results in white matter that is fragile and the nerve fibres loose their essential function later in development. There are different types of Canavan disease which include congenital, infantile, and late-onset forms.

What are the symptoms?

Babies with Canavan disease appear normal in the first few months of life. However, in early infancy they begin to lose previously acquired skills including seeing and hearing. The head becomes progressively enlarged (megalencephaly) as the brain swells and the bones of the skull fail to fuse. Babies lose control of their muscles and the muscles supporting the head become floppy and weak (see entry, hypotonia). Sitting, standing and walking are rarely achieved. Although speech is delayed, infants are able to interact socially. Learning difficulties become more severe over time. As children become older, floppiness of the muscles gives way to spasticity (stiffness of the limbs). After the first or second year of life, feeding difficulties become apparent and assisted feeding is required. Life expectancy is between three to ten years, although on average most babies die by eighteen months.

How is it diagnosed?

Canavan disease may be suspected on the basis of an MRI (magnetic resonance imaging) examination which will indicate swelling and spongy degeneration of the white matter of the brain which is characteristic of Canavan disease. Alternatively the less sensitive CT (computer tomography) scan may be used to aid diagnosis. The suspect diagnosis may be confirmed if individuals have an increased level of a specific chemical (N-acetyl-L-aspartic acid) in their urine, blood and spinal fluid and a biochemical test can be used to detect this.

How is it treated?

Although at present no definitive treatment has been established, Canavan disease remains an active focus of the forefront of neurosciences research and has been the subject of an approved trial in the USA for gene therapy. This trial has recently shown promising changes in some areas of the brain of affected children therefore giving the grounds for hope. Whether successful gene therapy alone or researched techniques including neural stem cell therapy will prove to be effective is a matter for active research in the field.

Although Canavan disease may occur in any ethnic group, it appears to be most prevalent among certain semitic cultures including Eastern European (Ashkenazi) Jewish individuals and Saudi Arabians.

Inheritance patterns and prenatal diagnosis

Inheritance patterns

Canavan disease is inherited as an autosomal recessive trait. It is now possible to identify the causative gene mutation which may provide the means for genetic counselling in those individuals or families who seek it.

Prenatal diagnosis

Identification in a given family of the causal mutation in the ASPA Gene may allow prenatal diagnosis to be carried out as DNA can be analysed for the specific gene changes (or mutations).

Medical text written April 2002 by Contact a Family. Approved April 2002 by Professor T Cox. **Last updated March 2007 by Professor T Cox, Professor of Medicine, University of Cambridge School of Clinical Medicine, Cambridge, UK.**

Further online resources

Medical texts in *The Contact a Family Directory* are designed to give a short, clear description of specific conditions and rare disorders. More extensive information on this condition can be found on a range of reliable, validated websites. Further information on these resources can be found in our **Medical Information on the Internet** article on page 21.

Support

While there is no specific support group for families of children in the UK for this condition, information is available from Climb (see entry, Metabolic disease) and support is available from a group of families under the umbrella of Climb.

There is currently no designated UK support group for adults with this metabolic disease. Support for dementia can be obtained from the Alzheimer's Society, see entry, Alzheimer's disease.

CANCER

Background

Cancer is the uncontrolled multiplication of body cells which form a tumour. Many specific conditions come under the term cancer.

Leukaemia (see also separate entry, Leukaemia and other allied blood disorders) is the condition in which the bone marrow is taken over by an excess number of immature white cells, which are unable to perform the normal function of white cells in protecting the body from infection. As a result of the proliferation of these primitive cells within the marrow, there is suppression of the production of normal blood cells, resulting in anaemia, susceptibility to infection and bleeding problems, the hallmarks of leukaemia.

Both conditions are potentially life threatening. The prognosis has been greatly altered in recent years due to treatment with chemotherapy and radiotherapy.

Inheritance patterns and prenatal diagnosis

Inheritance patterns

Genetic changes within a cell in the body may develop which allow uncontrolled multiplication of that cell and leads to the development of a cancer or leukaemia. The majority of cancers and leukaemias have no inherited component in their cause but some forms of cancer and leukaemia are associated with inherited conditions.

Prenatal diagnosis

None.

Further Information

There are a number of conditions that need to be monitored carefully for cancer involvement. These include:

Ataxia-Telangiectasia (see entry). The main cancers likely in Ataxia Telangiectasia are leukaemia and lymphoma but there is also a higher risk of solid tumours including brain tumours. Treatment needs to take into account an extreme sensitivity to radiotherapy and chemotherapy.

Beckwith-Wiedemann syndrome (see entry). The two most common tumours associated with this syndrome are: Wilms tumour and hepatoblastoma (tumour of the liver), the former being the more likely (five to seven per cent). Regular abdominal/pelvic ultra sound screening should take place.

Brain Tumours (see entry). These can be benign, causing damage by pressing on the brain, or malignant, growing and invading the brain.

Cowden disease (see entry). In Cowden disease there both non-cancerous tumour-like growths and an increased risk of a number of types of cancer including breast, thyroid and endometrial cancers.

Dancing Eye syndrome (see entry). In some cases of Dancing Eye syndrome the cause is an underlying cancer known as a neuroblastoma. This is often very small and may only be found by specific investigations for this type of tumour. If localised, the cancer can usually be successfully treated by surgery possibly with additional chemotherapy.

Down syndrome (see entry). In Down Syndrome there is a leukaemia risk of about twenty-fold compared to the non-Down Syndrome population or one to two per cent by the age of ten years. It can be either Acute Lymphoblastic Leukaemia (ALL) or Acute Myeloid Leukaemia (AML) (see entry, Leukaemia). Infants can also develop transient myeloproliferative disorder (TMD), a condition which is similar to leukaemia but often self limiting or needing minimal treatment. Approximately twenty-five per cent of children with TMD will go on to develop clinically evident AML.

Gorlin syndrome (see entry). The main cancer risk is the development of multiple basal cell carcinomas. Regular screening for skin lesions is important. It is thought that there is a risk of developing medulloblastoma (a malignant tumor of the central nervous system arising in the cerebellum especially in children) and this is estimated as four to five per cent with a mean age at diagnosis of two and a half years. It has been suggested that screening with clinical examination and even yearly MRI up to the age of seven years should take place. The avoidance of radiotherapy is strongly recommended (although difficult) in treating this malignant brain tumour due to the high incidence (one hundred per cent) of skin cancer in the radiotherapy field.

Klinefelter syndrome (see entry). Increased risk of breast cancer has been reported.

Li-Fraumeni syndrome (see entry). The syndrome is a rare heritable condition which predisposes many members of a family to a wide range of cancers.

Neurofibromatosis (see entry). Development of tumours is a hallmark of Neurofibromatosis (NF). The name comes from the development of neurofibromas which are benign tumours arising in the skin or from the coverings of nerves (they can occur almost anywhere in the body). There are two main types of neurofibromatosis: NF1 which affects ninety per cent of cases and NF2.

In NF1 plexiform neurofibromas are more complex benign tumours that can be difficult to treat needing multiple resections. At present drug therapy is experimental and there is a malignant potential. Optic gliomas (benign brain tumour) occur in up to fifteen per cent of children and thirty to fifty per cent of all optic nerve gliomas occur in children with NF1. They can affect the child's vision and therefore when a child is old enough regular visual tests are recommended. These benign tumours can spontaneously resolve or behave in a very indolent fashion with fifty per cent requiring no therapy. Chemotherapy or occasionally surgery can successfully treat these tumours. Gliomas can occur in other sites usually requiring surgery. Malignant Peripheral Nerve Sheath Tumours (MPNST's), sarcomas (soft tissue tumour) and Acute Myeloid Leukaemia (AML) have all been reported to occur in excess of the normal population.

NF2 is associated with acoustic neuromas (these benign tumours affect the nerve supplying the middle ear and can lead to hearing loss and balance problems). Another benign tumour known as a meningioma (benign tumour arising from the lining of the brains surface) is also more common in patients with NF2. Both acoustic neuromas and meningiomas are treated with surgery or occasionally radiotherapy. Gliomas can occur in NF2 as can neurofibromas but despite the name the latter are uncommon in NF2.

Retinoblastoma (see entry). Retinoblastoma is a malignant tumour which develops at the back of the eye. It affects babies and young children and is very rare after the age of five years.

Shwachman syndrome (see entry). Malignant transformation and leukaemia are associated with Shwachman syndrome as well as myelodysplasia (abnormality of blood cell production).

Tuberous Sclerosis (see entry). In Tuberous Sclerosis (TS), cardiac rhabdomyomas (benign tumours made up of stripes of nerve fibres) normally develop in utero and can be detected by prenatal scans. Typically these regress during life.

Subependymal Giant Cell Astrocytoma (SEGA), are tumours that almost exclusively occur in patients with TS. These are benign, slow growing tumours arising in the wall of the lateral ventricle (chamber of the brain). There is an incidence of SEGA in approximately fifteen per cent of TS patients. The presence of these tumours often shows with a worsening of epilepsy; they may cause hydrocephalus which can be treated surgically.

Cortical tumours (tumours on the outer part of an organ), hamartomas (a tumour like mass representing anomalous development of tissue natural to a part or organ rather than a true tumor) of the eye and liver and kidney angiomyolipoma (benign tumour containing blood vessels, muscle tissue and fat cells) are also found in TS.

Turcot syndrome (see entry). A rare syndrome of brain and colon tumours.

Von Hippel-Lindau syndrome (see entry). The most common tumours associated with Von Hippel-Lindau syndrome are:

- Cerebellar haemangioblastomas (benign tumours consiting of a mass of blood vessels appearing in the rear part of the brain) – multiple capillary haemangioblastomas appearing in the small blood vessels of the cerebellum or in the spine and Cysts in the cerebellum;
- Retinal angiomas (tumours of blood vessels appearing in the eye);
- There is a lifelong risk of development of Renal Carcinomas (kidney cancer). These malignant tumours often appear in association with renal cysts;
- Phaechromocytoma (vascular tumor of the adrenal gland). These can be single, multiple, benign or malignant tumours.

Wilms Tumour A cancerous tumour of the kidney. See entries, Beckwith-Wiedemann syndrome and Aniridia.

Xeroderma Pigmentosum (see entry). A condition of varying pigmentary changes which can be come malignant.

Medical text written November 1991 by Contact a Family. Approved November 1991 by Professor M Patton, Professor of Medical Genetics, St Georges Hospital Medical School, London UK and Dr J E Wraith, Consultant Paediatrician, Royal Manchester Children's Hospital. **Last updated September 2004 by Contact a Family and Dr D Hargrave. Approved September 2004 by Dr D Hargrave, Consultant Paediatric Oncologist, Royal Marsden Hospital, Sutton, UK.**

Support

Support Groups for children and families:
Christian Lewis Trust
62 Walter Road, Swansea SA1 4PT   Tel: 01792 480500 (Mon-Fri, 9.30am-4.30pm)
Fax: 01792 480700   e-mail: enquries@christianlewistrust.org
Web: http://www.christianlewistrust.org
The Trust is a National Registered Charity No. 801856, established in 1989. It offers a philosophy of child centred care focusing on 'quality of life' issues, a range of family support services, bereavement support, self-help support groups, play therapists and holidays. Group details last updated May 2007.

CLIC Sargent
Griffin House, 161 Hammersmith Road, London W6 8SG   Tel: 020 8752 2800
Tel: 0800 197 0068 Helpline (Mon-Fri, 9am-5pm)   Fax: 020 8752 2806
e-mail: info@clicsargent.org.uk   e-mail: helpline@clicsargent.org.uk
Web: http://www.clicsargent.org.uk
CLIC (Cancer and Leukaemia in Childhood) has joined with Sargent Cancer Care for Children to become CLIC Sargent, National Registered Charity No. 1107328. CLIC Sargent provides support to children and young people with cancer and leukaemia and their families through: clinical and care professionals (specialist doctors, nurses, social workers, family support workers, youth workers and play specialists to provide care, support and advocacy to children and young people with cancer and their families in hospital and at home); homes from home (homes allowing parents, children and siblings to stay together near the hospital); holidays (free opportunities for families to take a break from treatment

in supported settings); care grants (grants to help families cope financially); and research (research projects working to identify causes and treatments of childhood cancer and also looking at managing the many side effects that treatment impose on children which can have significant impact on their future lives).
Group details last updated February 2008.

Teenage Cancer Trust

3rd Floor, 98 Newman St, London W1T 3EZ   Tel: 020 7612 0370   Fax: 020 7612 0371
e-mail: tct@teenagecancertrust.org   Web: http://www.teenagecancertrust.org
The Trust is National Registered Charity No. 1062559, established in 1997. It focuses on the particular needs of UK teenagers and young adults with cancer, leukaemia, Hodgkin's and related diseases. The Charity designs and builds dedicated adolescent cancer units in hospitals. It funds and organises support and information services for patients, their families, schools and health professionals. It has a number of awareness and fundraising activities throughout the year and publishes 'TC Times' annually.
Group details last updated September 2007.

Children's Cancer and Leukaemia Group (CCLG)

University of Leicester, 3rd Floor, Hearts of Oak House, 9 Princess Road West,
Leicester LE1 6TH   Tel: 0116 249 4460   Fax: 0116 254 9504
e-mail: info@cclg.org.uk   Web: http://www.cclg.org.uk
The CCLG is a national professional body responsible for the organisation of the treatment and management of children with cancer in the UK. The Group's main remit is the co-ordination of national and international clinical trials, including biological studies. Other areas of activity include national cancer registration and provision of information for patients and families, details on request, including 'Contact', a quarterly, free magazine for families of children and young people with cancer.
Group details last confirmed October 2007.

National Childhood Cancer Group

NACCPO, PO Box 176, Bromley BR2 7YN   Tel/Fax: 01785 603763
e-mail: ro@naccpo.org.uk   Web: http://www.naccpo.org.uk
The National Alliance of Childhood Cancer Parent Organisations (NACCPO) is a National Registered Charity No. 1090871, established in 1989. It is an umbrella group which has twenty-four member groups around the UK supporting children with cancer and their families. The group has five associate member groups that support families whose children have cancer. They also advise charities and medical bodies on the needs of affected children and their families, advocates better facilities and helps to set up parent-run support groups.
Group details last updated February 2007.

Support Groups for adults:

Cancerbackup

3 Bath Place, Rivington Street, London EC2A 3JR
Tel: 0808 800 1234 Freephone Helpline   Tel: 020 7696 9003 (Administration)
Fax: 020 7696 9002   Tel: 0141 553 1553 (Cancerbackup Scotland)
e-mail: info@cancerbackup.org   Web: http://www.cancerbackup.org
Web: http://www.click4tic.org.uk Teen web site
Cancerbackup, formerly CancerBACUP, is a National Registered Charity No. 1019719. It is the UK's cancer information charity, providing information, support and details of support groups, services and products to help people live with cancer. Services include a national helpline staffed by cancer information nurse specialists, an e-mail service, eight local drop-in centres in hospitals around the UK, and over eighty patient-friendly booklets and two hundred and seventy factsheets on all aspects of cancer treatment and care, as well

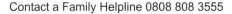

as an award-winning website and a new site for teenagers affected by cancer. A range of information is available on audiotape, and there's a Type talk service and an interpreting service for most languages spoken in the UK.
Group details last updated May 2007.

Macmillan Cancer Support
89 Albert Embankment, London SE1 7UQ
Tel: Tel: 0808 808 2020 Macmillan CancerLine (Mon-Fri, 9am-9pm)
Tel: 0808 808 0800 Youth line (12-21 year olds), Tel: 0808 808 0100 (Hindi)
Tel: 0808 808 0101 (Punjabi) Tel: 0808 808 0102 (Urdu)
Tel: 0808 808 0121 Text Language Line service available
Tel: 020 7840 7840   Fax: 020 7840 7841
e-mail: cancerline@macmillan.org.uk   Web: http://www.macmillan.org.uk
Macmillan Cancer Support is a National Registered Charity No. 261017, established in 1911. It works to help improve the quality of life for people living with cancer, and their families. It funds Macmillan nurses and doctors, who specialise in cancer care; builds cancer care units for inpatient and day care; and gives grants to patients in financial need (enquiries to Patient Grant Department). Macmillan also funds a medical support and education programme to improve doctors' and nurses' skills in cancer care, and funds four associated charities providing information and support for people with cancer.
Group details last updated November 2007.

Rarer Cancers Forum
The Great Barn, Godmersham Park, Canterbury CT4 7DT
Tel: 01227 738279 (Mon-Fri; 9.30 am to 5.30 pm)   e-mail: penny@rarercancers.org.uk
Web: http://www.rarercancers.org.uk
The Forum is a National Registered Charity No. 1109213, established in 2001. The Forum works to raise awareness of the rarer cancers to health professionals and the general public. It also aims to improve services and reduce isolation in affected individuals.
Group details last confirmed October 2007.

There are also support networks for Lymphoma, Neuroblastoma and Retinoblastoma (see entries).

There are a number of very supportive local self help groups around the country. If you want to contact one of these and have been unable to do so through the organisations in this Directory please get in touch with Contact a Family.

CARDIOFACIOCUTANEOUS SYNDROME

Cardiofaciocutaneous syndrome: CFC syndrome

Background

Cardiofaciocutaneous syndrome was first described independently by James Reynolds from the US and Michael Baraitser and Michael Patton from the UK in 1986. It is an infrequent congenital (present at birth) condition of multiple physical anomalies and learning disability. Less than 300 cases of CFC syndrome are known worldwide. CFC syndrome affects both sexes and all ethnic groups.

What are the symptoms?

There are a wide range of features of CFC syndrome including:

- Relatively macrocephaly (large head) with a high forehead;
- Hypertelorism (wide spaced eyes), short nose, low set ears and other facial abnormalities. These characteristics can resemble Noonan syndrome (see entry) to a great extent;
- Brittle and sparse hair together with skin problems such as scaly or thickened skin;
- Heart defects relating to valves and openings between the left and right chambers, and hypertrophic cardiomyopathy (see entry, Cardiomyopathies) (abnormal development of the muscle of the heart);
- Short stature;
- Motor and speech delay;
- Learning disability.

What are the causes?

CFC syndrome can be caused by mutations of at least four different genes located on chromosome 7, chromosome 12 and chromosome 15. It is thought that more genes are involved as in less than half of the patients an abnormality in one of the genes can be found.

How is it diagnosed?

Diagnosis of CFC syndrome is made by observation of the known features of the syndrome. Ultrasound imaging of the heart and brain and MRI (magnetic resonance imaging) may be used.

How is it treated?

CFC syndrome cannot be cured and treatment is symptomatic for the features of the syndrome affecting the individual. Speech therapy, appropriate special education and skin care can help. Surgical intervention for the heart defects and tube feeding, or in some cases gastrostomy (an opening through the stomach wall for feeding purposes), may be required.

Inheritance patterns and prenatal diagnosis

Inheritance patterns

Autosomal dominant. Most frequently a patient is the first one in the family to have the syndrome.

Prenatal diagnosis

This may be possible using DNA techniques for those families in which an earlier child with CFC syndrome has been born and the mutation in the DNA has been found.

Medical text written June 2006 by Contact a Family. Approved June 2006 by Professor R Hennekam, Professor of Clinical Dysmorphology, Institute of Child Health, London, UK.

Further online resources

Medical texts in *The Contact a Family Directory* are designed to give a short, clear description of specific conditions and rare disorders. More extensive information on this condition can be found on a range of reliable, validated websites. Further information on these resources can be found in our **Medical Information on the Internet** article on page 21.

Support

There is no support group for Cardiofaciocutaneous syndrome in the UK. However, details of the UK contact person for the world wide CFC International http://www.cfcsyndrome. org can be obtained from Contact a Family's Freephone Helpline. Cross referrals to other entries in the Contact a Family Directory are intended to provide relevant support for these particular features of the disorder. Organisations identified in those entries do not provide support specifically for Cardiofaciocutaneous syndrome. Families can use Contact a Family's Freephone Helpline for advice, information and, where possible, links to other families. Contact a Family's web-based linking service Making Contact.org can be accessed at http://www.makingcontact.org

CARDIOMYOPATHIES

Hypertrophic Cardiomyopathy

The condition was first recognised in the 1950's and has been known by the names Hypertrophic Obstructive Cardiomyopathy (HOCM), Idiopathic Hypertrophic Sub-aortic Stenosis (IHSS) and Muscular Sub-aortic Stenosis but the term Hypertrophic Cardiomyopathy (HCM) is now generally used.

HCM is an inherited condition which, in the majority of affected people, does not limit the quality and duration of life. It is a disorder of the heart consisting of excessive growth of the muscle, which may begin before birth when the fetal heart is developing. The natural history is characterised by slow progression of symptoms but a significant incidence of sudden death. Symptoms of chest pain, dizziness, loss of consciousness, palpitation and breathlessness can occur but some affected persons do not experience symptoms. Irregularity of the heartbeat can lead to palpitations but usually is only detected during ECG monitoring. Treatment is usually by drug therapy but surgery may be indicated where the thickening of the muscle causes obstruction to the outflow tract of the heart. Risk stratification to identify an affected individual's potential risk of sudden death is an important part of medical management to ensure appropriate preventative measures are taken. If the condition is diagnosed, intense competitive exercise should be avoided. Special monitoring during anaesthesia is required.

If the condition is diagnosed, violent exercise, prolonged standing in hot conditions and very hot baths/showers should be avoided. Special monitoring during anaesthesia is required.

Inheritance patterns
Autosomal dominant. Family screening is strongly recommended. Research shows 1 in 500 people are affected in the UK.
Prenatal diagnosis
None.

Dilated Cardiomyopathy

Dilated cardiomyopathy is a condition which was first recognised in the 1950s. It is characterised by dilation and impaired pumping function of the main chambers of the heart. The onset of the condition is genetically determined in the majority of patients. It may be triggered by viral infection, pregnancy, or excessive alcohol abuse. Symptoms of heart failure, in particular breathlessness and fatigue, are the usual presenting feature. Natural history is usually progressive though there have been recent improvements in the treatment of heart failure including newer drugs and the possibility of transplantation.

Inheritance patterns

Dilated cardiomyopathy is an autosomal dominant condition with incomplete penetrance and family screening is recommended. The condition is familial in at least fifty per cent of cases.

Prenatal diagnosis

Not applicable.

Medical text written November 1994 by Professor W J McKenna. **Last updated October 2004 by Professor W J McKenna, Clinical Director, Heart Hospital, London, UK.**

Support

Cardiomyopathy Association

Unit 10, Chiltern Court, Asheridge Road, Chesham HP5 2PX   Tel: 01494 791224
Tel: 0800 018 1024 Helpline   Fax: 01494 797199   e-mail: info@cardiomyopathy.org
Web: http://www.cardiomyopathy.org

The Association is a National Registered Charity No. 803262, established in 1989. It offers: advice and information for individuals and families; linking families where possible; raising awareness among doctors, nurses, health professionals, educational institutions and the general public; and a regional contact network. It publishes a quarterly newsletter and has a wide range of information available, details on request. The Association has approximately 2,000 members.

Group details last updated March 2007.

Further support for young people with Hypertrophic Cardiomyopathy is available from CRY - Cardiac Risk in the Young (see entry, Heart Defects)

Support for bereaved families of adults who have died as a result of Cardiomyopathy is provided by the Sudden Adult Death Trust (SADS UK) (see entry, Heart Defects)

CATARACTS

Background

About two hundred children a year are born in the UK with opacity of the lens of one or both eyes - a cataract.

Most children born with cataracts are otherwise healthy and many will have other family members born with cataract. However, in some cases, cataract is a sign of a syndrome: Down syndrome (see entry), Lowe syndrome (see entry), Nance-Horan syndrome, Deafblindness (see entry), Galactosaemia (see entry), Marinesco-Sjögren syndrome, Cockayne syndrome (see entry), Hallermann-Streiff-Francois syndrome, Pollitt syndrome, Werner syndrome, Rothmund-Thomson syndrome, Zellweger syndrome or Conradi-Hunermann syndrome (see entry).

If cataract is the only abnormality of the eye and the child is treated within the first few months of life, the prognosis for vision is good. It is expected that the child will attend mainstream school and read, although often will have difficulty with distance vision for the white board.

How is it treated?

In most cases the lens will be cloudy enough to prevent clear vision developing and the child will need surgery to have the lens removed. For the child to focus thick glasses or a contact lens will be needed. The strength of these will be regularly changed as the child's eye grows, unlike an artificial lens placed inside the eye, which cannot be altered. In a few cases, if the eye is of normal size, a lens implant can be considered particularly if only one eye is affected. In these cases the child has to wear glasses in addition.

It is most important that children born with cataracts in both eyes have regular eye examinations. In those cases with mild cataract, that does not need a surgical operation, glasses are often needed and the cataract may become denser with time. Children who have had cataract surgery require regular review of their vision development, glasses prescription, a check for glaucoma and examination of their retina.

Inheritance patterns and prenatal diagnosis

Inheritance patterns

The commonest inheritance pattern is autosomal dominant. However, X-linked and autosomal recessive inheritance of isolated cataract also occurs.

Prenatal diagnosis

This is not yet available for the majority of isolated congenital cataract

Medical text written December 1999 by Miss Isabelle Russell-Eggitt FRCS FRCOphth.
Last updated September 2004 by Miss Isabelle Russell-Eggitt FRCS FRCOphth, Consultant Ophthalmic Surgeon, Great Ormond Street Hospital, London, UK.

Contact a Family Helpline 0808 808 3555

Support

Childhood Cataract Network

c/o National Blind Children's Society, Shawton House, 792 Hagley Road West, Quinton, Birmingham, B68 0EP Tel c/o NBCS: 01278 764 770

e-mail c/o NBCS: FaFamilySupport@nbcs.org.uk

e-mail group/forum for Network: egroup@childhoodcataracts.org.uk

Web: http://www.childhoodcataracts.org.uk

This is a small network set up in 2007 supporting adults and parents of children with cataracts. The Group is currently offering web based support. All initial enquiries preferred through the website. Mail and telephone calls are being managed by the National Blind Children's Society. The Network works closely with ophthalmologist at Moorfields Eye Hospital to ensure accuracy of medical information.

Group details last updated March 2008

Our eight London borough-based projects provide long term one-to-one support to families, including those with complex needs.

CEREBELLAR ATAXIA

Background

Cerebellar Ataxia affects the cerebellum, which is the hind part of the brain responsible for the co-ordination of movement.

What are the symptoms?

People with this disorder have balance impairment in sitting, standing and walking, lack of co-ordination in their hands and a slurred speech. Eyes can also be affected and as a result cerebellar ataxic patients can complain of blurred or double vision.

Inheritance patterns and prenatal diagnosis

Inheritance patterns

There are many different causes of cerebellar ataxia some of which will be genetic in origin. Genetic counselling is indicated for affected families. Inheritance may be dominant, recessive, or rarely mitochondrial and X-linked.

Over the past few years there has been a tremendous increase in our understanding of the genetics of the autosomal dominant cerebellar ataxias. The genes are given the acronym SCA (Spino-Cerebellar Ataxia) and at the most recent count (October 2005) it is clear that there are over twenty-seven SCA genes. Some of these seem to be very rare and have only been reported in one or two families and for these there are no gene tests currently available. For others (SCA 1, 2, 3, 6, 7, 12 and 17) there are now genetic tests available. Interestingly all these different genes have a very similar mutation. This is an abnormally long repetition of a DNA fragment called CAG which can be detected relatively simply using molecular methods. These tests can be used to accurately define the genetic cause of cerebellar ataxia in families or in a single individual. Once the genetic diagnosis has been established it can lead to more accurate presymptomatic and prenatal testing if required.

Prenatal diagnosis

Both prenatal and presymptomatic diagnosis are available in families who have been proven to have mutations in SCA 1, 2, 3, 6, 7,12 and 17 after genetic tests. Chorionic villus sampling is available at ten to twelve weeks.

Medical text written November 1991 by Contact a Family. Approved November 1991 by Professor M Patton, Professor of Medical Genetics, St Georges Hospital Medical School, London, UK and Dr J E Wraith, Consultant Paediatrician, Royal Manchester Children's Hospital, Manchester, UK. **Last updated November 2005 by Dr P Giunti, Senior Clinical Fellow, University Department of Clinical Neurology, University College, London, UK.**

Support

Support for Cerebellar Ataxia can be obtained from Ataxia UK (see entry, Friedreich's Ataxia).

CEREBRAL PALSY

Background

Cerebral Palsy is a non progressive disorder of the areas of the developing brain which control movement.

Cerebral Palsy occurs in approximately 1 in 400 births and causes can be multiple and complex.

What are the symptoms?

The effects of cerebral palsy vary with each individual. In some people, cerebral palsy is barely noticeable; others will be more severely affected. No two people will be affected in the same way.

Cerebral Palsy is frequently categorised into three main types although many people will have a combination of these types:

- Spasticity (stiff and tight muscles);
- Athetoid or Dyskinetic (involuntary movements, change of tone in muscles from floppy to tense);
- Ataxic (unsteady, uncoordinated shaky movements and irregular speech).

Terms such as hemiplegia (one half of body) (see entry), diplegia (legs more affected than arms) and quadriplegia (all four limbs equally affected) indicate the parts of the body affected.

As cerebral palsy is such a wide ranging condition and individual effects vary, some children may have a learning difficulties (see entry, Learning Disability), behavioural problems, epilepsy (see entry) or sensory impairment.

What are the causes?

Recent studies suggest that cerebral palsy is mostly due to factors affecting the brain before birth. Known possible causes can include infection, difficult or premature birth, cerebral bleeds, infection or accident in early years and abnormal brain development.

How is it treated?

Cerebral Palsy is non progressive and cannot be cured. However, early support and therapeutic intervention can help development. Importantly, children with cerebral palsy are children first and foremost.

Inheritance patterns and prenatal diagnosis

Inheritance patterns

In a few cases, cerebral palsy may be caused by a genetic link. However, this is quite rare. Parents who may be concerned should ask their GP for referral to a genetic counsellor.

Prenatal diagnosis

None at present available.

Medical text written September 2003 by Dr Martin C O Bax, Emeritus Reader in Child Health, Chelsea & Westminster Hospital (Imperial College School of Medicine), London, UK.

Further online resources

Medical texts in *The Contact a Family Directory* are designed to give a short, clear description of specific conditions and rare disorders. More extensive information on this condition can be found on a range of reliable, validated websites. Further information on these resources can be found in our **Medical Information on the Internet** article on page 21.

Support

Cerebral Palsy Helpline (Scope)

P.O. Box 833, Milton Keynes MK12 5NY

Tel: 0808 800 3333 Scope response, Freephone (Mon-Fri, 9am-7pm; Sat, 10am-2pm)
Tel: 01908 321049 Publications   Fax: 01908 321051   e-mail: response@scope.org.uk
Web: http://www.scope.org.uk
Scope is a National Registered Charity No. 208231 with a focus on cerebral palsy. The aim of Scope is that all disabled people achieve equality. Scope's work is focussed on four main areas – Early Years, Employment, Education and Daily Living. In addition to a range of national and local services, Scope has over 250 affiliated local groups. In-depth information and advice is provided on all aspects of cerebral palsy and disability issues as well as information about and referral to Scope services as appropriate. A team of trained Counsellors provides clients with emotional support and initial counselling. Scope publishes 'Disability Now' monthly.
Group details last updated September 2007.

Capability Scotland

ASCS, 11 Ellersly Road, Edinburgh EH12 6HY   Tel: 0131 313 5510   Fax: 0131 313 7864
e-mail: ascs@capability-scotland.org.uk   Web: http://www.capability-scotland.org.uk
Capability Scotland is a Registered Charity No. SC 011330, established in 1946. It provides a diverse range of services to children, young people and adults with a range of disabilities and their families and carers. Services include a national disability information and advice service. For children it offers activities, education and learning, children's short breaks and family support services.
Group details last confirmed February 2008.

Scottish Centre for Children with Motor Impairments

1 Craighalbert Way, Cumbernauld, Glasgow G68 0LS   Tel: 01236 456100
Fax: 01236 736889   e-mail: sccmi@craighalbert.org.uk
Web: http://www.craighalbert.org.uk
The Centre is a National Registered Charity, registered under its Company No. 129291, established in April 1991. It offers conductive education within national guidelines on education within Scotland, education for children with cerebral palsy under the age of ten years, services for children with dyspraxia under the age of ten years, a free service to children under the age of two years, accommodation for families who do not live within daily travelling distance and a programme of Saturday and Summer schools. It has information available, details on request.
Group details last confirmed October 2007.

Additionally there are two organisations providing alternative types of help for children with cerebral palsy. These are:

The Bobath Centre for Children with Cerebral Palsy
250 East End Road, East Finchley, London N2 8AU   Tel: 020 8444 3355
Fax: 020 8444 3399   e-mail: info@bobathlondon.co.uk
Web: http://www.bobath.org.uk
The Bobath Centre specializes in individual therapy for children (and adults) with Cerebral Palsy using the Bobath/NDT approach to treatment and management. Therapy is based on a problem solving approach to this disorder of posture and movement, based on movement, analysis and systematic treatment facilitating the child to develop a greater repertoire of functional activities. The focus of therapy is helping the parents and carers to use and adapt play and everyday activities to help the children reach their functional potential. The Bobath Concept, which is used internationally, was developed at this Centre. The Centre runs an eight week postgraduate course in the treatment and management of Cerebral Palsy for doctors, physiotherapists, occupational therapists and speech & language therapists. In addition, short, practical courses are run for other professionals such as teachers and classroom assistants. The Bobath Centre has a wide range of information available, details on request.
Group details last updated March 2007.

The Foundation for Conductive Education
Cannon Hill House, Russell Road, Moseley, Birmingham B13 8RD   Tel: 0121 449 1569
Fax: 0121 449 1611   e-mail: foundation@conductive-education.org.uk
Web: http://www.conductive-education.org.uk
The Foundation is a National Registered Charity No. 295873, established in 1986 to develop and advance the science and skill of Conductive Education in the UK. The National Institute of Conductive Education provides direct services to children and adults with motor disabilities; cerebral palsy, multiple sclerosis, Parkinson's disease, children with dyspraxia and those who have suffered strokes and head injuries. Through a system of positive teaching and learning support, Conductive Education maximises their control over bodily movement in ways that are relevant to daily living. The National Institute also undertakes research and offers a comprehensive range of professionally oriented, skills-based training courses at all levels.
Group details last updated February 2007.

CHARCOT-MARIE-TOOTH DISEASE

Charcot-Marie-Tooth disease: CMT: Peroneal Muscular Atrophy: Hereditary Motor and Sensory Neuropathy

Background

This is a genetic disorder characterised by slowly progressive muscular weakness.

The onset of the condition may be from childhood to late middle or old age.

What are the symptoms?

Onset is in the lower limbs first causing weakness around the ankles and, often, an abnormality in the shape of the feet (high in-step.) After many years, weakness may develop in the hands and spread upwards in the lower limbs to affect the knees and thighs. Mild loss of sensation may be present in the feet and hands.

Inheritance patterns and prenatal diagnosis

Inheritance patterns

1. Autosomal dominant is the most common pattern of inheritance.
2. Autosomal recessive (least common)
3. X-linked passed to both sons and daughters. However, affected sons will usually display more severe symptoms.

Prenatal diagnosis

In families who have Type 1a prenatal diagnosis is now becoming available but is rarely requested.

Medical text written November 1991 by Contact a Family. Approved November 1991 by Professor M Patton, Professor of Medical Genetics, St Georges Hospital Medical School, London, UK and Dr J E Wraith, Consultant Paediatrician, Royal Manchester Children's Hospital, Manchester, UK. Last updated August 1999 by Dr David Hilton-Jones. **Last reviewed January 2004 by Dr David Hilton-Jones, Clinical Director, Muscle and Nerve Centre, Radcliffe Infirmary, Oxford, UK.**

Further online resources

Medical texts in *The Contact a Family Directory* are designed to give a short, clear description of specific conditions and rare disorders. More extensive information on this condition can be found on a range of reliable, validated websites. Further information on these resources can be found in our **Medical Information on the Internet** article on page 21.

Contact a Family Helpline 0808 808 3555

Support

CMT United Kingdom

PO Box 5089, Christchurch BH23 7ZX   Tel: 0800 652 6316 helpline (Mon-Fri, 8.30am-3pm) Tel: 01202 481 161 office (Mon-Fri, 8.30am-3pm) e-mail: secretary@cmt.org.uk
Web: http://www.cmt.org.uk

The organisation is a National Registered Charity No. 1112370, established in 1986. It offers support and advice to people with CMT and their families and a network of local groups. It publishes a newsletter three times a year and has around 1,200 members. Group details last updated October 2007.

During 2008 – 2011 the government intends to support the development of parent forums in every part of England as part of a programme called 'Aiming High for Disabled Children'.

CHROMOSOME DISORDERS

Background

The human body is made up of billions of individual cells. Apart from the red blood cells, each cell contains a structure called a nucleus. Inside each nucleus are found long, thread-like bodies, the chromosomes. Chromosomes are made up of a short arm (designated by the letter 'p') and a long arm ('q'), joined at a point, the centromere. The ends of the two arms are called the telomeres. Chromosomes are made up of deoxyribonucleic acid (DNA) and proteins. The DNA of each cell, when stretched out, is around 2 m long. In chromosomes the DNA is coiled and much condensed. Chromosomes contain genes, which are special stretches of DNA. The genes provide the instructions that tell our bodies how to develop and function properly.

Apart from the mother's egg cells (ova) and the father's sperm cells (spermatozoa), every cell in the human body normally contains twenty-three pairs of chromosomes, giving forty-six chromosomes in total. There are thought to be around thirty thousand genes in each cell. Of the twenty-three pairs of chromosomes in each of these cells, one member from each pair is normally inherited from the father and the other member of each pair is normally inherited from the mother. The first twenty-two pairs of chromosomes are called the autosomes and are numbered from one to twenty-two, generally in order of length, chromosome 1 being the longest. The chromosomes in the twenty-third pair are called the sex chromosomes. They are labelled X or Y. Males normally have one copy of the X chromosome and one copy of the Y chromosome while females normally have two copies of the X chromosome in their body cells.

A mother's egg cells each normally contain only twenty-three chromosomes, made up of one copy each of chromosomes 1 to 22 and one copy of the X chromosome. A father's sperm cells also normally contain only twenty-three chromosomes, again made up of one copy each of chromosomes 1 to 22 but also either one copy of the X chromosome or one copy of the Y chromosome. It is the father's sperm that determines whether a child will be a boy (XY) or a girl (XX).

A person's chromosomal make-up is called their karyotype which can be described by a code of letters and numbers.

Chromosome abnormalities

Chromosome abnormalities have, by tradition, been defined as those abnormalities large enough to be seen down a light microscope. With more recent and sophisticated analytical techniques, much smaller abnormalities that cause symptoms can now be detected. Chromosome abnormalities often involve many different genes and they can be classified into two main types, numerical abnormalities and structural abnormalities. If these arise during formation of an egg or sperm cell, then the abnormality would be passed on to every cell in the child's body. If the abnormality arises in one of the new cells produced soon after an egg has been fertilised by a sperm, then only a proportion of the child's cells will be affected and this is called mosaicism. When a person carries such an abnormality, they are at risk of displaying the symptoms of the associated chromosome disorder.

Numerical abnormalities

When cells carry complete extra sets of chromosomes, this is called polyploidy. When there is one extra complete set, to give sixty-nine chromosomes in total, then this is known as triploidy. Two extra sets of chromosomes, to give niney-two chromosomes in total, would be called tetraploidy.

When individual whole chromosomes are missing or extra, this is called aneuploidy. This can happen with any of the autosomal chromosomes (1 to 22) or the sex chromosome (X or Y).

If one extra complete chromosome is present, this is known as trisomy and the number of chromosomes in each affected cell would be 47. The most common disorder arising from a trisomy is Down syndrome (Trisomy 21). Two extra complete chromosomes would be called tetrasomy and the number of chromosomes would be 48. Three extra complete chromosomes would be called pentasomy and the number of chromosomes in each cell would be 49. If a complete chromosome is missing, this is known as monosomy and the number of chromosomes in each cell would be 45.

Examples of aneuploidy involving the sex chromosomes include XYY (male with one extra Y chromosome), XXY (male with one extra X chromosome), XXXY (male with two extra X chromosomes), XXXXY (male with three extra X chromosomes), XXYY (male with one extra X and one extra Y chromosome), XXX (female with one extra X chromosome), XXXX (female with two extra X chromosomes) and XXXXX (female with three extra X chromosomes).

Structural abnormalities

Structural chromosome abnormalities arise when there are breakages in chromosomes, leading to a net loss, gain or abnormal rearrangement of one or more chromosomes. Structural abnormalities include deletions and duplications, including those too small to be seen down the light microscope (microdeletions and microduplications) those near the end of the chromosome (subtelomeric deletions and duplications), ring chromosomes, reciprocal translocations (balanced or unbalanced), Robertsonian translocations (balanced or unbalanced), insertional translocations (balanced or unbalanced) and inversions (pericentric or paracentric). As analytical techniques improve, smaller and more subtle structural abnormalities can often be detected where previously a person's karyotype was thought to be normal.

Balanced and unbalanced reciprocal translocations

Balanced reciprocal translocations arise when breakages occur in two or more different (non-homologous) chromosomes with the resulting detached segments swapping places with each other. No chromosomal material has been lost or gained, just rearranged. Usually, carriers of a balanced reciprocal rearrangement will have no symptoms themselves. However, they run the risk of having problems at reproduction, e.g reduced fertility, miscarriage and/or the birth of a child with an unbalanced reciprocal translocation (in which there is both a net loss and gain of chromosomal material) and therefore symptoms. A small proportion of babies born with an apparently balanced reciprocal translocation will have symptoms. One of the reasons may be that the break has caused damage to a gene. Another may be that there is a microdeletion or microduplication that has caused the symptoms.

Robertsonian translocations

Balanced Robertsonian translocations arise when the short arms of two of the acrocentric chromosomes (chromosomes 13, 14, 15, 21 or 22) are lost and the remaining parts of the centromeres and the long arms fuse together. Although carriers of such balanced Robertsonian translocations would not be expected to have symptoms themselves, they run the risk of reduced fertility, miscarriage and/or producing babies with unbalanced chromosomes and therefore symptoms.

Balanced and unbalanced insertional rearrangements

Balanced insertions occur when a segment of one chromosome is inserted into a break in the arm of another chromosome. No chromosomal material has been lost or gained, just rearranged. Carriers of such balanced insertions should not have symptoms but they are at risk of fertility problems, miscarriage and/or the birth of a child with an extra or missing copy of the inserted chromosomal segment and therefore symptoms.

Deletions

A deletion (sometimes called a partial monosomy) involves loss of a segment of a chromosome. Deletions can occur near to the centromere (proximal deletion), nearer to the end of the chromosome (distal deletion), in the middle of a chromosome arm (interstitial deletion), at the end of the chromosome (terminal deletion) or as a tiny segment missing very near to the telomere (subtelomeric deletion). Deletions can cause symptoms due to loss of any genes contained within the deleted chromosomal segment.

Ring chromosomes

Ring chromosomes arise when the ends of both arms of a chromosome are lost and the remaining broken ends join together to form a ring shape.

Thus a ring chromosome is essentially a double deletion. However, if a ring chromosome exists as an extra, supernumerary chromosome, then it is the material contained within the ring that is in effect duplicated.

Duplications/triplications
A duplication (sometimes called a partial trisomy) occurs when an extra copy of a segment of a chromosome is present. If a person has two extra copies of a chromosomal segment, this is known as a triplication (or sometimes as a Partial tetrasomy). Duplications and triplications can cause symptoms due to gain of extra copies of any genes contained within the additional chromosomal segment.

Inversions
Inversions arise when a chromosome breaks in two places, the intervening segment flips around and is then re-inserted into the 'gap.' Inversions are known either as paracentric, if the two breaks are in the same chromosomal arm, or as pericentric if the breaks occur in different arms of the same chromosome. Inversions would not usually cause symptoms in the carrier but can lead to fertility problems, or miscarriage. In the case of pericentric inversions there is also a risk for the birth of an affected baby with duplications and deletions of the two end segments of the chromosome involved. Carriers of paracentric inversions very rarely give birth to children with symptoms.

Isochromosomes and extra structurally abnormal chromosomes
Sometimes people carry an extra or supernumerary chromosome made up of part of one or more chromosomes. They will effectively carry a duplication of the material forming this extra chromosome. If the origin of the extra chromosome is unknown, it is referred to as an extra structurally abnormal chromosome or an extra marker chromosome. If the extra chromosome is made up of two copies of the same segment of a chromosome, this is called an isochromosome. When these extra chromosomes carry two copies of the same centromere, they are called isodicentric chromosomes.

Uniparental disomy
Normally one member of each pair of chromosomes is inherited from the father and the other from the mother. In rare cases, a trisomy in an early embryo can 'correct' itself by losing one of the extra chromosomes. If the remaining two chromosomes are inherited from the same parent, then this is called uniparental disomy (mUPD for inheritance from the mother and pUPD for inheritance from the father). UPD will only cause problems when the chromosome involved is susceptible to imprinting (i.e. the expression of the genes is parent-specific).

Inheritance patterns and prenatal diagnosis

Inheritance patterns

Many chromosome abnormalities do not recur in families. However, since some abnormalities are due to a balanced chromosomal rearrangement in either parent, a child could display a chromosome disorder. Genetic advice should be sought to quantify the specific risks posed by individual chromosome abnormalities.

Prenatal diagnosis

Chorionic villus sampling (CVS) can be carried out usually around eleven to thirteen weeks of pregnancy and amniocentesis from around fifteen to seventeen weeks of pregnancy.

Medical text written October 2001 by Dr B Searle. Approved October 2001 by Professor M A Hultèn. Additional material on small Supernumerary Marker Chromosomes written July 2005 by Dr T Liehr, Institute of Human Genetics and Anthropology, Jena, Germany. **Last updated October 2006 by Dr B Searle, Unique - the Rare Chromosome Support Group. Approved October 2006 by Professor M A Hultèn, University of Warwick, Coventry, UK.**

Support

Unique - The Rare Chromosome Disorder Support Group
PO Box 2189, Caterham CR3 5GN   Tel/Fax: 01883 330766 (answerphone 24 hours)
e-mail: info@rarechromo.org   Web: http://www.rarechromo.org
The Group is a National Registered Charity No. 1110661, established in 1984. It offers contact with families with an affected member who has the same rare chromosome disorder or who has similar symptoms or practical concerns, irrespective of specific chromosome disorder. It produces a comprehensive range of family-friendly, medically-verified leaflets on various rare chromosome disorders. There is a network of local contacts and Unique promotes awareness of rare chromosome disorders to the public and professional workers. It co-ordinates families to assist in research and has a password-protected discussion forum on the website for registered members. It also has a telephone translation and interpretation service (UK only). It publishes a newsletter three times a year and has information available, details on request. The Group has nearly 5,000 affected families and many professional workers as members worldwide.
Group details last updated May 2007.

CHRONIC FATIGUE SYNDROME / MYALGIC ENCEPHALMIMYELITIS

Chronic Fatigue syndrome / Myalgic Encephalomyelitis: CFS/ME; Myalgic Encephalomyelitis or Encephalopathy; ME; Epidemic Neuromyasthenia; Post Viral Fatigue syndrome; PVFS; Chronic Fatigue and Immune Dysfunction syndrome - CFIDS (in USA and Canada)

Background

Myalgic Encephalomyelitis appears on the World Health Organisation's International Classification of diseases list (G93.3, ICD-10) as a neurological disease.

Myalgic Encephalomyelitis is a distinctive clinical syndrome first reported in patients after outbreaks of viral infections in 1950s and was characterised by persistent fatigue, muscle pain (myalgia), symptoms suggestive of brain and spinal cord dysfunction (encephalomyelitis) and conspicuous deterioration of symptoms after physical exertion. Only limited neuropathological studies have been possible in ME. There is no significant abnormality in muscles and peripheral nerves, but there are abnormal inclusion bodies in brain (corpora amylacea) and inflammatory changes in the dorsal root ganglion of spinal nerve root. Post-viral fatigue syndrome was used to describe a similar syndrome where patients could clearly trace the onset of their illness back to a viral infection. However, ME-type symptoms are also known to follow other infections (for example, Lyme disease and Q fever), post-infective neurologic diseases (such as Guillain-Barré syndrome - see entry) immunisation or exposure to neurotoxins (for example, ciguatera fish poisoning). The quality of fatigue in ME is disabling and comparable to fatigue in Multiple Sclerosis. The term chronic fatigue syndrome was introduced in 1988 by the Centers for disease Control (Atlanta, USA) to describe medically unexplained, persistent or relapsing fatigue of new onset. ME/PVFS was subsumed within this new designation. CFS is a broad diagnostic category and patients with psychiatric causes of chronic fatigue may be offered a diagnosis of CFS. The term chronic fatigue and immune dysfunction syndrome is still preferred in the USA and Canada because research studies in the 1980s showed subtle immunological changes in elevation of cytotoxic T cells, pro-inflammatory cytokines and low natural killer cell activity. In the absence of better pathologic data, CFS/ME is likely to be used as the most preferred clinical descriptor. Recent research on DNA microarray and gene profiling of patients with CFS/ME suggest changes due to increased oxidative stress, accelerated apoptosis (programmed cell death) and altered immune regulation.

The prevalence of CFS/ME is estimated to be at least 2 in 1,000 adult population (that is around 150,000 people in the UK). All age groups are affected although onset is rare below the age of seven and above the age of sixty years. The most common age of onset is between mid-teens and mid-forties, in previously fit and often, physically active individuals. ME is more prevalent in females than males (similar to multiple sclerosis) and may be one of the common medical reasons of long time school absenteeism in children.

What are the symptoms?
Common symptoms include:
- Persistent or relapsing fatigue unrelieved by rest or sleep;
- Cognitive dysfunction: impairments in short term memory, concentration and attention span, inability to name common objects (anomia);
- Muscle pain (present in approximately seventy-five per cent cases) and coarse twitching of muscles (myokymia or benign fasciculations);
- Exercise induced fatigability with a prolonged recovery time (post-exertional malaise), usually accompanied by muscle pain and slowing of speed in processing cognitive tasks;
- Unrefreshing sleep (excessive sleep in early phases and broken sleep pattern later);
- Light headedness, palpitations and/or fainting with sudden changes in position (orthostatic intolerance), especially in adolescents and young patients;
- Altered cutaneous sensations to pain and reversal of thermal sensations;
- Attacks of nervousness, anxiety and/ sweats (especially night time).
- Daily headache of a new type or pattern;
- Multi-joint pain (without redness or swelling);
- Recurrent sore throats and enlarged neck glands.

Some conditions are more frequently associated with CFS/ME. These are: new onset asthma or allergy; chest pain (cardiologic syndrome X); Gilbert's disease; idiopathic cyclic oedema (in women); or new onset alcohol intolerance.

What are the causes?
The cause of ME is unknown. However, neither depression nor physical deconditioning causes CFS/ME. There is also little evidence that the symptoms of CFS/ME are due to any persistent viral or bacterial infection. Chronic fatigue is a complex symptom and is probably best understood as the combined outcome of physical, neuropsychological and cognitive changes induced by the primary disease process (for example, viral infection).

How is it diagnosed?

A diagnosis of CFS/ME cannot be made in the presence of the following primary diagnoses: major depression; somatoform disorders; chronic viral infections (for example, chronic viral hepatitis or HIV infection); and known medical disorders of chronic fatigue (for example, post-polio fatigue, rheumatoid arthritis, anaemia, diabetes, thyroid disorder, sarcoidosis, systemic lupus, multiple sclerosis or cancer), substance abuse or withdrawal and eating disorders.

The diagnosis of CFS/ME is clinical and based on the exclusion of any other underlying medical or psychiatric condition that can sufficiently account for chronic fatigue. For research purposes, modified US Centers for disease Control criteria (1994) are commonly used to make a diagnosis of CFS. There is no specific or sensitive laboratory test for CFS/ME. The diagnosis is based on a combination of careful history taking, physical examination and, where indicated, a set of appropriate laboratory investigations to exclude other disorders of chronic fatigue.

How is it treated?

There is no pharmacologic or behavioural cure for CFS/ME. Pacing is the most effective strategy and offers the best approach to recovery in combination with symptomatic pharmacotherapy (such as that for sedation and muscle pain) and a flexible schedule of individualised physical and mental activity plan. The role of cognitive behaviour therapy in CFS/ME is debatable. Over-enthusiastic graded exercise therapy has been associated with worsening symptoms of muscle pain and fatigue. Immunological treatment (Ampligen or human immunoglobulin), steroid replacement (hydrocortisone and fludrocortisone), galantamine, antibiotics and antiviral drugs are generally not recommended. The cornerstone of management is still supportive and a positive outlook, pacing, attention to diet, avoidance of caffeinated drinks and a regular pattern of daily activity (physical as well as mental) are the best ingredients that aid recovery.

The clinical outcome in CFS/ME usually takes one of the three courses: complete recovery (more common in children but rare in adults), relapsing course (majority of adults) and permanent incapacity (approximately 25% of adult patients). Progressive and rapid deterioration of symptoms is highly uncharacteristic of CFS/ME.

The UK Royal College of Paediatrics and Child Health has published Evidence Based Guideline for the Management of CFS/ME (Chronic Fatigue Syndrome/ Myalgic Encephalopathy) in Children and Young People available from Web: http://www.rcpch.ac.uk/doc.aspx?id_Resource=1480 and a Young Person's Guide to CFS/ME which is available from Web: http://www.rcpch.ac.uk/doc. aspx?id_Resource=2013.

Inheritance patterns and prenatal diagnosis
Inheritance patterns
None known although cases involving more than one family member have been recognised.
Prenatal diagnosis
None available or required.

Medical text written October 2001 by Dr A Chaudhuri. **Last reviewed December 2007 by Dr A Chaudhuri, Consultant Neurologist, Essex Centre for Neurosciences, Queen's Hospital, Romford, UK.**

Support
ME (Myalgic Encephalomyelitis) Association
4 Top Angel, Buckingham Industrial Park, Buckingham MK18 1TH   Tel: 0870 444 1836
Fax: 01280 821602   e-mail: meconnect@meassociation.org.uk
Web: http://www.meassociation.org.uk
The ME Association is a National Registered Charity No 801279, established in 1976 which provides information and support to 240,000 people in the UK with ME/Chronic Fatigue Syndrome, their families and carers, through a quarterly magazine, literature, education and training. It also runs ME Connect, a helpline for people with ME/CFS. Through its Ramsay Research Fund, the charity supports research into the physical nature and causes of ME.
Group details last confirmed June 2007.

Action for M.E.
Third Floor, Canningford House, 38 Victoria Street, Bristol BS1 6BY
Tel: 0845 123 2314 Support Line   Tel: 0845 123 2380 Admin Lo-call line
Tel: 0117 927 9551 Admin   e-mail: admin@afme.org.uk   Web: http://www.afme.org.uk
Web: http://www.a4me.org.uk (for children and young people)
Action for M.E. is a National Registered Charity No. 1036419 working to improve the lives of people with M.E. It campaigns for more research, funding and services for people with M.E. It has a membership service which gives members access to a quarterly magazine 'InterAction', welfare rights helpline, and lending library. It produces a wide range of publications which are discounted to members. The Welfare Rights Helpline is available to members only. The telephone support line is available to non-members.
Group details last confirmed March 2007.

Association of Young People with ME
PO Box 5766, Milton Keynes MK10 1AQ   Tel: 08451 23 23 89   e-mail: info@ayme.org.uk
Web: http://www.ayme.org.uk
AYME is a National Registered Charity No. 1082059 providing information, advice and support across the UK to children and young people with ME aged 5-25 and their families. AYME publishes a free bi-monthly members' magazine "Cheers", a subscription news and research bulletin "Link" suitable for parents and professionals and an informative website. Membership and members services are free-of-charge there is a range of professional advisors from the medical, education, and child protection arenas. it's most popular services are the telephone helpline (local rate number) and their busy and informative website.
Group details last confirmed August 2007.

The Young ME Sufferers Trust (Tymes Trust)
PO Box 4347, Stock, Ingatestone CM4 9TE
Tel:0845 003 9002 (Advice Line: Mon-Fri, 11am-1pm & 5pm-7pm)
e-mail: access via the website   Web: http://www.tymestrust.org
The Trust is a National Registered Charity No.1080985 providing quality information and a personal approach for children and young people with ME, their families, doctors, teachers and other professionals. It is represented on the government Chief Medical Officer's Working Group on CFS/ME. It publishes a magazine available free of charge to those under 26 years old, and on subscription to those over 26. The Trust has a wide range of information available on their website at no charge. The Trust helps over 5,000 people per year.
Group details last updated August 2007.

"When our former organiser ceased running the group, it went into a period of decline. Thanks to Contact a Family, it is up and running. They empowered us, providing teleconferencing so the original members could make contact and locating a medical adviser interested in the condition. I cannot praise them enough." Group leader.

CHRONIC GRANULOMATOUS DISORDER

Background

Chronic Granulomatous Disorder (CGD) is a rare, inherited disorder of the immune system that affects 1 in 250,000 people. The basic defect lies in phagocytic cells which are made in the bone marrow (neutrophils and monocytes). These fail to effectively destroy certain invading bacteria and fungi.

What are the symptoms?

Affected individuals are susceptible to serious bacterial and fungal infection. They also experience symptoms associated with chronic inflammation, often granulomatous in nature.

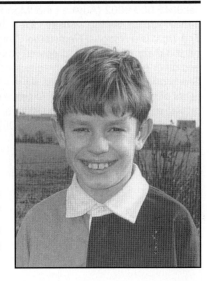

Infections may occur as abscesses in lymph glands. Other sites of infection include bones and joints, the liver, the bowels, the lungs and skin. However, individuals with the condition are able to combat viral infection normally.

How is it diagnosed?

CGD can be diagnosed by a simple blood test. If CGD is suspected it is important that referral is made to a specialist centre and diagnostic tests carried out in a laboratory that is familiar with doing these tests on a regular basis.

How is it treated?

Most CGD patients should be on daily antibacterial and antifungal prophylaxis (preventive drug therapy).

Bone marrow transplantation is a curative treatment option for some patients, but requires a fully matched donor. New treatments based on gene therapy are also being developed.

Early diagnosis and treatment of the symptoms with appropriate antibiotics as well as lifelong antibiotic and antifungal prophylaxis, has greatly mitigated the effects of this condition.

Inheritance patterns and prenatal diagnosis

Inheritance patterns

X-linked and autosomal recessive inheritance. Genetic advice is available.

Prenatal diagnosis

This is possible where the mother is a known carrier of the disease.

Contact a Family Helpline 0808 808 3555

Medical text written February 2006 by the CGD Research Trust. Approved February 2006 by Dr W Qasim, Specialist Registrar and Clinical Lecturer in Immunology, Institute of Child Health, London, UK.

Support

CGD Research Trust

Manor Farm, Wimborne St. Giles, Wimborne BH21 5NL   Tel: 01725 517977
e-mail: cgd@cgdrt.co.uk   Web: http://www.cgd.org.uk

The Trust is a National Registered Charity No. 1003425, established in 1991 to raise money and boost funds to find improved treatments and a cure for this rare genetic blood disorder, as well as to improve support services. It offers support and a point of contact between families. It funds a clinical nurse specialist based at Great Ormond Street Children's Hospital, London and it is about to employ a second specialist nurse based in the North of England. It is planning a clinical psychology service for families. The Trust runs conferences and workshops for health professionals and holds fun days and get-togethers for affected individuals and their families. It has twice yearly newsletters and has information available, details on request. The Trust is in touch with approximately 185 families. The CGD RT is the founder member of the annual Jeans for Genes Campaign. Group details last updated February 2007.

CHRONIC INFANTILE NEUROLOGIC CUTANEOUS AND ARTICULAR SYNDROME

Chronic infantile neurologic cutaneous and articular syndrome: CINCA; Neonatal Onset Multisystem Inflammatory Disease; NOMID

Background

Chronic infantile neurologic cutaneous and articular syndrome: CINCA; Neonatal Onset Multisystem Inflammatory Disease; NOMID

Chronic infantile neurologic cutaneous and articular syndrome (CINCA) is a severe chronic inflammatory disease starting shortly after birth. It is characterized by skin, central nervous system and joint problems with recurrent fever and inflammation. The syndrome progresses in a context of chronic inflammation with bouts of fever of varying intensity. The disease affects children of both sexes and all ethnic groups and was first described in 1987 by Dr A M Prieur and Dr C Griscelli. It is a rare condition but is becoming frequently more recognised by paediatricians.

What are the symptoms?

The main features of CINCA include:

- **Skin**. Persistent and migratory urticarial skin rashes (hives appearing in varying places) associated with infiltrates, are present, starting around birth;
- **Central nervous system**. Chronic meningitis (inflammation of the membranes covering the eyes) with headaches and seizures (see entry, Epilepsy) resulting in a progressive impairment and often leading to visual defects (see entry, Vision Disorders in Childhood) and perceptive deafness (see entry, Deafness);
- **Joints**. Recurrent joint flares with or without modifications of growth. A prominence of the knees is characteristic and is caused by overgrowth of the patella (knee cap) and distal (further part) femur.

Other features include:

- Eye inflammation, characteristic frontal bossing (protrusion of the forehead) and protruding eyes;
- Shortening of distal limbs giving rise to growth retardation;
- Muscle and tissue wasting.

How is it diagnosed?

CINCA is diagnosed by means of blood and spinal fluid tests together with x-rays to identify the bone effects of the disorder. Genetic analysis can be done but fifty per cent of the children do not have known genetic mutations.

Contact a Family Helpline 0808 808 3555

How is it treated?

Treatment for CINCA is symptomatic and supportive.

Inheritance patterns and prenatal diagnosis

Inheritance patterns

In most cases CINCA is sporadic but familial cases have been reported.

Prenatal diagnosis

None.

Medical text written January 2006 by Contact a Family. Approved January 2006 by Dr C Bredrup, Fellow in Ophthalmology, Institute of Child Health, London, UK.

Further online resources

Medical texts in *The Contact a Family Directory* are designed to give a short, clear description of specific conditions and rare disorders. More extensive information on this condition can be found on a range of reliable, validated websites. Further information on these resources can be found in our **Medical Information on the Internet** article on page 21.

Support

There is no support group for CINCA. Cross referrals to other entries in the Contact a Family Directory are intended to provide relevant support for these particular features of the disorder. Organisations identified in these entries do not provide support specifically for CINCA. Families can use Contact a Family's Freephone Helpline for advice, information and, where possible, links to other families. Contact a Family's web-based linking service MakingContact.org can be accessed at http://www.makingcontact.org

CLEFT LIP and/or PALATE

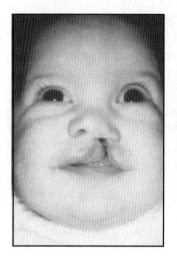 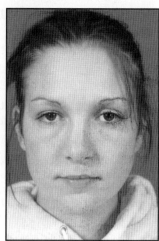

Background

A cleft of lip or palate occurs when there is a partial or total failure of the lip and palate to fuse during the early stages of pregnancy. Clefts may affect the lip (on one or both sides), the palate, or both. Surgery is carried out in the early weeks of life.

How is it treated?

Infants with clefts of the lip and/or palate should be referred to a recognised multi-disciplinary cleft team. Following the publication of the Clinical Standards Advisory Group report on cleft lip and/or palate in 1998, the number of cleft teams in the UK has been reduced. There are nine teams in England and Wales, one in Northern Ireland and three is Scotland and these new teams will provide comprehensive care from birth to maturity. Teams include surgeons, speech or language therapists, orthodontists, paediatricians and others. Early referral is encouraged.

Inheritance patterns and prenatal diagnosis

Inheritance patterns

Slight genetic predisposition. The risk of recurrence increases with the severity of the cleft, unless the condition is part of another inheritable syndrome.

Prenatal diagnosis

Clefts of the lip are often found on the eighteen to twenty week ultrasound during pregnancy. Referral should then be made to a cleft team for discussion.

Medical text written November 1991 by Contact a Family. Approved November 1991 by Professor M Patton, Professor of Medical Genetics, St Georges Hospital Medical School, London, UK and Dr J E Wraith, Consultant Paediatrician, Royal Manchester Children's Hospital, Manchester, UK. **Last updated November 2004 by Mr B Sommerlad, Consultant Plastic Surgeon, Cleft Lip and Palate Unit, Great Ormond Street Hospital, London, UK.**

Support

CLAPA

1st Floor, Green Man Tower, 332 Goswell Road, London EC1V 7LQ

Tel: 020 7833 4883

Fax: 020 7833 5999

e-mail: info@clapa.com

Web: http://www.clapa.com

The Association is a National Registered Charity No. 1108160, established in 1979. It offers local parent-to-parent support through a nationwide network of branches, a specialist service for parents and health professionals seeking help for feeding babies with clefts and encouragement and support of research into causes and treatment. It publishes an annual Newsletter and has information available, details on request. The organisation is in touch with approximately 7,000 people and has more than 40 groups and local contacts.

Group details last confirmed September 2007.

CLEIDOCRANIAL DYSOSTOSIS

Background

Cleidocranial Dysostosis is a condition characterised by varying degrees of hypoplasia (under-development) of membranous bones throughout the body, and is now regarded as a generalised skeletal dysplasia (disorder of bone growth affecting many bones in the body). It was first described by Marie and Sainton in 1898. The most significant and obvious abnormalities affect the head and face, although there is commonly involvement of many different bones.

What are the symptoms?

The seams between the skull bones, which are known as sutures, remain persistently open such that the vault of the skull continues to bulge (see entry, Craniofacial Conditions). This is part of the cause of the typical craniofacial deformity with micrognathia (small jaw), receding chin, narrow forehead, large anterior and posterior fontanelles (membranous junctions between the plates of the developing skull bone), and wide set bulging eyes.

The clavicles (collar bones) are commonly affected and may be malformed or completely absent This leads to an inward positioning of the shoulders and may result in difficulties with arm co-ordination. The pelvis may be involved, again being malformed, which, if severe, may result in difficulties with leg co-ordination. The middle bone of the fifth finger is commonly shorter than expected. The joints may be unusually flexible (hyperlaxity) leading to genu valgum (knock knees), again with resultant co-ordination difficulties. Vertebral (back bone) malformations may occur, and short stature is not uncommon.

There is significant involvement of tooth development affecting both baby and second dentition. The teeth are late to appear and develop, and are frequently misaligned or underdeveloped. The palate (roof of the mouth) may be affected, with a fissure (opening) through its midline, or there may be a high arched palate. This requires a specialised dental team approach to dental abnormality management with regular review to prevent and minimise oral deformity, and other complications, such as pain and decay.

Further complications of Cleidocranial Dysostosis which have been identified include upper respiratory (breathing) problems, sinus infections, recurrent otitis media (middle ear inflammation) and hearing loss. Therefore it has been recommended that a child with Cleidocranial Dysostosis should have a hearing evaluation at birth and regularly during childhood. They should also have medical and surgical evaluations for the consequences of delayed craniofacial development, including otitis, sinusitis and obstructive sleep apnoea (airflow restricted during sleep).

Although much is known about Cleidocranial Dysostosis, its various physical presentations and their managements, little has been written in relation to cognitive, emotional and behavioural consequences of having the condition. The developmental pathway of intelligence in Cleidocranial Dysostosis is inadequately documented, unlike other genetic syndromes e.g. Down syndrome, Prader-Willi syndrome, Williams syndrome and Fragile X syndrome (see entries), but there has been an acknowledgement and reporting of the existence of co-morbid intellectual (learning) difficulties. However the extent of the disability using standardised testing has not been quantified, and certainly, to our knowledge, the potential change in disability over time has not been examined. It is also not known whether Cleidocranial Dysostosis is more commonly associated with other developmental difficulties and delays, such as Attention Deficit Hyperactivity Disorder (see entry), but this may come to light in time.

Inheritance patterns and prenatal diagnosis
Inheritance patterns
Numerous genetic studies have concluded that inheritance is autosomal dominant and the Cleidocranial Dysostosis gene has been assigned to a locus (position) on the short arm of chromosome 6 (6p21).

Medical text written October 2003 by Dr H McBrien, Consultant Child and Adolescent Psychiatrist, Adolescent Outreach Service, Tottenham, London, UK.

Support
There is no support group for Cleidocranial Dysostosis in the UK. Cross referrals to other entries in The Contact a Family Directory are intended to provide relevant support for these particular features of the disorder. Organisations identified in these entries do not provide support specifically for Cleidocranial Dysostosis. Families can use Contact a Family's Freephone Helpline for advice, information and, where possible, links to other families. Contact a Family's web-based linking service Making Contact.org can be accessed at http://www.makingcontact.org

COATS DISEASE

Coats disease: Exudative retinopathy; Coats' retinitis; exudative retinitis; morbus Coats'

Background

Coats disease was first described by George Coats in 1908. The disease is an uncommon form of retinal telangiectasia. It is characterised by congenital dilation (widening) and malformation of the retinal capillaries (tiny blood vessels), usually in one eye. It is a progressive condition most often seen in boys before the age of ten. It may be severe.

What are the symptoms?

The symptoms of the disease can vary although strabismus (an eye turn or squint), leukocoria (white pupil), extensive exudative retinitis (fluid in the retina) and a reduction in either the central or peripheral (side) vision may be seen. Glaucoma may present with pain and loss of appetite.

What are the causes?

Currently there is no known cause. Coats disease is a blanket term used to describe a number of different types of retinal vascular disorder leading to the same final common clinical pathway.

The retina is the light-sensitive screen which lines the back of the eye. Light reaching the retina is converted into electric impulses which are transmitted to the brain via the optic nerve and converted to sight. The retinal capillaries carry blood, rich with oxygen and nutrients, to the retina. In Coats disease these capillaries exhibit localised dilation leading to leakage caused by an increase in permeability of the capillary walls and, occasionally, to haemorrhage (bleeding from ruptured blood vessels). This results in an accumulation of yellowish or white fluid (exudate) at the back of the eye that may extend to the macula (the centre of the retina). The accumulation of exudate can lead to impaired macular function and, in the worst cases, retinal detachment and complete, or near complete, loss of vision in the affected eye. Occasionally, a severe form of glaucoma may follow prolonged retinal detachment.

How is it diagnosed?

The diagnosis may be confirmed by examination of the back of the eye using an ophthalmoscope, aided by ultrasound examination and, occasionally, by angiography in which a dye is injected into the eye so that the structure of the capillaries can be better seen and photos can be taken to observe the retinal circulation.

How is it treated?

If caught early, treatment may stop the progression of the disease. Treatment can involve surgery using laser light (photocoagulation) or extreme cold (cryotherapy) to close the leaking blood vessels. If successful, the exudates may absorb over many months and retinal detachment may be prevented. If untreated there is a danger of progressive retinal detachment and loss of sight. Complete recovery of the retina is rare and, when it occurs, usually takes too long to prevent the eye becoming permanently amblyopic (lazy). Glaucoma is common in advanced cases. It can often be treated successfully with laser with preservation of the eye though not of vision. Occasionally, advanced glaucoma is resistant to treatment and warrants removal of the eye.

Inheritance patterns and prenatal diagnosis

Inheritance patterns

Usually sporadic (with no other affected family members).

Prenatal diagnosis

None.

Medical text written January 2007 by Contact a Family. Approved January 2007 by Mr John Hungerford, Consultant Ophthalmic Surgeon, St Bartholomew's Hospital and Moorfields Eye Hospital, London, UK.

Support

There is no support group for Coats disease. Cross referrals to other entries in The Contact a Family Directory are intended to provide relevant support for these particular features of the disorder. Organisations identified in these entries do not provide support specifically for Coats disease. Families can use Contact a Family's Freephone Helpline for advice, information and, where possible, links to other families. Contact a Family's web-based linking service Making Contact.org can be accessed at http://www.makingcontact.org

COCKAYNE SYNDROME

Background

This syndrome was described in 1936. In its classical form it presents with premature ageing and neurological deterioration.

The age of the onset of symptoms and the progression of the disease is variable. The early onset cases overlap with COFS (Cerebro-Oculo-Facio-Skeletal) syndrome.

What are the symptoms?

The facial features show progressive ageing with thinning of the skin, deep sunken eyes, hair loss and dental decay. There may be loss of motor and intellectual skills with changes in the white matter of brain (leukodystrophy) on an MRI brain scan. Deafness (see entry) and visual problems due to retinitis pigmentosa (see entry) will develop. The bones show thinning and the back becomes curved and there will be joint contractures.

One of the hallmarks of the syndrome is sensitivity to the sun leading to blistering and excessive reddening of the skin. This has lead to the recognition that in Cockayne syndrome ultra violet (UV) light can cause damage to the DNA.

What are the causes?

The underlying cause is known to be a defect in the enzymes that repair DNA after UV damage. There are several different enzymes involved and the diagnosis of the specific enzyme depends on cellular studies carried out from the cells grown from a skin biopsy (fibroblasts). This is carried out in highly specialised laboratories.

How is it treated?

The sun sensitivity can be reduced by avoiding exposure to UV light and the use of sun block creams. However, there is no treatment for the progressive neurological degeneration.

Inheritance patterns and prenatal diagnosis

Inheritance patterns

The disorder is inherited as an autosomal recessive trait. Clinical features are likely to be similar for affected children within the family but there may be considerable variation in the severity of this disorder between different families.

Prenatal diagnosis

This is available after the skin biopsy studies have been completed and the causative enzyme deficiency identified.

Medical text written February 2002 by Professor M Patton, **Last reviewed September 2007 by Professor M Patton, Professor of Medical Genetics, St. George's Hospital Medical School, London, UK**

Further online resources

Medical texts in *The Contact a Family Directory* are designed to give a short, clear description of specific conditions and rare disorders. More extensive information on this condition can be found on a range of reliable, validated websites. Further information on these resources can be found in our **Medical Information on the Internet** article on page 21.

Support

While there is no specific support group in the UK for this condition, information is available from Climb (see entry, Metabolic diseases) and support is available from a group of families under the umbrella of Climb.

A donation of £20 a month with Gift Aid would enable us to give detailed advice to ten families each year. A donation form is on page 1088

COELIAC DISEASE

Background

Coeliac disease affects the small intestine and is due to a sensitivity to gluten, which is a protein found in wheat. Similar proteins are found in rye, barley and, to a much smaller extent, oats.

Dermatitis Herpetiformis is an itchy skin rash which usually occurs on the elbows, buttocks and knees, although any area of skin may be affected. The condition is due to sensitivity to gluten and patients usually also have a small intestinal abnormality similar to that in coeliac disease. Dermatitis herpetiformis is rare, the prevalence being approximately 1 in 10,000 people. It is particularly rare in children.

What are the symptoms?

Symptoms may occur at any age and may include weight loss, vomiting and diarrhoea. Many patients, however, may have mild, long-standing, non-gastrointestinal symptoms such as tiredness, lethargy and breathlessness. A baby predisposed to coeliac disease could, after the introduction of gluten-containing solids, develop pale, bulky, offensive smelling stools, and become miserable, lethargic and generally fail to thrive.

How is it diagnosed?

The condition is diagnosed by means of an endoscopic small intestinal biopsy where the mucosal lining of the small intestine is seen to be damaged by inflammation, presumed to be a result of a reaction to the gluten in the diet. There is now a reasonably accurate blood test available for screening.

How is it treated?

Coeliac disease is treated with a gluten-free diet, which allows the mucosal lining to heal and return towards normal. Screening suggests that the prevalence of the disease in the general population may be as high as 1 in 100, but many cases often go undiagnosed so that the number of diagnosed cases is approximately 1 in 1,000.

Inheritance patterns and prenatal diagnosis

Inheritance patterns

Coeliac disease, though not inherited directly, does tend to run in families, there being a 1 in 10 chance of having an affected relative.

Prenatal diagnosis

None

Medical text written January 1995 by the Coeliac Society. Approved January 1995 by Dr P Howdle. **Last updated January 2004 by Professor P Howdle, Consultant Physician and Gastroenterologist, St James's University Hospital, Leeds, UK.**

Contact a Family Helpline 0808 808 3555

Support

Coeliac UK

Suites A-D, Octagon Court, High Wycombe HP11 2HS   Tel: 0870 444 8804 Helpline
Tel: 01494 437278 Office   Fax: 01494 474349   e-mail: adminsec@coeliac.org.uk
Web: http://www.coeliac.org.uk

Coeliac UK is a National Registered Charity No. 1048167, established in 1968. It offers advice on coping with a gluten-free diet and has a network of regional support groups. It funds research into Coeliac disease and Dermatitis Herpetiformis. It publishes a quarterly Magazine 'Crossed Grain' (free to members) and has a wide range of information available, details on request. Coeliac UK responds to the estimated 42,000 people in the UK with Coeliac disease.

Group details last updated March 2007.

"Children need to interact with other local children to ensure that they are part of their local community. Children with rare disorders feel isolated in many, many ways. You can help by positively encouraging children to attend your activities. Be pro-active and seek out these families – don't rely on them coming to you." Rare Matters. Contact a Family. 2004

COFFIN-LOWRY SYNDROME

Background
Coffin-Lowry syndrome (CLS) is a rare inherited disorder of craniofacial and skeletal abnormalities, short stature and learning disability. It was described separately by Dr G S Coffin in 1966 and by Dr R B Lowry in 1971. In 1975 the two descriptions were recognised as the same disorder and named Coffin-Lowry syndrome. CLS affects both males and females.

What are the symptoms?
CLS is characterised by a number of features some of which, to a greater or lesser degree of severity, are present in affected individuals, with females likely to be less severely affected. Manifestations include:
- Significant learning delay (see entry, Learning Disability);
- Mild to moderate restricted growth (see entry, Restricted Growth);
- Speech problems (see entry, Speech and Language Impairment);
- Facial features that may include abnormally prominent brow, unusually thick eyebrows, down slanting palpebral fissures (eyelid folds), hypertelorism (widely spaced eyes), a broad nose, protruding (nares) nostrils, maxillary hypoplasia (an underdeveloped upper jaw bone) and large ears;
- Progressive coarsening of the facial features;
- 'Puffy' hands and feet with tapering digits;
- Kyphoscoliosis (backward and lateral curvature of the spine) (see entry, Scoliosis);
- Stimulus-induced drop attacks (episodes of interruption to the cerebral (brain) blood flow affecting the balance and causing the individual to fall) affecting ten to twenty per cent of children and adolescents.

Although no clear pattern of behavioural or psychological features relating to CLS has been established, people with the syndrome seem to have a higher incidence of psychiatric difficulties.

What are the causes?
CLS is caused by a defective gene, RSK2, on the X chromosome (Xp22.2-p22.1). It is not clear how mutations (changes) in the DNA structure of the gene lead to the manifestations of the disorder.

How is it diagnosed?
CLS can be diagnosed due to the existence of learning disability, together with characteristic craniofacial and hand abnormalities. Molecular genetic testing of the RSK2 gene can confirm the diagnosis but mutations are only found in approximately fifty per cent of cases.

How is it treated?

Treatment of CLS is symptomatic including physiotherapy and speech therapy to improve the affected individual's abilities.

Inheritance patterns and prenatal diagnosis

Inheritance patterns

CLS is X-linked dominant. Carrier females are at risk of some learning disability and the physical features of the syndrome.

Prenatal diagnosis

This is possible where it is already known that there is an affected family member in whom a mutation has been identified. Alternatively, linkage analysis (a technique that traces patterns of heredity in at risk families, in an attempt to locate a disease-causing gene mutation by identifying traits that are co-inherited with it) can be used.

Medical text written August 2004 by Contact a Family. Approved August 2004 by Professor I Young, Department of Clinical Genetics, Leicester Royal Infirmary, Leicester, UK.

Further online resources

Medical texts in *The Contact a Family Directory* are designed to give a short, clear description of specific conditions and rare disorders. More extensive information on this condition can be found on a range of reliable, validated websites. Further information on these resources can be found in our **Medical Information on the Internet** article on page 21.

Support

While there is no specific support group in the UK for this condition, information is available from Climb (see entry, Metabolic diseases) and support is available from a group of families under the umbrella of Climb.

COHEN SYNDROME

Background

Cohen syndrome is a rare genetic disorder characterised by typical facial features including a smaller than average head, characteristic 'wave-shaped' eyes and a short upper lip which reveals the central teeth (incisors). The palate is often quite high and narrow.

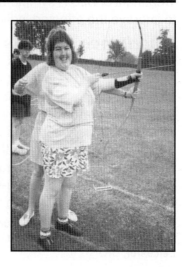

What are the symptoms?

From mid childhood onwards, there is a tendency for people with Cohen syndrome to develop obesity, most often around the trunk. The limbs, however, remain slender and the hands and feet are often small and tapering. Low muscle tone is common in Cohen syndrome and the joints are usually over extendible. Moderate learning difficulties are also a feature. Other features associated with the condition include eye problems such as short sight, poor night vision or changes on the retina at the back of the eye. A low white blood cell count may also be present, although this does not often cause any symptoms. The signs and symptoms of Cohen syndrome are variable from one person to another.

Inheritance patterns and prenatal diagnosis

Inheritance patterns

Autosomal recessive. The gene for Cohen syndrome, COH1 has now been identified and lies on chromosome 8. Changes within this gene have been found in many affected individuals.

Prenatal diagnosis

Prenatal diagnosis is possible in those families where a gene change has been identified.

Medical text written April 2000 by Dr J Clayton-Smith. **Last updated October 2005 by Dr J Clayton-Smith, Consultant Clinical Geneticist, St Mary's Hospital, Manchester, UK.**

Further online resources

Medical texts in *The Contact a Family Directory* are designed to give a short, clear description of specific conditions and rare disorders. More extensive information on this condition can be found on a range of reliable, validated websites. Further information on these resources can be found in our **Medical Information on the Internet** article on page 21.

Support

The support group for Cohen Syndrome is currently in abeyance. Families can use Contact a Family's Freephone Helpline for advice, information and, where possible, links to other families. Contact a Family's web-based linking service Making Contact.org can be accessed at http://www.makingcontact.org

COLOBOMA

Background

Coloboma means that there is a gap, or cleft, in one of the structures of the eye. This is the results of congenital malformation, with a portion of the eye failing to complete its growth and fuse together, so leaving a cleft. Different parts of the eye may be affected, including the lens, choroid and optic nerve, although the iris is most commonly involved, giving a keyhole shaped pupil.

What are the symptoms?

Vision may or may not be affected depending on the part of the eye involved. Coloboma may be unilateral (on one side) or bilateral (on both sides) and if bilateral, can be quite asymmetrical. It may be an isolated ocular finding or may be associated with other eye defects, such as Microphthalmia (small eye, see entry Anophthalmia) in the same or opposite eye and, extremely rarely, Anophthalmia (absent eye, see entry) in the opposite eye.

Inheritance patterns and prenatal diagnosis

Inheritance patterns

Coloboma may be isolated or associated with other systemic findings, or specific genetic disorders. The occurrence of Coloboma may be sporadic (with no other associated family members), or may be inherited. A few genes have been identified that give rise to isolated ocular Colobomas either with or without Microphthalmia. Dominant mutations in PAX2 and PAX6 cause optic nerve Colobomas, in the MAF gene result in iris Coloboma and in the SHH gene cause Coloboma and Microphthalmia. Further genes may have been identified in the case where Colobomas are part of a recognised syndrome.

Prenatal diagnosis

High resolution ultrasound or fetoscopy (observation of the fetus by introduction of a stethoscope through a small incision into the abdomen under local anaesthetic) could provide details of the fetal eye in the second trimester.

Genetic counselling is available in cases of specific genetic disorder, in familial cases of Coloboma, or if requested for isolated Coloboma. At present, genetic testing for isolated Coloboma is only carried out on a research basis.

Medical text written October 2004 by Miss Nicola Ragge MD FRCOphth FRCPCH, Honorary Consultant Ophthalmic Surgeon, Moorfields Eye Hospital, London, UK and Birmingham Children's Hospital, Birmingham, UK and Senior Surgical Scientist, University of Oxford, Oxford, UK.

Support

Coloboma is one of the eye conditions covered by M.A.C.S. (Micro & Anophthalmic Children's Society). Support and information is available from M.A.C.S. (see entry, Anophthalmia).

Contact a Family's web-based linking service, www.makingcontact.org which enables families with disabled children to link with one another across the world electronically, now has over 5,000 members

---

CONDUCT DISORDER and OPPOSITIONAL DEFIANT DISORDER

Background

Managing tantrums, arguments and other difficult behaviours in children and young people is a common experience for parents. However, for about five per cent of children their negative behaviour is severe, persistent and enormously challenging for parents and teachers. Family relationships become strained and school progress may be affected. Conduct disorder and Oppositional Defiant disorder (ODD) are the diagnostic terms for those types of long lasting, aggressive and defiant behaviours that are extreme and outside the range of normal.

These problems are more common in boys and may start at a very young age. Some children grow out of them but some do not. Those who have persistent problems are at risk of poor social functioning as adults and social exclusion. Antisocial behaviour at the age of ten years predicts increased use of services such as special educational provision, the criminal justice system, foster and other residential care and state benefits. Most young people with these severe behaviours leave school with no qualifications, a third become recurrent juvenile offenders and problems continue into adulthood.

Children who show such behaviours at a very early age (around two to three years) often have other problems such as a difficult temperament, hyperactivity and Attention Deficit Hyperactivity disorder (ADHD) (see entry), language disorders, some degree of learning disability and specific learning problems with reading. They often live in a family environment that leads to harsh, inconsistent and critical parenting. In contrast, behaviours that appear for the first time in adolescence are less likely to be associated with other problems and seem to be more influenced by environmental factors.

Some young people with difficult behaviour are depressed and may be using illicit substances. Self-esteem is often low despite the superficial appearance of bravado.

Parents understandably tend to end up stressed by their child's provocative and difficult behaviour but may unintentionally worsen it by giving attention (such as by shouting, smacking or other negative reactions) rather than ignoring it. Positive, co-operative behaviour in their child then becomes less and less likely as it is not rewarded with attention.

How is it diagnosed?

The International Classification of Diseases, 10th revision (ICD-10) describes Conduct disorder as including many of the following: severe fighting, aggressiveness, bullying, cruelty to animals or other people, theft, fire setting, severe destruction of property, persistent and severe lying, truancy from school, severe disobedience or extreme or very frequent tantrums. These behaviours must have persisted for six months or more.

Oppositional Defiant disorder

Oppositional Defiant disorder (ODD) is the term usually reserved for less severe, but equally persistent conduct problems in younger children. It describes behaviours such as aggression, defiance and disobedience rather than those that are severely antisocial or against the law. Children with ODD frequently defy adults, deliberately annoy people and seem angry and resentful. They may blame others for things that they themselves have done and will not take responsibility for their behaviour. They may be very provocative and rude, especially to those in authority.

How is it treated?

There are effective ways to treat Conduct disorder and ODD in younger children. Programmes aimed at teaching parents how to manage the difficult behaviours are effective if they provide specific behaviour management skills and they may be combined with social skills programmes for children. One example of such a well-evaluated and effective parenting programme is the Incredible Years Parenting Program, developed by Carolyn Webster Stratton. She has also developed Dinosaur School, a programme for children run in schools. The UK government has targeted services to reduce antisocial behaviour in areas of the country at most risk. Such initiatives include Sure Start programmes aimed at families with children up to the age of three years and On Track aimed at preventing antisocial behaviour in four to twelve year olds.

In contrast to parenting programmes for younger children, parenting programmes for antisocial behaviour in adolescence, on their own, have been less effective. Packages of help for the young person are usually required, involving individual, family and parenting interventions.

Parents and teachers can do a great deal to reduce negative and antisocial behaviour in children. It is important to play with children regularly in a warm, non-directive and interested way. Praise, verbal and through hugs and affectionate touches, are important to encourage positive behaviours. Instructions and commands given to children should be clear and specific. It is important to set limits and stick to these in a calm and predictable manner. These positive parenting strategies are helpful if used consistently from an early age and can help reduce antisocial behaviours in older children.

Medical text written October 2003 by Dr A York, Child and Adolescent Psyachiatrist, Child and Family Consultation Centre, Richmond, London, UK.

Support

Advice and information on Conduct Disorders and Oppositional Defiant Disorder for parents and professionals can be obtained from Young Minds (see entry, Mental Health).

For help with setting up or developing a local or national support group, phone the Contact a Family group development team on 020 7608 8700.

CONGENITAL ABSENCE OF THE TESTES

Congenital absence of the testes: Anorchia

Background

Congenital absence of the testes (anorchia) is a very rare condition with most paediatric endocrine specialists seeing only two or three boys at any particular time.

Although the testes are absent the male external genitalia is otherwise normal. This suggests that there was normal testicular function in early fetal life and normal male differentiation took place. The testes are presumed, therefore, to have regressed for some reason. Torsion of the testes (twisting) in fetal life has been suggested as a cause.

Boys may also present with rudimentary non-functioning testes, palpable in the scrotum. This is quite a different condition from anorchia. The importance of making sure that there is no testosterone response to a stimulus is firstly to document that the diagnosis is correct and secondly to make sure that there is no testicular tissue present. Testes may be absent from the scrotum but may be present within the abdomen which is where they come from in fetal life. It is important to look for a male sex hormone (testosterone) response. If present, the testicular tissue needs to be found because of the potential for development of malignancy within the tissue remnant.

What are the causes?

No defect in the genes which regulate male development has been documented so far in these patients. Ischaemic necrosis (tissue deterioration due to poor blood supply) during descent of the testes is thought to be the more common cause for anorchia. This occurs during testicular migration when the testis is mobile and vulnerable to torsion.

How is it diagnosed?

The boys often present because the parents have noticed that the bag in which the testes sit (the scrotum) is poorly developed or else their attention may be directed to the problem by some other event, for example, the presence of a hernia. It is often during the exploration and repair of herniae that the problem first comes to light. A number of blood tests are usually conducted at this stage to show that there is no male sex hormone production from the gonad. At the same time a blood sample is often taken to make absolutely sure that the genetic make up of the individual is male.

How is it treated?

In the long term the boys will need male sex hormone replacement. The introduction of testosterone pre-pubertally would need some age limitations. The defined onset of puberty in males occurs around the age of eleven and a half years. As a result, a very low dose of testosterone could be given at around ten years of age gradually increasing the dosage schedule. This would in part mimic the changes that occur in normal boys. In adulthood, testosterone preparations can be used as capsules, intramuscular injections, skin patches, subcutaneous pellets, gel or cream. Testicular prostheses should be considered pre-pubertally to overcome psychological problems related to anorchia.

Inheritance patterns and prenatal diagnosis
Inheritance patterns
None
Prenatal diagnosis
None

Medical text written August 1995 by Dr P Hindmarsh. Last updated November 2001 by Dr P Hindmarsh. **Last reviewed September 2005 by Professor P Hindmarsh, Professor of Paediatric Endocrinology, Middlesex Hospital, London, UK.**

Support
Anorchidism Support Group
PO Box 3025, Romford RM3 8GX   Tel: 01708 372597 (Mon-Sat, 9am-5pm)
e-mail: asg.uk@virgin.net   Web: http://freespace.virgin.net/asg.uk
This is a very small support group, established in 1995. It offers support by telephone, letter and e-mail for families and affected persons and attempts to link families if requested. It publishes a newsletter twice a year and has information available, details on request. The Group is in touch with over 100 families in the UK and abroad.
Group details last updated October 2007.

CONGENITAL ADRENAL HYPERPLASIA

Congenital Adrenal Hyperplasia: CAH

Background

Congenital Adrenal Hyperplasia is the name given to a group of enzyme disorders causing impaired production of cortisol (hydrocortisone) from the adrenal glands. By far the commonest type of CAH is 21 hydroxylase deficiency which occurs in roughly 1in 15,000 births. Production of cortisol and the salt-retaining steroid aldosterone is impaired but the androgen pathway (which produces the male hormone testosterone) is intact. The brain, sensing the low levels of cortisol, produces large amounts of adrenocorticotrophin hormone (ACTH) which stimulates the adrenal glands and causes enlargement (hyperplasia). Because of the enzyme block ACTH stimulation cannot normalise cortisol levels and instead results in over-production of androgen.

What are the symptoms?

The clinical presentation of 21 hydroxylase deficiency depends on the severity of the enzyme defect and the sex of the child. Boys with a severe defect will present at about ten days of age with vomiting, dehydration, and weight loss - the salt-losing crisis. Girls with a severe defect will have ambiguous genitalia at birth due to the effect of androgen over production in the fetus. Unless treated promptly these girls will also develop a salt-losing crisis. Boys and girls with a mild defect will present later in childhood with signs of androgen excess - tall stature, enlargement of penis or clitoris, and pubic hair - but no manifest salt loss.

How is it treated?

Children

Treatment consists of surgery in girls to reduce the size of the clitoris and open up the lower end of the vagina. Both sexes require hydrocortisone to suppress ACTH secretion and thus switch off androgen production, fludrocortisone to replace aldosterone and (during the first year of life) salt supplements.

The dose of hydrocortisone has to be carefully adjusted since under-treatment will result in over-production of androgen with excessive growth and virilisation, while over-treatment will cause slow growth and obesity. By adjusting the dose of hydrocortisone against the child's size, growth rate, skeletal maturity ('bone age') and adrenal steroid levels the treatment can be optimised and the general health of these children is good. It is important for parents to learn how to increase the hydrocortisone dose during acute illness, so as to mimic the normal cortisol response to stress. In particular, there is a need for an emergency regimen of hydrocortisone injection and salt replacement in severe illness.

Adults

The management of Congenital Adrenal Hyperplasia is very similar in adults. Treatment needs to be continued in men, particularly for them to maintain fertility. Women may have problems with excessive hair growth which requires specific treatment. It is important to have an assessment of their genitalia and vagina and additional surgery or non-surgical dilatation treatment may be need for comfortable sexual intercourse. Polycystic ovarian syndrome has an increased incidence and probably accounts for the increased risk of infertility. However, the infertility can usually be treated. There are several UK centres offering specialist Congenital Adrenal Hyperplasia clinics for adults.

Inheritance patterns and prenatal diagnosis

Inheritance patterns

Autosomal recessive.

Prenatal diagnosis

Once an affected child has been diagnosed, genetic testing can be carried out on the parents and patient. Diagnosis can then be done in the fetus by chorionic villus sampling (CVS) at nine to ten weeks gestation. If the mother starts taking the potent steroid dexamethasone as soon as she knows she is pregnant (ideally at four to six weeks gestation) virilisation in an affected female fetus will be prevented or greatly diminished. If CVS at nine to ten weeks shows that the fetus is an unaffected female, or a male (affected or not) then dexamethasone treatment is stopped. Prenatal dexamethasone treatment is controversial because it means exposing (on average) eight fetuses to steroids when only one will benefit. Dexamethasone can cause weight gain and striae (stretch marks) in the mother while the long-term effects of prenatal treatment on the child are unknown. However, the adverse effects of prenatal virilisation are all too well known and prevention is of enormous benefit to the individual concerned.

Medical text written August 1996 by Dr M Donaldson, Senior Lecturer in Child Health, Royal Hospital for Sick Children, Glasgow, UK and Dr R Stanhope. Material on Adults written October 2002 by Dr R Stanhope. **Last updated August 2006 by Dr R Stanhope, Consultant Paediatric Endocrinologist, Great Ormond Street Hospital, London, UK.**

Further online resources

Medical texts in *The Contact a Family Directory* are designed to give a short, clear description of specific conditions and rare disorders. More extensive information on this condition can be found on a range of reliable, validated websites. Further information on these resources can be found in our **Medical Information on the Internet** article on page 21.

Support

CAH Group (Climb)

2 Windrush Close, Flitwick, Bedford MK45 1PX   Tel: 01525 717536
e-mail: webmaster@cah.org.uk   Web: http://www.cah.org.uk
This is a self help group, established in 1993 under the umbrella of Climb which is a National Registered Charity No. 1089588. It offers support by telephone, e-mail and letter and organises home visits where possible. It publishes a quarterly newsletter and a free information pack is available on request. A national conference is held biennially and smaller local meetings are also arranged throughout the country at varying intervals. The Group has over 500 members including professional workers from the UK and overseas. Group details last confirmed February 2007.

Adrenal Hyperplasia Network

c/o 17 Newton Road, Lichfield WS13 7EF   Tel: 01543 252 961   Fax: 01543 411 761
e-mail: webmaster@ahn.org.uk   Web: http://www.ahn.org.uk
The Network is a support organisation, established in February 1999 primarily for adults and teenagers although it can cover all ages. It offers support by letter and e-mail and contact with others with Congenital Adrenal Hyperplasia. Support for research and research clinicians is a major part of AHN's work. Presentations given to medical conferences and medical study days on request. It has a website and has information available, details on request. Aims to improve treatment via liaison with clinicians, researchers, nurses, GP's, NHS, and Dept of Health and by raising awareness in society. Group details last updated July 2007.

CONGENITAL AND ACQUIRED BRAIN DAMAGE AND DYSFUNCTION IN CHILDHOOD

Background

The relationships between problems of learning, behaviour, epilepsy and motor function in children and the underlying disease in their brain are complex. Broadly speaking, there are three patterns that are recognised:

- Congenital, i.e. present from before birth;
- Acquired acutely, i.e. resulting from a sudden onset;
- Acquired slowly and progressively.

It is however the exceptions that tend to detain us and require explanation. Within each group there are conditions in which there is clear evidence of damage to the brain on imaging and others in which no such damage is evident and are perhaps better regarded as examples of brain dysfunction. The time of birth is arbitrary and acquired, acute and chronic processes may start before birth and this needs to be remembered both for children with problems from birth and at birth.

Even when we are sure that damage to the brain is static, there may be apparent deterioration in the child. Four examples of this are:

- Damage to the cerebral cortex may cause epilepsy (see entry) which because of either the severity of the attacks or an associated loss of cognitive function (epileptic encephalopathy) may resemble a progressive disease;
- A behaviour disorder may occur in a child who had not previously shown such problems, without any change in the underlying brain damage but the family perception of the child may change enormously;
- A problem may be revealed, like language disorder and specific reading difficulty, at the developmental stage at which it would have been expected, e.g. the developmental progress of many children with Down syndrome (see entry) appears faster in the first six to eight months than later when major difficulties with language may occur;
- In athetoid cerebral palsy, where there is damage to the basal ganglia, there may be an early phase of lack of movement with increasingly wild extra movements appearing during the latter part of the first and the second year.

Thus some children with non-progressive brain disease may look much more normal when young than later.

If we therefore look at each category and specific examples, some of the problems of definition come into focus and some conditions, which do not fit these simple schemata, can be illustrated. This structure forms the basis along which paediatric neurologists, paediatricians and geneticists work, to provide a diagnosis.

Congenital and acquired disorders

Congenital disorders i.e. present before birth

This broad category includes the following:

- Early genetic defects with fixed effects such as chromosome abnormalities, primary microcephaly, Prader Willi and Angelman syndromes (see entries) although in the latter plateauing or deterioration in development may occur with epilepsy;
- Acute intrauterine events such as the early death of a twin with damage to the surviving fetus, a stroke causing hemiplegia, an early lack of blood supply causing damage to selective areas, for example perisylvian polymicrogyria and some children with Worster-Drought syndrome (see entry). Intrauterine infection with Rubella (see entry), cytomegalovirus (CMV) and toxoplasmosis (see entries) come into this group but occasionally these may constitute a more long-term progressive illness, even going into extrauterine life, for example HIV (see entry HIV infection and AIDS) and some cases of CMV;
- Chronic intrauterine events such as Fetal Alcohol Spectrum disorder (see entry), anti-epileptic drugs, or maternal diabetes;
- Progressive diseases with intrauterine onset such as some peroxisomal disorders (Zellwegers syndrome), early spinal muscular atrophy (see entry) and Menkes disease, where although dysmorphic or motor abnormalities are present at birth the condition progresses, i.e. the child loses skills.

Acquired acutely in the perinatal period

This group includes the disorders that follow birth asphyxia, markedly pre-term birth, perinatal infection and haemorrhage i.e. causing a proportion of the cerebral palsies (see entry). It must however be emphasised that more causes of cerebral palsy are attributable to prenatal events and these causes are usually not identified. The conclusion that there was brain damage at the time of birth is often a very difficult one to be sure of. Quite often when a baby has prenatal abnormalities they will be associated with malpresentation and the baby may be in poor condition at birth, for example babies with dystrophia myotonica (see entry, Myotonic Dystrophy), with weak neck muscles, may produce a brow presentation which may cause a slow and difficult delivery.

In both congenital disorders and those acquired acutely in the perinatal period, the family predicament includes having to manage the sadness of not having the child they expected and also having to face uncertainties of diagnosis, prognosis and service provision.

Acquired acutely in childhood

This section includes children who suffer brain damage caused by meningitis, encephalitis (see entries), head injury (see entry, brain injury), lack of blood supply during and acute illness, very severe epilepsy, acute metabolic diseases and stroke (see entries). This group of disorders is relatively straightforward to diagnose, with a period of normal development, an acute illness with dramatic loss of skills and a slow process of recovery with varying degrees of residual impairments. Occasionally epilepsy may mimic such a process and infantile spasms and Lennox-Gastaut syndrome may present acutely with regression that resembles an acute encephalitic illness but in such illnesses there may or may not be evidence of brain damage on a scan. If there is, it will not change, despite what may be a dramatic change in the child's level and style of functioning.

The parental predicaments in this situation include:
- 'loss' of the child that they remember;
- uncertainty of the future;
- lack of facilities for rehabilitation;
- a changing pattern of impairments and skills that seem not to be educationally convenient;
- a mixed group of motor, cognitive and behavioural impairments, quite often with epilepsy and a lack of behavioural/mental health services that are experienced in either acute brain illnesses or multiple impairment;
- quite often there is a feeling of guilt and/or anger about the possible preventability of the acute illness.

In all of the above situations it is important to emphasise that scans of the brain, now mostly MRI scans, are much more helpful in leading to a cause, i.e. a diagnosis, than in predicting outcome. In some cases such as lissencephaly (see entry Cortical Malformations) or almost total loss of one cerebral hemisphere (see entry, hemiplegia), the clinical condition can be predicted but normally that is not the case. This is illustrated by the fact that some of the most severely impaired children that we see have normal MRI scans.

Three impairments tend to go together, cognitive, behavioural and epilepsy and we broadly relate these to damage to cerebral cortical grey matter. Within the cerebral palsies different weighting of these impairments occurs so that when damage is to mainly cerebral white matter in diplegic cerebral of pre-term babies there is a relatively pure motor disorder. In contrast, some types of congenital hemiplegia, which have extensive cortical grey matter damage, the clinical picture is dominated by cognitive, behavioural and seizure impairments.

Epilepsy is a major influence upon cognitive, behavioural and sometimes motor outcome, which confounds attempts to predict the outcome from the pattern of brain damage seen on scanning. For example, in tuberous sclerosis (see entry) there may be two children with similar scan appearances: one who had very early onset epilepsy with infantile spasms and the other who did not suffer epilepsy in the first two years of life. The former child has a high chance of moderate/severe cognitive impairment and autistic features and the latter is not at such risk. This process, by which epilepsy, particularly sub-clinical epilepsy in sleep, causes loss of skills and deviant behaviour, both of which may be permanent, is not well understood. It is known as an epileptic encephalopathy, meaning brain dysfunction caused by epilepsy and it may be partially or totally reversible by treatment or may be permanent. Such intercurrent events in any of the above groups of diseases can change the child's developmental trajectory without any change in the scan appearances, i.e. without evidence of additional brain damage. In some disorders, for example hemimegalencephaly (see entry) and pyridoxine dependent epilepsy, the seizures and encephalopathy may start in the last trimester of pregnancy so that the stage for long-term impairments has already been set by the time the child is born.

Progressive brain diseases

These conditions are many in number and diverse in their manifestations. The difficulty in recognising them as progressive diseases include the following:

- They may start very early, especially prenatally, for example Zellweger's disease;
- They may show loss of skills in one area of development, such as motor, with continuing improvement in other areas like cognition, for example spinal muscular atrophy (see entry);
- Progression may be sufficiently slow that despite active disease the child gains skills in the area affected by the disease for some of the early years, for example Duchenne muscular dystrophy;
- Some manifestations of the disease, such as myoclonic epilepsy in late infantile Batten disease (see entry), may be treatable;
- The disease may have a tendency to show episodic deterioration with some incomplete recovery, for example adrenoleukodystrophy, ataxia-telangiectasia, mitochondrial diseases and some other metabolic disorders (see entries) in which a (stepwise) deterioration may occur.

Recognition of these disorders is often on the presence of specific characteristic features, which are beyond the scope of this text. Otherwise careful assessment, follow-up and review of early data, including family videotapes, are the main methods used in trying to answer the question: is this a static or progressive disease? The majority of progressive conditions are genetically determined and although it is now possible to look for many of these conditions by genetic means the main diagnostic tools remain careful parental, educational and medical observations. We have to recognise that a 'diagnosis' which is in problem form (for example, moderate learning impairment with myoclonic epilepsy) is provisional and may stay that way for years. Only a limited amount of treatment is currently available for this group of conditions but more treatments will be coming into use, which will require objective methods of assessing outcome.

Overview of Diagnosis

The assembling and analysis of developmental trajectories is the main diagnostic tool of paediatric neurology. Even having described the main pathways above and the potential variations upon them, there are some conditions, which do not fit any of the models. Rett syndrome (see entry) is a good example: girls, with classical Rett syndrome, develop normally, or nearly so, until the latter part of the first year, when skills are lost in cognition and manual function, behaviour changes and abnormal movements of the hands appear. There is then a phase of plateauing of development, followed by slow progress, acquiring skills along a deviant line. Then later there is increasing evidence of a motor disorder and scoliosis tends to progress. Understanding how such a process comes about remains difficult despite the identification of the gene defect.

This short article is intended to map out the main structure of diagnosis in developmental neurology and how clinical history and examination remains the cornerstone of this process. Detailed analysis of the clinical history and examination will continue to be cornerstone of diagnosis. It is hoped that this illustrates how diagnoses may be provisional and change over time despite the best endeavours of paediatric neurologists and how parental perceptions may vary from that of their doctors in children with brain damage and dysfunction.

Medical text written January 2002 by Professor B Neville. **Last updated February 2007 by Professor B Neville, Professor of Childhood Epilepsy, Institute of Child Health, London, UK.**

Support

Families can use Contact a Family's Freephone Helpline for advice, information and, where possible, links to other families. Contact a Family's web-based linking service Making Contact.org can be accessed at http://www.makingcontact.org

CONGENITAL BILATERAL PERISYLVIAN SYNDROME

Background

The term Congenital Bilateral Perisylvian syndrome (CBPS) describes a structural malformation of the brain. The underlying anomaly is Polymicrogyria, a malformation of the cerebral cortex (outer layer of the brain). The term polymicrogyria designates an excessive number of small and prominent convolutions spaced out by shallow and enlarged sulci (grooves), giving the surface of the brain a lumpy aspect. Although it may be difficult to recognise mild forms of polymicrogyria on a magnetic resonance imaging (MRI) scan, infolding of the outer layer of the brain and secondary, irregular, thickening due to packing of microgyri (small folds) represent quite distinctive MRI characteristics.

Polymicrogyria may have a focal or regional distribution or involve the whole cortical mantle (covering of the brain). There are consequently a wide spectrum of clinical manifestations which include children with severe encephalopathies (brain impairments) and intractable epilepsy, or normal individuals with selective impairment of cognitive functions (mental processes) in whom the mild cortical abnormality is only detected on pathological brain study.

Several malformation syndromes featuring bilateral polymicrogyria have been described, including bilateral perisylvian polymicrogyria (the most frequent form), bilateral parasagittal parietooccipital polymicrogyria, bilateral frontal polymicrogyria and unilateral perisylvian or multilobar polymicrogyria. Several distinct entities might exist with regional distribution in which contiguous, non overlapping areas of the cerebral cortex are involved, possibly under the influence of regionally expressed developmental genes.

What are the symptoms?

Patients have paralysis of the face, throat, tongue and the chewing process, with dysarthria (speech difficulties) and drooling. Most have cognitive deficit and epilepsy (see entry). Fixed deformity of the ankle joints (arthrogryposis) has been described in some patients. Seizures usually begin between the ages of four to twelve years and are poorly controlled in about sixty per cent of patients. The most frequent seizure types are atypical absences, tonic or atonic drop attacks and tonic-clonic seizures, often occurring as Lennox-Gastaut syndrome (see entry). A minority of patients (twenty-six per cent) have partial seizures.

What are the causes?

Consistent familial recurrence has been reported only for bilateral perisylvian polymicrogyria, which is sporadic in the great majority of patients. A genetic basis is also possible for unilateral polymicrogyria, at least in some cases.

Bilateral perisylvian polymicrogyria has been reported in children born from identical twin pregnancies which were complicated by twin-twin transfusion syndrome.

Inheritance patterns and prenatal diagnosis

Inheritance patterns

Several families with multiple affected members have been reported with possible autosomal recessive, X-linked dominant and X-linked recessive inheritance. Some families have been linked to the Xq28 chromosomal region but the causative gene is not known at present.

Prenatal diagnosis

Prenatal diagnosis using fetal ultrasound or magnetic resonance imaging may be particularly difficult as the regions of the brain that are involved in this malformation may not have reached their final folding until birth.

Medical text written January 2003 by Contact a Family based on a text provided by Professor R Guerrini. Approved January 2003 by Professor R Guerrini, Istituto Scientifico per la Neuropsichiatria dell'Infanzia e dell'Adolescenza, Pisa, Italy.

Support

Congenital Bilateral Perisylvian syndrome is now known to be similar to Worster-Drought syndrome (see entry) and support for CBPS is given by the Worster-Drought syndrome Support Group.

CONGENITAL CENTRAL HYPOVENTILATION SYNDROME

Congenital Central Hypoventilation syndrome: Central Hypoventilation syndrome; Ondine's

Background

Congenital Central Hypoventilation syndrome (CCHS) is a rare genetic condition of under-breathing involving the failure of automatic control of breathing in the brain. The incidence of CCHS is currently unknown.

The breathing abnormalities are always present during sleep, but may occur to a milder degree during wakefulness. Thus the condition may range in severity from being relatively mild during quiet sleep, with normal breathing when awake, to a complete cessation of breathing during sleep and severe under-breathing when awake. The latter may be particularly evident when feeding (particularly in infancy) or when concentrating.

What are the Symptoms?

Some babies do not breathe at birth and need assisted ventilation in the delivery room and on the neonatal or special care baby unit. Many of these infants may not breathe at all during the first few months of life, but may mature to a better pattern of breathing when awake, with under-breathing or stopping breathing persisting during sleep. Sometimes it is thought that babies may have a congenital heart problem when they first present, because the low oxygen levels caused by inadequate breathing in CCHS leads to high blood pressure in the lungs, which places strain on the heart which may lead to heart failure.

Some infants present solely because of an observation by a parent or health professional that the baby appears to often stop breathing. If this is severe, needing vigorous stimulation or resuscitation to bring recovery, this is termed an 'apparent life threatening event'. It is known that some children may not present until a few months or years of age, because they have a very mild form of the condition.

Children with CCHS may also present with:
- Hirschsprung's disease (see entry);
- blue breath holding episodes;
- fainting episodes;
- epileptic or absence seizures (see entry, Epilepsy);
- heart rhythm disorders (see entry, Heart defects);
- swallowing difficulties;
- learning difficulties (see entry, Learning disability);

- eye problems such as squints;
- unusual responses to anaesthesia;
- increased sweating.

Rarely, Neuroblastomas (see entry) and ganglioneuromas - abnormal growths of nerve cells alongside the spine – may present. These need surgery and treatment if malignant.

How is it diagnosed?

The diagnosis of CCHS depends on documenting that under-breathing occurs during sleep, and that this is not due to a muscle, nerve or lung disease. Measured breathing can be done without discomfort to the baby by using skin sensors to monitor carbon dioxide and oxygen saturation. The diagnosis can be confirmed in over ninety-five per cent of cases by finding the genetic abnormality. In the UK, this is carried out by the South Western Regional Genetic Laboratory based at Southmead Hospital, Bristol.

How is it treated?

The treatment of CCHS involves ensuring adequate ventilation when the child is unable to breathe on their own. No medication has been shown to be effective and mechanical ventilation is needed. This blows air/oxygen at pressure intermittently through a tracheostomy (see entry) or face mask into the lungs (positive pressure ventilators). For those with daytime ventilation, special pacemakers can be implanted to stimulate the nerves to the diaphragm, the main breathing muscle.

As children with CCHS may under-breathe or stop breathing as soon as they fall asleep, it is important that they receive continuous observation or monitoring so that ventilation may be started at the beginning of sleep. Oxygen monitoring is required as a minimum, although giving additional oxygen to breathe would be inadequate treatment alone. Hospital discharge usually takes place once patients are set up with their home ventilator and monitors and are stable. Parents and any other carers at home need training in how to look after the child's ventilation. The biggest delays to hospital discharge include alterations to housing and employment of carers - these can take many months to achieve.

As children grow, their need for ventilation may change and hence regular assessment is required. The condition appears to be life-long, as no patient with CCHS has been documented to outgrow this disorder. Despite this, many children do well, and may attend a regular school and have a normal lifestyle while awake. They should be wary of swimming under water, as they do not have a normal sense of asphyxia.

Inheritance patterns and prenatal diagnosis

Inheritance patterns

CCHS usually arises early in the formation of the new embryo, due to a spontaneous genetic mutation found on Chromosome 4, but in five to ten per cent of cases, one parent may carry the mutated (damaged) gene PHOX2b and pass this on to the child. As this is a 'dominant' gene, such children will always be affected.

Prenatal diagnosis

Possible.

Medical text written October 1996 by Dr M Samuels. **Last updated August 2006 by Dr M Samuels, Consultant Paediatrician/Senior Lecturer in Paediatrics, North Staffordshire Hospital/Keele University, Stoke-on-Trent, UK.**

Further online resources

Medical texts in *The Contact a Family Directory* are designed to give a short, clear description of specific conditions and rare disorders. More extensive information on this condition can be found on a range of reliable, validated websites. Further information on these resources can be found in our **Medical Information on the Internet** article on page 21.

Support

CCHS Support Group
24 Larners Road, Toftwood, Dereham NR19 1LE   Tel: 01362 696509
e-mail: cchssupp@hotmail.com
This is a support network, established in 1995 for the families of children with Congenital Central Hypoventilation syndrome. It offers support by telephone and letter and attempts to link families where possible. It has information available, details on request, please send SAE. There are thought to be up to 30 affected families in the UK.
Group details last confirmed February 2008.

CONGENITAL DISLOCATION AND DEVELOPMENTAL DYSPLASIA OF THE HIP

Background

The hip is a 'ball and socket' joint. The top of the thigh bone (femur) is shaped like a ball and fits into a matching cup (acetabulum) on the outer side of the pelvis. Various problems can affect the baby's hip as it develops. Sometimes the ball does not lie safely in the socket and is displaced from it: this is what is meant by dislocation. Sometimes, although the ball is in the socket it can slip in and out of place. This is what is meant by the hip being dislocatable. Sometimes although the hip is in the socket it is not deeply in place and we call this hip 'subluxated.' Finally in some children although the hip is in the right place the socket does not grow properly and is too shallow. If the hip socket is shallow this may allow the ball to move from the position it should occupy.

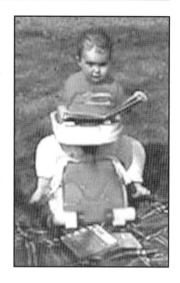

1 to 2 in 1,000 babies born may have a hip that is dislocated at birth. A slightly larger group of children have hips which are not safely in the socket or in whom the socket is shallower than it should be. In general girls are more likely to be affected that boys. The left hip is more often affected than the right.

What are the symptoms?

The condition is not painful and there are no definite signs that a child may have a problem with hip development, but the following are associated with the condition:

- One leg appears shorter than the other;
- An extra deep crease is present on the inside of the thigh;
- One hip joint moves differently from the other and the knee may appear to face outwards;
- When a baby's nappy is changed one leg does not seem to move outwards as fully as the other one;
- The child crawls with one leg dragging.

After walking age it may be noticed that:

- a child stands and walks with one foot on tiptoes with the heel up off the floor. (The child walks this way in an attempt to accommodate the

difference in leg length);
- the child walks with a limp (or waddling gait if both hips are affected).

What are the causes?

In many instances the causes of hip dislocation are not known. It is more common in babies who are born by breech and it is more common if the baby has been a little squashed inside the womb. Special care is taken in the examination of babies when there is a special risk factor. In many centres in the UK children who have risk factors are examined not only clinically but by ultrasound. The ultrasound improves the chance of diagnosing the hip problem and is very helpful in checking to see that hips grow better after treatment. Ultrasound is most useful, however, in the first few weeks of life. Thereafter x-rays are more reliable in seeing how a baby's hip is growing.

How is it diagnosed?

Babies undergo routine examination of their hips at different ages. At birth they are checked by two tests called the Ortolani and Barlow tests. The baby is laid on his or her back and the hips are gently taken sideways. It is usually possible for a baby's hips to be takenfully out sideways. If the baby's hip does not move as fully as this it may be that the hip is not developing properly and further investigations and checks are necessary. In a young baby further investigation is usually by ultrasound but in an older child x-rays are more commonly helpful in establishing the diagnosis. The GP or clinic doctor will check the hips again at around six to eight weeks.

The Ortolani and Barlow Tests are not one hundred per cent accurate. This means that sometimes there is a false alarm, where the baby appears to have a hip condition. However, further tests may show that in fact she or he does not have the condition.

It also means that sometimes a problem may not be picked up even if it is present. So even if a baby has had a hip check and was found to be OK, there may still be a problem; any concerns should be brought to the attention of a health visitor or GP. Do not assume that because the check was 'normal', there cannot be a problem.

Research has shown that parents are good at detecting hip problems, but often delay seeking advice because of uncertainty. However, treatment is usually less complex the earlier it is started, so if there are concerns parents should talk to the Health Visitor or GP as soon as possible.

How is it treated?

Most children who have slight instability of the hip at birth will get better on their own without the need for specific treatment. Nonetheless it is important to try to identify these children to ensure that the expected improvement occurs.

If developmental dysplasia of the hip is recognised early it can nearly always be treated simply by a splint which may need to be worn for six to twelve weeks. This keeps the baby's hips flexed and out sideways. This is a position in which the hip is most likely to develop satisfactorily.

Sometimes, however, these simple splints do not work and the baby's hip does not become stable and grow normally. Some children's hip problems are not detectable at birth or in early infancy and it is not until they begin to walk that a limp is detected which highlights the problem. For older children treatment is usually a little more difficult. Sometimes it is possible to put the hip safely into joint and hold it in a plaster cast. Sometimes it is necessary to release some slightly tight tendons in the groin through a small incision and occasionally it is necessary for an operation to put the hip safely in the socket. After such an operation it is usual to put the child in a plaster of Paris or fibre glass plaster which extends from the waist down to the ankles or feet.

Whenever children have been treated for Congenital Dislocation of the Hip (CDH) or Developmental Dysplasia of the Hip (DDH) it is very important that they are carefully followed up for a long time to make sure the hip grows properly. Occasionally another operation is necessary as they grow older if the socket fails to grow properly.

Inheritance patterns and prenatal diagnosis

Inheritance patterns

In some families there may be an hereditary element but this is unusual.

Prenatal diagnosis

There is no prenatal diagnosis for Congenital Dislocation of the Hip or Developmental Dysplasia of the Hip.

Medical text written May 2000 by Mr M K D Benson. **Last updated May 2005 by Mr M K D Benson, Consultant Orthopaedic Surgeon, Nuffield Orthopaedic Hospital, Oxford, UK.**

Support

As Congenital Dislocation and Developmental Dysplasia of the Hip is a lower limb disorder, information, support and advice is available from STEPS (see entry, Lower Limb Abnormalities).

CONGENITAL DISORDERS OF GLYCOSYLATION

Background

Congenital disorders of glycosylation (CDG) are a group of inherited metabolic disorders which affect all parts of the body, particularly the brain. Other organs may be affected to some degree including the liver, intestines, pancreas, kidney, heart and gonads. Different problems are found in the different forms of CDG. These disorders were previously known as Carbohydrate Deficient Glycoprotein syndromes

What are the symptoms?

CDG Ia is the commonest type currently recognised. These patients all have neurological problems such as developmental delay, squint, visual problems (retinitis pigmentosa) and abnormalities on brain scans (cerebellar hypoplasia). Some patients also have liver disease, kidney cysts, diarrhoea, an abnormal facial appearance or an abnormal fat distribution under the skin.

A similar range of problems are seen in most other forms of CDG except CDG Ib and CDG IIc. Patients with CDG Ib have liver disease, diarrhoea and a tendency to low blood sugar levels due to too much insulin but they do not have neurological problems. CDG IIc causes recurrent infections as well as neurological impairment and poor growth and was previously known as Leukocyte Adhesion Defect type II.

What are the causes?

In all forms of CDG, the chemical abnormality involves glycoproteins. These are proteins with a short chain of sugar molecules attached to them. Glycoproteins are commonly found on the surface of cells (for example, blood groups) or secreted into the blood (such as some hormones). A number of enzymes are involved in attaching sugars to glycoproteins. In each type of CDG, a different one of these enzymes is faulty, leading to abnormalities in the sugar part of the glycoproteins.

How is it diagnosed?

Most forms of CDG can be diagnosed by electrophoresis of transferrin, a glycoprotein present in blood.

How is it treated?

Most forms of CDG cannot be treated but patients with CDG Ib do improve if given mannose by mouth.

Inheritance patterns and prenatal diagnosis

Inheritance patterns

All forms of CDG show an autosomal recessive pattern of inheritance.

Prenatal diagnosis

This can be undertaken by enzyme assay in forms of CDG for which the enzyme defect is known. Molecular genetic techniques can be used if the mutations are known in the index case.

Medical text last updated June 2002 by Dr A Morris, Consultant Paediatrician with Special Interest in Metabolic disease, Willink Biochemical Genetics Unit, Royal Manchester Children's Hospital, Manchester, UK.

Further online resources

Medical texts in *The Contact a Family Directory* are designed to give a short, clear description of specific conditions and rare disorders. More extensive information on this condition can be found on a range of reliable, validated websites. Further information on these resources can be found in our **Medical Information on the Internet** article on page 21.

Support

As Congenital Disorders of Glycosylation are metabolic diseases, information and advice is available from Climb (see entry, Metabolic diseases).

CONGENITAL HYPERINSULINISM

Congenital Hyperinsulinism: Persistent Hyperinsulinaemic Hypoglycaemia of Infancy; PHHI; Nesidioblastosis (old name)

Background

Congenital Hyperinsulinism (CH) is a rare inherited disorder in which the regulation of the secretion of insulin is faulty and there is an over production of insulin from the beta cell of the pancreas. Insulin is the most important hormone that controls the blood glucose (sugar) level. Too much insulin leads to hypoglycaemia (low blood glucose levels). If the hypoglycaemia is not treated it can cause brain damage, learning disability and even death. It is thought that CH occurs in about 1 in 40,000 live births with a male to female ratio of 1.3 to 1. Neonatal onset CH shows in the first days or weeks after birth and is the most severe form. Infant onset CH shows in the first few months, or even years, of life and is milder. A rare adult onset form of CH has been documented. CH occurs in all ethnic groups.

What are the symptoms?

Features of hypoglycaemia in neonatal onset CH include:
- Hunger;
- Lethargy;
- Seizures;
- Apnoea;
- Agitation/restlessness;
- Pallor;
- Poor feeding;
- Irritability;
- Sweating.

Features of infant onset CH may show:
- Any of the above symptoms;
- Confusion;
- Mood or behaviour changes;
- Excessive perspiration.

Features of the rare adult onset CH have been reported as:
- Confusion;
- Headaches, fainting;
- Loss of consciousness;
- Dizziness.

What are the causes?

A number of gene mutations are now known to be involved in CH. However, in about sixty per cent of patients the genetic basis of the disease is not known.

How is it diagnosed?

Fast diagnosis of CH can be made if blood and urine samples are taken while in an episode of hypoglycaemia. Following diagnosis, children should be referred to a specialist centre.

How is it treated?

Treatment of CH in the short term is by immediate correction of the hypoglycaemia by intravenous glucose to prevent further hypoglycaemia and brain damage. In the longer term other medications are used. A pancreatectomy (surgical intervention to remove a large or small part of the pancreas) has to be carried out where medication does not maintain proper regulation of the production of insulin.

Inheritance patterns and prenatal diagnosis

Inheritance patterns

Autosomal recessive in the case of three of the currently known mutations and autosomal dominant in the case of the remaining two known mutations. Genetic counselling should be sought in families known to be at risk of CH.

Prenatal diagnosis

In some forms of CH, amniocentesis at fifteen to eighteen weeks of pregnancy may be possible where there is already an affected family member. However, this is not possible in all forms of CH.

Medical text written December 2005 by Contact a Family. Approved December 2005 by Dr K Hussain, Consultant Paediatric Endocrinologist, Great Ormond Street Hospital and Institute of Child Health, London, UK.

Further online resources

Medical texts in *The Contact a Family Directory* are designed to give a short, clear description of specific conditions and rare disorders. More extensive information on this condition can be found on a range of reliable, validated websites. Further information on these resources can be found in our **Medical Information on the Internet** article on page 21.

Support

PHHI Support Group

17 Bridge End Lane, Great Notley, Braintree CM77 7GN   Tel: 01376 528569
e-mail: juliakill@tiscali.co.uk   Web: http://www.hi-fund.org
The group works under the Children's Hyperinsulinism Fund which is a special trustee fund of the GOSH (Great Ormond Street Hospital) children's charity and was, established in 2003 as no research was being carried out in the UK into the condition. The group offers a listening ear to families, an occasional newsletter and has information about the condition, details on request. It is advised by a consultant at the Institute of Child Health/Great Ormond Street Hospital and has over thirty families in contact.
Group details last confirmed February 2007.

CONGENITAL INSENSITIVITY/ INDIFFERENCE TO PAIN

Congenital Insensitivity to Pain: Congenital Indifference to Pain; Hereditary and Sensory Autonomic Neuropathy Types I-IV; HSAN Types I-IV

Background

In Congenital Insensitivity to Pain, there are structural abnormalities in peripheral nerves which are the peripheral pathways carrying electrical impulses from pain sensitive nerve endings in both superficial and deep tissues.

In Congenital Indifference to Pain, the peripheral nerves are intact and the defect is apparently in the central structures such as the thalamus where painful impulses are normally interpreted. However, it is now thought that some individuals, formerly given a diagnosis of Congenital Indifference to Pain, have been shown by refined histological techniques, which look at the minute structures of bodies, to also have peripheral nerve abnormalities and are therefore examples of Congenital Insensitivity to Pain. Nevertheless, Congenital Indifference to Pain almost certainly exists as an independent condition, but is very rare.

Congenital Insensitivity to Pain (of which types I to IV are generally accepted, with some other very rare conditions) is usually classified under the more general heading of Hereditary and Sensory Autonomic Neuropathy (HSAN). The various categories are distinguished according to clinical features, including age of onset, progressive or non-progressive, presence or absence of abnormalities of the autonomic nervous system, if the system is sympathetic (augmenting actions) or parasympathetic (inhibiting actions) and also according to the nature of structural abnormalities in peripheral nerves.

Abnormalities of peripheral nerves complicate many hereditary neurological and neurometabolic diseases, but they are incidental findings, whereas absent or reduced pain sensation is the hallmark presenting feature in Congenital Insensitivity to Pain.

This classification of hereditary sensory neuropathies overlaps with classifications of hereditary sensory neuropathies in which there are varying degrees of impairment of tactile sensation, with or without impairment of pain sensation. There are also other very rare HSAN which have been identified, mostly as single families, since the original classification was proposed by Dr P J Dyck in 1984. This almost certainly reflects the number of genes which are responsible for the development and maintenance of healthy nerve function, defects in any one of which can lead to impairment of one or many sensory modalities (senses).

HSAN Type I
Sensory and Autonomic Neuropathies - HSAN Type I

HSAN Type I has late onset in late childhood or adolescence. The nerve fibres subserving pain sensation and their connections to the spinal cord degenerate. Impaired pain sensation starts distally (the furthest point) in the legs and ultimately involves the arms. Due to the unawareness of pain, damage to skin, nails, joints etc occurs without the affected person being aware until they see the bruise, or the spreading skin infection, abscess, or see the deformity at a site of fracture. Thus pain provides a valuable protection.

Inheritance patterns
Autosomal Dominant.
Prenatal diagnosis
This is possible. The change in a gene, SPTLC1 on chromosome 9 is responsible for HSAN Type I.

HSAN Type II
Sensory and Autonomic Neuropathies - HSAN Type II

HSAN Type II is congenital (present at birth) or very early onset. There is universal absence of pain in most, and defective tactile sensation in many, resulting in burns, mutilation of finger tips, painless fractures, painless arthritis with joint destruction, and leprosy-like damage to the extremities. In some people there are areas of normal sensation on the trunk. There may be impaired bladder sensation with overdistention. There is deafness in some affected individuals. In most, the condition does not progress, or progresses very slowly. Rarely there is rapid progression. HSAN Type II is almost certainly produced by different genes or combinations of genes. Microscopically there is degeneration of peripheral nerves.

Inheritance patterns
Autosomal recessive.
Prenatal diagnosis
This is not possible as the gene defect has not been identified nor a test developed

HSAN Type III
Sensory and Autonomic Neuropathies - HSAN Type III

HSAN Type III is present at birth. It is also known as the Riley-Day syndrome or Familial Dysautonomia (see entry). While FD occurs almost exclusively in Ashkenazi Jews, Riley-Day Syndrome occurs in the wider community. There are marked degenerative abnormalities in the peripheral and central autonomic nervous system. The symptoms and signs are those of disturbed autonomic function - floppy, feeding difficulties with cyclical vomiting, no overflow tears, blotchy skin, unstable temperature and blood pressure control, poor co-ordination. There is indifference to pain. Intelligence is normal. Only fifty per cent reach adult life (pneumonia is a common cause of death in childhood.)

Inheritance patterns

Autosomal recessive.

Prenatal diagnosis

This is possible. The gene change in HSAN Type III has been localised to a gene (IKBKAP) on chromosome 9q31-q33.

HSAN Type IV

Sensory and Autonomic Neuropathies - HSAN Type IV

HSAN IV is also known as Congenital Insensitivity to Pain and Anhidrosis (absence of sweating). It is present at birth and there is an absence of identifiable pain-conducting nerve fibres in peripheral nerves, and in their connections to spinal cord. The clinical features are similar to HSAN Type II, except that learning disability is the rule.

Inheritance patterns

Autosomal recessive.

Pre-natal diagnosis

This is possible. The gene change in HSAN Type IV is NTRK1 on Chromosome 1q21-q22

Medical text written September 2003 by Dr J Wilson. **Last reviewed July 2005 by Dr J Wilson, Honorary Consultant Paediatric Neurologist, Great Ormond Street Hospital, London, UK.**

Support

There is no specific support group for Hereditary and Sensory Autonomic Neuropathies. However, support for Familial Dysautonomia (HSAN Type III) may be obtained from the Dysautonomia Society of Great Britain (see entry, Familial Dysautonomia) and Climb (see entry, Metabolic Diseases) provides support for Riley-Day Syndrome (HSAN Type III). Families can use Contact a Family's Freephone Helpline for advice, information and, where possible, links to other families, or to organisations providing support for individual features of the different types of HSAN.

CONGENITAL MELANOCYTIC NAEVI

Background

A congenital melanocytic naevus (CMN) is one of many different types of birthmark that may be found in newborn babies:

- *congenital* indicates that the abnormality is present at birth;
- *melanocytic* is the adjective derived from the word *melanocyte*, a type of cell present in normal skin and in certain other organs, whose function is to produce *melanin* - a brown pigment;
- *naevus* is the technical (Greek) word that dermatologists (skin specialists) and paediatricians use to describe any type of birthmark that occurs in the skin, the plural is *naevi*.

CMNs are classified according to size. A 'small' CMN measures less than 2.5cm across; a 'medium'-sized CMN measures 2.5-20cm across, and a 'large' (sometimes called 'giant') CMN will measure over 20cm across. Small CMNs are found in about 1 in 100 newborn babies: it is one of the most common types of birthmark. Medium CMNs occur in approximately 1 in 1,000 newborns; whereas large CMNs only occur in about 1 in 10,000 newborns.

Characteristics of CMNs

Although a CMN is primarily an abnormally large accumulation of melanocytes and melanocyte precursor cells in the skin, CMNs show a number of characteristics which vary considerably, and which may change somewhat in any CMN over a period of time. These include:

- **Size**. CMNs vary greatly in their size (see above);
- **Site**. CMNs occur most commonly on the head and neck followed by the trunk, although they can occur at any site on the skin;
- **Pigmentation**. The colour of a CMN depends on the skin colour of the child, lighter brown in fair-skinned children and almost black in dark-skinned children. Colour is often uneven and can vary over the years, generally becoming lighter in the first two years. Very rarely they can disappear altogether. Although darker areas may appear, they are of little significance;
- **Texture**. The texture of large CMNs tends to be different from that of normal skin, being softer, looser and more wrinkled. The skin tends to be more fragile than normal, tearing rather easily if traumatised;
- **Hairiness**. CMNs are usually hairier than normal areas of skin, but this is very variable. The colour of the hair over a CMN is generally relatively dark. They can occasionally be completely hairless, even ones on the scalp;

- **Lumpiness**. In large CMNs, quite often there are raised or lumpy areas. This doesn't imply any special medical problem. Some lumps are paler and softer than the rest of the CMN, and some are firmer and darker;
- **Eczema** (see entry). The skin overlying a CMN is often rather dry and itchy, and may sometimes develop eczema. If eczema becomes a problem, you may need to see your GP or speak to a dermatologist;
- **Underlying absence of fat**. The presence of many melanocytes interferes with the development of the layer of fat which is normally present between the skin and underlying muscle and bone. In large CMNs, this can result in the CMN actually appearing to be depressed below the general skin surface, or it may cause a noticeable thinness in an affected leg, for example. This has no special significance other than its aesthetic effect;
- **'Satellites'**. Often children with an extensive CMN will have a scattering of smaller pigmented spots elsewhere on the skin. These are known as 'satellites.' While these usually look quite similar to ordinary 'moles', they tend to be bigger. Although most frequently about 0.5-1cm across they become progressively, but proportionately, larger as the child grows: some ending up at 10cm across. The number of satellites can increase over the years, but it is impossible to predict how many are likely to appear. Their final number may be as many as a few hundred. Sunlight may increase the rate of their appearance locally, and this is one of the reasons why anyone with a large CMN should minimise sun exposure.

Are there complications?

There is a malignancy risk involved but the scale is at present unknown.

Similar accumulations of melanocytes can be present on the surface of the brain. This is called intracranial melanosis and will generally occur in combination with CMNs in the skin. This combination is called neurocutaneous melanosis (NCM).

Intracranial melanosis may interfere with the brain's function, and the principal problems that may result are fits and developmental delay. The fits may have their onset at any age, but is most likely to happen during the first few years of life. In a young child, slow attainment of developmental milestones might provide an important clue, or educational difficulties in an older child. Other symptoms that might be provoked by intracranial melanosis include unsteadiness or clumsiness, but the wide variety of possible locations of the accumulations of melanocytes is reflected in an equally wide variety of possible consequences.

When a CMN is very close to an eye, there is a small risk of an abnormality in the eye - glaucoma (see entry). It is most likely that the glaucoma occasionally seen in this situation is due to interference with the drainage process, but the exact cause is unknown.

What are the causes?

Birthmarks are the visible effect of errors that have occurred during a child's development before birth. The causes of these errors are not known for certain, but may include exposure to radiation during pregnancy, infections during pregnancy, and exposure to certain drugs and, perhaps, certain chemicals including some that may sometimes be present in food.

A CMN is a type of benign tumour composed of a large collection of melanocytes. Why such a collection develops is still unknown. Melanocytes originate near the developing spine, and migrate along nerves that connect the spinal cord with the skin. As they arrive in the skin, they are normally evenly and thinly distributed among the other skin cells. Their function is to produce pigment, which protects the skin from damage by ultraviolet rays in sunlight. The amount of pigment produced depends on skin colour and the degree of exposure to sunlight. It seems likely that a CMN reflects a failure of the normal process and many melanocytes gather at the same spot. This might happen because their progress is somehow impeded, or because they are actually attracted to this site and collect there voluntarily.

How is it treated?

There are surgical treatment options available which should be discussed with a paediatric dermatologist.

Inheritance patterns and prenatal diagnosis

Inheritance patterns

CMNs are sporadic events and there appears to be very little risk for further children.

Prenatal diagnosis

It is extremely unlikely that the presence of a CMN could be identified currently by ultra sound scanning or any other method.

Medical text written October 2001 by Dr D Atherton. **Last updated November 2006 by Dr D Atherton, Consultant in Paediatric Dermatology, Great Ormond Street Hospital, London, UK.**

Support

Support and information for Congenital Melanocytic Naevi is provided by the Birthmark Support Group (see entry, Vascular Birthmarks).

CONGENITAL MUSCULAR DYSTROPHY

Background

Congenital Muscular Dystrophies are an heterogenous group of disorders which show at birth or within the first six months of life.

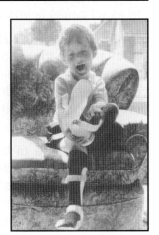

Forms of Congenital Muscular Dystrophy that occur in western countries are:

- The merosin deficient form (also know as MDC1A);
- The merosin positive form with rigidity (stiffness) of the spine (also know as RSMD1);
- One form with significant distal joint laxity (also known as Ullrich variant);
- One form with large muscles (also known as MDC1C);
- The muscle-eye brain disease (also known as MEB);
- The Walker-Warburg variant with severe eye and brain involvement.

It should be noted that congenital muscular dystrophy is not the same disorder as congenital myopathy.

What are the symptoms?

Symptoms include floppiness, poor head control, muscle weakness and contractures (tightness) in the limbs although these symptoms are not specific to congenital muscular dystrophy.

Most of the cases affected by Congenital Muscular Dystrophy only have weakness of the muscles; in some instances learning difficulties, epilepsy and abnormality of the eye can be present. In these latter cases, the learning difficulties may be subtle, moderate or severe but are not progressive.

How is it diagnosed?

A blood test, muscle biopsy and, often, a brain scan would be performed to make an accurate diagnosis.

Inheritance patterns and prenatal diagnosis

Inheritance patterns

Autosomal recessive in most instances; rare de-novo dominant mutations have been reported in Ullrich Congenital Muscular Dystrophy

Prenatal diagnosis

At present this is possible in approximately forty per cent of cases.

Medical text written May 2000 by Professor F Muntoni. **Last updated December 2004 by Professor F Muntoni, Professor and Consultant in Paediatric Neurology, Hammersmith Hospital, Neuromuscular Centre, London, UK.**

Support

The support group covering Congenital Muscular Dystrophy is currently unavailable. This medical description is retained for information purposes. Further information in the form of a detailed fact sheet can be obtained from the Muscular Dystrophy Group (see entry, Muscular Dystrophy and neuromuscular disorders) who act as an umbrella organisation for research in all neuromuscular diseases. Families can use Contact a Family's Freephone Helpline for advice, information and, where possible, links to other families. Contact a Family's web-based linking service Making Contact.org can be accessed at http://www.makingcontact.org

We distribute over 98,000 guides, leaflets and booklets for parents each year.

CONGENITAL OCULAR MOTOR APRAXIA

Congenital Ocular Motor Apraxia: Saccade Initiation Failure; Cogan's Apraxia

Background

This disorder is characterised by an inability to make horizontal fast eye movements from birth.

The congenital condition may occur in isolation (idiopathic), but can be associated with a wide range of brain malformations, metabolic disorders, and perinatal problems. It is also associated with various clinical syndromes. The condition may also be acquired at school-age, secondary to progressive neurological and metabolic diseases.

What are the symptoms?

Infants may at first appear blind but later develop characteristic head movements to shift gaze (head thrusts). Infants may be hypotonic with mild motor delay. Ataxia may persist. Speech development may be slow requiring speech therapy, and reading problems may occur. Typically the abnormal head movements subside, as the child learns to make blinks, to help move the eyes which can make detection of the condition difficult in the older child. Eye movement recordings confirm the condition.

How is it treated?

The congenital condition is not progressive. There is no treatment and educational support may be needed.

Inheritance patterns and prenatal diagnosis

Inheritance patterns

May be familial in rare cases but is usually sporadic.

Prenatal diagnosis

None

Medical text written March 1997 by Dr C Harris. **Last updated December 2007 by Professor C Harris, Professor of Neurosciences, Institute of Neurosciences, Plymouth University, Plymouth, UK**

Support

COA Support Group

c/o Contact a Family, 209-211 City Road, London EC1V 1JN
Tel: 0808 808 3555 Freephone Helpline   Tel: 0808 808 3556 Text
Tel: 020 7608 8700 Admin   Fax: 020 7608 8701   e-mail: helpline@cafamily.org.uk
This is a self help group, established in 1996. It offers support by e-mail but offers telephone support for parents without internet access. The group attempts to link families where possible. It publishes a newsletter and has information available, details on request.
Group details last updated June 2007.

CONGENITAL TALIPES EQUINOVARUS

Background

Congenital refers to a condition that is present at birth. Talipes refers to an abnormality of the ankle and foot. Equinovarus refers to the position of the foot, pointing downwards and inwards. One or both feet may be affected. It is commonly called clubfoot and can be recognized in the infant by examination. The foot is turned inwards, is stiff and cannot be brought to a normal position.

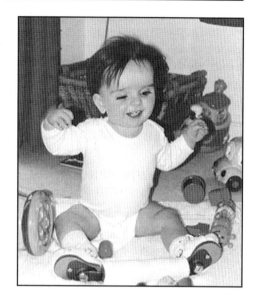

How is it treated?

There are various treatment options and the aim is to obtain a mobile, pain free foot that will fit into normal shoes. The Ponseti Method of treatment, involving specific manipulation and serial plaster casts and Foot Abduction Braces (FABs), minimises the need for extensive surgery, though up to eighty per cent of children may need a small operation to the tendon at the back of the heel. Other treatment options may include gentle manipulation, manipulation with adhesive strapping, splints or plaster casts to hold the foot in the corrected position or soft tissue surgery to release the tight ligaments, tendons and joint capsules. Older children may need bone surgery or tendon transfers. Extensive surgery is more likely to result in a stiffer foot than minimal surgical treatment, particularly as the years pass by. Some children may wear special boots for a time.

Without any treatment, clubfoot will result in severe functional disability; with treatment, most children should have a nearly normal foot. However the corrected clubfoot will still not be perfect. It could be up to one to two sizes smaller and somewhat less mobile than the normal foot. The calf muscles on the clubfoot leg will also stay smaller.

Inheritance patterns and prenatal diagnosis

Inheritance patterns

Clubfoot can be associated with other conditions such as spina bifida (see entry) or arthrogryposis (see entry). An isolated or idiopathic clubfoot is one that is not related to another condition or syndrome. Between 1 to 2 in 1,000 live births have an isolated clubfoot or feet. There is no single cause of isolated clubfoot, however there is quite a lot of evidence to suggest there is a strong genetic component. Twice as many boys are affected as girls. Research into detecting the gene or genes associated with clubfoot is being undertaking in the both the UK and the USA.

Prenatal diagnosis

Clubfoot can be detected by prenatal ultrasound scan, though it cannot be treated before birth.As Congenital Talipes Equinovarus is a lower limb disorder, information, support and advice is available from STEPS (see entry, Lower Limb Abnormalities).

Medical text written June 2005 by Contact a Family. Approved June 2005 by Ms N Davis, Consultant Paediatric Orthopaedic Surgeon, Booth Hall Children's Hospital, Manchester, UK.

Further online resources

Medical texts in *The Contact a Family Directory* are designed to give a short, clear description of specific conditions and rare disorders. More extensive information on this condition can be found on a range of reliable, validated websites. Further information on these resources can be found in our **Medical Information on the Internet** article on page 21.

Support

As Congenital Talipes Equinovarus is a lower limb disorder, information, support and advice is available from STEPS (see entry, Lower Limb Abnormalities).

CONRADI-HUNERMANN SYNDROME

Background

Conradi-Hunermann syndrome is a term used to describe at least two different conditions. These conditions are part of the group which together are called chondrodysplasia punctata. This name describes an unusual pattern which can be seen in the X-rays of babies and young children where the ends of the bones appear 'stippled' or 'punctate.'

What are the symptoms?

In Conradi-Hunermann syndrome the bones of the arms and legs are short causing short stature (see entry, Restricted Growth). The bones of the face (see entry, Craniofacial Conditions) may also be involved. Some children with this condition have eye changes including cataracts. Babies may be born with a skin rash (see entry, Ichthyosis) and can later develop thickening of the skin. The hair may be sparse or absent in patches.

It can be difficult to differentiate the various forms of this condition.

Inheritance patterns and prenatal diagnosis

Inheritance patterns

There is an autosomal dominant and X-linked dominant form of Conradi-Hunermann syndrome. In addition there are autosomal recessive and X-linked recessive forms of chondrodysplasia punctata which can be sometimes be mistaken for Conradi-Hunermann syndrome. The genes which cause some of these conditions are known and can be tested for.

Prenatal diagnosis

This may be possible if the exact cause of the condition is known. In other cases ultrasound scanning may be helpful.

Medical text written March 2002 by Dr M Wright. **Last updated October 2003 by Dr M Wright, Consultant Clinical Geneticist, Institute of Medical Genetics, International Centre for Life, Newcastle upon Tyne, UK.**

Further online resources

Medical texts in *The Contact a Family Directory* are designed to give a short, clear description of specific conditions and rare disorders. More extensive information on this condition can be found on a range of reliable, validated websites. Further information on these resources can be found in our **Medical Information on the Internet** article on page 21.

Support

There is no support group for Conradi-Hunermann syndrome in the UK. Cross referrals to other entries in The Contact a Family Directory are intended to provide information and advice for these particular features of the disorder. Organisations identified in these entries do not provide support specifically for Conradi-Hunermann syndrome. Families can use Contact a Family's Freephone Helpline for advice, information and, where possible, links to other families. Contact a Family's web-based linking service Making Contact.org can be accessed at http://www.makingcontact.org

CORNELIA DE LANGE SYNDROME

Cornelia de Lange: Brachman de Lange; De Lange I syndrome; Amsterdam dwarfism

Background

Cornelia de Lange syndrome (CdLS) is rare and affects between 1 in 15,000 and 1 in 50,000 babies born.

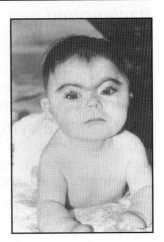

Children with the syndrome are small at birth and remain small compared to children of the same age. There are now growth charts specifically for children with CdLS and these can be downloaded from Web: http://www.cdlsusa.org/growthcharts.htm

What are the symptoms?

The children will have slow or very slow development, usually associated with significant learning problems that are of variable severity. Some children have psychological and behavioural problems including autistic-like features and self injury. Most children have some form of limb abnormality but these can range from having small hands and particularly short thumbs in mild cases to almost complete absence of the forearms in severe cases. Almost all children will have an unusual marbled appearance to the skin on their arms and legs, particularly when they are cold. The most striking feature of the syndrome is that all the children look alike, like brothers and sisters.

Some medical complications are very common in CdLS including feeding and bowel problems (particularly gastro-oesophageal reflux) and hearing problems. Other complications that are seen in a minority of cases are congenital heart problems and seizures.

Psychological and behavioural characteristics

The Psychological and behavioural characteristics information below was last updated March 2004 by Dr O Udwin, Consultant Clinical Child Psychologist, West London Mental Health NHS Trust, London, UK and Dr A Kuczynski, Child Clinical Psychologist, South London & Maudsley NHS Trust, London, UK with further information provided by Professor C Oliver, School of Psychology,University of Birmingham, Birmingham, UK.

Most of the children with Cornelia de Lange syndrome have moderate or severe learning difficulties, but some have borderline or low average cognitive abilities. All have delayed or limited speech development and perhaps as many as a third never develop more than a few words. In contrast, nonverbal visuospatial and fine motor skills are relative strengths. As they develop, many individuals are able to cope with their everyday needs, including eating, toileting and dressing, and they continue to acquire new skills into their late teens. Some adults are able to live in relatively independent settings.

Individuals with Cornelia de Lange syndrome show great variability in their behaviour, but there are common features. Some are placid and good-natured, but many are described as restless, overactive, distractible and irritable. Often, even those with well-developed vocabularies are not talkative. Many show autistic features, including diminished ability to relate socially, infrequent facial expression of emotion, rejection of physical contact, little reaction to sounds or to pain, and repetitive and stereotypic movements such as twirling. Some also display rigidity and inflexibility to change, and prefer a consistent and structured environment.

Self-injurious behaviour is common, although this may reflect the severity of general developmental difficulties rather than being a specific feature of the syndrome. The self-injury takes various forms, such as eye-pressing and poking, head-slapping, scratching and hand-biting. The latter is particularly common in Cornelia de Lange syndrome; it tends to be stereotyped and repetitive for a given individual and may have a compulsive quality. Aggression towards others may be less common. There is some evidence that hyperactive and self-injurious behaviours are related to pain from gastrointestinal reflux which is common in people with the syndrome.

Inheritance patterns and prenatal diagnosis
Inheritance patterns
Although CdLS is a genetic disorder, it is rare for this condition to occur twice in the same family. At least one appointment at a genetics clinic is recommended. One gene that causes CdLS, NIPBL, has now been identified and this accounts for half of the cases.
Prenatal diagnosis
Prenatal testing of subsequent pregnancies in an affected family is possible using either genetic testing or detailed ultrasound scanning.

Medical text written August 2002 by Dr D Fitzpatrick. **Last updated October 2005 by Dr D Fitzpatrick, Senior Clinical Scientist and Hon. Consultant Geneticist, MRC Human Genetics Unit, Western General Hospital, Edinburgh, UK.** Psychological and behavioural characteristics last updated March 2004 by Dr O Udwin, Consultant Clinical Child Psychologist, West London Mental Health NHS Trust, London, UK and Dr A Kuczynski, Child Clinical Psychologist, South London & Maudsley NHS Trust, London, UK with further information provided by Professor C Oliver, School of Psychology,University of Birmingham, Birmingham, UK.

Further online resources

Medical texts in *The Contact a Family Directory* are designed to give a short, clear description of specific conditions and rare disorders. More extensive information on this condition can be found on a range of reliable, validated websites. Further information on these resources can be found in our **Medical Information on the Internet** article on page 21.

Support

CDLS Foundation UK

The Gate House, 104 Lodge Lane, Grays RM16 2UL   Tel: 01375 376439
Fax: 01375 427 014   e-mail: info@cdls.org.uk   Web: http://www.cdls.org.uk
The Foundation is a National Registered Charity No. 1054033, established in 1984.
It offers telephone support, regional contacts and meetings. It publishes a quarterly
newsletter and has a wide range of information available, details on request. The
Foundation is in touch with over 400 families.
Group details last updated September 2007.

It is estimated that around five million children and adults are affected by rare disorders in the UK.

CORTICAL MALFORMATIONS

Lissencephaly

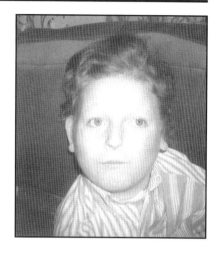

Lissencephaly

Neuronal migration describes the journey the nerve cells make from the inner to the outer surface of the brain during development to form the cortex (grey matter). Lissencephaly is a neuronal migration disorder, and the name 'lissencephaly' is derived from the Greek words 'lissos' - smooth and 'encephalos' - brain. The convolutions (folds) of the brain can be absent, giving the surface the 'smooth' appearance. Two major types are distinguished: classical lissencephaly (also known as type I) and cobblestone lissencephaly (also known as type II). Several syndromes are recognised with each type. General problems include developmental delay, seizures, and feeding difficulties. Life expectancy is often reduced.

Classical lissencephaly can be associated with agyria (absent convolutions) or pachygyria (reduced and thickened convolutions) of the brain and subcortical band heterotopia (SBH) - a band of nerve cells located in the white matter instead of the grey matter. Syndromes with classical lissencephaly include Miller-Dieker syndrome (MDS) associated with distinct facial features and occasional heart or abdominal defects, and Isolated Lissencephaly Sequence (ILS), where associated features are uncommon.

Cobblestone lissencephaly syndromes include Walker-Warburg syndrome (WWS), Muscle-Eye-Brain disease (MEB) and Fukuyama Congenital Muscular Dystrophy (FCMD). These conditions are also associated with developmental eye problems and muscular dystrophy.

Related neuronal migration disorders

Variant lissencephalies: describes conditions associated with classical lissencephaly, but also additional distinguishing abnormalities, like severe cerebellar hypoplasia (Lissencephaly with Cerebellar Hypoplasia, LCH) or absence of the corpus callosum (Lissencephaly with Agenesis of the Corpus Callosum, LACC). Autosomal recessive inheritance has been reported. Mutations in the RELN and VLDLR genes have been found in a few families with LCH.

X-linked lissencephaly with abnormal genitalia: this condition only affects males and is characterized by lissencephaly, absence of the corpus callosum and small basal ganglia associated with underdeveloped genitalia. The prognosis is poor. Mutations in the ARX gene have been identified.

Periventricular nodular heterotopia (PVNH): this condition is also a neuronal migration disorder. Nerve cells, which have failed to migrate to the cortex, line the ventricle in a nodular fashion. Mutations in the FLNA gene on the X-chromosome have been predominantly identified in women with PVNH. An autosomal recessive form of PVNH has been associated with mutations in ARFGEF2.

Other cortical malformations

Polymicrogyria (PMG): this may also be a neuronal migration disorder, but the exact nature of the condition is unclear. It is likely to be more common than lissencephaly. PMG is characterised by more frequent and smaller convolutions on the surface of the brain. It often appears in distinct patterns, and the most common is Perisylvian Polymicrogyria. Intrauterine infection (cytomegalovirus - CMV) is a known cause for PMG; intrauterine hypoperfusion has also been implicated. Familial occurrences and association with a number of different chromosome anomalies also point to a genetic aetiology in some cases. PMG is associated with a number of different chromosome anomalies; 22q11 deletions are the most common. A rare form of PMG has been associated with mutations in the GPR56 gene; causes for a number of syndromes with PMG as a feature have also be identified (Goldberg-Shprintzen syndrome (see entry), Joubert syndrome (see entry).

Schizencephaly (SCH): this describes a cleft from the cerebral cortex to ventricle, usually lined with polymicrogyria. The causes for SCH are thought to be similar to PMG; familial occurrences appear uncommon.

Congenital microcephaly and cortical malformations: Lissencephaly, polymicrogyria, or simplified (not fully formed) gyri (SG) can also be seen in association with severe congenital microcephaly (very, very small head at birth). In these conditions autosomal recessive inheritance has been observed The general term 'Microlissencephaly' is often used, but is unfortunately inadequate to describe the variation in cortical anomalies mentioned above (like PMG and SG).

Inheritance patterns and prenatal diagnosis

Inheritance patterns

Although the inheritance pattern is well, established in some of the conditions described above, counselling in individual cases depends on the precise diagnosis, family history and laboratory investigations where available.

Classical lissencephaly/subcortical band heterotopia is commonly caused by deletions/mutations of the LIS1 gene on chromosome 17p, or the DCX gene on the X-chromosome. Recently mutations in the TUBA1A gene have been identified in some patients.

The inheritance observed in cobblestone lissencephaly and associated syndromes is autosomal recessive. WWS has been associated with mutations in the POMT1, POMT2 and FKRP genes, MEB with mutations in the POMGnT1 gene, and FCMD with mutations in the Fukutin gene.

Prenatal diagnosis

Prenatal diagnosis using molecular (genetic) tests is available in some cases. In certain circumstances ultrasound or MRI investigations during pregnancy may be helpful.

Medical text written September 2001 by Dr D Pilz, Last updated by Dr D Pilz, Consultant Clinical Geneticist, Institute of Medical Genetics, University Hospital of Wales, Cardiff, UK.

Further online resources

Medical texts in *The Contact a Family Directory* are designed to give a short, clear description of specific conditions and rare disorders. More extensive information on this condition can be found on a range of reliable, validated websites. Further information on these resources can be found in our **Medical Information on the Internet** article on page 21.

Support

Lissencephaly Contact Group

c/o Contact a Family, 209-211 City Road, London EC1V 1JN
Tel: 0808 808 3555 Freephone Helpline   e-mail: info@lissencephaly.org.uk
Web: http://www.lissencephaly.org.uk
The Group was, established in 1989. It offers contact with others where possible and mutual support through newsletters and telephone, e-mail or letter. It publishes a newsletter and has information available, details on request. The Group has over 200 members.
Group details last confirmed November 2007.

CORTICOBASAL DEGENERATION

Corticobasal Degeneration: CBD

Background

CBD is a rare form of dementia. It is an heterogeneous disease (i.e. composed of different elements), and is characterised by a combination of cognitive impairment and movement disorder.

In a review by Rinne in 1994 the authors found only forty cases. However, CBD is difficult to diagnose. Studies have shown that a clinical diagnosis may be different from neuropathology, i.e. a diagnosis made after examining brain tissue damage which would be revealed at autopsy.

What are the symptoms?

Symptoms of the disease can be cognitive (relating to comprehension, judgement, memory and reason) or motor. A range of cognitive skills, including memory and concentration, are affected by CBD.

Motor symptoms (problems with co-ordination of movement) are asymmetrical - i.e. they are on one side or the other. They are often described as a stiff hand or arm, or difficulty with writing.

How is it diagnosed?

It is a difficult disease to diagnose with accuracy and so CBD is sometimes diagnosed as something else, most commonly Parkinson's disease, vascular dementia, Alzheimer's disease or Pick's disease.

As the first symptoms a person develops could be cognitive or motor, some patients are referred to neurologists or geriatricians with an interest in movement disorders, whilst other patients may be referred to neurologists or psychiatrists with an interest in dementia.

There is no medical test for CBD. The clinical diagnosis is differential in that it is made by excluding other conditions that have similar symptoms such Alzheimer's disease or Parkinson's disease, by observing the person carefully and by talking to them and to those who know them well.

A conclusive diagnosis requires an autopsy. This is carried out after death, when brain tissue can be examined under a microscope. The characteristic hallmarks of the disease in the brain of someone who has died of CBD include:

- death of neurones (brain cells) in a particular area of the brain;
- degeneration of the substantia nigra (a small part of the brain described as the 'gearbox of the brain'); if the substantia negra is not working properly there may be difficulty with leg and arm movements;

- an absence of Lewy bodies (abnormal structures found in certain areas of the brain);
- the presence of swollen, 'ballooned' cells in the substantia nigra;
- gliosis in the brain (a type of brain scar tissue which can be seen under a microscope) caused by glial cells multiplying. This also occurs in Alzheimer's disease.

Inheritance patterns and prenatal diagnosis
Inheritance patterns
None
Prenatal diagnosis
None

Medical text written November 2001 by the Alzheimer's Society. **Last reviewed December 2004 by Dr N Fox, Dementia Research Society and Alzheimer's Society Medical & Scientific Advisory Committee.**

Support
Support for Corticobasal Degeneration is available from the PSP Association (see entry, Progressive Supranuclear Palsy). As CBD gives rise to dementia, further information and support is available from the Alzheimer's Society (see entry, Alzheimer's disease) and from the Pick's Disease Support Group (see entry, Frontotemporal Lobar degeneration including Frontotemporal Dementia).

COSTELLO SYNDROME

Costello syndrome: Faciocutaneoskeletal syndrome; FCS syndrome

Background

Costello syndrome (CS) is a rare genetic condition, first described in 1977 by Dr J M Costello. Approximately one hundred and fifty individuals worldwide are known to be affected. CS may affect many different body systems, but the range and severity of health problems varies widely. Developmental delay is always present, but the degree of this is also highly variable.

Babies with CS are usually of normal birth weight. Polyhydramnios (excessive amniotic fluid in pregnancy) may have been present. From birth, children with CS have feeding difficulties, which include a severe aversion to taking solids or fluids orally and reflux (vomiting after feeding). Some babies require tube or gastrostomy feeding. Infants may be significantly irritable and hypersensitive to sound and tactile stimuli, and this may cause disturbed sleep. These features tend to resolve between the ages of two to four years.

There is an increased incidence of congenital abnormalities of the heart (see entry, Heart defects). The range of heart problems associated with CS includes Hypertrophic Cardiomyopathy (see entry, Cardiomyopathies), Pulmonic Stenosis, Mitral Valve Prolapse, Ventricular Septal defect and abnormalities of heart rhythm.

What are the symptoms?

Children and adults with CS resemble one another facially. Facial features include Macrocephaly (a relatively large head), low-set ears with large, thick lobes and thick lips. Excessive loose skin on the palms, fingers and soles, which may become thickened over time, is very characteristic. Many children develop Papillomata (small wartlike growths) around the mouth, nostrils and other moist body areas.

Joint abnormalities are relatively common. For example, there may be increased movement at the small joints of the hand, unusual posturing at the wrist and restriction of movement at the elbow. Tightening of the tendon at the ankle may require surgery. Scoliosis (see entry) is also relatively common.

Despite supplemental feeding, failure to grow normally is usual in CS and children and adults will be short. Growth hormone treatment has been used in some cases.

Delayed developmental milestones include sitting, crawling, talking and walking. Most children will walk. Speech and language skills are usually acquired but not all children will acquire age appropriate skills. Memory skills are good. Most children will require special schooling and supervised living

© Copyright Contact a Family 2008

in adult life. After the first years of life, people with CS are described as very sociable and affectionate with a good sense of humour.

Some individuals with CS have developed cancer including rhabdomysarcoma and neuroblastoma (see entry). The cancer risk appears to be greatest in the first years of life.

How is it diagnosed?

A number of syndromes including Cardio-facio-cutaneous syndrome (CFC), Noonan syndrome (see entry), Simpson-Golabi-Behmel syndrome (SGB) and storage diseases especially Mucopolysaccharidosis (see entry, Mucopolysaccharide diseases and associated diseases), share certain features with CS and therefore need to be excluded in the process of making a diagnosis.

Inheritance patterns and prenatal diagnosis

Inheritance patterns

Most cases of Costello syndrome are sporadic (isolated with no other affected family members). The cause of CS is unknown. It is thought to be a new genetic change, either in a single genetic instruction or gene or a sub-microscopic missing piece of chromosome.

Prenatal diagnosis

None available.

Medical text written August 2004 by Contact a Family. Approved August 2004 by Dr Bronwyn Kerr, Consultant Clinical Geneticist, Royal Manchester Children's Hospital, Manchester, UK.

Further online resources

Medical texts in *The Contact a Family Directory* are designed to give a short, clear description of specific conditions and rare disorders. More extensive information on this condition can be found on a range of reliable, validated websites. Further information on these resources can be found in our **Medical Information on the Internet** article on page 21.

Support

International Costello Syndrome Support Group
90 Parkfield Road North, Manchester M40 3RQ   Tel: 0161 682 2479
e-mail: c.stone8@ntlworld.com (UK)   e-mail: lschoyer@ladhs.org (US)
Web: http://www.costellokids.org.uk
The UK section of the International Costello Syndrome Support Group is a National Registered Charity No. 1085605, established in 2001. It offers support by phone, e-mail and letter. They also link families by e-mail, through their internet Listserv. It has a large amount of information available online or by request. The group is in touch with over 160 families around the world and organises international conferences bi-annually. The US section, Costello Syndrome Family Network (CSFN), is a registered non-profit organisation.
Group details last confirmed October 2007.

COT DEATH

Background

Cot death is the sudden and unexpected death of a baby for no obvious reason. The post-mortem examination may explain some deaths. Those that remain unexplained after post-mortem examination may be registered as sudden infant death syndrome (SIDS), sudden infant death, sudden unexpected death in infancy or cot death.

What are the causes?

No one knows yet why these babies die. Researchers think there are likely to be a number of different causes, or that a combination of factors affect a baby at a vulnerable stage of development.

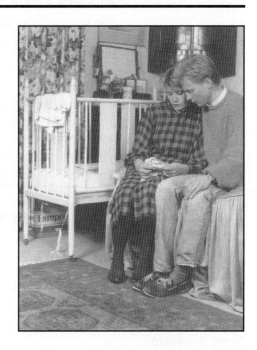

Research has shown that certain babies are more at risk, namely boys, premature and low birth-weight babies. The vast majority of cot death happens to babies aged under six months and there is a peak occurrence at two to three months. Cot death can happen to any family but it is more likely to happen in families living in difficult circumstances.

Since the introduction of the Reduce the Risk of Cot Death campaign in 1991 the numbers of babies dying has fallen by around seventy per cent. However, cot death still claims the lives of seven babies every week in the UK.

To reduce the risk of cot death:

- Place your baby on the back to sleep;
- Cut smoking in pregnancy – fathers too!;
- Do not let anyone smoke in the same room as your baby;
- Keep your baby's head uncovered – place your baby with feet to the foot of the cot to prevent wriggling down under the covers;
- If your baby is unwell seek medical advice promptly;
- Parents should not sleep with their baby in their bed if either partner:
    - is a smoker, even if they never smoked in bed or in their home;
    - has been drinking alcohol;
    - takes medication or drugs that make them drowsy;

-     —   feels very tired.
- Bed sharing should be avoided if a baby was born prematurely, with a low birth weight or has a high temperature.

The safest place for a baby to sleep is in a cot in the parents' bedroom for the first six months.

Inheritance patterns and prenatal diagnosis

Inheritance patterns

None.

Prenatal diagnosis

None.

Medical text written April 2000 by Dr Sarah Levine, Medical Adviser to the Foundation for the Study of Infant Death, London, UK. **Last updated October 2005 by Professor Peter Fleming, Professor of Infant Health and Developmental Physiology, Institute of Child Health, Bristol, UK and the Foundation for the Study of Infant Death, London, UK.**

Support

Foundation for the Study of Infant Deaths
Artillery House, 11-19 Artillery Row, London SW1P 1RT   Tel: 020 7233 2090 Helpline
Tel: 020 7222 8001 General   Fax: 020 7222 8002   e-mail: support@fsid.org.uk
Web: http://www.fsid.org.uk
The Foundation is a National Registered Charity No. 262191, established in 1971. It is the UK's leading baby charity working to prevent sudden infant deaths and promote baby health. FSID achieves its aims through funding research, supporting families, promoting safe infant care advice to parents and professionals and working with professionals to improve investigations when a baby dies. In particular, FSID runs CONI (Care Of the Next Infant) with the NHS, to support bereaved families when they have subsequent babies. The Foundation has a network of trained befrienders and produces a range of publications including the leaflet 'When a baby dies suddenly and unexpectedly'.
Group details last updated February 2008.

The Scottish Cot Death Trust
Royal Hospital for Sick Children, Yorkhill, Glasgow G3 8SJ
Tel: 0141 357 3946 (Mon-Fri, 9am-5pm)
e-mail: contact@sidscotland.org.uk   Web: http://www.sidscotland.org.uk
The Trust is a Scottish Charity No. SC003458, established in 1985. It offers support to bereaved families and awards research grants. It publishes a newsletter twice a year and acts as a centre for advice, information and education about sudden infant death. Details on request. The Trust has a mailing list of 1,200.
Group details last updated June 2007.

COWDEN DISEASE

Cowden disease: Cowden syndrome; Multiple Hamartoma syndrome

Background

Cowden disease (CD) is a rare inherited disorder of multiple hamartomas (non-cancerous tumour like growths) and an increased risk of a number of types of cancer (see entry). CD is named after the family of Rachel Cowden in whom the disorder was described in 1963. CD's mode of inheritance was identified in 1972 and the alternative name of Multiple Hamartoma syndrome was suggested.

It is estimated that CD affects 1 in 300,000 individuals but is underdiagnosed. Both males and females are affected by CD. Onset is usually by the late twenties. CD is caused by mutations of the PTEN tumour suppressor gene on chromosome10.

What are the symptoms?

Features of CD may include:

- Hamartomas most commonly to be found on the skin and mucous membranes such as the lining of the mouth and nose but also in the intestines and other parts of the body;
- Non-cancerous tumours of the breast and thyroid;
- Increased likelihood of breast, thyroid and endometrial (mucous membrane lining of the uterus) cancers. Males are more likely to develop thyroid cancer and females are more likely to develop breast cancer;
- Macrocephaly (increased head size);
- Learning disability (see entry);
- Lhermitte-Duclos disease - presence of a cerebellar dysplastic gangliocytoma (a type of benign brain tumour).

How is it diagnosed?

Diagnosis of CD is based on identification of the distinctive skin features of the disorder. The International Cowden Syndrome Consortium has proposed diagnostic criteria for the syndrome (Operational Criteria for the Diagnosis of CS. Daly, M. NCCN practice guidelines: Genetics/familial high-risk cancer screening. Oncology 1999:13:161-86).

Individuals with CD need to be regularly screened for cancers.

Inheritance patterns and prenatal diagnosis

Inheritance patterns

Autosomal dominant.

Prenatal diagnosis

This is possible by Chorionic Villus Sampling (CVS) at about ten to twelve weeks or amniocentesis at sixteen to eighteen weeks if the version of the PTEN gene affecting the family is known.

Medical text written September 2004 by Contact a Family. Approved September 2004 by Dr D Hargrave, Consultant Paediatric Oncologist, Royal Marsden Hospital, Sutton, UK.

Further online resources

Medical texts in *The Contact a Family Directory* are designed to give a short, clear description of specific conditions and rare disorders. More extensive information on this condition can be found on a range of reliable, validated websites. Further information on these resources can be found in our **Medical Information on the Internet** article on page 21.

Support

There is no support group for Cowden disease. Cross referrals to other entries in The Contact a Family Directory are intended to provide relevant support for those particular features of the disorder. Organisations identified in those entries do not provide support specifically for Cowden disease. Families can use Contact a Family's Freephone Helpline for advice, information and, where possible, links to other families. Contact a Family's web-based linking service Making Contact.org can be accessed at http://www.makingcontact.org

CRANIOFACIAL CONDITIONS

Background

Abnormalities of skull shape can arise either from external pressure exerted on the head in early life, or from intrinsic abnormalities of growth. The most common intrinsic abnormality of skull growth is called craniosynostosis, which affects about 1 in 2,500 children. Craniosynostosis is the medical term for the premature closure of one or more of the seams between the skull bones. As the brain grows during fetal life and childhood, the overlying skull also enlarges by adding new bone at these seams, which are termed sutures. The major sutures are the midline metopic (at the front) and sagittal (at the top) sutures,

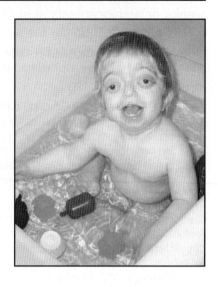

and the paired coronal and lambdoid sutures. The coronal sutures run across the skull in front of the ears, crossing the junction of the metopic and sagittal sutures; the lambdoid sutures divide from the back end of the sagittal suture and run obliquely forwards to end up behind the each ear.

What are the symptoms?

Craniosynostosis causes distortion of the shape of the skull owing both to failure of bone growth at the prematurely closed suture, and to compensatory overgrowth at the sutures that remain open. The different types of craniosynostosis are classified by which sutures have closed prematurely. Most common (forty-five per cent) is sagittal synostosis, which gives a long, narrow head; next most frequent is coronal synostosis (twenty per cent), which may affect one side (unilateral) or both sides (bilateral) and gives a broad, flat head that is asymmetric in unilateral cases; metopic synostosis (fifteen per cent) causes a triangular-shaped forehead. Lambdoid synostosis is rare. However, not all abnormalities of skull shape are caused by craniosynostosis; a consequence of the 'back to sleep' campaign to reduce the occurrence of cot death has been a marked increase in the frequency of babies who have flat backs to their heads due to sleeping on their backs. In the absence of craniosynostosis, this condition, termed 'deformational plagiocephaly' slowly improves with age and does not require surgery.

The remaining twenty per cent of craniosynostosis is more complex and either involves the fusion of multiple sutures (five per cent), and/or is combined with additional changes in the face, limbs or other parts of the body, indicating a 'syndrome' (fifteen per cent). Over one hundred craniosynostosis syndromes have been described, most of which are extremely rare; the most common syndromes are Crouzon, Pfeiffer, Apert, Muenke, Saethre-Chotzen and craniofrontonasal syndromes. In these complex cases, there may be additional problems with the vision, breathing, hearing, teeth, learning development, facial appearance and malformation of the limbs and other organs.

What are the causes?

Craniosynostosis has a diversity of causes, the most important of which are abnormal pressure on the fetal skull inside the womb (intrauterine factors), and alterations in the genetic makeup (mutations). Intrauterine factors that predispose to craniosynostosis include having twins, reduced amniotic fluid, an abnormally shaped womb and breech position; commonly the mother reports that there was persistent discomfort during the pregnancy or that she had a feeling of the fetal head being stuck. These factors are believed to be especially important in sagittal and metopic synostosis, for which there is usually a low risk of the condition recurring in further children.

How is it diagnosed?

The diagnosis, assessment and surgical/medical management of craniosynostosis requires a multidisciplinary team approach, involving plastic, maxillofacial, and neurological surgeons, eye and ear/nose/throat specialists, geneticists, psychologists and speech therapists. In England and Wales, four centres located at Birmingham, Liverpool, London (Great Ormond Street Hospital) and Oxford are accredited to undertake this work. These centres also specialise in distinguishing true craniosynostosis from deformational plagiocephaly, which can sometimes be difficult.

Inheritance patterns and prenatal diagnosis

Inheritance patterns

Genetic mutations can be identified in about twenty-five per cent of cases, including many of the specific syndromes and also in some children with apparently non-syndromic coronal synostosis. The important genes identified to date are three of the fibroblast growth factor receptors (FGFR1, FGFR2 and FGFR3) and other genes called TWIST1 and EFNB1. Cases with a genetic cause are more likely to recur within the family. Genetic testing is available in the UK at two centres (Great Ormond Street Hospital, London and Churchill Hospital, Oxford).

Prenatal diagnosis

Prenatal diagnosis for craniosynostosis is generally only possible when a specific mutation has been identified.

Medical text written February 1994 by Dr W Reardon, Senior Registrar in Clinical Genetics, Institute of Child Health, London, UK. **Last updated December 2006 by Professor A Wilkie, Nuffield Professor of Pathology, Weatherall Institute of Molecular Medicine, Oxford University, Oxford, UK.**

Further online resources

Medical texts in *The Contact a Family Directory* are designed to give a short, clear description of specific conditions and rare disorders. More extensive information on this condition can be found on a range of reliable, validated websites. Further information on these resources can be found in our **Medical Information on the Internet** article on page 21.

Support

Headlines – Craniofacial Support

128 Beesmoor Road, Frampton Cotterell, Bristol BS36 2JP   Tel: 01454 850557
e-mail: info@headlines.org.uk   Web: http://www.headlines.org.uk

Originally, established in 1993 as the Craniofacial Support Group, the Group is a National Registered Charity No. 1058461 established by Contact a Family working with parents of affected children. It acts as an umbrella group for all the conditions associated with Craniosynostosis, many of which are individually listed in the index. Headlines has a full list of conditions coming under the Craniosynostosis umbrella that have been checked and approved by medical experts. It offers contact with other families with the same or similar condition where possible and has information and advice about the practical aspects of hospital visits and surgery. For UK residents, it can offer help and guidance in being referred to one of the four designated Craniofacial units. It publishes a newsletter 'Headlines' and has information available, details on request. The Group is in touch with over 1,000 people including professional workers, overseas members and over 500 families.

Group details last confirmed November 2007.

CREUTZFELDT-JAKOB DISEASE

Creutzfeldt-Jakob disease: CJD

Background

Creutzfeldt-Jakob disease is a rare, untreatable, fatal illness affecting the brain resulting in progressive neurological symptoms including dementia, involuntary movements, ataxia (incoordination and unsteadiness) and speech disturbances. It is a member of the group of Transmissible Spongiform Encephalopathies (TSEs) that are caused by an incompletely understood change in a normal cellular protein (designated PrPC) to an abnormal form (designated PrPSc). The manufacture of the normal protein (PrPC) is governed by a gene designated the PRNP gene (on human chromosome 20). The accumulation of the abnormal PrPSc in brain tissue is an essential underlying feature of CJD. Under certain, very specific, circumstances, CJD can be transmitted from one individual to another. The nature of this infectivity is not fully understood.

CJD is divided into four different forms (sporadic, genetic, iatrogenic, variant), partly on differences in symptoms and pathological changes in the brain, but essentially on differences in causation.

Sporadic CJD is the commonest form and is of unknown cause, apparently occurring randomly, mainly in the middle-aged and elderly. Most countries (including the UK) report incidences around 1 to 2 in 1,000,000 persons per year. A small number of cases are genetic, due to inherited defects in the PRNP gene. A minority of cases (iatrogenic CJD) are due to transmission of disease via medical or surgical treatments.

In 1996, a new variant of CJD, affecting relatively young people, was reported. Now called 'variant CJD', it is believed to be due to dietary contamination of food with Bovine Spongiform Encephalopathy (BSE). The number of cases of this form of CJD are in decline in the UK. Other countries, especially France, have also identified cases. In the UK, accidental transmissions of variant CJD by blood has been reported; this has not been reported for other forms of CJD.

How is it diagnosed?

There is, at present, no absolutely specific diagnostic test for CJD in life, aside from brain biopsy. However, a reasonably confident diagnosis of all forms of CJD is generally possible on purely clinical grounds, with the support of medical investigations including brain MRI (Magnetic Resonance Imaging) scans, EEG (electro-encephalogram recordings) and CSF (cerebro-spinal fluid) examinations. A genetic cause can be determined by PRNP gene analysis performed on a simple blood sample.

There is continuing surveillance of CJD in the UK, undertaken by the National CJD Surveillance Unit at Edinburgh. The Unit also has a Care Team who advise on, and help to co-ordinate, care of people with all forms of CJD.

Inheritance patterns and prenatal diagnosis

Inheritance patterns

A minority of cases is inherited with an autosomal dominant pattern.

Prenatal diagnosis

A test is available in the case of genetic CJD.

Medical text written December 1997 by Dr R Knight. **Last updated June 2007 by Dr R Knight, Consultant Neurologist, National Creutzfeldt-Jakob disease Surveillance Unit, Western General Hospital, Edinburgh, UK.**

Support

The National CJD Surveillance Unit
Bryan Matthews Building, Western General Hospital, Crewe Road, Edinburgh EH4 2XU
Tel: 0131 537 2128   Web: http://www.cjd.ed.ac.uk
The National CJD Surveillance Unit covering the UK is based in Edinburgh and can answer general queries on CJD.
Group details last updated July 2007.

CJD Support Network
PO Box 346, Market Drayton TF9 4WN   Tel/Fax: 01630 673993 Tel: 01630 673973 CJD Helpline   e-mail: support@cjdsupport.net Web: http://www.cjdsupport.net
The Network is a National Registered Charity No. 1097173. It offers support and advice on all forms of CJD and links families where possible. It also offers support to those who have been told they have an increased risk of CJD and to people who have been told that they are at a higher risk of CJD through blood transfusions or surgical instruments. It publishes a newsletter twice yearly and has information available, details on request. The Network has approximately 400 members.
Group details last updated March 2007.

Families of Human BSE
c/o Contact a Family, 209-211 City Road, London EC1V 1JN
Tel: 0808 808 3555 Helpline Tel: 020 7608 8700 Fax: 020 7608 8701
e-mail: info@cafamily.org.uk Web: http://www.cafamily.org.uk
The Families of Human BSE is a group established in 1997, all of whom have personal experience of the tragedy of variant CJD. They offer support to families of victims through family days, memorial events, a newsletter and an opportunity to talk to others. They had a formative role in gaining official recognition for the disease and believe their experience may be useful for concerned individuals.
Group details last updated February 2008.

National Prion Clinic
Box 98, National Hospital for Neurology and Neurosurgery, Queen Square, London WC1N 3BG Tel: 020 7405 0755   Fax: 020 7061 9889
e-mail: help.prion@uclh.org   Web: http://www.nationalprionclinic.org
The National Prion Clinic is a specialist service of the National Hospital for Neurology and Neurosurgery. Assessment, diagnosis, information, advice and support are available for patients, families, and health care professionals. A referral is not necessary for families or professionals to contact the clinic to discuss any CJD or Prion related issues.
Group details last confirmed October 2007.

CRI DU CHAT SYNDROME

Cri du Chat syndrome: Deletion 5p- syndrome; chromosome 5 short arm deletion

Background

Cri du Chat syndrome was first described by Lejeune et al (1963). Early research described the prevalence of Cri Du Chat syndrome as about 1 in 50,000 live births (Neibhur, 1978), although more recent estimates suggest a greater incidence of 1 in 37,000 live births (Higurashi, Masaaki et al 1990).

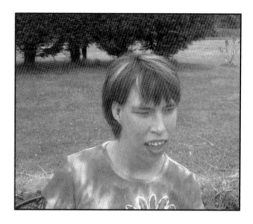

What are the symptoms?

The hallmark cat-cry is a core feature of Cri du Chat syndrome and is still regarded as an important early clinical diagnostic feature in most but not all individuals. Many infants tend to be of low birthweight and show marked hypotonia (see entry). Feeding difficulties are common and the associated failure to thrive may be the initial clinical presentation. Some infants may require enteral feeding, a process which may have to continue for several years. Certain facial and head abnormalities are also over represented: microcephaly (see entry), micrognathia, rounded face, macrostomia, hypertelorism with downward sloping palpebral fissures, low set ears, broad nasal ridge and short neck. Structural laryngeal abnormality and hypotonia are thought to be responsible for the cat-like cry.

The phenotype tends to become less striking with advancing age which may result in diagnostic difficulty in these circumstances; conversely, other features tend to become more apparent: long face, scoliosis (see entry) and macrostomia (Van Buggenhout et al 2000). In addition to the major health problems already described, children with Cri du Chat syndrome are very prone to develop recurrent upper respiratory tract infections, otitis media and dental problems. In contrast, the prevalence of epilepsy is very low compared to heterogeneous samples of people with severe learning disabilities (Cornish and Pigram 1996). Once patients manage to negotiate childhood, they can probably expect to live a normal life-span.

Psychological and behavioural characteristics

The early reports on the syndrome suggested that profound learning disability was a cardinal feature of the syndrome, presenting in all individuals with a 5p deletion. However, recent findings indicate that in children with typical Cri du

Chat, IQ predominantly falls into the moderate to severe learning disability range but that there is a crucial discrepancy in the pattern of language functioning with children displaying better receptive than expressive language (Cornish, Bramble et al 1999; Cornish and Munir 1998). These findings extend previous research that discovered 'language delay' to be a deviant feature of the syndrome by highlighting a particular strength within their cognitive profile. Even in children with very minimal speech, studies have shown that many can use basic sign or gestural language for communication (Carlin 1990).

Self-injurious behaviour appears to be very common in Cri du Chat syndrome (Dykens and Clarke 1997; Collins and Cornish 2001) most notably head banging, hitting the head against body parts, and self-biting all reaching a plateau in late childhood and then remaining constant throughout early adulthood. Clinical hyperactivity is also known to be over represented in children with the syndrome (Dykens and Clark 1997) and is further compounded by a high incidence of chronic sleep problems and restlessness.

Inheritance patterns and prenatal diagnosis

Inheritance patterns

Most cases of Cri du Chat syndrome are sporadic (eighty-five per cent) while ten to fifteen per cent of cases are familial with the overwhelming majority due to parental translocations.

Prenatal diagnosis

Chorionic Villus Sampling at ten to twelve weeks and amniocentesis at fifteen to sixteen weeks are available.

Medical text written July 2001 by Dr K Cornish and Dr D Bramble, Consultant Child and Adolescent Psychiatrist, Nottingham University, Nottingham, UK. **Last reviewed October 2005 by Professor K Cornish, Canada Research Chair in Neuropsychology and Education, McGill University, Montreal, Canada.**

Further online resources

Medical texts in *The Contact a Family Directory* are designed to give a short, clear description of specific conditions and rare disorders. More extensive information on this condition can be found on a range of reliable, validated websites. Further information on these resources can be found in our **Medical Information on the Internet** article on page 21.

Support

Cri du Chat Syndrome Support Group
5 Latimer Drive, Basildon SS15 4AD Tel: 0845 094 2725
e-mail: info@criduchat.co.uk Web: http://www.criduchat.co.uk
The Group is a National Registered Charity No. 1044942, established in 1987. It aims to provide support and friendship to families and carers throughout the UK and Ireland. The Group also seeks to raise awareness of the syndrome amongst the medical profession, parents, carers and the public. It organises an annual family weekend conference for families and professionals, encourages local area gatherings and produces two newsletters per annum. The Group is in touch with over 200 families.
Group details last confirmed October 2007.

CROHN'S DISEASE AND ULCERATIVE COLITIS

Background

Collectively known as Inflammatory Bowel disease (IBD), these chronic illnesses both involve severe inflammation of the digestive tract. Although they are different illnesses they are sometimes difficult to tell apart.

What are the symptoms?

Crohn's disease

Crohn's disease is usually characterised by inflammation of one or more areas of the digestive tract, with normal areas of gut in between. It can occur anywhere from the mouth to the anus but most commonly in the small and large intestine. This inflammation may lead to ulceration, abscesses and strictures in the bowel. It is a chronic (long lasting) condition which can wax and wane over a period of months and years. So far there is no cure but treatment can produce a symptom-free remission.

Oral Crohn's affecting the mouth and lips, occurs quite frequently in children and may occur with or without any involvement of the digestive tract.

With Crohn's disease the symptoms are extremely variable and can include severe abdominal pain (sometimes mistaken for appendicitis), vomiting, nausea, persistent diarrhoea (possibly with blood and/or mucus), constipation, dramatic weight loss, tiredness, anaemia and mouth ulceration. Sometimes the symptoms may not initially suggest bowel disease at all, with the child or young adult feeling very lethargic with a loss of appetite, joint pains, skin rash or even a failure to grow or develop pubertally.

Ulcerative Colitis

Ulcerative Colitis involves inflammation of the colon (large bowel) causing ulceration and bleeding. It may affect only the rectum or may spread along the whole length of the colon (universal or total Colitis). It is characterised by periodic relapses where the symptoms recur and periods of remission where the patient is symptom free.

With Ulcerative Colitis the symptoms are usually more acute with severe abdominal pain, persistent diarrhoea, usually with blood and mucus (slime) in the stools, and joint pains.

Inheritance patterns and prenatal diagnosis

Inheritance patterns

No definitive inheritance patterns have been scientifically established although there appears to be a familial tendency to develop the conditions and considerable evidence of inflammatory bowel disease running in families and even with siblings of the same parents.

Prenatal diagnosis

None.

Medical text written September 2000 by the Crohn's in Childhood Research Association. Approved September 2000 by Professor I Sanderson. **Last reviewed October 2005 by Professor I Sanderson, Professor of Paediatric Gastroenterology, St Bartholomew's and Royal London School of Medicine and Dentistry, London, UK.**

Further online resources

Medical texts in *The Contact a Family Directory* are designed to give a short, clear description of specific conditions and rare disorders. More extensive information on this condition can be found on a range of reliable, validated websites. Further information on these resources can be found in our **Medical Information on the Internet** article on page 21.

Support

Crohn's in Childhood Research Association
Parkgate House, 356 West Barnes Lane, Motspur Park KT3 6NB
Tel: 020 8949 6209 Administration, Information & Helpline   Fax: 020 8942 2044
e-mail: support@cicra.org   Web: http://www.cicra.org
The Association is a National Registered Charity No. 278212, established in 1978. It offers an advisory and support service for affected children, their families and carers and contact with other families where possible. It has several Regional Support Groups. It publishes a quarterly newsletter and has a wide range of information available, details on request.
Group details last confirmed October 2007.

National Association for Colitis and Crohn's Disease
4 Beaumont House, Sutton Road, St Albans AL1 5HH   Tel: 0845 130 2233 Information
Tel: 01727 830038 Office   Fax: 01727 862550   e-mail: nacc@nacc.org.uk
Web: http://www.nacc.org.uk
The Association is a National Registered Charity No. 1117148, established in 1979. It offers information and support. It publishes a newsletter: 'NACC News' and has a wide range of information available, details on request. The Association has over 30,000 members - affected people, their families and friends and health professionals.
Group details last updated August 2007.

CROUZON SYNDROME

Background

Crouzon syndrome was first described by Octave Crouzon in 1912. It is an inherited disorder of abnormal craniofacial (skull and face) appearance. The condition is thought to occur in about 1 in 50,000 births in the UK.

What are the symptoms?

A child with Crouzon syndrome may have the following symptoms with varying severity: facial problems (possibly causing cosmetic concern); and severe malformation of skull and face (bone or tissue) which can affect breathing, feeding, vision, hearing, dental and brain development.

The skull is made up of a number of flat plate-like bones (cranial bones) which are connected by seam-like joints (sutures). These joints allow neighbouring cranial bones to be mobile, so that they can slide over each other during birth and allow the growth of the brain without restriction during childhood. In adulthood these sutures fuse, becoming rigid and protecting the brain within. The growth of the face and the skull are closely related with similar sutures or joints of the facial bones, which also fuse through life.

In Crouzon syndrome the face, skull or both can be affected. Usually during pregnancy or within the first year of life the cranial (or facial) sutures begin to fuse early (craniosynostosis). The early fusion alters the normal pattern of skull growth and therefore the shape of the skull which can raise pressure within the skull (intracranial pressure) and have consequences for the brain. Characteristic skull shapes result from the pattern of the sutural fusion. Common terms for the resulting head shapes are brachycephaly (flat forehead and back of head, broad from side to side), scaphocephaly (a long narrow skull) and turricephaly or acrocephaly (a high, tower-shaped or pointed skull).

As well as the altered shape of the top of the head, the mid-face is often under-developed and the eye sockets are shallow. This can be present at birth or become more evident over time. The arrangement of teeth is also affected and, rarely, there can be palate problems. Seen from the side the face has a concave appearance and the shallow eye sockets can result in bulging eyes (exorbitism, also sometimes termed proptosis). Exorbitism can lead to problems with damage to the surface of the eyeball and it is important to protect the eyes. Characteristically in Crouzon syndrome there are no significant problems with the hands and feet, which helps doctors to distinguish it from related conditions such as Apert and Pfeiffer syndromes.

Although affected children may have a range of clinical problems, the head shape is often seen as the most striking initial feature, at the outset the major concerns are the ease of breathing and potential feeding problems. The under-developed mid-face can be associated with a small larynx (voice box) and restrict air supply to the windpipe and lungs causing respiratory distress. Similarly the passage of food can be affected and regurgitation can result in food going down the windpipe.

How is it treated?

The abnormal skull shape may require surgery to help relieve raised intracranial pressure (commonly revealed by headaches or visual changes identified by the ophthalmologist), and to reshape the abnormally formed skull and midface. Surgical decisions are made in the light of circumstances as they arise in the individual.

A child with Crouzon syndrome usually enters a co-ordinated programme of care involving many different clinical specialities integrating their diverse expertise, from birth to later teenage years. These include plastic-, maxillofacial- and neuro-surgeons, ophthalmologists, geneticists, orthodontists, orthoptists, psychologists and speech therapists. However, provided that the potential complications are treated and the child is regularly monitored, the majority of individuals with Crouzon syndrome have normal development and intelligence.

Inheritance patterns and prenatel diagnosis

Inheritance patterns

Most affected children are born to healthy parents ('new mutations') and increased age of the father may often be a related factor. The risk for such healthy parents of having another affected child is generally low (under one per cent). However, individuals who are themselves affected with Crouzon syndrome have autosomal dominant inheritance.

Prenatal diagnosis

The skull changes of Crouzon syndrome cannot reliably be detected by ultrasound scanning in pregnancy, because they develop too late on, and are usually too mild. However, where a specific genetic alteration has been identified in one of the parents, prenatal diagnosis is possible. Preimplantation genetic diagnosis (analysis of the fertilised egg in the test tube, followed by introduction of unaffected eggs) has also been successfully undertaken.

Medical text written March 2007 by Professor A Wilkie, Nuffield Professor of Pathology, Weatherall Institute of Molecular Medicine, Oxford University, Oxford, UK.

Support

There is no support group for Crouzon syndrome. Families can use Contact a Family's Freephone Helpline for advice, information and, where possible, links to other families. Contact a Family's web-based linking service Making Contact.org can be accessed at http://www.makingcontact.org

CUSHING SYNDROME/DISEASE

Before treatment   9 months after treatment

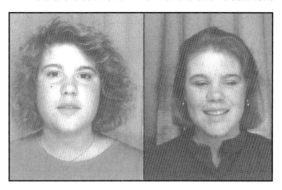

Background

Cushing syndrome is characterised by a 'moon' face, obesity of the trunk allied to muscular wastage of the limbs, Diabetes (see entry, Diabetes Mellitus), Osteoporosis (fragility of the bones) see entry Osteoporosis (Adult), hypertension (blood pressure), polycythaemia (an abnormal increase in circulating red cells in the blood), bruising and amenorrhoea (cessation of periods in girls and women). All characteristics may not be present in every case. The differential diagnosis may be difficult to elucidate and such patients may require intensive investigations for several weeks.

What are the causes?

Cushing syndrome is due to the effect of overproduction by the adrenal glands (small glands that sit on top of the kidneys). It is mostly commonly caused by hyperstimulation of the adrenal glands by a hormone called ACTH released by benign tumours of the pituitary gland (a pea size gland at the base of the brain) or rarely by tumours (ectopic ACTH syndrome) elsewhere in the body, such as the lungs or pancreas. Cushing syndrome caused by a pituitary tumour is called Cushing disease. Cushing syndrome can also be caused by tumours of the adrenal glands that can be benign or malignant.

Generally, young children have an adrenal tumour, whereas in adolescents this is usually a pituitary tumour.

However, a common cause of the syndrome is iatrogenic (the result of treatment), due to prolonged therapy with steroids prescribed for other disorders such as asthma.

The condition may arise at any age but most typically occurs in middle age and is more common in women.

How is it treated?

Treatment is predominantly surgical and directed at the site of the tumour.

Inheritance patterns and prenatal diagnosis

Inheritance patterns

None

Prenatal diagnosis

None

Medical text written September 2006 by Dr Peter Traine, Consultant Endocrinologist, Christie Hospital, Manchester, UK.

Further online resources

Medical texts in *The Contact a Family Directory* are designed to give a short, clear description of specific conditions and rare disorders. More extensive information on this condition can be found on a range of reliable, validated websites. Further information on these resources can be found in our **Medical Information on the Internet** article on page 21.

Support

ACTH

54 Powney Road, Maidenhead SL6 6EQ   Tel: 01628 670389
e-mail: cushingsacth@btinternet.com   Web: http://www.cushingsacth.co.uk
ACTH is a patient led and patient run self help support group, established in 1993. It offers telephone and e-mail support and an information pack. ACTH has the support of a medical panel.
Group details last confirmed June 2007.

CUTIS LAXA

Background

Cutis Laxa is an uncommon disorder that is usually hereditary and present either at birth or later in life. It is a disorder of very loose skin hanging in folds resulting from faults in the connective tissue which acts to bind together other tissues. Internally, the lungs, heart, intestines and arteries may be severely affected in some forms. Cutis Laxa affects both sexes equally and all ethnic groups.

There are a number of forms of Cutis Laxa caused by varying types of inheritance. Mutations of genes on Chromosomes 7,14 and the X chromosome have been identified or suggested. Cutis Laxa may also occur with a number of other inherited syndromes. Rarely, it can be acquired following illnesses in which fever or severe skin rash is present.

What are the symptoms?

There are a large number of features of the different types of Cutis Laxa as so many body organs can be affected. These include:

- Autosomal Dominant Cutis Laxa (Isolated skin laxity)
    - Loose skin;
    - Premature ageing.
- Autosomal Recessive Cutis Laxa - Type 1
    - Generalised loose skin from birth;
    - Breathing difficulties due to emphysema;
    - Defect in one of the connective tissues called fibrillin has been reported.
- Autosomal Recessive Cutis Laxa - Type 2
    - Generalised loose skin from birth;
    - Joint laxity including dislocation of hips;
    - Delayed closure of the skull sutures (seams between the skull bones);
    - Developmental delay;
    - Growth failure.
- Autosomal Recessive Cutis Laxa - Type 3 (De Barsy)
    - Generalised loose skin from birth;
    - Joint laxity;
    - Abnormal movements (athetosis);
    - Developmental delay;
    - Clouding of front of eye (corneal opacity).
- X-Linked Cutis Laxa/Ehlers-Danlos syndrome (see entry, Ehlers-Danlos syndrome) (Lysyl oxidase deficiency)
    - Loose skin;
    - Joint laxity;

- Abnormal scarring of skin;
- Deficiency of the enzyme that is vital to the development of the connective tissue.
- Acquired Cutis Laxa
  - Cutis Laxa may rarely occur following fever or skin disorders. The acquired form can be serious if it involves the blood vessels or lungs.

How is it diagnosed?

Diagnosis of Cutis Laxa can be made by observation of the known features of the disorder. Skin biopsies (tissue examination) and pulmonary tests may be carried out.

How is it treated?

There is no cure for Cutis Laxa and treatment is symptomatic for the features of the condition. Surgical intervention may help to manage loose folds of skin, prolapses (the slipping out or fall of an organ) and hernias but these procedures may be of temporary benefit.

Inheritance patterns and prenatal diagnosis

Inheritance patterns

Cutis Laxa can be autosomal recessive, autosomal dominant or X-linked.

Prenatal diagnosis

None

Medical text written July 2006 by Contact a Family. Approved September 2006 by Professor Michael Patton, Professor of Medical Genetics, St George's Hospital Medical School, London, UK.

Further online resources

Medical texts in *The Contact a Family Directory* are designed to give a short, clear description of specific conditions and rare disorders. More extensive information on this condition can be found on a range of reliable, validated websites. Further information on these resources can be found in our **Medical Information on the Internet** article on page 21.

Support

There is no UK based support group for Cutis Laxa but Cutis Laxa Internationale, Web: http://www.orpha.net/nestasso/cutislax has contacts in a number of countries. Contact a Family's Freephone Helpline has contact details for the UK representative. Families can use Contact a Family's Freephone Helpline for advice, information and, where possible, links to other families. Contact a Family's web-based linking service Making Contact.org can be accessed at http://www.makingcontact.org

CYCLICAL VOMITING

Cyclical Vomiting: CVS; Cyclic Vomiting syndrome (USA)

Background

Cyclical Vomiting syndrome is a condition of recurrent episodic attacks of vomiting and intense nausea. CVS typically has an on-off pattern which is stereotypical within individuals. The episodes are similar, in time of onset, duration and symptomatology, for each patient.

CVS is usually a disease of children with an average age of onset of five years but onset may be at any age and CVS can affect both children and adults. Children with CVS have a strong predisposition to develop migraine headache. This most commonly occurs around puberty but about one third of children with cyclical vomiting will continue to suffer from cyclical vomiting attacks well into their teens. In many but not all patients, the cyclical vomiting attacks will subside as migraine headaches develop. In a number of patients the onset of symptoms may be during the teens or even in adult life and some patients will continue to have symptoms of cyclical vomiting as adults.

Cyclical vomiting is probably not a single condition. Most children probably have a condition related to migraine, but similar symptoms may be secondary to a number of other conditions including renal pelvi-ureteric junction obstruction, intracranial space occupying lesions and a number of rare metabolic disorders. It is not known if the syndrome in adults has the same relation to migraine as that in children

What are the symptoms?

Before the attacks some patients experience early signs of an attack minutes to hours in length and consisting usually of malaise, anxiety and mild nausea. The onset of the attack is more frequently seen during the night or on awakening in the morning. The principal feature of the condition is recurrent discreet episodes of vomiting lasting hours or days with frequent retching. If prolonged and untreated the attack may cause life-threatening dehydration. Nausea is constant throughout the episode and is frequently intense, although the intensity varies from patient to patient. There is a high frequency of vomiting at the peak of the attack with vomiting every ten to fifteen minutes. The average attack duration is twenty-four hours but some patients have considerably longer attacks lasting for several days. Most patients become intensely pale although some may become flushed. Other associated problems include headache, abdominal pain, photophobia and dizziness. The attacks are self-limited and at the end of the attack there is rapid resolution to normality. Shortly after the attack stops the patient is likely to be completely well and demanding food. Between attacks the patient is completely well and free of nausea and vomiting.

The frequency of attacks ranges from one to seventy per year with an average of twelve attacks per year. They occur at regular intervals in about half of patients and sporadically in others. Most patients can identify experiences or conditions which may precipitate attacks, the most common being heightened emotional states and infections. Both unpleasant emotional stress and pleasant excitements such as birthdays, parties and holidays may trigger episodes. Other reported triggers include tiredness, hot weather, motion sickness, fasting and specific foods.

How is it diagnosed?

Individual attacks of CVS are often diagnosed as gastroenteritis and it is only when a pattern emerges over time that they can be identified as CVS. Many patients with milder symptoms have not sought medical attention or the condition has not been recognised.

How is it treated?

There is no good evidence-based treatment for cyclical vomiting based on controlled clinical trials. Attack frequency may be reduced by the use of migraine prophylactic drugs such as Propranolol and Pizotifen. Acute attacks are usually treated with intravenous fluids (usually ten per cent Dextrose) and Ondansetron. Sedation with Lorazepam may be required.

Inheritance patterns and prenatal diagnosis

Inheritance patterns

A family history of migraine is frequently seen in Cyclical Vomiting syndrome and, as with other forms of migraine, the condition appears more commonly to be inherited from the mother. It has been suggested that cyclical vomiting may be a mitochondrial disease.

Prenatal diagnosis

None.

Medical text written October 2002 by Dr D N K Symon. **Additional material written August 2005 by Contact a Family. Last updated June 2007 by Dr D.N.K. Symon, Consultant Paediatrician, University Hospital of Hartlepool, Hartlepool, UK.**

Support

CVSA

77 Wilbury Hills Road, Letchworth SG6 4LD   Tel: 0151 342 1660
e-mail: info@cvsa.org.uk   Web: http://www.cvsa.org.uk
The CVSA is a National Registered Charity No. 1045723, established in 1991. It offers support for families of affected children and adults and contact between families where possible. The group holds an annual family day/conference, publishes a biannual newsletter and has information available, details on request. The CVSA has over 240 family, affected adult, professional and overseas members.
Group details last updated August 2007.

CYSTIC FIBROSIS

Background

Cystic Fibrosis causes the mucous glands to produce abnormally thick, adherent mucus and the sweat glands to produce excess salt. The two main areas of the body involved are the lungs and the pancreas (part of the digestive system). The mucus is responsible for the principal complications.

What are the symptoms?

As well as Diabetes, later complications can include liver disease (see entry) and Osteoporosis - see entry, Osteoporosis (Adult). The lung problems of Cystic Fibrosis result from the pressure of thick sticky mucus which attracts infection. This is controlled by physiotherapy and drugs to help clear the mucus and antibiotics to tackle the infections.

Cystic fibrosis is a life-threatening condition. seventy-five per cent of affected children now survive to young adulthood and the average survival is around thirty years.

What are the causes?

In cystic fibrosis the lungs are normal at birth but become susceptible to bacterial infection and damage. The thick mucus collects in the lungs blocking some airways and resulting in damage caused by the infection. Much of this damage can be prevented through adequate treatment of infections.

In the pancreas the small channels (through which the enzymes produced in the pancreas flow to reach the intestines) become blocked with mucus. This results in cysts being formed and these lead to fibrosis in the pancreas. The enzymes produced by the pancreas are vital to normal digestion. Digestive enzyme preparations can replace most of the digestive enzymes produced by the pancreas.

Insulin is also produced in the pancreas. However, in most cases of cystic fibrosis, the pancreas usually manages to produce enough insulin in childhood but diabetes (see entry, Diabetes Mellitus) is increasingly common in adults.

How is it diagnosed?

A simple mouthwash test can determine if an individual is a carrier. Testing is important if a relative is known to have Cystic Fibrosis or is a carrier. It is particularly important if a partner is known to be a carrier.

Less than a quarter of babies in the UK are tested for Cystic Fibrosis at birth using a heel-prick blood test. Neo-natal testing for all babies has been approved and should be available in 2004.

Inheritance patterns and prenatel diagnosis

Inheritance patterns

Cystic fibrosis is the commonest inherited life-threatening disorder amongst Caucasians in the UK today. Inheritance is autosomal recessive.

Prenatal diagnosis

Diagnosis can be made by chorionic villus sampling about the tenth to twelfth week of pregnancy. A later test (amniocentesis) is available at sixteen weeks. These tests are usually offered to mothers recognised as being at high risk of having a child with Cystic Fibrosis. Screening for carriers of the CF gene is now possible.

Medical text written November 1991 by Contact a Family. Approved November 1991 by Professor M Patton, Professor of Medical Genetics, St Georges Hospital Medical School, London, UK and Dr J E Wraith, Consultant Paediatrician, Royal Manchester Children's Hospital, Manchester, UK. **Last updated January 2003 by the Cystic Fibrosis Trust. Approved January 2003 by Dr J Littlewood, Chairman of the Cystic Fibrosis Trust Research and Medical Advisory Committee, Bromley, UK.**

Support

Cystic Fibrosis Trust

11 London Road, Bromley BR1 1BY   Tel: 0845 859 1000 CF Trust Helpline
Tel: 020 8464 7211 CF Trust   Fax: 020 8313 0472   e-mail: enquiries@cftrust.org.uk
Web: http://www.cftrust.org.uk
The Trust is a national registered charity No. 1079049, established in 1964. It offers support and information to anyone affected by Cystic Fibrosis. It funds research, offers some financial support to families and campaigns for improved services. It publishes CF Today, CF Talk (for adults with CF) and Focus on Fundraising, distributed free of charge, and has a wide range of information available, including publications and consensus documents on Cystic Fibrosis. Details on request or via the website.
Group details last updated June 2007.

Barnardos Sherwood Project
2 Clinton Avenue, Nottingham NG5 1AW   Tel: 0115 969 1177
Barnardos Orchard Service (Cystic Fibrosis)
Orchard House, Buston Terrace, Jesmond, Newcastle on Tyne NE2 2JL
Tel: 0191 240 4813   e-mail: orchard.project@barnardos.org.uk
Barnardos also run some regional services for children and young people with cystic fibrosis. Each service varies slightly in the support it offers. Referral varies slightly according to the support offered.
Group details last updated August 2006.

Butterfly Trust

Forth House, 28 Rutland Square, Edinburgh EH1 2BW   Tel: 0131 221 6556
Fax: 0131 221 6557   e-mail: info@butterflytrust.org.uk
Web: http://www.butterflytrust.org.uk

The Butterfly Trust is a Scottish Charity No. SC 033174, established in 2002. The Trust offers emotional and practical support to people with Cystic Fibrosis including supporting statements on a range of issues, help to obtain benefits and grants, and advocacy and representation at Disability Appeals Tribunals. They also offer transport to hospital appointments and a youth befriending service. The Butterfly Trust's services are delivered by a national team of trained volunteer support workers. The Trust responds to the estimated 700 people in Scotland with Cystic Fibrosis.
Group details last updated October 2006.

Research by Contact a Family Wales found that support groups offered a variety of services including: play and leisure facilities; mutual support; information; and training. Parent Support Groups - from Parent Support to Providing Services. Sally Rees. Contact a Family. 2002.

CYSTIC HYGROMA

Background

Cystic Hygromas are non-malignant malformations of lymphatic vessels, usually occurring around the head and neck region. They are usually evident by three years of age. They may be single or multiple. If they are large they may be detected on antenatal ultrasound scans. They are usually slow-growing and may spontaneously resolve or reduce in size. Rapid growth does occasionally occur if there is internal bleeding into the cysts or if there is a complicating infection.

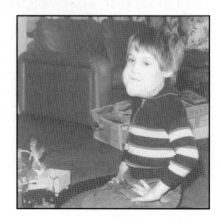

How is it treated?

Large cysts present at birth may necessitate a tracheostomy (see entry) if there is pressure on the airway, though this is rare. Small cysts may not require any specific treatment except to wait and see how they develop. Larger cysts which continue to grow may need to be actively treated. Laser treatment to cystic hygromas in the mouth can help to reduce their bulk to help eating. Surgical reduction of these lesions in either the mouth or neck may also be helpful. An alternative treatment has been to use an attenuated bacteria (OK432) as an injection into the cysts, which causes a local sclerosing reaction which may help to reduce the size of the lesions.

Inheritance patterns and prenatal diagnosis

Inheritance patterns

No hereditary association has been identified

Prenatal diagnosis

In some cases the condition has been diagnosed through ultrasound scanning while in others it has remained undetected. This is because there is a wide variation in the extent of the condition which ranges from a small growth on the neck to a very extensive mass of growths.

Medical text written July 1999 by Mr J Harcourt. **Last reviewed November 2004 by Mr J Harcourt, Consultant Paediatric Ear Nose and Throat Surgeon, Chelsea and Westminster Hospital, London, UK.**

Support

Cystic Hygroma Support Group

55 Jewel Walk, Bewbush, Crawley RH11 8BH   Tel: 01293 571545 (24 hour answerphone)
This is a Contact Group started in 1983. It offers contact with other parents where possible. The group represents around 200 families in the UK, mainly with affected children. The group also has contact with families in Australia and the USA.
Group details last confirmed June 2007.

"I searched for information on the condition for over two years and your e-mail contained more information than I had been able to find in all that time. I cannot thank you enough." Parent.

CYTOMEGALOVIRUS (CMV)

Background

Cytomegalovirus (the large cell virus) is a common virus and about fifty per cent of the population of Britain have been infected with it at some time. Frequently the infection passes unnoticed or there may be mild flu-like symptoms. The virus belongs to the herpes family, which includes the chicken-pox, cold sore and glandular fever viruses. Once infection has taken place, the virus remains dormant within the body, usually with no ill effects. However, recurrences of the virus in body fluids may occur at intervals.

In the UK about forty per cent of women are susceptible to CMV at the time of pregnancy. The main risk is when women catch the viral infection for the first time in pregnancy. Women are usually only mildly unwell with a sore throat and flu-like illness. The chance of the baby becoming infected is about forty per cent. Over ninety per cent of infected babies have no signs of anything wrong at birth.

What are the symptoms?

Some of the infected infants may go on to develop sensorineural hearing loss (SNHL) over the first five years of life. CMV is probably one of the main causes of isolated bilateral SNHL in childhood. A small proportion of vertically infected children will be symptomatic at birth and they can have pneumonia, liver disease, or neurological problems. The central nervous system problems include microcephaly, cerebral palsy, and developmental delay.

Some or all of these symptoms may occur in individual cases.

How is it treated?

Trials are ongoing for the treatment of infected children in the newborn period with antiviral medication. There is no prenatal therapy at present, but trials are starting in this area also.

Inheritance patterns and prenatal diagnosis

Inheritance patterns

None

Prenatal diagnosis

Infections can be diagnosed in pregnancy, and women should be encouraged to seek medical advice for minor flu like illnesses during pregnancy.

Medical text written November 1991 by Contact a Family. Approved November 1991 by Professor M Patton, Professor of Medical Genetics, St Georges Hospital Medical School, London, UK and Dr J E Wraith, Consultant Paediatrician, Royal Manchester Children's Hospital, Manchester, UK. **Last updated December 2004 by Dr M Sharland, Consultant Paediatrician in Paediatric Infectious diseases, St George's Hospital, London, UK.**

Contact a Family Helpline 0808 808 3555

Further online resources

Medical texts in *The Contact a Family Directory* are designed to give a short, clear description of specific conditions and rare disorders. More extensive information on this condition can be found on a range of reliable, validated websites. Further information on these resources can be found in our **Medical Information on the Internet** article on page 21.

Support

The Congenital Cytomegalovirus Association
11 Windmill Hill Lane, Kingsway, Derby DE22 3BN Tel: 01332 365528
e-mail: support@cmvsupport.org   Web: http://www.cmvsupport.org
The Association is a Self Help Group, established in 1986. It offers contact between families and campaigns for further research. It publishes a newsletter and has information available, details on request. The Association represents approximately 100 families.
Group details last updated February 2008.

If you are a parent caring for a disabled child who receives the middle or highest rate of Disability Living Allowance care component you may also be entitled to receive Carer's Allowance as their carer. For more information, and a copy of the guide 'Benefits, Tax Credits and other financial assistance' call the Contact a Family Helpline.

DANCING EYE SYNDROME

Dancing eye syndrome: Kinsbourne syndrome; Myoclonic encephalopathy; Opsoclonus-Myoclonus syndrome

Background

This is a very rare neurological condition which develops over days or a week or two. The features are unsteadiness (ataxia) jerky movements of the trunk and limbs (myoclonus), rapid involuntary eye movements in all directions (opsoclonus) and usually marked irritability with sleep disturbance. As with many other diseases, there is considerable variation in severity.

Most children develop the condition in the second or third year of life but rarely it may occur earlier or later in childhood.

What are the causes?

There is also an adult variant of the condition which is almost always associated with particular cancers. In children the condition may occur with no clear trigger or it may follow a viral illness or it may be associated with a tumour called a neuroblastoma (see entry). Whenever Dancing Eye syndrome is diagnosed it is therefore important that tests are undertaken to exclude neuroblastoma. If neuroblastoma is present it is usually, but not always, a benign variant of the tumour. Treatment of the neuroblastoma, whilst important in its own right, does not appear to alter the outcome of the Dancing Eye syndrome.

Because of the association with preceding infection and with neuroblastoma, it is thought likely that Dancing Eye syndrome is the result of an immune or allergic cross-reaction in the brain although there is no definite proof of this as yet.

How is it treated?

The treatments used have been those used to suppress the immune response. Steroids given by mouth or injection have been the main drugs used. More recently, intravenous immunoglobulin infusions have been used with benefit either instead of, or in addition to, steroids. Other treatments which may help include azathioprine, cyclophosphamide, plasma exchange and rituximab. Because the condition is very rare and variable in the way it develops, it has been very difficult to collect enough children to formally evaluate different treatment options in a controlled and scientific fashion. Currently such a study is under way in the USA but will probably take some time to reach a conclusion.

The longer term outcome of this condition is very variable. Occasional children fully recover very quickly without treatment. Others respond to treatment partially or completely. Some of these children may relapse either as the treatment is withdrawn or following a viral infection which may have stimulated the immune response. More severely affected children often have longer-term problems with learning, co-ordination, behaviour and sleep.

Inheritance patterns and prenatal diagnosis

Inheritance patterns

No familial trend has been identified.

Prenatal diagnosis

Not applicable.

Medical text written August 1996 by Dr J Wilson, Honorary Consultant Paediatric Neurologist, Great Ormond Street Hospital, London, UK. **Last Updated January 2007 by Dr M Pike, Consultant Paediatric Neurologist, Children's Hospital, Oxford. UK.**

Further online resources

Medical texts in *The Contact a Family Directory* are designed to give a short, clear description of specific conditions and rare disorders. More extensive information on this condition can be found on a range of reliable, validated websites. Further information on these resources can be found in our **Medical Information on the Internet** article on page 21.

Support

Dancing Eye Syndrome Support Trust

78 Quantock Road, Worthing BN13 2HQ   Tel/Fax: 01903 532383
e-mail: support@dancingeyes.org.uk   Web: http://www.dancingeyes.org.uk
The Trust is a National Registered Charity No. 1060181, established in 1988. It offers telephone contact and a summer outing for families. It publishes a newsletter twice a year and has information available, details on request. The Trust represents over 65 families. Group details last confirmed January 2007.

DANDY-WALKER SYNDROME

Background

This is a condition whereby there is probably abnormal development of the foraminae (holes) through which the cerebrospinal fluid (CSF) exits from inside the brain to the outside surface. The foraminae, not having properly opened during fetal development cause a blockage of the flow of the CSF and so produce an abnormal enlargement of the fourth ventricle (fluid cavity between the brainstem and the cerebellum). This results in failure of parts of the cerebellum to develop correctly. A large cyst is then visible on scans of the back of the brain. These are severe abnormalities with hydrocephalus (see entry) being present in ninety per cent of cases. Dandy-Walker causes two to four per cent of all hydrocephalus cases. Conditions with similar appearances are called Dandy-Walker variant. Most commonly, however, there is no obvious explanation for its presence.

There are often many associated brain abnormalities including agenesis of the corpus callosum (see entry) in seventeen per cent of cases, occipital encephalocoele (failure of fusion of the bones at the back of the head) in seven per cent, spina bifida (see entry), syringomyelia (cysts in the spinal cord) (see entry), or small heads and bone abnormalities of the neck (Klippel-Feil syndrome). Other associated abnormalities include facial, ocular (eye) and cardiac.

How is it treated?

With treatment, prognosis is generally good with a seventy-five to one hundred per cent chance of survival, but only fifty per cent of cases will develop a normal IQ. Balance, co-ordination and mobility problems are common, reflecting problems with the cerebellum and brain stem. Up to fifteen per cent of cases will have seizures.

Inheritance patterns and prenatal diagnosis

Inheritance patterns

Most cases are sporadic but there is one per cent chance of recurrence in further pregnancies.

Prenatal diagnosis

Ultrasound scan may detect the Dandy-Walker syndrome cysts.

Medical text written November 2002 by Mr Neil Buxton, **Last updated June 2007 by Mr Neil Buxton, Consultant Paediatric Neurosurgeon, Alder Hey Children's Hospital, Liverpool, UK.**

Further online resources

Medical texts in *The Contact a Family Directory* are designed to give a short, clear description of specific conditions and rare disorders. More extensive information on this condition can be found on a range of reliable, validated websites. Further information on these resources can be found in our **Medical Information on the Internet** article on page 21.

Support

Support and advice about Dandy-Walker syndrome is available from ASBAH (Association for Spina Bifida and Hydrocephalus (see entry, Spina Bifida).

Local Authorities can give payments, instead of services, to allow disabled people and carers to buy in the services they have been assessed as needing. To find out more about direct payments, and for a copy of a guide on this, call the Contact a Family Helpline.

DARIER DISEASE

Darier disease: Darier's disease; Keratosis Follicularis

Background

Darier disease is characterised by itchy, warty, skin-coloured bumps (known as papules) and characteristic nail abnormalities. The features and severity of Darier disease vary enormously from isolated nail changes or a few warty bumps to disfiguring involvement.

What are the symptoms?

The characteristic features of Darier disease are firm, rather greasy, rough papules, which are skin coloured, yellow-brown or brown. The papules may join up in certain moist areas of the body such as the armpits, groin, or under the breasts to form large, sometimes thick plaques. When this occurs, the affected skin may smell unpleasant. The smell is caused by bacteria growing in the rash and does not mean that the skin has not been washed. In some individuals large warty masses cause embarrassment. The psychosocial consequences of the papules may be one of the main difficulties faced by individuals with Darier disease.

Many individuals become aware of the signs of Darier disease before the age of thirty years and in the majority, it starts between the ages of ten to twenty years. At first papules tend to appear on an individual's chest, neck or upper back and many papules are freckle-like. In addition, an individual's scalp, forehead, neck and the skin around the ears may be scaly and itchy. Occasionally, small spots may form in the mouth, which gives the roof or sides of the mouth a rough feeling.

Papules are initially skin-coloured but become darker and more greasy and crusted over time. Darier disease tends to worsen with exposure to sunlight, typically in the summer. Thus affected regions may improve during the winter. The itch of Darier disease may be exacerbated by wool or nylon clothing. Some women may notice that it worsens around the time of their period.

Individuals with Darier disease may have dry and brittle fingernails that sometimes appear 'bitten'. The nails often have red and white longitudinal bands with a V-shaped nick at the free margin of the nail. Wart-like bumps on the backs of the hands may be present in childhood and pits or small 'corns' may appear on the palms of the hands or on the soles of the feet. Some individuals notice that the condition improves or stabilises as they get older, whilst others report that the condition slowly gets worse.

Individuals may be susceptible to skin infections with the herpes simplex virus, otherwise known as the 'cold sore' virus. This does not mean that Darier disease is contagious - it is not. If the condition suddenly worsens and becomes more painful, then this may be a sign of herpes simplex infection. In these instances, it is recommended that individuals contact their GP or dermatologist.

Darier disease may cause depression and in some families has been linked to learning difficulties.

What are the causes?

Normally, the cells that form the epidermis (top layer of the skin) are held together by special 'glues' and 'cables', like bricks cemented in a wall. In Darier disease, the skin cells are not held together properly and subsequently the skin becomes scaly, lumpy and may blister. Darier disease is caused by a mutation (change) in a gene on chromosome 12 that makes a calcium pump within the skin cells. This pump produces signals that control the complicated operations of the cells. In Darier disease the pump does not work properly leading to faulty signalling in the skin cells.

Inheritance patterns and prenatal diagnosis

Inheritance patterns

Darier disease is inherited as an autosomal dominant trait and affects both men and women. People with the condition have a fifty per cent chance of passing Darier disease on to their children. Sometimes Darier disease appears 'out of the blue' in families without a history of the condition.

Prenatal diagnosis

Not available.

Medical text written November 2003 by Contact a Family. Approved November 2003 by Dr S Burge. **Last updated April 2006 by Dr S Burge, Assistant Director of Clinical Studies and Consultant Dermatologist, Churchill Hospital, Oxford, UK.**

Support

There is no effective support group for Darier Disease. Families can use Contact a Family's Freephone Helpline for advice, information and, where possible, links to other families. Contact a Family's web-based linking service Making Contact.org can be accessed at http://www.makingcontact.org

DEAFBLINDNESS

Background

Deafblindness - sometimes known as dual sensory impairment or multi-sensory impairment - is a combination of sight (see entry, Vision Disorders in Childhood) and hearing difficulties (see entry, Deafness). Some individuals will be literally deaf and blind; many others will have some sight and/or hearing that they can make use of. Most deafblind people will have difficulties with communication, mobility and access to information.

An individual may be born deafblind (called congenital deafblindness) or acquire deafblindness later in life, and the needs and problems of these two groups are different. People born deafblind will often have other difficulties to cope with. They may have physical disabilities, learning difficulties, experience delays in learning, or have challenging behaviour.

What are the causes?

In the past, the predominant cause of congenital deafblindness was rubella. If a woman catches rubella in early pregnancy, it can be passed on and cause damage to the unborn child - including vision and hearing impairment, heart defects (see entry) and damage to the central nervous system. Today, deafblindness is caused by a wide range of factors including premature birth, plus a range of syndromes and conditions such as CHARGE syndrome (see entry). Deafblindness may also be acquired as a result of infection after birth, for example, meningitis (see entry).

There are many causes of acquired deafblindness. The genetic condition Usher syndrome (see entry) and hearing. Some people who have been born deaf or blind, may also lose their sight or hearing through accident or illness.

Inheritance patterns and prenatal diagnosis

Inheritance patterns

Some causes of deafblindness such as Usher syndrome are inherited. Some such as Joubert syndrome (see entry) may be inherited or sporadic. Some causes such as CHARGE Association are a sporadic event the cause of which is often unknown.

Prenatal diagnosis

Where deafblindness is associated with a specific condition, prenatal diagnosis may be available.

Medical text written October 2004 by Dr T Best, Chief Executive, Sense, London, UK.

Support

Sense

11-13 Clifton Terrace, London N4 3SR   Tel: 0845 127 0060   Tel: 0845 127 0062 Text
Fax: 0845 127 0061   e-mail: info@sense.org.uk   Web: http://www.sense.org.uk

Sense Northern Ireland

Family Centre, Manor House, 51 Mallusk Road, Newtonabbey BT36 4RU.
Tel: 028 9083 3430 (querty text phone)   Fax: 028 9084 4232
e-mail: nienquiries@sense.org.uk

Sense Scotland

42 Middlesex Street, Kinning Park, Glasgow G41 1EE   Tel: 0141 429 0294
Tel: 0141 418 7170 Querty text phone   Fax: 0141 429 0295
e-mail: info@sensescotland.org.uk   Web: http://www.sensescotland.org.uk

Sense Cymru

5 Raleigh Walk, Brigantine Place, Atlantic Wharf, Cardiff CF10 4LN   Tel: 029 2045 7641
Text: 029 2046 4125   Fax: 029 2049 9644   e-mail: cymruenquiries@sense.org.uk
Sense is a National Registered Charity No: 289868, established in 1955. Sense supports and campaigns for children and adults who are deafblind. Sense provides specialist information, advice and services to deafblind people, their families, carers and the professionals who work with them. In addition, it supports people who have sensory impairments with additional disabilities. Services include support for families, help for deafblind people living in their own homes, day services where deafblind people can build confidence and learn new skills, and small group homes in the community - where people are supported to live as independently as possible. It publishes a journal 'Talking Sense' three times a year and has a wide range of information available, details on request. Over 5,000 families and professionals are in touch with Sense.
Group details last updated August 2007.

DEAFNESS

Background

The human ear and its central connections are well developed and help us to hear a range of sounds in complex listening conditions, have a sense of direction and movement of sounds and also help to maintain our balance. In some ways it is probably the most developed sensory organ we have.

The outer hair cell system within the inner ear help us to hear a vast range of sounds from very quiet to very loud by dampening down the loud and amplifying the quiet sounds. The whole auditory system is capable of "filtering out" unwanted background noise. When this system fails, not surprisingly, the first symptom we experience is difficulty in hearing speech when there is background noise. Similarly if the balance organ within the inner ear is not functioning well we experience dizziness or vertigo and a sense of motion, and in a child, this may manifest as delayed physical milestones e.g. delay in walking.

Hearing is extremely important for the development of spoken language. Those with a pre-lingual (prior to development of speech) profound hearing loss will not have access to speech sounds and hence will not develop oral language, while those with a severe pre-lingual hearing loss will not develop normal speech. Moderate hearing loss may affect speech and (oral) language development and will have a considerable effect on mainstream education of children. Mild hearing losses also may affect the ability to learn depending on a number of other factors.

Permanent hearing impairment

The incidence of significant permanent congenital hearing impairment (PCHI) is about 1 in 1,000 live births in most developed countries although this may be 3-4 times higher in certain communities or parts of the UK. The incidence almost doubles by ten years of age because of acquired hearing loss from meningitis (see entry), mumps, measles, trauma and other causes. The most common reason for PCHI is loss of hair cells in the inner ear but it is sometimes due to malformation of the middle ear ossicles (small bones that transmit vibrations of the ear drum) or the ear canal (tube from the outer to the inner ear). If the hearing loss is due to a problem within the inner ear (sensory), or occasionally due to abnormalities in the hearing nerve (neural), the term sensorineural hearing loss is used. Hearing loss due to a problem within the middle ear or the outer ear is called a conductive hearing loss while a combination of sensorineural and conductive hearing loss is called a mixed loss.

Glue Ear

In addition to PCHI and postnatally acquired permanent hearing loss, almost 40 – 60% of children develop 'glue ear' (synonyms: otitis media with effusion, fluid in the middle ear, middle ear effusion) during the first 6 years of life due to dysfunction of the Eustachian tube (tube that links path of the throat to the ear) with the incidence reducing as the child gets older. Otitis media with effusion (OME) is usually a temporary condition with mucus-like fluid accumulated within the middle ear (behind the ear drum) becoming thick with time (hence the name 'glue ear'). Glue ear during the first few critical developmental years of life, may lead to some speech and language delay and sometimes auditory processing difficulties. Persistent glue ear, with a significant hearing loss or other associated problems such as frequent ear infections, is normally treated by draining the middle ear fluid and inserting a tube called a 'grommet' to ventilate the middle ear. Hearing aids are also recommended as an alternative or while waiting for grommets, or when surgery is not possible. The hearing loss with glue ear is never severe or profound unless there is an additional permanent sensorineural hearing loss. Hence 'glue ear' alone is unlikely to cause severe speech and language delay.

Auditory Neuropathy/ Auditory Dys-syncrony

A form of deafness that has attracted interest of audiologists and clinicians more recently is Auditory Neuropathy/ Dys-synchrony. This is a condition where there is often a mis-match between objective tests of hearing and the behavioural tests. This group belongs to the "neural" component of sensorineural deafness and is estimated to be up to 10% of all SNHL. The dys-synchronous firing of the hearing nerve fibres can be due to a number of reasons including dysfunction of the (1) inner hair cells, (2) synapse (the junction between the IHC and the hearing nerve), (3) hearing nerve itself, (4) VIIIth nerve nucleus in the brainstem and (5) brainstem pathways themselves. The pathology / aetiology may vary from genetic (otoferlin mutation that leads to absent or malfunctioning IHC) and, jaundice and hypoxia at birth, to delayed maturation of the hearing pathway. Diagnosis of this condition entails specific testing and multidisciplinary assessments with management requiring an experienced team.

Some of the aetiological investigations need to be carried out within the first few months of life and others repeated later to maximise the potential for arriving at a diagnosis. Amongst the causes of congenital hearing loss are: maternal infections such as Rubella which is now very rare because of immunisation; cytomegalovirus which is probably the commonest infective aetiology that can cause a progressive hearing loss; prematurity; severe lack of oxygen to the fetus; severe jaundice; some drugs that are harmful to inner ears; and genetic inheritance.

How is it diagnosed?

NHS Newborn hearing screening program was launched to cover the whole of England in April 2005 and this gives an opportunity for all parents to have their newborn baby's hearing screened at birth, leading to early diagnosis of hearing loss and any associated medical conditions, giving a chance to make an informed choice for their child, intervene early, leading to better hearing, speech and educational outcomes.

How is it treated?

Interventions include introducing a communication medium of parental choice, hearing aid fitting and cochlear implants when hearing aids do not help. Those children with absent ear canals or significant middle ear abnormalities may be helped with specialised devices such as bone conduction or bone anchored hearing aids.

Once confirmed it is also important to find the reason for the hearing loss for the following reasons:

- For prevention of progression of hearing loss by treating the cause e.g. CMV infections;
- Hearing loss may be only a part of a general condition or may be the first symptom of such a condition. Identifying this will help to manage other associated medical problems and also may help to prevent complications;
- Knowing the cause of the hearing loss and hence the natural history will help to better plan the needs of the child;
- Knowing the diagnosis, both audiological and medical, will lead to better counselling for the parents especially if they are planning to have more children. Also, the child may eventually want to know the diagnosis and chances of passing it on to his/her children.

Inheritance patterns and prenatal diagnosis

Inheritance patterns

About 50% of all PCHI is due to a genetic cause. Of this 75-80% show an autosomal recessive (AR) inheritance. In this form of inheritance each parent passes on one copy of the gene responsible for deafness and therefore the baby has two copies of the same gene thus manifesting the condition while the parents are asymptomatic as they also have a copy of the normal gene. AR hearing loss can be part of a syndrome such as Usher syndrome (see entry) and Pendred syndrome (see entry), or non-syndromic (NS). The commonest AR gene responsible for non syndromic deafness (NS) is Connexin 26. This accounts for 40-50% of all AR NS deafness and can be tested for.

About 20% of PCHI is due to an autosomal dominant (AD) inheritance, where the child needs only one copy of the dominant gene to be affected. Often there is deafness on one side of the family with each baby carrying approximately 50% chance of having the dominant gene responsible for deafness. Examples of dominant syndromic deafness include Treacher Collin syndrome (see entry), Branchio Otorenal (BOR) syndrome and Waadenburg Syndrome. Often in AD syndromic hearing loss the degree of symptoms and signs may vary from member to member because of variability of penetrance and expressivity of the gene responsible.

Other forms of inheritance include X-linked and mitochondrial. Inheritance of X-linked deafness e.g. Alport syndrome (hearing loss and kidney involvement) is from affected father to daughters (because the father passes on the Y chromosome to his sons) and from affected mother to approximately 50% of all children irrespective of the sex. As mitochondria are in the cytoplasm, and it is only the ovum that contains cytoplasm (sperm has only the nucleus and no cytoplasm) the inheritance of mitochondrial deafness is from mother to children. Often in mitochondrial deafness there is more than one system/organ involved. A1555G is one such mitochondrial mutation that makes individuals more susceptible to ototoxicity from aminoglycoside drugs such as gentamicin.

It must be remembered that more than one gene could be responsible for a given syndrome and some syndromes may show more than one pattern of inheritance.

Your geneticist should be able to tell you more about the small number of genes that can be tested for, but as new mutations are identified it is expected that this number will increase.

Prenatal diagnosis

Where deafness is part of a specific syndrome or condition with major abnormalities prenatal diagnosis may be available.

Medical text written January 2003 by Dr Tony Sirimanna. **Last updated December 2007 by Dr Tony Sirimanna, Consultant Audiological Physician, Great Ormond Street Hospital for NHS Trust, London, UK**

Support

The National Deaf Children's Society (NDCS)
15 Dufferin Street, London EC1Y 8UR
Tel: 0808 800 8880 Freephone Helpline & Minicom (Mon-Fri, 10am-5pm)
Tel: 020 7490 8656 Switchboard   Fax: 020 7251 5020
e-mail: helpline@ndcs.org.uk   Web: http://www.ndcs.org.uk
The Society is a National Registered Charity No. 1016532. It is the only UK charity solely dedicated to the support of all deaf children and young deaf people, their families and professionals working with them. NDCS services include a Freephone helpline giving clear, balanced information and support on many issues relating to childhood deafness with specialist advice on audiology and technology. When calling the helpline, if you prefer to speak a language other than English, tell us the language of your choice and your phone

number (in English). An interpreter will ring you back within a few minutes. The NDCS also provides a network of family officers, who offer advice on education and welfare benefits.
Group details last confirmed August 2007.

RNID for deaf and hard of hearing people

19-23 Featherstone Street, London EC1Y 8SL   Tel: 0808 808 0123
Tel: 0808 808 9000 Text   Fax: 020 7296 8199
e-mail: informationline@rnid.org.uk   Web: http://www.rnid.org.uk
The organisation is a National Registered Charity No. 207720. It offers equipment and employment services. It has a network of regional offices and a national telephone relay service through RNID Typetalk. It holds Disability and Deaf Awareness Training and campaigns on issues ranging from subtitling to audiology services. It publishes a membership magazine 'One in Seven' and has a wide range of information available, details on request. Over 25,000 use the services of the RNID.
Group details last confirmed November 2007.

Deafness Research UK

330-332 Gray's Inn Road, London WC1X 8EE
Tel: 0808 808 2222 Freephone Information Service (Mon-Fri 9am-5pm)
Tel: 020 7915 1412 Textphone   Tel: 020 7833 1733   Fax: 020 7278 0404
e-mail: info@deafnessresearch.org.uk   Web: http://www.deafnessresearch.org.uk
Deafness Research UK, formerly Defeating Deafness, is a National Registered Charity No. 326915, established in 1985. It is the medical charity for deaf and hard of hearing people. Supported entirely by voluntary contributions, Deafness Research UK aims to educate people about hearing problems and their treatments, offering information and advice based upon the most up-to-date evidence available. It also aims to encourage and finance research into the prevention, diagnosis, treatment and cure of hearing difficulties.
Group details last updated October 2007.

deafPLUS

National Office, Trinity Centre, Key Close, Whitechapel, London E1 4HG
Tel/Fax: 020 7790 6147   Tel: 020 7790 5999 Textphone   e-mail: info@deafplus.org
Web: http://www.deafplus.org
deafPLUS is a National Registered Charity No. 1073468, established in 1970 as Breakthrough. It is committed to deaf/hearing integration for those 18 plus and delivers essential services through its regional structure across England, covering the North, South, Midlands, London and Eastern regions. deafPLUS operates a Mobile Advisory Service providing demonstrations of equipment across the range of deafness for use in the home, at work or in the community. Information, advice and support is provided through drop in centres, advocacy work and peer group support. deafPLUS provides employment, sports and healthy living advice, internet cafes, equipment assessment, an interpreting agency and works with ethnic communities. It delivers a wide array of training to the public and private sector on deafness issues.
Group details last updated October 2007.

Hearing Concern

95 Gray's Inn Road, London WC1X 8TX   Tel: 08450 744 600 HelpDesk (voice & text)
Tel: 020 7440 9871   Fax: 020 7440 9872   e-mail: info@hearingconcern.org.uk
Web: http://www.hearingconcern.org.uk
Hearing Concern is a National Registered Charity No. 1094497, established in 1947. It supports deaf and hard of hearing people, in the UK, whose main mode of communication is speech.
Group details last updated April 2007.

DEGOS DISEASE

Degos disease: Malignant Atrophic Papulosis: Kohlmeier-Degos disease

Background

Degos disease is a rare inherited condition first described by Kohlmeier in 1941 and Degos in 1942. There are thought to have been about one hundred and fifty cases of the condition reported in medical literature. The most severe form is Systemic Degos disease affecting children and adolescents with most cases occurring in young adults. Benign Degos disease also affects adults.

What are the symptoms?

Systemic Degos disease affects a number of body systems:

- **Skin** – pink or red papules (solid raised lesions) primarily on the trunk and limbs healing to leave white scars;
- **Gastrointestinal** – abdominal pain, nausea, vomiting, diarrhoea or constipation and, in the later stages, intestinal perforation and haemorrhage may occur;
- **Neurological** – manifestations involve the peripheral and central nervous systems leading to headaches, dizziness, seizures, hemiplegia (total or partial paralysis of one side of the body), aphasia (loss or impairment of the power to use or comprehend words), paraplegia (paralysis of the lower half of the body), and gaze palsy (partial or complete inability to move the eyes to all directions of gaze);
- **Ocular** – ptosis (drooping of the upper eyelid), optic neuritis (inflammation of optic nerves), diplopia (double vision) and visual field defects may occur.

Benign Degos disease usually only produces the typical skin lesions of the condition.

How is it diagnosed?

Degos disease is usually diagnosed by endoscopy (an instrument for visualizing the interior of a hollow organ) or skin biopsy (examination of tissue).

Affected individuals need to be carefully monitored for symptoms of Systemic Degos disease.

How is it treated?

There is only symptomatic treatment for the condition although research continues to try to find effective drugs. Surgical intervention may be needed for gastrointestinal bleeding, gastrointestinal perforation, bowel infarction (death of tissue) or intracranial bleeding.

Inheritance patterns and prenatal diagnosis
Inheritance patterns
Degos disease is familial (tending to occur in a number of members of a family). It has been suggested that it has autosomal dominant inheritance but this has not been confirmed.
Prenatal diagnosis
Not applicable.

Medical text written September 2004 by Contact a Family. Approved September 2004 by Dr A Theodoridis, Department of Dermatology, Charité - Universitaetsmedizin Berlin, Germany.

Further online resources
Medical texts in *The Contact a Family Directory* are designed to give a short, clear description of specific conditions and rare disorders. More extensive information on this condition can be found on a range of reliable, validated websites. Further information on these resources can be found in our **Medical Information on the Internet** article on page 21.

Support
Degos Patient's Support Network
53 Mill Road Avenue, Angmering BN16 4HX   Tel: 01903 787737
e-mail: judith@degosdisease.com   Web: http://www.degosdisease.com
The Degos Patients' Support Network is a contact group, a support group and an information hub for those affected by Degos disease. Medical professionals who are seeking help will find information, links to medical sites and to ongoing research. As Degos disease is an extremely rare disease, the Network welcome input from those affected by it. Group details last updated August 2007.

DEMENTIA IN CHILDREN

Dementia in Children: Neurodevelopmental Regression in Children

Background

Dementia is the more common term for neurodevelopmental regression. The majority of people with dementia are elderly people with such disorders as Alzheimer's disease (see entry), Frontotemporal Lobar degeneration including Frontotemporal Dementia (see entry) and Multi-infarct Dementia (see entry, Dementias)

Conditions that involve dementia include:

- **Adrenoleukodystrophy** (see entry). Except in extremely rare cases, only boys have Adrenoleukodystrophy, a life limiting disorder, which leads to progressive dementia;
- **Alexander disease** (see entry). The infantile form of the disease leads to delayed development and dementia;
- **Autism (Infantile)** see entry Autism Spectrum disorders including Asperger syndrome. Within the first three years, children have a triad of poor social communication; delayed acquisition of speech or unusual use of language; circumscribed interests or repetitive behaviours. In a small proportion of children with autism, regression and loss of previously acquired skills occur. Usually not progressive;
- **Batten disease** (see entry) **(infantile): Neuronal Ceroid Lipofuscinosis 1**. With an onset of between six months and two years, rapidly progresses with seizures, dementia, blindness and a severe loss of neurones;
- **Batten disease** (see entry) **(late infantile): Neuronal Ceroid Lipofuscinosis Type 2**. With an onset of between two and four years, leads to seizures, blindness, loss of muscle co-ordination, mental deterioration and dementia;
- **Batten disease** (see entry) **(Juvenile): Neuronal Ceroid Lipofuscinosis Type 3**. With an onset of between five and nine years, characterised by visual loss initially, and later seizures, loss of motor abilities and dementia;
- **Brain injuries** (see entry). Depending on the severity of the injury, there can be many possible long-term problems, such as permanent memory problems, speech problems, weakness of the limbs, fits, cognitive, developmental and emotional problems and occasionally dementia;
- **Canavan disease** (see entry). In early infancy, children begin to lose previously acquired skills including vision and hearing;
- **Creutzfeldt-Jacob disease** (see entry) **(CJD)**. Results in progressive neurological symptoms including dementia;

- **Disintegrative disorder**. Children usually develop normally in the first three years of age, but then gradually develop significant social communication difficulties and lose previously acquired skills, including cognitive, motor and social skills. Often progressive;
- **Huntington's disease** (see entry) **(Juvenile)**. The cognitive impairment is selective so, despite their difficulties with speech, patients may have a considerable degree of comprehension throughout the illness;
- **Metabolic diseases** (see entry). Dementia can be associated with a number of the very rare metabolic disorders not separately described in this list;
- **Niemann-Pick disease** (see entry) **Type C**. Onset of dementia in a very varied life expectancy of between five and forty years;
- **Rett syndrome** (see entry). Although signs may not be initially obvious, it is present at birth but usually becomes more evident during the second year. Children with Rett syndrome are almost always profoundly and multiply disabled and dependent on others for all their needs throughout their lives but severity may vary considerably;
- **Subacute-sclerosing Panencephalitis** (see entry) **(SSPE)**. SSPE is a rare consequence of measles leading to a rapid or, in some cases, lengthy decline in function;
- **Tay Sachs disease** (see entry). A baby usually develops normally until about six months of age but the nervous system is progressively affected.

For support and information, relating to these disorders, refer to the separate entries.

What are the symptoms?
Symptoms may include:
- loss of memory, inability to concentrate and poor sense of time and place;
- difficulty in finding the right words, or understanding what people are saying;
- difficulty in completing simple tasks and solving minor problems;
- mood changes and emotional upsets, sometimes with depression.

It is important that professionals involved with families of children with conditions that include dementia are aware of these aspects of the condition. Great distress can be caused to families if professionals without this knowledge consider such conduct as forgetfulness and mood change as bad or disobedient behaviour. Information about possible dementia in a child as a result of their condition should be given clearly and sensitively to families.

What are the causes?

In children, dementia mainly arises from genetic, often metabolic, disorders that affect the brain and cause loss of learnt skills. Other causes of dementia in children include AIDS related dementia, brain injury and subacute-sclerosing panencephalitis (SSPE). The term pseudo-dementia is used where loss of skills is temporary, such as during the spasms of some rare epilepsies, or when a temporary dementia-like picture occurs during severe depression.

Dementia may involve loss of memory, the ability to think clearly, to understand words and to recognise people. Children with dementia can show personality changes and unusual or distressing behaviour.

Medical text written April 2006 by Contact a Family. Approved April 2006 by Dr P Santos, Consultant in Developmental Neuropsychiatry and Neuropharmacology, Great Ormond Street Hospital, London, UK.

Support

For support and information, relating to these disorders, refer to the separate entries.

There is no support group for Childhood Disintegrative disorder, also known as Heller syndrome. A description of the disorder can be found at Web: http://www.nlm.nih.gov/medlineplus/ency/article/001535.htm .

DEMENTIAS

Background

Dementia is caused by different illnesses which affect the brain. It may involve loss of memory, the ability to think clearly, to understand words and to recognise people. People with dementia can show personality changes and unusual or distressing behaviour. There are currently seven hundred and fifty people in the UK with some form of dementia. Mostly they are over sixty-five, but eighteen thousand people under sixty-five also suffer from dementia.

What are the symptoms?

Symptoms may include:

- loss of memory, inability to concentrate and poor sense of time and place;
- difficulty in finding the right words, or understanding what people are saying;
- difficulty in completing simple tasks and solving minor problems;
- mood changes and emotional upsets, sometimes with depression.

Often people forget what they meant to do, lose their way in places they know and become confused when using a telephone or working out change. Some people change their eating habits, get dressed in the middle of the night or wander off.

Early in the disease the affected person, their friends and family can help by writing things down and using reminders. Later people often lose the skills they need for everyday life, and may fail to recognise family members. Eventually the brain ceases to direct activities and they become dependent on others. People may become bed-bound and unable to resist infection. The most common cause of death is pneumonia.

What are the causes?

The most common cause of dementia is Alzheimer's disease (see entry), closely followed by vascular dementia and dementia with Lewy bodies. Other conditions which can cause dementia include Frontotemporal Lobar degeneration including Frontotemporal Dementia, Down syndrome (see entries), HIV (see entry, HIV infection and AIDS) and many others.

Inheritance patterns

This varies according the type of dementia.

Prenatal diagnosis

None.

Contact a Family Helpline 0808 808 3555

Vascular Dementia

Vascular Dementia (VaD) also including Multi-infarct Dementia

This can be caused by a single stroke that is either large or affects very important areas of the brain; by repeated very small strokes that accumulate over time; or by extensive changes around the very small blood vessels in the white matter of the deep part of the brain (which in an extreme form is sometimes called Binswanger's disease). Large strokes are obvious but, because of the physical problems that can develop, the related difficulties with memory or other higher cognitive functions are often not recognised. As many as twenty-five per cent of older people can develop VaD after a stroke. Smaller strokes in the brain and changes around the very small blood vessels are less obvious and may just result in gradual progression of symptoms or may be experienced as 'dizzy spells' , but they do lead to cumulative damage to important areas of the brain. VaD is the most common cause of dementia after Alzheimer's disease.

Symptoms can sometimes be distinguished from Alzheimer's - the decline in higher brain function is more likely to have a clear start date, and symptoms often progress in a series of steps following small strokes. Symptoms may include:

- difficulties with planning and slowed thinking;
- memory problems;
- depression and mood swings;
- epilepsy.

Some areas of the brain may be more affected than others and, as a result, some cognitive abilities may be relatively unaffected. The person is more likely to be aware of their impairments than in Alzheimer's disease. This can increase depression.

Anyone who has had a stroke is at greater risk of another, and someone with VaD is usually at high risk of further damage.

There is no specific treatment for VaD, but the underlying risk factors and stroke disease can be treated. Proper control of blood pressure and other risk factors such as high cholesterol, diabetes and irregular heart rhythm will reduce the rate of progression and improve outcome. Treatment with an antiplatelet drug like aspirin will also reduce the risk of further stroke. Half of the people with VaD will also have some changes similar to Alzheimer's disease in the brain. There is some evidence that these people benefit from treatment with cholinesterase inhibitor drugs.

Inheritance patterns

Unclear, but a number of genes have been identified as risk factors for vascular disease.

Prenatal diagnosis
None.

Dementia with Lewy bodies

Dementia with Lewy bodies (DLB) is a cause of dementia very similar to Alzheimer's disease. A very similar dementia can develop in people who have had Parkinson's disease (see entry) for a number of years. DLB differs both in the precise nature of the symptoms and in the damage that is found in the brain after death from Alzheimer's disease. The disease gets its name because of the deposits which are found in the brain after death (named after the doctor who first wrote about them). Lewy bodies are round deposits which contain damaged nerve cells. They are probably formed as the cells try to protect themselves from attack.

Dementia with Lewy bodies can result in:

- problems with attention and concentration ;
- impairments of language;
- difficulties with memory;
- impaired consciousness, a bit like delirium;
- visual hallucinations;
- symptoms of Parkinson's disease;
- falls.

For people with this form of dementia, hallucinations, for example seeing a person or pet on a bed or a chair when nothing is there, can be particularly distressing and problematic.

They usually develop some Parkinson's disease-type symptoms such as slowness of movement, stiffness and tremor. In a few cases heart rate and blood pressure are affected. The abilities of the affected person often fluctuate from hour to hour, and over weeks and months. This sometimes causes carers to think that the person is putting on their confusion.

It is possible that some people suffer from both Alzheimer's disease and Dementia with Lewy bodies.

Similarly to what happens in Alzheimer's disease, production of numerous chemical messengers, including acetylcholine and glutamate, are disrupted as nerve ends are attacked and cells die. The loss of the cholinergic system (nerves with acetylcholine as the messenger) is particularly pronounced in DLB patients. DLB patients also have a loss of the messenger dopamine in one of the parts of the brain that controls motor movement.

Several studies (mostly using the drug exelon) show that people with DLB and with dementia developing after Parkinson's Disease respond very well to cholinesterase inhibitor treatment. Drugs given to improve symptoms of Parkinson's disease may help the motor symptoms, but have to be used cautiously as they can worsen hallucinations in some people. It is also important to avoid harm, as people with DLB are particularly sensitive to neuroleptic tranquilliser drugs (which are often prescribed for visual hallucinations or behavioural symptoms), which can cause severe side-effects, or even death.

Inheritance patterns

A lot is now known about genetic factors which may be important for the development of Parkinson's disease. These are now being investigated to see whether they are also important for the development of DLB. As is the case for Alzheimer's disease, in the wider community there is a genetic risk linked to the ApoE4 gene.

Prenatal diagnosis

None.

Medical text written November 2004 by the Alzheimer's Society. Approved November 2004 by Professor C Ballard, Director of Research, Alzheimer's Society, London, UK.

Further online resources

Medical texts in *The Contact a Family Directory* are designed to give a short, clear description of specific conditions and rare disorders. More extensive information on this condition can be found on a range of reliable, validated websites. Further information on these resources can be found in our **Medical Information on the Internet** article on page 21.

Support

Support and information about dementia can be obtained from the Alzheimer's Society (see entry, Alzheimer's disease).

DEPRESSION IN CHILDREN AND YOUNG PEOPLE

Background

Depression is an illness that affects people of all ages including children and young people.

It is thought that about one per cent of children and three per cent of teenagers are affected by depression.

The rate rises sharply at puberty. Before puberty, as many boys as girls are affected but after puberty twice as many girls are affected as boys. There is little good evidence about depression in children in various ethnic groups but is it thought that under the age of ten it is similar in all ethnic groups. However in teenagers it is thought that emotional problems, including depression, are much higher in the Pakistani and Bangladeshi communities but this is not reflected in the black and Indian communities. There is evidence that adults who have depression first experienced this before the age of twenty years.

What are the symptoms?

The symptoms of depression in children and young people, as with adults, include changes in mood, thinking and behaviour. The key symptoms are:
- persistent sadness or low (irritable) mood;
- loss of interests and/or pleasure;
- fatigue or low energy levels.

These core symptoms may also be accompanied by:
- Change in sleeping patterns – poor or increased sleep;
- Agitation or slowing of movement;
- Change in eating habits – poor or increased appetite;
- Low self-confidence and indecisiveness;
- Feelings of guilt, self blame or worthlessness;
- Lack of concentration leading to lower school performance;
- Self harm and possible suicidal feelings;
- Withdrawal from communication with other children and young people.

Children and young people may find it difficult to voice or describe their feelings and the stigma associated with mental illness can also make diagnosis difficult. The onset of symptoms may be masked by what are thought of by adults as some of the usual aspects of childhood and adolescence such as irritability and changes in enjoyment of, or participation in, previously liked activities.

What are the causes?

Depression usually has multiple causes. Most episodes of depression arise in young people where there is a background of longstanding psychosocial difficulties, for example, family disharmony, divorce, separation, domestic violence, child abuse, and school difficulties such as bullying academic problems and/or isolation. The majority of episodes of depression also occur acutely after a life event such as the breakdown of an important relationship.

One way to make sense of the different theories of causation is to think of children and young people as being made more vulnerable to depression because of genetic and biological factors, and early adverse experiences and then having their depression 'triggered' by a combination of current social circumstances and adverse life events. Possible biological factors include changes in monoamine transmitter levels in the brain and also changes in cortisol metabolism.

How is it diagnosed?

A diagnosis will usually be made after a health care professional talks with the child or teenager both with and without his/her parents. Information from others such as a teacher who knows the child or teenager may be sought. Occasionally, a physical condition can lead to symptoms similar to those of depression. For this reason a physical examination may be needed to eliminate conditions such as glandular fever, anaemia, breathing problems such as sleep apnoea or thyroid disorders. If a diagnosis of depression is made, it may be described as mild, moderate or severe according to the number of symptoms that are identified.

How is it treated?

Treatment of depression in children and young people falls into two categories: psychological treatments (psychotherapy or counselling - talking treatments); and physical treatments (medication). Psychological treatments should be suggested first. For mild depression, referral to a specialist may not be necessary and the health care professional may advise 'watchful waiting' - monitoring the progress of the young person accompanied by sensible advice about diet, exercise and encouraging the child to take part in normal activities.

If there is no progress or if the depression is more severe, psychological treatments such as cognitive behaviour therapy and interpersonal therapy will be suggested. Other psychological treatments that may be suggested include family therapy and more intensive individual child psychotherapies. If psychological treatments are not bringing about improvement then, in teenagers, antidepressant medication will be suggested (and considered even in children) in addition to the psychological treatment. Where medication is prescribed children and young people should be monitored carefully in the first few weeks as there is evidence that the use of anti-depressants could lead to feelings of agitation and suicide when first prescribed. Hospital treatment may be indicated if the child or young person is at serious risk because of self harm or self neglect.

About ten per cent of children and young people will recover spontaneously within a few months and forty per cent within a year. The average length of depression referred for treatment is about six months but relapses are common and about one third will have a further episode within five years. There is evidence that if medication has helped treat depression it should be continued for at least six months after symptoms have gone in order to prevent recurrence.

The National Institute for Health and Clinical Excellence (NICE) has produced guidelines on the treatment of depression in children and young people for healthcare professionals, children and young people themselves, parents and carers, Web: http://www.nice.org.uk/CG028. More information can be found at Web: http://www.besttreatments.co.uk/btuk/conditions/35261.html which carries information for both doctors and lay people. It is produced by the British Medical Journal and endorsed by NHS Direct.

Inheritance patterns and prenatal diagnosis
Inheritance patterns
None.
Prenatal diagnosis
None.

Medical text written March 2006 by Contact a Family and Professor D Cottrell, Professor of Child and Adolescent Psychiatry, Leeds University, Leeds, UK.

Support
Support and information relating to Depression in children and young people can be obtained from Young Minds and the Scottish Mental Health Association. Details of these organisations can be found in the Mental Health entry.

DERMATOMYOSITIS and POLYMYOSITIS

Background

These conditions are manifestations of a very rare auto-immune inflammatory disease of the muscles and skin. **Dermatomyositis (DM)** usually affects the skin with a rash, and the muscles, which become weak; while **Polymyositis (PM)** generally affects the muscles but not the skin. The rash of DM is typically on the face and knuckles but can be on other parts of the body. The weakness of DM and PM typically starts in the large muscles of the arms and legs. In adults, both DM and PM may be associated with cancer, which can become apparent after the onset of the muscle problem.

Juvenile Dermatomyositis (JDM) can develop in children at any age but typically children with JDM get their illness between the ages of four and ten. JDM is rare, affecting about 3 or 4 in 1,000,000 each year. JDM is more common than **Juvenile Polymyositis (JPM)**.

What are the symptoms?

The onset of the disease may be sudden but more usually it develops over a period. Lethargy is often the first symptom and, in young children, parents may notice that the child is miserable or irritable. They may have a rash, often on the knuckles, hands and face, but it also may occur on other parts of the body, such as elbows, knees or ears. The child may gradually become weak and may also have fever, joint pain, tummy ache and headaches.

What are the causes?

These diseases are thought to be due to inflammation of the muscle and small blood vessels which can show invasion of the tissues by lymphocytes (white blood cells). The reason for this is not known.

How is it treated?

The progress of the disease is unpredictable and may include relapses. However most children with JDM will respond well to treatment which usually includes using steroids and other medications such as methotrexate. Children with JDM or JPM also need physiotherapy and an exercise programme, to help them regain strength in their muscles, as the disease is controlled by the treatment. A major difference between affected children and adults is that in children there is no association between JDM and cancer.

Inheritance patterns and prenatal diagnosis

Inheritance patterns

Some research has shown that certain parts of our genetic make-up may make Dermatomyositis and Polymyositis slightly more likely. However these diseases are not "inherited" and it is very rare indeed to have two patients with myositis in any one family. JDM and JPM are more common in girls than boys; while DM and PM are more common in women than in men.

Prenatal diagnosis

The condition is extremely rare under one year and therefore is not diagnosed before birth.

Medical text written September 2006 by Dr Lucy Wedderburn, Reader and Consultant in Paediatric Rheumatology, Institute of Child Health and Great Ormond Street Hospital, London, UK.

Further online resources

Medical texts in *The Contact a Family Directory* are designed to give a short, clear description of specific conditions and rare disorders. More extensive information on this condition can be found on a range of reliable, validated websites. Further information on these resources can be found in our **Medical Information on the Internet** article on page 21.

Support

Myositis Support Group

146 Newtown Road, Woolston, Southampton SO19 9HR

Tel: 023 8044 9708 (Mon-Fri, 10am-3pm)   Fax: 023 8039 6402

e-mail: enquiries@myositis.org.uk   Web: http://www.myositis.org.uk

The Group is a National Registered Charity No. 327791, established in 1985. It offers support for families and affected persons together with advice and information about problems such as welfare rights. It publishes a bi-annual newsletter and has information available, details on request. It also raises funds for research. The Group has over 500 members including over 250 affected adults and the families of over 80 affected children. Group details last updated November 2007.

DIABETES - MATURITY ONSET DIABETES OF THE YOUNG

Background

Maturity Onset Diabetes of the Young (MODY) is a rare, genetic form of diabetes accounting for one per cent of diabetes (twenty thousand people) in the UK, although it often goes unrecognised. It is familial and is characterised by a young age of onset (often diagnosed under twenty-five years of age) and non-insulin dependent diabetes.

What are the causes?

It runs in families as the diabetes is caused by a change in a single gene which may be inherited from an affected parent. Six genes have been identified in which changes may cause MODY. The two most common are called glucokinase (GCK) and hepatocyte nuclear factor 1 alpha (HNF1 alpha).

How is it diagnosed?

Diagnostic genetic testing for patients thought to have MODY is now available at the Royal Devon and Exeter Hospital which is the UK referral centre for MODY. This may confirm the diagnosis of MODY and the specific subtype which allows specific decisions regarding treatment to be made, such as the use of a sulphonyurea in those with HNF1 alpha. It also allows guidelines to be given about the likely clinical course of the diabetes.

In families where MODY has been confirmed by genetic testing a predictive genetic test may be offered to those family members who have shown no signs of diabetes. This would reveal whether they have inherited a normal gene and have the same chance of developing diabetes as the general population or whether they have inherited an affected gene and therefore have a seventy-four per cent chance of developing diabetes before the age of 30.

Further information regarding MODY and genetic testing may be obtained from the website http://www.diabetesgenes.org which is run by the Department of Diabetes and the Centre for Molecular Genetics at the University of Exeter and Royal Devon and Exeter Hospital, Exeter, UK.

How is it treated?

People with MODY due to a change in the GCK gene have a slightly raised blood glucose from birth which may go undetected. This remains stable throughout life and is usually managed by diet alone. The complications of diabetes are rare in this group.

HNF1 alpha accounts for sixty-five per cent of UK MODY and this type of diabetes usually presents during adolescence or early adult life. This type of diabetes is progressive with diet treatment frequently being replaced by tablets or insulin. However these patients are known to be particularly sensitive to tablets called sulphonylureas which help the body produce more insulin and this is considered the most appropriate form of treatment for this group.

Inheritance patterns and prenatal diagnosis

Each child has a fifty per cent chance of inheriting the affected gene from their parent with MODY and if they inherit the affected gene their lifetime risk of developing diabetes is greater than ninety-nine per cent.

Medical text written April 2003 by Dr M Shepherd, Senior Clinical Research Fellow, Peninsula Medical School, Exeter, UK.

Support

Support for Maturity Onset Diabetes of the Young can be obtained from Diabetes UK, see entry, Diabetes Mellitus.

DIABETES MELLITUS

Background

Diabetes mellitus is a condition in which the amount of glucose (sugar) in the blood is too high because the body cannot use it properly. Glucose comes from the digestion of starchy foods such as bread, rice, potatoes, chapatis, yams and plantain, from sugar and other sweet foods, and from the liver which makes glucose.

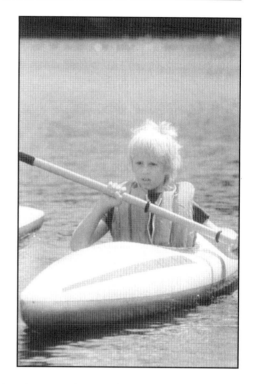

Insulin is vital for life. It is a hormone produced by the pancreas, which helps the glucose to enter the cells where it is used as fuel by the body.

Type 1 diabetes develops if the body is unable to produce any insulin. This type of diabetes usually appears before the age of forty. It is treated by insulin injections and diet.

Type 2 diabetes develops when the body can still make some insulin, but not enough, or when the insulin that is produced does not work properly (known as insulin resistance). This type of diabetes usually appears in people over the age of forty, though often appears before the age of forty in South Asian and African-Caribbean people. It is treated by diet alone or by diet and tablets or, sometimes, by diet and insulin injections.

What are the symptoms?

The main symptoms of untreated diabetes are increased thirst, going to the loo all the time (especially at night), extreme tiredness, weight loss, genital itching or regular episodes of thrush, and blurred vision.

What are the causes?

Type 2 diabetes in children

The number of children developing Type 2 diabetes continues to rise and spread through all cultures as children become less active and more overweight.

Insulin resistance is strongly associated with obesity. The importance of prevention of Type 2 diabetes in children cannot be overstated, as this is a chronic lifelong condition with the possibility of serious complications. The most effective prevention is to keep a child's weight at the right level for their height, the 'centile' lines can be found in the child's health record book and the family doctor or health visitor will be able to explain what these are. Active hobbies such as brisk walking, swimming and cycle riding should be encouraged as well as ones which do not involve too much physical exertion such as going for a stroll.

Families who are concerned about the risk of developing diabetes should talk to their GP for further advice and support.

How is it treated?

The main aim of treatment of both types of diabetes is to achieve near normal blood glucose and blood pressure levels. This, together with a healthy lifestyle, will help to improve well being and protect against long-term damage to the eyes, kidneys, nerves, heart and major arteries.

Once diagnosis has been made, referral to a registered dietitian and close monitoring by the healthcare team is necessary to give help to make the changes in lifestyle. In Children it is very important that the whole family is involved as increasing the level of physical activity to the recommended one hour per day and a healthy eating plan are at the top of the list of changes that can make a big difference in managing weight control and achieving optimum blood glucose levels. Intake of saturated fats should be reduced and intake of fibre should be increased. Sometimes medication is necessary to help achieve blood glucose control too

Inheritance patterns and prenatal diagnosis

Inheritance patterns

Both types of diabetes run in families and emerge in individuals in whom genetic susceptibility is triggered by environmental determinants. Genetic susceptibility to Type 1 resides largely in the genes encoding the HLA (human leukocyte antigen) molecules of the MHC (major histocompatibility complex) located on the short arm of chromosome 6. Relatives sharing these genes are more likely to develop Type 1 but even in identical twins, only about forty per cent share the disease. Type 1 occurs substantially more frequently in people of European than non-European origin, but its incidence varies greatly between national groups and over the course of time within them. Environmental trigger factors are uncertain.

Identical twins are much more likely both to have Type 2. No single genetic locus for susceptibility has yet been located though in rare subtypes of Type 2, occurring atypically in young people (see entry, Diabetes - Maturity Onset Diabetes of the Young), a clear pattern of Mendelian dominant inheritance is seen and, in some, the genetic variant characterised. Environmental determinants include increasing age, central obesity and physical inactivity. Some drugs may provoke glucose intolerance. Intrauterine and early life environment may 'programme' liability to diabetes in adult life.

Prenatal diagnosis

Inapplicable

Medical text written October 2000 by Diabetes UK. Approved October 2000 by Dr A C F Burden, Consultant Physician and Hon. Senior Lecturer, Chair of the Diabetes Care Advisory Committee of Diabetes UK, London, UK. **Last updated August 2005 by Diabetes UK. Approved August 2005 by Dr R I G Holt, Senior Lecturer in Endocrinology and Metabolism, University of Southampton, Southampton, UK.**

Support

Diabetes UK

10 Parkway, London NW1 7AA   Tel: 0845 120 2960 Careline
Tel: 020 7424 1000   Fax: 020 7424 1001
e-mail: info@diabetes.org.uk
Web: http://www.diabetes.org.uk
Formerly known as the British Diabetic Association, Diabetes UK is a National Registered Charity No. 215199, established in 1934 by Dr R D Lawrence and H G Wells. It offers a confidential help and support service for people with diabetes, their carers and health care professionals. It has a nationwide support network and funds research into diabetes. It campaigns for improvements for people who live with diabetes. It publishes: 'Link Up' a quarterly newsletter for parents; 'Tadpole Times' and 'On The Level' quarterly newsletters for children and teenagers with diabetes; 'Balance' a magazine published two monthly; 'Diabetic Medicine' a monthly publication for health care professionals containing research papers on diabetes; and 'Diabetes Update' a quarterly publication for health care professionals with an interest in diabetes. It also has a wide range of information available, details on request. Diabetes UK has around 200,000 members.
Group details last updated 2007.

DIAMOND BLACKFAN ANAEMIA SYNDROME

Diamond Blackfan anaemia: DBA; Diamond Blackfan anemia (US); Congenital Red Cell Aplasia

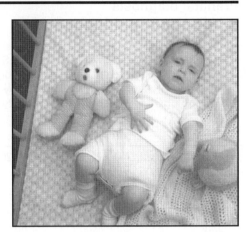

Background

Diamond Blackfan anaemia is a rare disorder. It is usually identified in the first few months of life when a young child becomes severely anaemic. Some children, however, may not develop anaemia until later on in childhood.

DBA occurs in around 5 to 10 in 1,000,000 births. This means that each year in the UK there will be an average of seven babies born with DBA.

What are the symptoms?

Some children with DBA may show physical features such as an extra thumb joint, cleft palate or a characteristic facial appearance. Many affected children are very short for their age, and may have delayed puberty. Children with DBA otherwise develop normally, and it is unusual for affected children to have learning difficulties.

What are the causes?

The anaemia is caused by a failure of the bone marrow to produce red blood cells ('red cell aplasia'). The exact cause is not clear, but the problem seems to be a fault in one of the early steps of red blood cell production. In up to twenty-five per cent of affected children there is a fault within a gene called RPS19 (short for 'small ribosomal protein 19'). There is a lot of research looking for the genes that are damaged in the other seventy-five per cent, with some promising leads, but no definite answers as yet.

Infection with a particular virus (parvovirus) can cause a switch off of red blood cell production. Nearly always this lasts for such a short time that it goes unnoticed, but infection during pregnancy can sometimes cause severe anaemia in the baby. There is also a condition known as 'transient erythroblastopenia of childhood' in which red cell production is temporarily switched off, usually following a viral infection. This is rare in babies, being most common in toddlers and pre-school children. This gets better on its own within a few months, and can sometimes be difficult to tell apart from DBA, except by waiting to see if the anaemia improves on its own.

How is it diagnosed?

The diagnosis is easy if there is already an affected child within the family, or the baby has a physical feature of DBA. Otherwise, it is a matter of confirming that the problem lies in a red blood cell production failure, and then to exclude parvovirus infection. Preliminary blood tests will show if too few red blood cells are being produced. The next step is for a small sample of bone marrow to be taken, to confirm that the anaemia is caused by production failure. Tests on the marrow will also include checking for evidence of infection with parvovirus. There is an additional test which measures the level of an enzyme, adenosine deaminase (eADA), in the red blood cells. The eADA level is usually raised in DBA, and can provide further evidence that the anaemia is due to DBA. The red blood cells in DBA are often larger than average (they are said to have a 'high MCV'), which can give further support to a probable diagnosis of DBA.

How is it treated?

Rarely, some individuals will have a spontaneous remission, in which the red cell production switches back on, but this is uncommon, and is impossible to predict.

Treatment for DBA can be with medication (steroids), blood transfusion, bone marrow transplantation or use of cord blood which is a rich source of the bone marrow stem cells from an unaffected sibling identified prenatally. However, these options need to be discussed in detail with the child's specialist.

Inheritance patterns and prenatel diagnosis

Inheritance patterns

In most cases DBA occurs sporadically. In subsequent generations the pattern of inheritance is typically autosomal dominant, although there may be variable severity within the family.

Prenatal diagnosis

Prenatal diagnosis is currently only possible if there is a mutation affecting RPS19, as DBA is usually clinically silent until early infancy.

Medical text written October 2003 by Dr S Ball, Consultant Paediatric Haematologist, St George's Hospital Medical School, London, UK.

UK DBA registry

The DBA Study Group, based at St George's Hospital, London SW17 0QT, has established a UK based registry of children with DBA to help learn more about the cause and treatment of this rare anaemia. For further information on the registry, please contact Dr Sarah Ball, Tel: 020 8725 3921.

Support

DBA.UK

71-73 Main Street, Palterton, Chesterfield S44 6UR   Tel: 0845 0941 548
e-mail: info@diamondblackfan.org.uk   Web: http://www.diamondblackfan.org.uk
The Group is a National Registered Charity No. 1083179, established in 1997. It offers support by telephone and letter and attempts to link families where possible. It publishes a newsletter twice a year and has information available, details on request. The Group is in touch with approximately 50 families.
Group details last updated March 2006.

A donation of £5 a month with Gift Aid would enable us to print another 300 free guides for parents each year. A donation form is on page 1088.

DIAPHRAGMATIC HERNIA

Background

The diaphragm is the muscular sheet which separates the chest from the abdomen. A congenital diaphragmatic hernia (CDH) is a defect or hole in the diaphragm which the bowel can pass through. Usually the diaphragm is fully formed by ten weeks of gestation, so any problem can be picked up on an eighteen week ultrasound scan. The commonest hole is on the left side, though they can occur on the right or at the front. Usually only part of the diaphragm is deficient, though an entire half-diaphragm may be missing.

Because of the hole, the bowel can go up through the diaphragm into the chest. This squashes the heart and both lungs. While in the womb, the placenta provides the oxygen for the baby, who will grow normally. However, the lungs may not develop normally, depending on how squashed they are and how long the bowel is in the chest. In some babies, the bowel only goes into the chest at delivery and so the lungs are normal. Other babies have lungs which are so poorly developed that they cannot keep the baby alive after delivery and the baby dies very quickly. Most affected babies are in between and have a degree of breathing difficulty.

Up to fifty per cent of babies with CDH have major associated problems, either with their heart, spinal cord, brain or chromosomes. These problems may be lethal.

How is it treated?

Most UK units stabilise the baby in Intensive Care on a ventilator, so that the lungs and heart can be assessed. The baby is often kept for several days until the optimal moment for surgical repair is reached.

Most surgeons repair the hole in the diaphragm via the abdomen. If there is enough diaphragm, the two edges of the hole are stitched together. If not, then a patch has to be inserted. Depending on the material used for the patch, this may not grow and may need replacement. Post operatively, the baby will be more ill than before, because of the stress of the operation. After several days, or even weeks, if the lungs are good enough, then the baby can be weaned off the ventilator and will go home.

There has been some success with prenatal surgery in one unit in the USA, but it will probably never be routine, even in the USA.

Inheritance patterns and prenatal diagnosis

Inheritance patterns

There is a recurrence risk of two per cent based on an incidence of 1 in 2,000 live births.

Prenatal diagnosis

Most babies with CDH are diagnosed antenatally on routine scan. If termination is considered, then amniocentesis for chromosomal abnormality should be done, together with a detailed anomaly scan. Polyhydramnios (excess fluid around the baby) and the presence of the stomach in the chest are poor prognostic features. If there are no associated abnormalities, continuation to term is often recommended, as there is a fifty per cent chance of the baby's lungs being adequate.

Antenatal diagnosis allows transfer of the mother for assessment and delivery at a regional centre. The baby can then be electively delivered, resuscitated and undergo surgery, by a fully prepared team of neonatologists and surgeons. Babies are usually delivered normally, though some babies need a caesarian section.

Medical text written December 1999 by Mr M Griffiths MCh FRCS. **Last updated September 2004 by Mr M Griffiths MCh FRCS, Consultant Paediatric & Neonatal Surgeon, Wessex Regional Centre for Paediatric Surgery, Southampton General Hospital, Southampton, UK.**

Further online resources

Medical texts in *The Contact a Family Directory* are designed to give a short, clear description of specific conditions and rare disorders. More extensive information on this condition can be found on a range of reliable, validated websites. Further information on these resources can be found in our **Medical Information on the Internet** article on page 21.

Support

Cherubs UK
43 Vancouver Avenue, Kings Lynn PE30 5RD   Tel: 0800 731 6991
e-mail: brakha88@hotmail.com   Web: http://www.uk-cherubs.org.uk
The group is a National Registered Charity No. 1106065 providing support and contact between families. Information is available on request. The group has over 130 members. Group details last updated October 2007.

DIASTROPHIC DYSPLASIA

Diastrophic Dysplasia: Diastrophic Dwarfism

Background

Diastrophic Dysplasia (DTD) is a rare, inherited skeletal dysplasia (a condition of abnormal bone growth or development) affecting both females and males equally. It was first described in 1960 by French doctors, Dr M. Lamy and Dr P. Maroteaux, as Le nanisme diastrophique. DTD is a disorder of restricted growth, spinal curvature and abnormalities of the fingers and toes. Intelligence is normal. The average height of adults is 118 cm (males: 86-127 cm; females 104-122 cm). Respiratory complications can cause an increase in infant mortality, but individuals who survive infancy have a normal life span.

The incidence is thought to be 1 in 110,000 births and it is caused by mutations in the SLC26A2 (DTDST) gene on chromosome 5q31-q34.

What are the symptoms?

The ways and severity that individuals with DTD are affected vary. The features of DTD include:

- shortening of the limbs but with a normal sized skull;
- small chest;
- protuberant abdomen;
- cleft palate in about thirty-three per cent of cases (see entry, Cleft Lip and/or Palate);
- swelling of the ears giving a 'cauliflower' appearance;
- joint contractures;
- shortening of the bones of the hands including hitchhiker thumbs (short bones cause the thumb to take up the typical hitchhiker position);
- club feet, varying from mild to severe due to bone abnormalities;
- progressive Scoliosis (sideways curvature of the spine, see entry), lumbar lordosis (forward curvature of the lower spine) and cervical kyphosis (outward curvature of the upper spine).

How is it diagnosed?

DTD is diagnosed by recognition of the clinical features of the disorder, radiographic (x-ray) findings and in some cases by molecular genetic testing of the SLC26A2 gene.

How is it treated?

DTD is not a curable condition and treatment will be symptomatic for specific features. It important to maintain joint positioning and mobility as much as possible using physiotherapy and surgical correction for club feet to allow walking. This is often extremely difficult and ideally should be performed by a surgeon with experience of other children with diastrophic dysplasia. This is true of any surgical intervention in children with diastrophic dysplasia. Monitoring of abnormalities of the bones of the limbs and particularly of the spine is important since surgical intervention may be necessary. Progressive abnormality of the bones of the spine in the neck is an important complication and should be looked for specifically. This may also require surgical treatment. Surgical intervention to release joint contracture is not usually recommended since these tend to recur.

A range of support for families, based on the practical and psychological effects of being of short stature at school and in the wider community, is available. Families can obtain information about aids to ameliorate difficulties in access and operation of equipment from local and national statutory and support organisations.

Inheritance patterns and prenatal diagnosis
Inheritance patterns
DTD is inherited in autosomal recessive manner.
Prenatal diagnosis
A range of testing is available. Where DTD is known in a family and the mutations in the SLC26A2 gene in the affected individual are known, chorionic villus sampling can be used at about ten to twelve weeks or amniocentesis at about fifteen to eighteen weeks. Ultrasound examination may identify typical skeletal abnormalities.

Medical text written January 2005 by Contact a Family. Approved January 2005 by Dr M Wright, Consultant Clinical Geneticist, Institute of Medical Genetics, International Centre for Life, Newcastle upon Tyne, UK.

Further online resources
Medical texts in *The Contact a Family Directory* are designed to give a short, clear description of specific conditions and rare disorders. More extensive information on this condition can be found on a range of reliable, validated websites. Further information on these resources can be found in our **Medical Information on the Internet** article on page 21.

Support
As Diastrophic Dysplasia is a restricted growth condition, information and advice for adults and the families of children is available from the Restricted Growth Association (see entry, Restricted Growth).

DOWN SYNDROME

Down syndrome: Down's syndrome; Trisomy 21

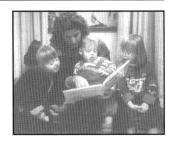

Background

Down syndrome, a chromosomal disorder, occurs when, instead of the normal complement of two copies of chromosome 21, there is a whole, or sometimes part of an, additional chromosome 21.

A chromosome is a rod-like structure present in the nucleus of all body cells, with the exception of the red blood cells, and which stores genetic information. Normally humans have twenty-three pairs of chromosomes, the unfertilised ova and each sperm carrying a set of twenty-three chromosomes. On fertilisation the chromosomes combine to give a total of forty-six (twenty-three pairs). A normal female has an XX pair and a normal male an XY pair.

What are the causes?

Chromosome abnormalities give rise to specific physical features seen in Down syndrome. The range of cognitive disabilities as well as other attributes is enormously wide in Down syndrome. The majority are in the mild range of cognitive ability. Associated defects may include ear and/or eye defects, an increased propensity for infections and heart defects.

A few individuals have the mosaic form of trisomy 21. This means that some body cells have forty-six chromosomes while others have forty-seven. In this form the severity and extent of the condition is dependent upon the proportional relation of normal to abnormal cells.

Inheritance patterns and prenatal diagnosis

Inheritance patterns

Most cases of Down syndrome are sporadic but there is a small risk of recurrence in further pregnancies. The incidence of Down syndrome is related to maternal age. The older the mother the higher the risk of an affected child, though the majority of children with Down syndrome are born to younger mothers.

However, in a minority of cases (three to four per cent) a mother or father may have a balanced translocation of chromosome 21. In these cases the condition is inheritable. Genetic counselling should be sought in all cases.

An ante-natal screening test, the 'Triple Test,' is sometimes used. It involves taking a small sample of blood from the mother, but it is not a definitive test; it is a screening process, the aim of which is to calculate whether the likelihood of having a Down syndrome fetus is sufficiently high to warrant the performance of an amniocentesis. This screening test has a rather high false positive rate, and it is only the amniocentesis which provides a definitive answer.

Prenatal diagnosis

Amniocentesis is usually offered at sixteen weeks. Chorionic villus sampling is usually available at ten to twelve weeks. Fetal scans for 'neck translucency' are also used.

Medical text written November 1991 by Contact a Family. Approved November 1991 by Professor M Patton, Professor of Medical Genetics, St Georges Hospital Medical School, London, UK and Dr J E Wraith, Consultant Paediatrician, Royal Manchester Children's Hospital, Manchester, UK. **Last reviewed August 2004 by Professor Ben Sacks, Down Syndrome Educational Trust, Portsmouth, UK. Additional genetic information provided June 2005 by Dr L Devlin, Senior Registrar in Genetics, Belfast City Hospital, Belfast, UK.**

Support

Down's Syndrome Association
Langdon Down Centre, 2a Langdon Park, Teddington TW11 9PS   Tel: 0845 230 0372
Fax: 0845 230 0373   e-mail: info@downs-syndrome.org.uk
Web: http://www.downs-syndrome.org.uk
The Association is a National Registered Charity No. 1061474, established in 1970. It offers information and support to people with Down Syndrome, their families, carers and professional workers. The Association champions the rights of people with the condition and strives to improve knowledge and understanding of Down Syndrome. The Association publishes a newsletter, 'Down's Syndrome Association Journal', and a wide range of information, details on request. There are approximately 19,000 members and 100 affiliated volunteer support groups in the UK.
Group details last confirmed March 2007.

Down's Syndrome Scotland
158/160 Balgreen Road, Edinburgh EH11 3AU   Tel: 0131 313 4225   Fax: 0131 313 4285
e-mail: info@dsscotland.org.uk   Web: http://www.dsscotland.org.uk
Down's Syndrome Scotland is a Scottish Registered Charity No. SCO11012, established in 1982. It provides advice, support and information to people with Down's syndrome, parents, carers, professionals and students. Specialist staff in health and education produce resources and literature and provide training on all aspects of Down's syndrome. A wide range of booklets are available plus a quarterly newsletter and lending library. Down's Syndrome Scotland responds to around 6,000 enquiries a year.
Group details last confirmed February 2008.

Mosaic Down Syndrome UK
26 Sandhills Avenue, Blackpool FY4 1QQ   Tel: 01253 313124 (after 6pm)
e-mail: judy.green@blueyonder.co.uk   Web: http://www.mosaicdownsyndrome.org
A web based support group for families of affected children, but which welcomes contact via phone and letter. The group currently has over 90 members worldwide. Information is available through the website and there is a related e-mail support group. Group members meet monthly on-line for mutual support.
Group details last confirmed October 2007.

Contact a Family Helpline 0808 808 3555

Down Syndrome Educational Trust
Sarah Duffen Centre, Belmont Street, Southsea PO5 1NA   Tel: 023 92 855330
Fax: 023 92 855320   e-mail: enquiries@downsed.org   Web: http://www.downsed.org
Web: http://www.down-syndrome.org
The Down Syndrome Educational Trust undertakes innovative research, provides expert advice and support, publishes information resources and provides hands-on services to deliver real benefits to the lives of people with Down syndrome in the UK and worldwide.
Group details last updated October 2007.

Every year new entries are added to the Directory, and many existing entries are substantially rewritten.

DOWN SYNDROME WITH HEART DEFECT

Background

Down syndrome (see entry) is caused by trisomy of chromosome 21 (the child carries an extra chromosome 21). Forty per cent of children with Down syndrome have an associated heart defect. These heart conditions vary from small holes in the heart to more complex problems which may require major open heart surgery. In a small number of children the condition is so severe that they are inoperable, but the majority are suitable for surgery and their prognosis is very good.

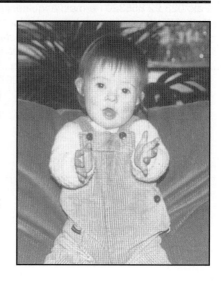

What are the symptoms?

Early failure to thrive may be indicative of a heart problem, but some babies may not show symptoms for several months and it is not always possible to detect a heart defect purely by clinical examination. Therefore all babies with Down syndrome should have an echocardiogram performed.

Inheritance patterns and prenatal diagnosis

Inheritance patterns

Most cases of Down syndrome are sporadic but there is a small risk of recurrence in further pregnancies. The incidence of Down syndrome is related to maternal age. The older the mother the higher the risk of an affected child, although it is possible for a mother of any age to have a baby with Down syndrome.

However, in a minority (thre to four per cent) of cases a mother may have a balanced translocation of chromosome 21. This means that the condition is inheritable.

Genetic advice may be sought in all cases. Amniocentesis is normally offered to all mothers over thirty-seven years of age. Recently a blood test in pregnancy (known as the Barts test) has been used for screening where there is no family history of Down syndrome.

Prenatal diagnosis

Amniocentesis usually at sixteen weeks but results may not be available until twenty weeks. Chorionic villus sampling usually available at ten to twelve weeks. Fetal heart scans should be perestablished in all cases where Down syndrome is diagnosed prenatally.

Medical text written November 1991 by Contact a Family. Approved November 1991 by Professor M Patton, Professor of Medical Genetics, St Georges Hospital Medical School, London, UK and Dr J E Wraith, Consultant Paediatrician, Royal Manchester Children's Hospital, Manchester, UK. **Last updated June 2003 by Dr P E F Daubenay, Consultant Paediatric and Fetal Cardiologist, Royal Brompton Hospital, London, UK.**

Support

The Down's Heart Group
PO Box 4260, Dunstable LU6 2ZT   Tel/Fax: 0845 166 8061   e-mail: info@dhg.org.uk
Web: http://www.dhg.org.uk
The Group is a National Registered Charity No. 1011413, established in 1989. It offers support and contact between families. It encourages research into heart defects, publishes a newsletter and has a wide range of information available, details on request. The Group represents over 1,100 families.
Group details last confirmed October 2007.

If you need to adapt your home to make it easier for you and/or your child to manage then you may be entitled to a grant. Call the Contact a family Helpline for more information.

DUANE RETRACTION SYNDROME

Duane Retraction syndrome: Duane syndrome; DRS

Background

Duane Retraction syndrome is a congenital disorder of ocular movements which was first described in 1905. There are three types of DRS that share common features. The condition may affect one or both eyes. DRS more commonly affects the left eye and is more common in girls. The reasons for this are not yet known.

What are the symptoms?

In DRS there is an abnormality of horizontal eye movements resulting in restriction of the affected eye from turning outwards or inwards or in both directions. As the eye is turned in toward the nose (called adduction) the eyelids narrow as the eye is apparently drawn back (retracted). As the affected eye is turned outwards (abducted), the eye lids widen. There may be associated vertical eye movement changes causing an up shoot or down shoot.

Individuals who are affected with DRS may also have a squint (strabismus) when they look straight ahead. It is possible to have good vision in each eye with stereo vision. However, in order to maintain stereo vision, individuals with DRS may adopt a face turn.

How is it caused?

The features associated with DRS are thought to be due to an abnormal nerve supply to the muscles that control eye movement. There may also be some scarring changes in the muscles themselves. Abnormal development occurs early in development approximately three weeks after conception.

How is it treated?

Treatment of the condition is aimed at achieving straight eyes when an individual looks straight ahead. If there is an unsightly narrowing of the eye, then surgery to relax the eye muscles may help. It is unlikely to make the eye movements normal but where there is a cosmetic problem, improvement can usually be achieved.

There a number of other clinical features which may be associated with DRS including hearing problems (see entry, Deafness), spinal and skeletal abnormalities.

Inheritance patterns and prenatal diagnosis

Inheritance patterns

Some forms of DRS run in families but these are extremely rare. Errors in a number of genes have been associated with DRS. It is possible that different genes run in different families and in many cases the cause may be multi-factorial.

Prenatal diagnosis

None

Medical written November 2001 by Miss R J Leitch. **Last reviewed October 2005 by Miss R J Leitch, Consultant Ophthalmic Surgeon, Sutton Hospital, Sutton, UK.**

Further online resources

Medical texts in *The Contact a Family Directory* are designed to give a short, clear description of specific conditions and rare disorders. More extensive information on this condition can be found on a range of reliable, validated websites. Further information on these resources can be found in our **Medical Information on the Internet** article on page 21.

Support

There is no support group for Duane Retraction syndrome. Cross referrals to other entries in The Contact a Family Directory are intended to provide relevant support for these particular features of the disorder. Organisations identified in these entries do not provide support specifically for Duane Retraction syndrome. Families can use Contact a Family's Freephone Helpline for advice, information and, where possible, links to other families. Contact a Family's web-based linking service Making Contact.org can be accessed at http://www.makingcontact.org

DUBOWITZ SYNDROME

Background

The features associated with Dubowitz syndrome include Microcephaly (see entry), delayed development, short stature, mild learning difficulties with behaviour problems and Eczema (see entry). Individuals with Dubowitz syndrome may show some or all of these features and furthermore may be differently affected by the severity of their symptoms. Symptoms may be so mild that they elude a diagnosis of Dubowitz syndrome in these individuals.

What are the symptoms?

Some degree of intellectual impairment is usually present in individuals with Dubowitz syndrome. Levels range from profound learning difficulties (see entry) to normal ability. Characteristic behaviour patterns include hyperactivity, shyness and stubbornness. There is anecdotal evidence of an association between Autism and Dubowitz syndrome. However, no formal psychological studies have been undertaken to confirm or refute this association.

Individuals with Dubowitz syndrome have normally proportioned bodies although they may be shorter than average for their age. Babies born with a normal weight are commonly severely delayed in their growth.

A characteristic facial appearance is probably the most typical feature of Dubowitz syndrome. The features include: a small, narrow and asymmetrical face; a high, broad and sloping forehead; widely spaced eyes; broad nasal bridge; and short, webbed neck.

A range of other features associated with Dubowitz syndrome may include Eczema, frequent infections (primarily viral), allergies (see entry), vomiting, and chronic diarrhoea or constipation.

Inheritance patterns and prenatal diagnosis

Inheritance patterns

Dubowitz syndrome is inherited as an autosomal recessive trait. However, the gene or genes associated with the clinical features of this condition have not yet been identified. There is currently no genetic or biochemical test to confirm a diagnosis of Dubowitz syndrome.

Prenatal diagnosis

None available.

Medical text written October 2003 by Contact a Family. Appoved October 2003 by Professor M Patton, Professor of Medical Genetics, St George's Hospital Medical School, London, UK.

Further online resources

Medical texts in *The Contact a Family Directory* are designed to give a short, clear description of specific conditions and rare disorders. More extensive information on this condition can be found on a range of reliable, validated websites. Further information on these resources can be found in our **Medical Information on the Internet** article on page 21.

Support

There is no support group for Dubowitz Syndrome. Cross referrals to other entries in the Contact a Family Directory are intended to provide relevant support for these particular features of the disorder. Organisations identified in these entries do not provide support specifically for Dubowitz Syndrome . Families can use Contact a Family's Freephone Helpline for advice, information and, where possible, links to other families. Contact a Family's web-based linking service Making Contact.org can be accessed at http://www.makingcontact.org

---

"We were just told the name of her condition. There was no other information offered to us; no prognosis; no treatment; no nothing. We had just been told our child had a critical rare disorder and we didn't know what to ask. We walked out of that hospital feeling stunned and alone." Parent.

DUCHENNE MUSCULAR DYSTROPHY

Background

Duchenne Muscular Dystrophy (DMD) is a relatively common and severe neuromuscular disorder, affecting approximately 1 in 3,000 or 1 in 4,000 male live births.

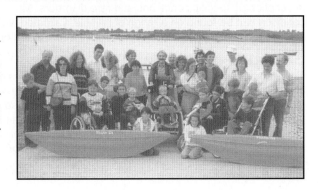

What are the symptoms?

The hallmark of the disease is the progressive weakness of all muscles; proximal muscles of the limbs are most severely affected. Children usually present with mild delay of the motor milestones such as walking and with tip-toe and unsteady gait. Difficulties rising from the floor, going upstairs and running are usually evident in the first two to three years of life. Enlarged calves can be seen in most children especially in the early phases of the disease.

A frequently associated feature (thirty per cent of cases) is mild learning disability. The presentation with predominantly cognitive problems is not uncommon (speech delay, for example). This is not progressive.

The weakness, however, is progressive and children with DMD will lose ambulation by the age of thirteen years; the mean age being approximately nine years. This is due to a combination of weakness and contractures affecting the ankles, knees and hips.

Affected children confined to a wheelchair are at high risk of developing spinal curvature; more than ninety per cent will eventually develop a significant scoliosis. Appropriate management (bracing) reduces the rate but very often spinal surgery is required to stop the progression of the scoliosis.

Respiratory muscles are also affected and this becomes a clinical problem usually in the late teens; respiratory failure causing night time hypoventilation is common at this age and is often followed by death after a few months if not treated. However with appropriate management using night time ventilatory support (facial or nasal mask ventilation) this complication can be helped considerably and this has resulted in a significant improvement of the mean age of survival of DMD individuals. While thirty years ago the mean age at death was fourteen and a half years, it is now twenty-five to thirty years. Cardiac muscle is also affected; however, because of the immobility, patients with DMD rarely develop signs of cardiac failure.

Psychological and behavioural characteristics

The information below has been drawn up by Dr Orlee Udwin of the Society for the Study of Behavioural Phenotypes.

Boys with DMD exhibit a range of intellectual deficits which are non-progressive. They typically have general developmental delay, especially in the acquisition of language and in gross motor development. Although the intellectual abilities of boys with Duchenne Muscular Dystrophy tend to be in the low average range, some may have moderate or severe learning difficulties. In adolescence some boys overcome early difficulties and proceed to higher education with appropriate support. Language and communication abilities, and especially spoken language, are usually more severely impaired than visuo-spatial abilities and manual skills. This is an unexpected finding in a disorder that is associated with severe and progressive physical disabilities. There is also a high prevalence of specific learning difficulties, with three-quarters of affected boys who are of normal intelligence having specific problems in reading, spelling and/or numeracy. Deficits in memory and concentration have also been highlighted.

Emotional difficulties are common, particularly anxiety and depressed mood, which is not surprising in young people with a disabling, progressive and life-threatening disorder. Affected boys are also often described as having poor peer relationships and being solitary and withdrawn.

How is it diagnosed?

Diagnosis is perestablished in centres where there is an expertise to deal with these conditions but serum creatine kinase (CK) is a very useful initial screening test. If the CK is normal, the diagnosis of DMD is excluded as affected children invariably have markedly elevated serum levels. A muscle biopsy (preferably with a needle) is often take to confirm the diagnosis and a genetic test will also help in establishing the diagnosis and in providing genetic counselling to the family.

Inheritance patterns and prenatal diagnosis

Inheritance patterns

DMD is a genetic condition inherited as an X-linked trait. Often there are no other members of the family affected. This is usually the result of a de-novo genetic event that has occurred in the affected child; or the fact that the mother, if she is a carrier of the genetic defect, usually does not manifest any sign of the disease (because of the X-linked inheritance). The gene responsible for DMD is known and mutations can be relatively easily found in approximately two thirds of affected children.

Prenatal diagnosis

This and carrier detection is available through Clinical Genetic Centres.

Medical text written June 2000 by Professor F Muntoni. **Last updated December 2004 by Professor F Muntoni, Professor and Consultant in Paediatric Neurology, Hammersmith Hospital, Neuromuscular Centre, London, UK. Psychological and behavioural characteristics written by Dr Orlee Udwin of the Society for the Study of Behavioural Phenotypes.**

Further online resources

Medical texts in *The Contact a Family Directory* are designed to give a short, clear description of specific conditions and rare disorders. More extensive information on this condition can be found on a range of reliable, validated websites. Further information on these resources can be found in our **Medical Information on the Internet** article on page 21.

Support

Duchenne Family Support Group
78 York Street, London W1H 1DP   Tel: 0870 606 1604 Family Helpline
Tel: 0870 241 1857 Office   e-mail: dfsg@duchenne.demon.co.uk
Web: http://www.dfsg.org.uk
The Group is a National Registered Charity No. 328220, established in 1987. It offers support and advice and has a network of families. It publishes a regular newsletter and has information available, details on request. The Group has over 200 member families.
Group details last confirmed March 2007.

Support for Duchenne Muscular Dystrophy is also available from the Muscular Dystrophy Group (see entry, Muscular Dystrophy and neuromuscular disorders).

DYSCALCULIA

Background

Dyscalculia is a developmental, or acquired, disorder which results in specific, major difficulties when learning mathematics, particularly numeracy. Some people with dyslexia experience problems with number skills because they have problems with the language of maths or with the short-term memory and retrieval skills needed for computational work. Dyscalculia can, however, be found in pure form and appears to relate to a specific deficit in the ability to rapidly assess number quantities.

What are the symptoms?

Difficulties in some or all of the following may occur:

- mastering simple number concepts;
- understanding number relationships;
- understanding spatial relationships;
- learning algorithms and applying them.

What are the causes?

Brain scanning studies in humans suggest that Intraparietal Sulcus is responsible for the abstract representation of numerical quantities and lowered activation is seen in these areas in those with dyscalculia.

Inheritance patterns and prenatal diagnosis

Inheritance patterns

There is some evidence for heritability.

Prenatal diagnosis

None.

Medical text written October 2005 by John Rack PhD, Director of Assessment and Research, The Dyslexia Institute, Egham, UK.

Further online resources

Medical texts in *The Contact a Family Directory* are designed to give a short, clear description of specific conditions and rare disorders. More extensive information on this condition can be found on a range of reliable, validated websites. Further information on these resources can be found in our **Medical Information on the Internet** article on page 21.

Support

Information and advice about Dyscalculia is available from organisations covering Dyslexia (see entry).

DYSKERATOSIS CONGENITA

Background

A variety of other abnormalities have been reported. These include abnormalities of the eyes, teeth, skeletal, gastrointestinal (bowel), genitourinary (kidneys, bladder) and respiratory systems. There is also an increased incidence of malignancy particularly of the skin and gastrointestinal system.

What are the symptoms?

Clinical manifestations of Dyskeratosis Congenita often appear during childhood. The skin pigmentation and nail changes typically appear first, usually by the age of ten years. The more serious complications of bone marrow failure (aplastic anaemia) and malignancy develop in the second and third decades of life. However, there is considerable variability in the age at which these develop in different patients.

How is it diagnosed?

The majority (eighty per cent) of patients are male and show X-linked recessive patterns of inheritance. The gene responsible for this has been identified and this now provides an accurate diagnostic test for the majority of patients.

How is it treated?

Patients who develop abnormalities in their bone marrow are at risk of life threatening infections and bleeding. Some patients may respond to drugs such as oxymetholone. If the bone marrow failure is severe and there is a compatible bone marrow donor, treatment by bone marrow transplantation is possible.

Inheritance patterns and prenatal diagnosis

Inheritance patterns

The most common pattern of inheritance is X-linked recessive where the gene responsible for Dyskeratosis Congenita is carried on the X- chromosome. The gene (DKCI) was identified in 1998. Autosomal dominant and autosomal recessive forms also exist. The gene (TERC-RNA component of telomerase) mutated in autosomal dominant DC was identified in 2001.

Prenatal diagnosis

DNA testing can be carried out for the genes responsible for the X-linked and autosomal dominant forms of Dyskeratosis Congenita. It is available in the UK as part of the Dyskeratosis Congenita Registry at the Department of Haematology, Imperial College School of Medicine, Hammersmith Hospital, London, UK.

Medical text written August 1996 by Dr I Dokal. **Last updated October 2005 by Professor I Dokal, Professor of Haematology, Hammersmith Hospital, London, UK.**

Support

Dyskeratosis Congenita Society

Professor Inderjeet Dokal, Chair of Paediatrics and Child Health, Academic Department of Paediatrics, Institute of Cell and Molecular Science, Barts and The London, Queen Mary's School of Medicine and Dentistry, 4 Newark Street, London E1 2AT

Tel: 020 7882 2205   Fax: 020 78822185   e-mail: i.dokal@qmul.ac.uk

The Society is a family contact group started in 1996. It offers contact between affected families by telephone and letter. It promotes the Dyskeratosis Congenita Registry, an international registry of affected persons with the aim of co-ordinating a clinical service and expediting research. It has information available, details on request.

Group details last updated June 2007

"They are absolutely brilliant. The staff are hard-working, kind, professional and above all able to work with parents and professionals at just the right level." Health care professional describing the work of Contact a Family's West Midlands office.

DYSLEXIA

Background

Dyslexia is a specific learning difficulty primarily affecting reading, writing, spelling and sometimes mathematics (see entry, Dyscalculia). It occurs at all levels of intellectual ability, but is harder to detect where there are other problems in learning. For the child who is otherwise quite capable, the frustrations of difficulties expressing themselves in writing and understanding printed words can be a source of stress and may sometimes lead to behavioural difficulties.

What are the symptoms?

Typical characteristics of dyslexia include a lack of phonological awareness and poor phonic decoding skills, poor short-term memory and difficulties with verbal labelling.

PET and Functional MRI studies show that there are differences in the language processing areas in the brains of dyslexic people in the left hemisphere temporo-parietal structures, particularly the angular gyrus.

How is it diagnosed?

Dyslexia is a complex, specific learning difficulty whose boundaries are not always clear in clinical practice. A significant difficulty in diagnosing dyslexia is that it often occurs alongside other specific difficulties such as Attention Deficit Hyperactivity Disorder, Dyspraxia and/or with a mild Specific Language Impairment (SLI), although it often occurs in a relatively pure form too.

How is it treated?

Early language-based intervention, focusing on developing awareness of sound pattern in words and their links to letter patterns is effective. It is harder to improve the skills of older children and adults, but this can be done with one-to-one multisensory teaching.

Inheritance patterns and prenatal diagnosis

Inheritance patterns

Dyslexia is strongly heritable. Candidate genes have been identified on Chromosomes 6, 15 and 1 and the two genes associated with dyslexia have been identified. Dyslexia is more apparent in males than females, although genetic factors seem to increase the risk of difficulties equally for both sexes.

Prenatal diagnosis

None.

Medical text written October 2005 by John Rack PhD, Director of Assessment and Research, The Dyslexia Institute, Egham, UK.

Further online resources

Medical texts in *The Contact a Family Directory* are designed to give a short, clear description of specific conditions and rare disorders. More extensive information on this condition can be found on a range of reliable, validated websites. Further information on these resources can be found in our **Medical Information on the Internet** article on page 21.

Support

The British Dyslexia Association

98 London Road, Reading RG1 5AU   Tel: 0118 966 8271   Fax: 0118 935 1927
e-mail: helpline@bdadyslexia.org.uk   Web: http://www.bdadyslexia.org.uk
The Association is a National Registered Charity No. 289243. It offers support for families and adults through its helpline and its local groups throughout England, Wales and Northern Ireland. It runs conferences, seminars and workshops for parents, adults, teachers and other professionals covering aspects of dyslexia at any age. It publishes a magazine 'Dyslexia Contact' three times a year and an International Journal of Research and Practice 'Dyslexia' quarterly. It has a wide range of information available, details on request.
Group details last updated March 2007.

Dyslexia Action

Park House, Wick Road, Egham TW20 0HH   Tel: 01784 222300   Fax: 01784 222333
e-mail: info@dyslexiaaction.org.uk   Web: http://www.dyslexiaaction.org.uk
Dyslexia Action is a National Registered Charity No. 268502. Previously The Dyslexia Institute, it is the UK's leading provider of services and support for people with dyslexia and literacy difficulties. It specialises in assessments, teaching and training. They also develop and distribute teaching materials and undertake research. Dyslexia Action is committed to improving public policy and practice. They partner with schools, LEAs, colleges, universities, employers, voluntary sector organisations and Government to improve the quality and quantity of help for people with dyslexia and specific learning difficulties. Dyslexia Action services are available through our 26 centres and 160 teaching locations around the UK.
Group details last updated September 2007.

Dyslexia Scotland

Stirling Business Centre, Wellgreen, Stirling FK8 2DZ   Tel: 0844 800 8484 (10am - 4pm)
Fax: 01786 471235   e-mail: info@dyslexiascotland.org.uk
Web: http://www.dyslexiascotland.org.uk
Dyslexia Scotland is a Registered Charity No. SC000951, established in 1968. It offers advice, information and support to people with dyslexia and operates a national tutor list. It conducts screening tests for both children and adults and workplace assessments. It organises workshops, conferences and seminars to raise awareness of dyslexia and attempts to influence the educational policy of both central and local government. It has a wide range of information available, details on request.
Group details last confirmed March 2007.

DYSPRAXIA

Dyspraxia: Developmental Co-ordination Disorder; Clumsy child syndrome; Perceptuo-Motor Dysfunction; Motor Learning Difficulty

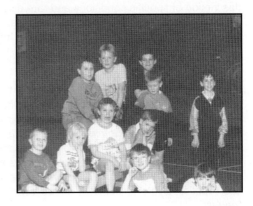

Background

Dyspraxia is a developmental disorder of organisation and planning of physical movement. The essential feature is the impairment of motor function that significantly interferes with academic achievement or activities of daily living, and is not due to a general medical condition, such as cerebral palsy or muscular dystrophy. Performance in daily activities that require motor co-ordination is substantially below that expected given the person's chronological age and general intelligence. This may be manifested in marked delays in achieving the main motor milestones of sitting, crawling and walking, or such problems as difficulty in self help skills, knocking over or dropping things, poor performance in sport or poor handwriting.

What are the symptoms?

Dyspraxia is a disorder with great variation between one child and another. In severe cases there is global dysfunction affecting gross, fine and oro-motor skills. These children are likely to present early in the pre-school period with gross and fine motor delay, hypotonia (see entry) and clumsiness with poor speech articulation. At the other end of the spectrum, problems become apparent at school age, with more subtle impairments in fine motor skills affecting buttoning, tying laces and poor handwriting.

Neuro-developmental examination may reveal signs such as left/right confusion, poor balance and postural maintenance, as well as hypotonia and weakness, poor rhythm and timing, and unusual patterns of sensory processing. Psychological assessment may show considerable discrepancies, typically with satisfactory verbal skills and relatively poor visual skills.

Besides the problems of motor control, there is usually significant impairment in skills relating to sequencing, organisation and planning as well as difficulties in attention control. These problems also contribute to the practical difficulties with skills such as dressing, and can have a major impact on written output and recording abilities at school.

The overall result is discrepant academic performance. The child shows ability by having good oral skills but is unable to achieve literacy or recording skills at the same level. Poor concentration and attention control and physical restlessness or over activity may be an additional problem. It is not uncommon for such children to be described by teachers as lazy or poorly motivated.

In older children and adolescents, there may be progressive educational underachievement for expected ability, avoidance of difficult tasks and disengagement from school life. Secondary emotional problems with low self esteem are more likely and this may be apparent from a young age.

In the past, dyspraxia was sometimes held to be a delay in maturation with motor problems resolving in the teen years. Recent longitudinal studies suggest that rather than resolving, dyspraxia may have important long term sequelae that persist into adult life. Motor problems may become ameliorated with therapy in childhood and practice, as well as with increasing neurological maturity. The organisational problems may continue to be a major impairment into adult life.

The risk of mental health problems, substance abuse and disruptive behaviour disorders are all increased.

How is it diagnosed?

Neuro-developmental disorders as a group do tend to show a great deal of overlap and therefore tend to have features in common. So problems seen in Dyspraxia may be also seen in other disorders. Common to many of these disorders are such problems of concentration, short term (especially auditory) memory, organisation and planning, specific learning difficulties, sensory processing abnormalities, language and communication, socialisation difficulties, motor tics and emotional disorders.

Sometimes these associated problems are severe enough to fulfil the criteria for a separate clinical diagnosis for example, Attention Deficit Hyperactivity Disorder, Autism Spectrum disorders, Dyslexia or Tourette syndrome (see entries). Because of these common associations, some practitioners have adopted the term 'DAMP', used in the Nordic countries, to describe those children with **D**eficits in **A**ttention, **M**otor control and **P**erception. The complexity of presentation, use of different terms and the possibility of multiple diagnostic labels can lead to difficulties or delays in families getting a satisfactory diagnosis. For these reasons, a child presenting with features suggestive of Dyspraxia ideally should have access to a comprehensive multidisciplinary assessment.

Inheritance patterns and prenatal diagnosis
Inheritance patterns
This has not been fully researched.
Prenatal diagnosis
None

Medical text written June 2001 by Dr D Keen. **Last reviewed October 2005 by Dr D Keen, Consultant Paediatrician, St George's Hospital, London, UK.**

Support
The Dyspraxia Foundation
8 West Alley, Hitchin SG5 1EG   Tel: 01462 454986 Helpline (Mon-Fri, 10am-1pm)
Fax: 01462 455052   e-mail: admin@dyspraxiafoundation.org.uk
Web: http://www.dyspraxiafoundation.org.uk
The Foundation is a National Registered Charity No. 1058352, established in 1987. It offers contact with other members locally and nationally. It publishes a regular newsletter and a twice yearly magazine. It has information available, details on request, please send SAE. The Foundation has over 2,000 members.
Group details last confirmed October 2007.

Direct services for children with Dyspraxia are also provided by the National Institute of Conductive Education (see Foundation for Conductive Education, under separate entry, Cerebral Palsy).

DYSTONIA

Background

Dystonia is a term for a group of neurological disorders in which involuntary muscle spasm leads to abnormal movements and postures. These postures tend to change from moment to moment especially during attempts to carry out a movement and may be most evident during walking or performing specific tasks. The dystonias are one of several movement disorders caused by impaired or altered function in large groups of nerve cells in the centre of the brain called the basal ganglia.

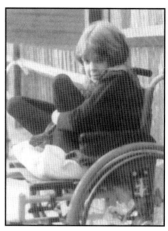

Dystonia can be classified as primary or secondary. Dystonia can also be classified by how much of the body is involved. Focal dystonia affects one body part such as the neck in spasmodic torticollis or cervical dystonia, or the eyes in blepharospasm. More severe dystonia can be described as segmental if it involves two adjacent body parts, for example the neck and an arm, and if the legs and trunk are also affected it is described as generalised. In general, the more severe forms of dystonia have onset in childhood whilst focal dystonia is a condition with onset in adulthood.

What are the symptoms?

Primary Focal Dystonia

These are the commonest forms of dystonia. For instance cervical dystonia or spasmodic torticollis affects around 12,000 people in the UK and blepharospasm, some 5-6,000.

- **Spasmodic Torticollis or Cervical Dystonia** affects the neck muscles. The neck and head can be twisted forward, backwards, to one side or even held in one specific position. Head tremor can also occur.
- **Blepharospasm** affects the muscles around the eyes leading to constant blinking or closure of the eyes, especially in strong light. In some cases the frequency of the spasm can be such that the eye remain shut resulting in the affected person being unable to see despite having normal vision.
- **Writer's Cramp** affects the muscles of the hand and arm when writing. Other dystonias of the hand muscles are typist's cramp and sport and musician's cramps.
- **Oromandibular Dystonia** affects the mouth, jaw and tongue muscles. Speech and swallowing are sometimes affected as the dystonia causes

the mouth to remain closed or open.

- **Cranial Dystonia** (also known as Breughel or Meige syndrome) is a combination of Oromandibular Dystonia and Blepharospasm.
- **Laryngeal Dystonia** affects the speech muscles of the throat and can lead to the voice becoming strained or forced, or in some cases only being able to speak in a whisper.

Generalised and Segmental Dystonia

Generalised dystonia usually starts in childhood, with onset in a limb which spreads to other parts of the body. It is often familial and can be very disabling. The commonest form has been shown to be caused by a mutation in a specific gene known as DYT1.

- **DYT1 Dystonia** is inherited in an autosomal dominant fashion, although many family members who carry the abnormal gene may only be mildly affected or not at all. Typically the condition causes onset of dystonia in an arm or leg in childhood or early teens which then spreads to involve the trunk and other limbs (generalised dystonia). Drug therapy is not particularly helpful but in recent years there have been reports of useful benefit from the neurosurgical procedure known as deep brain stimulation. Identification of the common mutation in the DYT1 gene means that genetic testing is available with appropriate counselling.
- **Dopa-responsive Dystonia** (aka **Segawa's syndrome)** is another genetic condition that can cause more widespread dystonia. In this condition dystonia tends to affect walking more than other activities and characteristically worsens towards the end of the day. Other members of the family may be affected, and can also show symptoms similar to Parkinson's disease. The commonest genetic cause in the UK is GTP-cyclohydrolase 1 deficiency which is usually dominantly inherited. The key point is that it usually responds well to treatment with the drug levodopa.
- **Secondary or Symptomatic Dystonia** is often characterised by the presence of other clinical features in addition to dystonia. Dystonia in childhood can be due to secondary causes such as a form of cerebral palsy, thought to be due to lack of oxygen to the brain around the time of birth, which damages the basal ganglia. Rare biochemical and metabolic disorders can also cause dystonia along with other cognitive and neurological features. In children and adults it is also important to exclude the possibility of drug induced dystonia. Drugs that interfere with the chemical neurotransmitter dopamine (such as anti-emetics and anti-psychotics) can cause what is referred to as tardive dystonia. Other secondary causes include structural damage to the basal ganglia from strokes, tumours and trauma.

Inheritance patterns and prenatal diagnosis

Inheritance patterns

It is mainly the more severe childhood onset forms that are genetic in origin. Both DYT1 dystonia and dopa-responsive dystonia are inherited in an autosomal dominant pattern. This means that any child of an affected parent has a 50/50 chance of inheriting the abnormal gene. However, it is clear that even if an individual inherits the abnormal gene, this does not always mean that they develop dystonia. Thus for DYT1 dystonia the risk to a child of an affected parent of developing dystonia is around twenty per cent.

Prenatal diagnosis

None.

Medical text written January 2003 by Dr T Warner, Reader in Clinical Neurosciences, Royal Free Hospital, London, UK.

Further online resources

Medical texts in *The Contact a Family Directory* are designed to give a short, clear description of specific conditions and rare disorders. More extensive information on this condition can be found on a range of reliable, validated websites. Further information on these resources can be found in our **Medical Information on the Internet** article on page 21.

Support

The Dystonia Society

1st Floor, Camelford House, 89 Albert Embankment, London SE1 7TP
Tel: 0845 458 6322 Helpline   Tel: 0845 458 6311 Office   Fax: 0845 458 6311
e-mail: support@dystonia.org.uk   Web: http://www.dystonia.org.uk
The Society is a National Registered Charity No. 1062595, established in 1983. It offers contact between affected individuals through local self help groups and area contacts in the UK and the Republic of Ireland. It also runs 'Young Dystonia' a support group for young people and their families. It publishes a newsletter 3 times a year and a Young Dystonia newsletter. It has a wide range of information available, details on request. The Society has over 3,500 members who are mostly affected individuals.
Group details last confirmed January 2007.

EATING DISORDERS

Background

Anorexia Nervosa is a potentially life threatening psychological disorder. Its main symptom is the relentless pursuit of thinness through self starvation.

Bulimia Nervosa is characterised by over eating followed by self induced vomiting or purging through the use of laxatives.

Eating disorders are conditions where disturbed eating behaviour is a primary characteristic. They indicate and express a disturbed perception of the self. Thus anorexia and bulimia are emotional disorders which focus on food and its consumption. The conditions are a method through which the individual attempts to cope with life as they see it.

The typical sufferer from these disorders is female aged 15-25. Males account for approximately ten per cent of the total affected persons.

Medical text last reviewed February 2004 by the Medical Advisory Group, Eating Disorders Association, Norwich, UK.

Support

BEAT

103 Prince of Wales Road, Norwich NR1 1DW

Tel: 0845 634 1414 Adults (Mon-Fri, 10.30am-8.30pm; Sat, 1pm-4.30pm)

Tel: 0845 634 7650 Youthline - 18 and under (Mon-Fri, 4.30pm-8.30pm; Sat, 1pm-4.30pm)

Fax: 01603 664915   e-mail: info@b-eat.co.uk   Web: http://www.b-eat.co.uk

The Association is a National Registered Charity No. 801343, established in 1989. It offers support and information, has a network of locally based self help groups and campaigns for improved standards of treatment and care. It publishes a quarterly magazine, 'Upbeat'. It has a wide range of information available, details on request. The Association represents approximately 3,500 members.

Group details last updated October 2007.

ECTODERMAL DYSPLASIA

Background

Ectodermal Dysplasia (ED) is not a single disorder, but a group of closely related conditions of which more than one hundred and sixty different syndromes have been identified. The Ectodermal Dysplasias (EDs) are genetic disorders affecting the development or function of the teeth, hair, nails and sweat glands. Depending on the particular syndrome ED can also affect the skin, the lens or retina of the eye, parts of the inner ear, the development of fingers and toes, the nerves and other parts of the body. The prevalence of the various types of ED is thought to be about 7 in 10,000 live births. EDs have been reported most often in caucasians, but they occur in all population groups. Hidrotic ED has been reported in an extensive kindred of French extraction. X-linked hypohidrotic ED has full expression predominantly in males. Female carriers outnumber affected men, but most show few, if any, signs of the condition although some do manifest it very clearly. Most of the other EDs affect males and females equally.

What are the symptoms?

Each syndrome usually involves a different combination of symptoms, which can range from mild to severe, such as:

- Absence or abnormality of hair growth;
- Absence or malformation of some or all teeth;
- Inability to perspire, which causes overheating;
- Abnormalities of the nails – which may be brittle and grow slowly or be thickened or ridged;
- Frequent infections due to immune system deficiencies or, in some cases, the inability of cracked or eroded skin to keep out disease-causing bacteria;
- Absence or malformation of some fingers or toes;
- Cleft lip and/or palate;
- Irregular skin pigmentation.

In addition to the above they may have:

- Sensitivity to light;
- Respiratory infections and allergies;
- A lack of breast development;
- Impairment or loss of hearing or vision;
- Constipation;
- A host of other challenges.

Individuals affected by ED face a lifetime of special needs which may include:

- Dentures at a young age with frequent adjustments and

replacements;
- Special diets to meet dental/nutritional needs;
- Air conditioned environments;
- Wigs to conceal hair and scalp conditions;
- Genetic testing to confirm the precise diagnosis and identify carriers;
- Protective devices from direct sunlight;
- Osseointegrated dental implants;
- Respiratory therapies.

Eye Problems and Ectodermal Dysplasia

The ectodermal dysplasias cause four main ocular problems:

- **Tears Deficiency.** Tears are composed of a mucus layer, water or aqueous layer and an oil layer, and ED can affect any of these layers. Defects in the tear film can predispose to infection, lead to corneal ulceration and delay healing. Treatment for tear deficiency includes tear replacement eye drops and punctal plugs (plugs that prevent tears being lost from the eyes through drainage through the nose) or occlusion (blockage) that reduce the loss.

- **Tear drainage.** The tear drainage system drains tears from the eye into the nose. Obstruction in this system can cause watery eyes especially from birth and dacryocystitis (infection of the tear drainage sac). Surgery may be required for blockage of the nasolacrimal duct (tear/drainage path) and this includes syringing and probing the system (usually done in childhood) and dacryocystorhinostomy or DCR (operation to 're-plumb' the duct into the nose).

- **Cornea.** The health of the cornea is essential for vision and corneal ulceration and scarring can result from dry eyes, recurrent infections, stem cell failure and misdirection of the eyelashes. Corneal problems are commonly seen in ectrodactyly-ectodermal dysplasia and ectrodactyly, ectodermal dysplasia and cleft lip/palate syndrome (EEC syndrome). Corneal ulcers are treated by a variety of measures – antibiotics, tear supplements, patching and special contact lens termed bandage contact lenses. Corneal transplantation and ocular surface reconstruction may be concerned in some cases of corneal scarring to restore vision.

- **Lens.** The lens forms from the ectoderm (surface skin). A cataract (cloudiness of the lens) results in defects in focus and clarity of vision. These cataracts (see entry) can be congenital (present at birth) and, if dense, result in poor vision from birth, wobbly eyes or nystagmus (see entry) and loss of the red reflex. Congenital cataract surgery is a complex procedure requiring careful visual rehabilitation.

How is it diagnosed?

In some cases, an ED is apparent at birth. In other cases, it may become evident when teeth fail to develop normally. Different types of ED are diagnosed according to the grouping of features. Complex forms of ED may affect the development or function of other body structures, as well.

It is important to remember that not all individuals affected by the EDs will have physical features that fit the description of a specific syndrome. There may be a great deal of variation in the physical appearance of the same type of ED from one affected person to the next. It is also conceivable for a person to have a type of ED that has not yet been described. Nonetheless, the EDs share certain features, an understanding of which makes it possible to appreciate the ramifications for most affected individuals and allows everyone involved to respond appropriately to the individual's needs.

Inheritance patterns and prenatal diagnosis

Inheritance patterns

These are variable according to the specific type of ED. Patterns include autosomal dominant, autosomal recessive, X-linked dominant, X-linked recessive. For hypohidrotic ED, inheritance is usually X-linked but can be autosomal dominant or autosomal recessive. Cases can arise as isolated (sporadic) cases within a family, when the mode of inheritance may be unclear.

Genetic counselling is available for families.

Prenatal diagnosis

This is available for some families with X-linked hypohidrotic ectodermal dysplasia using molecular genetic methods including mutational testing or linkage analysis but is not possible for all families.

A gene has been identified on chromosome 2 which is involved in some cases of autosomal hypohidrotic ED, and testing for this has recently become available as a regular diagnostic service.

Medical text written October 2005 by the Ectodermal Dysplasia Society and Contact a Family. **Approved October 2005 by Professor A Clarke, Professor in Clinical Genetics,Institute of Medical Genetics, University of Wales College of Medicine, Cardiff, UK. Additional material on Eye Problems and Ectodermal Dysplasia written July 2006 by Dr C Willoughby, Consultant Ophthalmic Surgeon and Senior Lecturer in Ophthalmology, Royal Victoria Hospital, Belfast, UK.**

Support

Ectodermal Dysplasia Society
108 Charlton Lane, Cheltenham, GL53 9EA   Tel: 01242 261332
e-mail: diana@ectodermaldysplasia.org   Web: http://www.ectodermaldysplasia.org
*The Society is a National Registered Charity No. 1089135, established in 1996. It provides
information, advice and support to those affected by an ectodermal dysplasia, promotes
the education of the medical profession and general public, supports research, encourages
a network for mutual support and produces a newsletter. The society has a medical
advisory board.*
Group details last confirmed April 2007.

"The group wouldn't exist without
Contact a Family's help." Group leader.

ECZEMA

Background

Eczema is a non-contagious inflammatory condition of the skin. The term 'eczema' comes from the Greek word ekzein meaning 'to boil over.' This makes sense when one considers the most common features of eczema are very itchy, dry, red skin. The itching and scratching, commonly known as the 'itch-scratch-itch cycle', are seen as the most distressing part of eczema, causing disturbed sleep for the person with eczema and also their families and carers.

There are various types of eczema including atopic, contact, seborrhoeic and varicose. The most common form of the condition is atopic eczema, which affects fifteen to twenty per cent of school children and one to two per cent of adults in the UK. Atopic eczema is often associated with asthma and hay fever. In most cases, the eczema lessens with age. Factors known to make the condition worse are woollen clothing, soaps, skin infections, dust mites, pet dander, pollen, sweating, stress and excessive heat. Sometimes certain foods may aggravate eczema. These include cow's milk, eggs and nuts. Professional advice should be taken before altering a child's diet.

Inheritance patterns and prenatal diagnosis

Inheritance patterns

Although the exact causes are not known, a combination of genetic and environmental irritant factors may be important. These environmental factors may be irritant as well as allergic.

Prenatal diagnosis

None

Medical text written November 1991 by Contact a Family. Approved November 1991 by Professor M Patton, Professor of Medical Genetics, St Georges Hospital Medical School, London, UK and Dr J E Wraith, Consultant Paediatrician, Royal Manchester Children's Hospital, Manchester, UK. **Last updated November 2004 by Professor Hywel Williams FRCP MSc PhD, Professor in Dermato-Epidemiology, University Hospital, Nottingham, UK.**

Support

National Eczema Society
Hill House, Highgate Hill, London N19 5NA
Tel: 0870 241 3604 Helpline (Mon-Fri, 8am-8pm)
Tel: 020 7281 3553 main office and membership   Fax: 020 7281 6395
e-mail: helpline@eczema.org   Web: http://www.eczema.org
The Society is a National Registered Charity No. 1009671, established in 1975. It offers advice and information by telephone, e-mail and through a network of local support groups. It has a wide range of information available. The Society has approximately 13,000 members.
Group details last updated August 2007.

EDWARDS SYNDROME

Edwards syndrome: trisomy 18; 18+ syndrome

Background

Edwards syndrome is a severe chromosome abnormality where the child has an extra chromosome 18 in every cell. A chromosome is a rod-like structure present in the nucleus of all body cells, with the exception of the red blood cells,and which stores genetic information. Normally humans have twenty-three pairs of chromosomes, the unfertilised ova and each sperm carrying a set of twenty-three chromosomes. On fertilisation the chromosomes combine to give a total of forty-six (twenty-three pairs). A normal female has an XX pair and a normal male an XY pair.

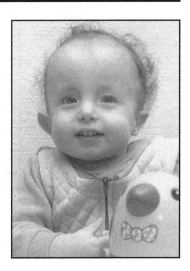

There are three types of the syndrome:

Full form (severe) – in this every cell in the body has three chromosome 18's instead of two.

Mosaic form (less severe) – in this some cells have two chromosome 18's while others have three. The extent and severity of the condition will depend upon the ratio of normal to abnormal cells.

Partial form – in some cases there may be an extra copy of part of chromosome 18. This is referred to as partial trisomy 18. The effects of this may be milder and would require further medical advice.

Children with all their cells affected do not normally survive beyond infancy. T hose affected by the mosaic and partial forms may survive to adulthood.

What are the symptoms?

Characteristic features include growth deficiency, low-set and malformed ears, clenched hands, bone abnormalities, hernias, skin mottling, heart defects, feeding and breathing problems in infancy and learning disability.

Psychological and behavioural characteristics

The information below has been drawn up by Dr Orlee Udwin of the Society for the Study of Behavioural Phenotypes.

Surviving children with Edwards' syndrome have marked developmental and motor delays. Their verbal communication is severely impaired, and is limited to a few single words at best; but they are mostly aware of their environment and are able to communicate some of their needs non-verbally. They continue to acquire new skills over time and develop some understanding of language. A few can walk with assistance. Overall, their skills in daily living, receptive language and social interaction tend to be higher than their motor and expressive language abilities.

Children with trisomy 18 mosaicism or partial trisomy 18 tend to be less severely handicapped; they are able to walk, and have moderate or mild learning difficulties or normal intelligence.

Inheritance patterns and prenatal diagnosis
Inheritance patterns
This is seen as being sporadic. In rare cases a balanced translocation in a parent can give rise to an unbalanced translocation in their child.
Prenatal diagnosis
Chorionic villus sampling at ten to twelve weeks and amniocentesis at sixteen weeks. The 'triple test' will detect approximately fifty per cent of cases. Routine detailed ultrasound scanning at eighteen weeks can detect up to eighty per cent of cases. A suspected diagnosis of Edwards syndrome can only be confirmed by amniocentesis or placental biopsy.

Medical text written November 1991 by Contact a Family. Approved November 1991 by Professor M Patton, Professor of Medical Genetics, St Georges Hospital Medical School, London, UK and Dr J E Wraith, Consultant Paediatrician, Royal Manchester Children's Hospital, Manchester, UK. **Last updated September 2003 by Contact a Family . Approved September 2003 by Professor I Young, Department of Clinical Genetics, Leicester Royal Infirmary, Leicester, UK.**

Support
SOFT UK
48 Froggatts Ride, Walmley, Sutton Coldfield B76 2TQ   Tel: 0121 351 3122 (Helpline) e-mail: enquiries@soft.org.uk   Web: http://www.soft.org.uk
SOFT UK is a National Registered Charity No. 1002918, established in 1990. It offers support and information to enable informed choices and contact with other families where possible. It also offers bereavement support and prenatal befrienders. It encourages research into causes, cures, new medical procedures and breakthroughs in care and support. It publishes a biannual newsletter and has information available, details on request. SOFT UK has over 500 member families.
Group details last confirmed February 2007.

EHLERS-DANLOS SYNDROME

Ehlers-Danlos: Arthrochalasis-Multiplex Congenita; Cutis Hyperelastica; EDS

Background

Ehlers-Danlos syndrome consists of several types of genetic connective tissue disorders. In general, these are due to collagen (a naturally occurring protein) abnormality. Common characteristics include abnormalities of the skin, ligaments and, in some instances, internal organs. Problems include fragile andlor stretchy skin, bruising, poor wound healing and loose joints, which are prone to dislocation and subluxation (partial dislocation). Chronic joint and limb pain is 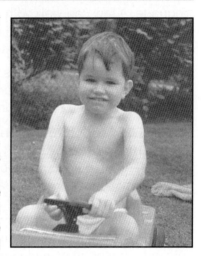 common even when skeletal radiographs are normal. Early degenerative arthritis, mitral valve prolapse and hernias may also present problems. Prematurity due to rupture of the fetal membranes can occur in pregnancy. When bruising presents in a child it may be incorrectly attributed to non-accidental injury.

These problems form the major difficulties bringing patients to the notice of Medical and Surgical Specialists. Many patients will be directed to Physiotherapy and Occupational Therapy for help with the musculoskeletal and ergonomic aspects.

The following issues are reported less frequently in those with EDS. However, they occur more frequently than in the non-EDS population. Hearing loss, ruptured ear drums, problems of making and maintaining voice alongside difficulties with articulatory development and maintenance of clarity are not uncommon. Difficulties with chewing and effective swallowing occur. Language development can be delayed. Many of these areas are affected by early ageing. Affected individuals will be directed to Speech & Language Therapists.

Types of Ehlers-Danlos syndrome

The different types of the syndrome are not graded in order of severity of the condition but each is a distinct type. Severe forms of the condition may be life threatening.

The re-categorisation of the Ehlers-Danlos syndromes appeared in the Revised Nosology, Villefranche, 1997.

Classical type (Formerly EDS I & II, gravis and mitis type).
Major clinical features: Skin hyperextensibility; widened thin scars; joint hypermobility.
Minor clinical features: Smooth velvety skin; complications of loose joints; muscle hypotonia (see entry, Hypotonia); easy bruising; manifestations of tissue extensibility (hernia, cervical insufficiency, etc); positive family history of EDS.
Basic defect: Abnormality of the pro alpha 1 (V) or pro alpha 2 (V) chain of the type V collagen encoded by COL5A1 and COL5A2 genes (in some but not all families).

Hypermobility type (Formerly EDS III hypermobile type).
Major clinical features: Generalised joint hypermobility; skin hyperextensible and smooth or velvety.
Minor clinical features: Recurrent joint dislocations; chronic limb and joint pains; positive family history of EDS.
Basic defect: Unknown.

Vascular type (Formerly EDS type IV arterial or ecchymotic type).
Major clinical features: Arterial/intestinal/uterine fragility or rupture; easy bruising; characteristic facial appearance.
Minor clinical features: Hypermobility of small joints; tendon and muscle rupture; clubfeet; varicose veins; positive family history of EDS; sudden death of close relative.
Basic defect: Structural defects in the proa I(III) chain of collagen type III, encoded by the COL3A1 gene.

Kyphoscoliosis type (Formerly EDS VI ocular or scoliosis type).
Major clinical features: Generalised joint laxity; severe muscle hypotonia in infancy; scoliosis present at birth and progressive; fragility of the sclera of the eye.
Minor clinical features: Tissue fragility; easy bruising; arterial rupture; marfanoid body shape; microcornea; skeletal osteopenia on X-ray; positive family history of affected siblings.
Basic defect: Deficiency of lysyl hydroxylase, a collagen modifying enzyme.

Arthrochalasia type (Formerly EDS VIIB type).
Major clinical features: Severe generalised joint hypermobility with dislocations; congenital bilateral hip dislocations.
Minor clinical features: Skin hyperextensibility; tissue fragility and scarring; easy bruising; muscle hypotonia; kyphoscoliosis; skeletal osteopenia on X-ray; positive family history of EDS.
Basic defect: Deficiencies of the proa (I) or proa 2(I) chains of collagen type I due to skipping of exon 6 in the COL1A1 or COL1A2 gene.

Dermatosparaxis type (Formerly EDS VII type).

Major clinical features: Severe skin fragility; sagging, redundant skin.

Minor clinical features: Soft, doughy skin texture; easy bruising; premature rupture of fetal membranes; hernias.

Basic defect: Deficiency of procollagen 1 N-terminal peptidase in collagen type I.

Inheritance patterns and prenatal diagnosis

Inheritance patterns

Typically autosomal dominant: Classical type; Hypermobility type; Vascular type; Arthrochalasia type.

Autosomal recessive: Kyphoscoliosis type; Dermatosparaxis type.

Prenatal diagnosis

Gene marker tests are available at present for a few types of Ehlers-Danlos syndrome. Further details should be obtained from your physician.

Medical text written by Professor P Beighton, Department of Human Genetics, University of Cape Town, Cape Town, South Africa. **Last updated April 2004 by Professor H A Bird, Professor of Pharmacological Rheumatology, Leeds General Infirmary, Leeds, UK.**

Further online resources

Medical texts in *The Contact a Family Directory* are designed to give a short, clear description of specific conditions and rare disorders. More extensive information on this condition can be found on a range of reliable, validated websites. Further information on these resources can be found in our **Medical Information on the Internet** article on page 21.

Support

Ehlers-Danlos Support Group

PO Box 337, Aldershot GU12 6WZ   Tel: 01252 690940   e-mail: info@ehlers-danlos.org
Web: http://www.ehlers-danlos.org

The Group is a National Registered Charity No. 1014641 established in 1988. It offers individual support by phone, letter and e-mail and attempts to link members for mutal support where possible. It maintains a list of specialists with particular interest in and experience of the condition. It publishes a six monthly newsletter for members and has a wide range of information available, details on request.

Group details last confirmed October 2007.

ELLIS-VAN CREVELD SYNDROME

Background

Ellis-van Creveld syndrome (EvC) is a rare inherited condition that causes a number of different problems. These include:

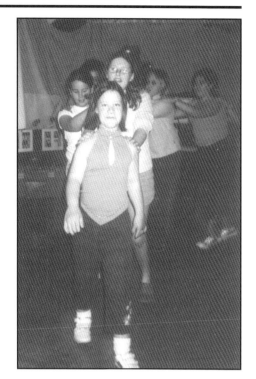

- Short arms and legs causing disproportionate short stature;
- Short ribs resulting in a narrow chest;
- Heart defects (see entry), most commonly an atrial or an atrioventricular septal defect;
- Extra fingers and or toes (Polydactyly);
- Small finger and toe nails;
- Small or absent teeth;
- Abnormal knee joints causing knock knees in older children and adults.

Not all of these features are present in everyone with EvC.

What are the symptoms?

Common problems that occur in adolescents and young adults include: knee pain due to the knock knee deformity sometimes requiring an operation to correct it and orthodontic problems due to small or missing teeth.

Some children have very small chests which can cause severe breathing problems in the first few months of life but this is unusual. Approximately half of children with EvC have a heart defect. In most cases this can be repaired by surgery. If these problems are treated successfully most children and adults with EvC have a normal life expectancy.

Most people with EvC have normal intelligence.

How is it diagnosed?

The diagnosis is normally made based on the features that a person has and the appearance of the bones on x-ray.

Inheritance patterns and prenatal diagnosis

Inheritance patterns

EvC is inherited in an autosomal recessive manner. It is cause by a change in one of two different genes that are both located on chromosome 4.

Prenatal diagnosis

This is normally made by ultrasound scan. Short limbs, extra fingers and a heart defect may be visible in the baby with EvC. If a mutation in one of the genes causing EvC can be found in an affected member of the family it may be possible to perform prenatal testing by chorionic villus biopsy at twelve weeks. This is not widely available.

Medical text written October 2005 by Dr M Wright, Consultant Clinical Geneticist, Institute of Medical Genetics, International Centre for Life, Newcastle upon Tyne, UK.

Support

Ellis-Van Creveld Foundation
Farthingale Farm, Hackmans Lane, Purleigh, Chelmsford CM3 6RW
Tel: 01621 829675 (evenings)
The Foundation is a self help group, established in 1991. It offers support and advice to the families of affected children. It raises awareness of the condition through contact with professionals and compiles data on affected children to support research into the condition. The Foundation has information available, details on request. There are 14 known affected families in the UK.
Group details last confirmed October 2007.

Web: http://www.ellisvancreveld.co.uk
An independent web site providing information and facilitating parent-parent networking.

ENCEPHALITIS

Background

Encephalitis comes from the Greek enkephalos meaning brain and itis meaning inflammation. The effects of Encephalitis can range in severity from having little or no long term results to being life-threatening. Children and adults of both sexes and all ethnic groups can be affected at any age. It is thought that the annual incidence in the UK and Republic of Ireland is 4 in 100,000 or two thousand five hundred people per year.

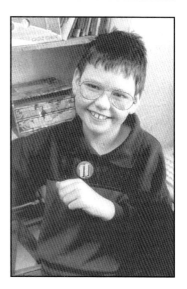

Specific forms of Encephalitis include Acute Disseminated Encephalomyelitis, Rasmussen's Encephalitis, Hashimoto's Encephalitis, Subacute-Sclerosing Panencephalitis (see entries), West Nile Encephalitis, Japanese encephalitis and Tick-borne encephalitis (see entry Arboviral Encephalitides).

What are the symptoms?

Symptoms of Encephalitis include:

- Fever or flu-like illness;
- Headache;
- Vomiting;
- Light-sensitivity of the eyes;
- Stiff neck and back (occasionally);
- Confusion, disorientation;
- Behaviour that is out of character;
- Drowsiness;
- Clumsiness, unsteady gait.

More serious acute symptoms that require immediate investigation include:

- Loss of consciousness, poor responsiveness, stupor, coma;
- Seizures;
- Muscle weakness or paralysis.

What are the causes?

Encephalitis is usually caused by a viral infection. Exposure to viruses can occur through insect bites, food or drink contamination, inhalation of respiratory droplets from an infected person, or skin contact. Common illnesses such as measles and mumps can lead to Encephalitis. The virus reaches the brain causing an infection. Infected nerves may become damaged or destroyed. Although viruses infecting the brain are a major cause of encephalitis, the body's reaction to a virus itself can lead to encephalitis. This occurs when the immune system tries to fight off the virus and by mistake, attacks the nerves in the brain at the same time. This condition is called Post Infectious or autoimmune Encephalitis.

How is it diagnosed?

A diagnosis of Encephalitis is made following a range of tests which can include:

- Lumbar puncture in which the cerebrospinal fluid is tested for viral particles, especially herpes simplex virus. These tests can also exclude bacterial meningitis;
- Brain scans (CT or MRI) - to exclude brain tumours, aneurysms and strokes and show the extent of any inflammation;
- An electroencephalogram (EEG) will help confirm a diagnosis of encephalitis by recording any unusual patterns of electrical activity in the brain.

It should be noted that it is not unusual for the results of some tests to be 'normal'. It is important to initially exclude some more common and treatable diseases.

How is it treated?

An antiviral medication, Acyclovir, will be prescribed. Acyclovir has significantly improved the outlook in cases of herpes simplex encephalitis but is not as effective against other viruses. Steroids may be prescribed for Post Infectious encephalitis. Other treatment for Encephalitis is symptomatic.

Provision of nutrition, fluids and rest will allow the body to fight the infection. Emotional support of agitated or confused persons is helpful.

After the acute phase of Encephalitis, which may last from one to two weeks, physiotherapy and speech therapy may be necessary and an assessment by a neuropsychologist is advised.

A proportion of people will be left with highly variable and often permanent consequences of the illness (acquired brain injury). These difficulties may include cognitive, physical, emotional or behavioural consequences. Specialist clinical support and rehabilitation are needed to help the person adjust to, and cope with, such difficulties.

Inheritance patterns and prenatal diagnosis
Inheritance patterns
None.
Prenatal diagnosis
None.

Medical text written November 2005 by the Encephalitis Society and Contact a Family. Approved November 2005 by Professor Hawkins, Professor of Clinical Neurology, Keele University and Consultant Neurologist to the Regional Neuroscience Centre, Stoke-on-Trent, UK.

Further online resources

Medical texts in *The Contact a Family Directory* are designed to give a short, clear description of specific conditions and rare disorders. More extensive information on this condition can be found on a range of reliable, validated websites. Further information on these resources can be found in our **Medical Information on the Internet** article on page 21.

Support

Encephalitis Society

Encephalitis Resource Centre, 7b Saville Street, Malton YO17 7LL   Tel: 01653 699599
Fax: 01653 604369   e-mail: mail@encephalitis.info   Web: http://www.encephalitis.info
The Society is a National Registered Charity No. 1087843, established in 1991. It offers support and contact by telephone, e-mail, letter and linking with other families where possible. The Society publishes a newsletter three times a year and two books specifically for families with children affected by encephalitis: "Encephalitis - a parents handbook" and "Gilley the Giraffe ...who changed", a storybook for children. It also produces a comic strip for teenagers. The Society has around 800 members. Each year the children's home page receives over 40,000 web hits and the society responds to approximately 100 child related enquiries.
Group details last confirmed August 2007.

EPIDERMOLYSIS BULLOSA

Background

Epidermolysis Bullosa (EB) is the term used to describe a number of genetically determined disorders whose principal characteristic is skin and/or mucous membrane fragility (for example in the mouth and oesophagus). The skin has a tendency to blister in response to mechanical trauma (for example any friction between the skin and clothing). Though a large number of distinct types of epidermolysis bullosa have been identified, in practice most cases can be placed in one of three categories: EB simplex, junctional EB and dystrophic EB. These are defined by the level at which there is a split between the epidermis (outer layer) and the dermis (inner layer) of the skin, which results in the characteristic fragility of EB.

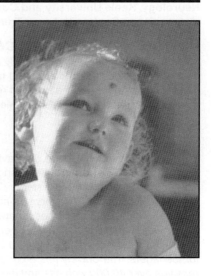

What are the symptoms?

Symptoms within each category will vary from mild to severe. In severe forms the condition can be life threatening.

How is it treated?

Treatment can range from simply avoiding triggering factors such as walking for long distances in warm weather which causes blistering on the soles of the feet in EB Simplex; eating harsh foods such as crisps which causes oral blistering, and avoiding knocks and scratching in the case of Junctional and Dystrophic EB; to daily regimes of applying creams and dressings depending on the type and severity of EB.

Inheritance patterns and prenatal diagnosis

Inheritance patterns

All forms of EB are autosomally inherited. In some cases inheritance is autosomal dominant in others autosomal recessive. The genes responsible for all the major forms of EB have now been identified.

Prenatal diagnosis

This is possible for the more severe forms of EB where a couple have previously had an affected child. Tests usually involve analysis of fetal DNA from chorionic villus sampling at ten to twelve weeks, but in some cases a fetal skin biopsy at sixteen to eighteen weeks may be necessary.

Medical text written March 2002 by Dr Raj Mallipeddi, DEBRA Research Fellow, St John's Institute of Dermatology, St Thomas' Hospital, London, UK.

Contact a Family Helpline 0808 808 3555

Further online resources

Medical texts in *The Contact a Family Directory* are designed to give a short, clear description of specific conditions and rare disorders. More extensive information on this condition can be found on a range of reliable, validated websites. Further information on these resources can be found in our **Medical Information on the Internet** article on page 21.

Support

DebRA

DebRA House, 13 Wellington Business Park, Dukes Ride, Crowthorne RG24 6LS
Tel: 01344 771961   Fax: 01344 762661   e-mail: debra@debra.org.uk
Web: http://www.debra.org.uk   Web: http://www.debra-international.org
The Association is a National Registered Charity No. 1084958, established in 1978. The Organisation has encouraged the establishment of DebRA in over 30 other countries. It offers support and advice for affected persons, families, carers and professional workers. It also offers a visiting service from eleven Nurse Consultants and Clinical Nurse Specialists and eleven social workers. It publishes a quarterly newsletter and has a wide range of information available, details on request. The Association has over 1,000 member families. There are thought to be 5,000 affected people in the UK.
Group details last updated April 2007.

EPILEPSY

Background

Epilepsy is the tendency to have recurrent seizures originating in the brain as a result of excessive or disordered discharge of brain cells.

Seizures are divided into two categories:

- In the **generalised seizures** both hemispheres of the brain are involved and consciousness is lost. The seizures include major convulsive episodes with jerking of all limbs and unconsciousness (tonic clonic seizures), seizures when the body goes stiff (tonic) or floppy (atonic), jerks of the limbs (myoclonic jerks) and momentary lapses of consciousness (absences);
- In **partial (or focal) seizures** the disturbance of brain activity starts in, or involves, a specific part of the brain. The nature of such seizures depends upon the area of the brain involved. Partial seizures may be simple or complex. Consciousness is not lost in a simple partial seizure, but is impaired in a complex partial seizure.

What are the causes?

Causes of epilepsy are variable and may be:

- **Idiopathic epilepsy** often starts in childhood or adolescence and is largely due to genetic causes;
- **Symptomatic epilepsy** may be due to brain damage or anomaly from any cause for example, infection, tumours, brain damage, or specific syndromes such as Sturge-Weber (see entry), Tuberous Sclerosis (see entry), or some metabolic disorders;
- **Cryptogenic epilepsy** is where no known cause may be found (such as structural change or lesions in the brain) for the epilepsy and may begin at any time in the individual's life.

Inheritance patterns and prenatal diagnosis

Inheritance patterns

People with idiopathic epilepsy may inherit a low seizure threshold. This would mean that given certain conditions (individual to each person) they may have a greater susceptibility to having a seizure. In cases of symptomatic epilepsy the inheritance pattern will depend upon the underlying cause of the condition.

In the case of Sturge-Weber syndrome the event is sporadic; whereas in Tuberous Sclerosis inheritance is either autosomal dominant or a sporadic event.

Genetic advice is available.

Prenatal diagnosis

This is rarely available unless the cause is metabolic.

Contact a Family Helpline 0808 808 3555

Medical text written October 1999 by Professor John Duncan. **Last reviewed February 2006 by Professor John Duncan, Medical Director, National Society for Epilepsy, Chalfont St Peter, UK.**

Support

The National Society for Epilepsy (NSE)
Chesham Lane, Chalfont St. Peter, Gerrards Cross SL9 0RJ
Tel: 01494 601400 Helpline (Mon-Fri, 10am-4pm)   Tel: 01494 601300
Fax: 01494 871927   Web: http://www.epilepsynse.org.uk
NSE is a National Registered Charity No. 206186, established in 1892. It provides medical services through out-patient clinics and in-patient assessment; short breaks and residential care services for adults with epilepsy. It has a comprehensive research programme into epilepsy, offers a membership scheme, epilepsy training services and information services. The latter include leaflets, books and videos, a helpline that gives information and listening support, and a network of epilepsy information services in hospital settings nationwide.
Group details last confirmed May 2007.

Epilepsy Action
New Anstey House, Gate Way Drive, Yeadon, Leeds LS19 7XY
Tel: 0808 800 5050 Helpline (9.00am-4.30pm, Mon-Thurs; 9.00am - 4.00pm, Fri)
Fax: 0808 800 5555 Helpline   Tel: 0113 210 8800 Admin   Fax: 0113 242 8804 Admin
e-mail: helpline@epilepsy.org.uk   Web: http://www.epilepsy.org.uk
Epilepsy Action is a National Registered Charity No. 234343, established in 1950. It offers a nationwide network of branches. It publishes a members' quarterly newsletter and has a wide range of information available, details on request. Epilepsy Action has nearly 16,000 members.
Group details last updated June 2007.

Epilepsy Scotland
48 Govan Road, Glasgow G51 1JL   Tel: 0808 800 2200 Helpline
(Mon-Wed & Fri, 10am-4pm; Thurs 10am-6pm)   Tel: 0141 427 4911   Fax: 0141 419 1709
e-mail: enquiries@epilepsyscotland.org.uk   Web: http://www.epilepsyscotland.org.uk
Epilepsy Scotland is a Scottish Registered Charity No. SC 000067, established in 1954. Epilepsy Scotland helps people of all ages who are affected by epilepsy. It campaigns for improved healthcare, better support and greater understanding of Epilepsy. It has a network of self-help groups and branches. It publishes a regular newsletter and provides a wide range of information through the freephone helpline, website and Epilepsy Scotland information leaflets. Epilepsy Scotland provides training throughout Scotland.
Group details last updated April 2007.

Epilepsy Wales
P.O.Box 4168, Cardiff CF14 0WZ   Tel: 08457 413 774 Helpline
Tel: 029 20 755 515   Fax: 02920 755515
e-mail: helpline@epilepsy-wales.co.uk   Web: http://www.epilepsy-wales.co.uk
Epilepsy Wales is a National Registered Charity No. 1059067, established in 1996. It aims to help people with epilepsy in Wales, their families and carers by offering a bi-lingual service wherever possible, non-medical support ,field workers and branches throughout Wales. A chat room is hosted on Epilepsy Wales' web site.
Group details last confirmed January 2007.

David Lewis Centre For Epilepsy
Mill Lane, Warford, Alderley Edge SK9 7UD   Tel: 01565 640000   Fax: 01565 640100
e-mail: enquiries@davidlewis.org.uk   Web: http://www.davidlewis.org.uk
The Centre is a National Registered Charity No. 1000392, established in 1904. It offers
a multi-disciplinary approach to assessment, treatment, education and care of adults and
children with complicated epilepsy and associated special needs.
Group details last confirmed February 2008.

For support for Epilepsy in childhood, see entry, Epilepsy syndromes in Childhood.

Make 2008 a year to remember by
scaling the heights of Kilimanjaro in aid
of Contact a Family. To take part in this
amazing adventure, call our fundraising
team, Tel: 020 7608 8731.

EPILEPSY SYNDROMES IN CHILDHOOD

Background

The epilepsy syndromes of infancy and childhood broadly separate into benign and more severe. The benign conditions usually occur in an otherwise normal child and are of one type of attack, normally easily treated and tending to show natural remission over time. Benign syndromes, including febrile seizures and benign epilepsy with centro-temporal spikes, quite often don't need treatment.

What are the symptoms?

Seizures are of many types:

- Tonic (stiffening);
- Clonic (jerking);
- Combinations of both tonic and clonic;
- Loss of awareness;
- Myoclonus (sudden jerks of the whole body or limb);
- Abnormal feelings of fear, smell, taste, vision and/or feeling in a part of the body with or without impairment of consciousness, all pointing to a focal onset (specific part of the brain from which the cause of the feelings originate);
- Automatic movements.

All types of epilepsy have a small risk of sudden unexplained death which is difficult to anticipate but has brought about the development of epilepsy networks and guidelines for effective diagnosis investigation and treatment.

The more severe syndromes include a number of conditions which may be difficult to treat and which cause severe regression of learning, social functioning and behaviour. Thus learning impairments (see entry, Learning disability), Autistic Spectrum disorder (see entry, Autism Spectrum disorders including Asperger syndrome), Attention Deficit Hyperactivity disorder (see entry) and other behavioural disorders are very common in children with intractable seizures. The regression in development particularly caused by early onset epilepsy is known as an epileptic encephalopathy and is particularly related to sub-clinical epileptic activity rather than the rate of obvious seizures.

What are the causes?

Epilepsy in childhood has a wide range of causes including a large number of specific syndromes and illnesses involving the brain, infection, trauma and metabolic abnormalities. Epileptic seizures are therefore a symptom of very many conditions that involve the brain and these require investigation by a paediatrician.

Brain damage or anomalies from other causes, for example infection, tumours, brain damage or specific syndromes such as Sturge-Weber syndrome , Tuberous Sclerosis (see entries) or some metabolic disorders may give rise to epilepsy.

How is it treated?

The treatment of severe conditions is difficult and sometimes the drug treatments are not those normally used in epilepsy, e.g. corticosteroids, see entries: West syndrome, Lennox-Gastaut syndrome, Ohtahara syndrome, Landau-Kleffner syndrome and Worster-Drought syndrome.

Many children with epilepsy don't fit into one syndrome and management is along the lines of the closest epilepsy type. Surgery is being increasingly used as early as possible for those with a clear removable source of the seizures in order to minimise secondary impairments.

The additional impairments require diagnosis and treatment in their own right. They are often much more disabling than the seizures and have educational implications. In a recent study about half of the children with epilepsy in childhood had problems with either behaviour, educational progress or both. Most children with epilepsy (about seventy-five per cent) become seizure free on antiepileptic drugs but in the rest the above problems are common.

Inheritance patterns and prenatal diagnosis

Inheritance patterns

The genetics of epilepsy are a mixture of specific genetic and non-genetic conditions and those without such clear diagnosis in which a small increased susceptibility for siblings is seen.

Prenatal diagnosis

This is only available for a limited number of genetically determined conditions.

Medical text written January 2006 by Professor B Neville, Professor of Childhood Epilepsy, Institute of Child Health, London, UK.

Support

National Centre For Young People With Epilepsy (NCYPE)
St Piers Lane, Lingfield RH7 6PW   Tel: 01342 832243   Fax: 01342 834639
e-mail: info@ncype.org.uk   Web: http://www.ncype.org.uk
NCYPE is a National Registered Charity No. 311877, established in 1963. It is the UK's major provider of specialised services to young people who are profoundly affected by epilepsy, as well as other neurological conditions. It provides a day and residential school and further education college, an on-site medical centre, epilepsy assessment and rehabilitation outreach service. It works in partnership with Great Ormond Street Hospital and the Institute of Child Health. (Together the three organisations founded the first professor in childhood epilepsy – The Prince of Wales's Chair of Childhood Epilepsy).
Group details last updated May 2006.

Contact a Family Helpline 0808 808 3555

There are a number support groups for specific epilepsy syndromes of childhood or conditions that commonly cause epilepsy, details of which can be found in the entries detailed above. For more general support organisations see entry, Epilepsy.

Disability Living Allowance (DLA) is the main benefit for disabled children. To find out more about this and other benefits you may be entitled to, call the Contact a Family Helpline for a copy of the guide 'Benefits, tax credits and other financial assistance'.

ERB'S PALSY

Erb's Palsy: Obstetric Brachial Plexus Palsy

Background

Erb's Palsy describes a paralysis mainly from birth of the nerves supplying the arm. There are three main types of paralysis:

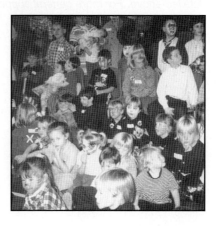

Erb's Palsy is a paralysis of the shoulder and elbow, involving the 5th and 6th cervical nerves. This manifests itself with the arm being turned towards the body, the elbow unable to bend and the hand being in the 'waiters tip' position.

Klumpke's Paralysis involves the 7th and 8th cervical and 1st thoracic nerves. The result is a flaccid paralysis of the hand which is often associated with Horner syndrome - drooping of the eyelid, the cheek does not sweat and the pupil may be smaller than the unaffected side.

Complete paralysis of the arm occurs when all the above five nerves are affected. The entire arm is paralysed and there is demonstrable sensory loss. Horner syndrome is often present as is Torticollis.

The incidence of Erb's Palsy is now established at 1 in 2,000 live births.

What are the causes?

Erb's Palsy is mainly caused by birth trauma when traction of the head or arm, or twisting the arm or shoulder down and backward, results in paralysis of the nerves supplying the arm.

How is it treated?

It is now possible to say that over half of children born with Erb's Palsy make a complete recovery and another thirty to thirty-five per cent make very useful recovery as relates to nerve injuries, but that between twenty-five to thirty per cent of the children face difficulties due to contracture at the shoulder leading to posterior dislocation of that joint. Properly conducted neurophysiological investigations are most helpful in determining the likelihood of recovery. The indication for an urgent operation can be restricted to a relatively small number of children who have complete and severe injuries or those who have suffered major injury to the plexus from breech delivery.

Inheritance patterns and prenatal diagnosis

Inheritance patterns

None

Prenatal diagnosis
None

Medical text written November 1992 by Dr R Birch. **Last updated January 2004 by Professor R Birch, Consultant Orthopaedic Surgeon, Royal National Orthopaedic Hospital, Stanmore, UK.**

Further online resources
Medical texts in *The Contact a Family Directory* are designed to give a short, clear description of specific conditions and rare disorders. More extensive information on this condition can be found on a range of reliable, validated websites. Further information on these resources can be found in our **Medical Information on the Internet** article on page 21.

Support
Erb's Palsy Group
60 Anchor Way Road, Coventry CV3 6JJ   Tel: 024 7641 3293
e-mail: info@erbspalsygroup.com   Web: http://www.erbspalsygroup.co.uk
The Group is a National Registered Charity No. 1036423, established in 1992. It offers support to parents and professional workers and contact between parents where possible. It gives advice on benefits and aids for affected children and aims to raise public & professional awareness of the condition. It publishes a quarterly newsletter and has information available, details on request. The families of over 1,000 children and 125 professional workers are in membership.
Group details last updated August 2007.

EVANS SYNDROME

Background

Evans syndrome is an uncommon, but not rare, condition first described by Dr R S Evans and colleagues in 1951. It is a syndrome characterised by immune thrombocytopenia (see entry, Immune (Idiopathic) Thrombocytopenic Purpura) and autoimmune haemolytic anaemia. Onset is variable as is the course and duration of the syndrome. Evans syndrome affects people of all ages but is usually first diagnosed in young children. Individually, immune thrombocytopaenia and autoimmune haemolytic anaemia affect people of all ethnic groups but Evans syndrome may affect white people more than other ethnic groups.

What are the symptoms?

There are a number of features found in people with Evans syndrome including:

- Purpura (patches of purplish discoloration resulting from leaking of blood into the skin);
- Petechiae (tiny localized haemorrhages from the small blood vessels just beneath the surface of the skin);
- Ecchymoses (discoloured spots or patches appearing in large irregularly formed areas of the skin);
- Pallor, fatigue and light-headedness which are signs of anaemia;
- Jaundice (yellowish pigmentation of the skin and tissues).

What are the causes?

The cause of Evans syndrome has not been identified but it is known that many people diagnosed with the syndrome have associated disorders such as Systemic Lupus Erythematosus (SLE) (see entry, Lupus) and other autoimmune disorders.

How is it diagnosed?

Diagnosis of the syndrome is made after other possible conditions are ruled out; these include rheumatological conditions, malignancies that first present with autoimmune cytopenias (deficiency of some specific cellular elements of the blood) and infections.

How is it treated?

Treatment involves medication (steroids or other immunosuppressives) and possibly surgical intervention such as a splenectomy (removal of the spleen). Children with the syndrome need to be monitored carefully after a splenectomy as there appears to be an increased risk of sepsis (infection) in some children.

Contact a Family Helpline 0808 808 3555

Inheritance patterns and prenatal diagnosis

Inheritance patterns

None.

Prenatal diagnosis

None.

Medical text written July 2006 by Contact a Family. Approved July 2006 by Dr A B Provan, Senior Lecturer in Haematology, Royal London Hospital, London, UK.

Further online resources

Medical texts in *The Contact a Family Directory* are designed to give a short, clear description of specific conditions and rare disorders. More extensive information on this condition can be found on a range of reliable, validated websites. Further information on these resources can be found in our **Medical Information on the Internet** article on page 21.

Support

There is no support group for Evans syndrome. Families can use Contact a Family's Freephone Helpline for advice, information and, where possible, links to other families. Contact a Family's web-based linking service Making Contact.org can be accessed at http://www.makingcontact.org

FABRY DISEASE

Anderson-Fabry: Angiokeratoma Corporis Diffusum; Haemorrhagic Nodular Glycolipid Lipidosis

Background

Fabry disease is a rare inherited metabolic disorder. It results from reduced activity of the enzyme alpha-galactosidase (α-Gal A) and progressive accumulation of a fatty substance, globotriaosylceramide (GL-3 or GB-3), in cells throughout the body.

What are the symptoms?

The classic form, occurring in males with very low levels of α-Gal A activity, usually has its onset in childhood or adolescence with periodic crises of severe pain in the hands and feet (acroparesthesias), the appearance of a skin rash (angiokeratomas), reduced sweating, eye changes bowel disturbance and protein in the urine. Gradual deterioration of kidney function usually occurs in men. Males may also develop heart problems such as an enlarged heart and neurological problems including stroke. Males with a higher level of enzyme activity often present later in life with predominantly heart or kidney problems with few of the other symptoms.

Females typically have milder symptoms at a later age of onset than males. However this is very variable; they may be relatively asymptomatic throughout a normal life span or may have symptoms as severe as those observed in males.

How is it diagnosed?

In males, the most efficient method for the diagnosis of Fabry disease is the demonstration of low α-Gal A activity in blood, and/or cultured skin cells. In females, measurement of α-Gal A activity is unreliable; molecular genetic testing of the gene encoding the α-Gal A enzyme is the most reliable method for identification of females with Fabry disease.

How is it treated?

Until relatively recently the only treatments available for Fabry disease were symptomatic. Nerve pain is treated using anti-epileptic drugs such as gabapentin and carbamezapine; angiokeratomas may be removed or treated with laser therapy. Standard therapies such as aspirin, antihypertensives and anti-cholesterol agents are used to treat the renal, cardiovascular and cerebrovascular manifestations of the disease. More recently, the introduction of enzyme replacement therapy has offered the opportunity to treat the underlying cause of Fabry disease. Intravenous infusion of recombinant α-Gal A enzyme has been shown to clear deposits of GB3, stabilise renal function, reduce heart size and significantly improve pain scores and quality of life. Enzyme is administered intravenously every 2 weeks. In the UK most patients receive enzyme replacement at home.

Inheritance patterns and prenatal diagnosis

Inheritance patterns

Fabry disease is inherited in an X-linked manner. A female with Fabry disease has a 50% chance of transmitting the mutation in each pregnancy. An affected male transmits his mutation to all his daughters but not his sons.

Prenatal diagnosis

Chorionic villus sampling at ten to 12 weeks gestation or by amniocentesis performed at about 15-18 weeks gestation is possible for pregnancies of women who have Fabry disease. Preimplantation genetic diagnosis may be available for families in which the disease-causing mutation has been identified.

Medical text written November 1991 by Contact a Family. Approved November 1991 by Professor M Patton, Professor of Medical Genetics, St Georges Hospital Medical School, London, UK and Dr J E Wraith, Consultant Paediatrician, Royal Manchester Children's Hospital, Manchester, UK. **Last updated January 2008 by Dr Derralyn Hughes, Lecturer in Haematology, Royal Free and University College Medical School, London, UK.**

Further online resources

Medical texts in *The Contact a Family Directory* are designed to give a short, clear description of specific conditions and rare disorders. More extensive information on this condition can be found on a range of reliable, validated websites. Further information on these resources can be found in our **Medical Information on the Internet** article on page 21.

Support

Information, support and advice for Fabry disease is available from the MPS Society (see entry, Mucopolysaccharide diseases and associated diseases).

FACIAL DIFFERENCE

Background

Facial disfigurement can have many causes including road accidents, burns, cancer, skin conditions, birthmarks and other congenital anomalies. Amongst congenital causes are a number of specific syndromes which include some form of facial abnormality as a characteristic feature of the condition. Facial disfigurement in varying degree may be a feature of chromosome abnormalities. Additionally, some genetic enzyme deficiency diseases result in facial abnormalities.

Examples of specific syndromes are Sturge-Weber syndrome (see entry) where the disfigurement is in the form of a port wine stain; hemifacial microsomia (Goldenhar syndrome, see entry) where there is under development of one side of the face. Cri du Chat syndrome (see entry) is a chromosome (5p-) abnormality, which includes facial asymmetry and poorly formed ears. In Treacher-Collins syndrome (see entry) malformations may include cheekbones, chin, jaw and temples, while ears may be malformed or absent.

How is it treated?

Whatever the underlying cause of the facial difference, the majority of people experience problems which are psycho-social in nature. Adjustment is not predicted by the physical or functional characteristics of the disfigurement (e.g. the severity, location or cause). Research has shown that high levels of self esteem, good social skills and an effective support network are powerful mediators of problems associated with looking different.

Inheritance patterns and prenatal diagnosis

Inheritance patterns

These will depend upon the cause of the facial disfigurement.

Prenatal diagnosis

This will depend on the cause of the disfigurement.

Medical text written November 1991 by Contact a Family. Approved by Dr M Patton, Consultant Clinical Geneticist, St George's Hospital Medical School London and Dr J E Wraith, Consultant Paediatrician, Royal Manchester Children's Hospital. Last updated June 2000 by Professor N Rumsey. **Last reviewed April 2005 by Professor N Rumsey, Centre for Appearance and Disfigurement Research, University of the West of England, Bristol, UK.**

Contact a Family Helpline 0808 808 3555

Support

Let's Face It

72 Victoria Avenue, Westgate-on-Sea CT8 8BH   Tel: 01843 833724   Fax: 01843 835695
e-mail: chrisletsfaceit@aol.com   Web: http://www.lets-face-it.org.uk
*Let's Face It is a National Registered Charity No. 1043461, established in 1984. It offers
support and advice to individuals and children with a facial disfigurement, their families
and professional workers and linking with others where possible. It gives help in rebuilding
lives and provides education for medical, nursing and health professionals. It publishes
a newsletter three times a year and has a wide range of information leaflets, details on
request. Let's Face It has over 1,000 members including over 100 children.*
Group details last confirmed August 2007.

Changing Faces

The Squire Centre, 33-37 University Street, London WC1E 6JN   Tel: 0845 4500 275
Fax: 0845 4500 276   e-mail: info@changingfaces.org.uk
Web: http://www.changingfaces.org.uk
Web: http://www.iface.org.uk (young people's forum)
*Changing Faces is a National Registered Charity No. 1011222, established in 1992.
It provides information, support and advice to anyone with a disfigurement and their
family. It has information and advice for employers to encourage equal opportunities in
the workplace and for schools to promote awareness. It offers advice for health-care
professionals in developing new models of health-care and build coping strategies
and self-confidence for patients. It publishes a twice yearly newsletter and has a wide
range of information available, details on request. Changing Faces has over 10,000
individuals, families, health and social care, educational and other professional workers in
membership.*
Group details last updated October 2007.

FACIOSCAPULOHUMERAL MUSCULAR DYSTROPHY

Facioscapulohumeral Muscular Dystrophy: FSH Muscular Dystrophy; FSHD; FSH MD

Background

Facioscapulohumeral Muscular Dystrophy is a muscle wasting condition, caused by a genetic fault present at, or soon after, conception. This fault probably affects the regulation of the level of several of the different proteins in muscles. Particular muscles are typically affected first, and the name reflects the usual distribution of these weakened muscles: 'facio' (facial); 'scapulo' (shoulder blade); 'humeral' (upper arm), as originally described in the 1880s by two doctors from Paris, Landouzy & Dejerine. However, in many people other muscles are also weakened.

FSHD is believed to be the third most common muscular dystrophy (after Duchenne and Myotonic Dystrophies - see entries). It occurs in all racial groups, although may be more common in some populations than others. In the UK, with an estimated frequency of 1 in 20,000, there are probably around three thousand cases in all.

What are the symptoms?

The age at which symptoms first develop and the severity of weakness can vary quite widely between people in different families, with symptoms generally increasing in severity with the fewer copies of the DNA sequence present. FSHD can also vary quite widely between different affected members in the family. For some, it can result in weakness not only of facial muscles and shoulders/upper arms, but also of additional combinations from the neck, forearms, wrists, fingers, hips, legs, ankles and the back muscles. Others may have mild weakness of facial or shoulder muscles only, and some may even be unaware of any problem.

Overall, around ten to twenty per cent of all people with FSHD eventually require a wheelchair but, by contrast, up to one third remain unaware of symptoms at least into old age, although they may have subtle detectable clinical signs. The majority of people come between these two extremes.

On average, men tend to show more weakness and from a slightly earlier age than women. Within large families, and therefore excluding the most severe cases, women may be the ones least obviously affected, and it has been estimated that thirty per cent of women who carry an FSHD DNA fault may not show any sign of the condition.

For someone, particularly a child, with a family history of FSHD, weakness of facial muscles can be suspected if the eyes remain slightly open when asleep, or if the eyelids cannot be screwed tightly enough to bury the eyelashes. Difficulties in pursing the lips to whistle or in blowing up balloons, are also suggestive of the condition. During the teenage years or in adulthood, difficulty raising an arm above the head, excessive aching around the shoulders, rounded shoulders and thin upper arms, or excessive winging of the shoulder blades, may be the first presenting signs or symptoms.

Many people find that their weakness, particularly when first noticed, affects one side of the body more than the other. This is often evident in the shoulders, usually with the right side to be the first one involved in right-handed people. Increasing weakness in the arms can be anticipated in most people.

Early weakness at the ankles causing 'foot drop' is not uncommon. Some degree of weakness at the knees or hips develops by middle age in over fifty per cent of people. Together with weakness in the back muscles, this can result in a typical backward-leaning and high-stepping gait. However, weakness in the upper legs is usually already present by early adulthood in those who will eventually require a wheelchair.

Life span is not usually affected, except in the most severe cases with greatly impaired mobility and consequent greater risk of chest infections. In some of the earliest childhood onset cases, with the greatest muscle involvement, learning difficulties and epilepsy (see entries) have been reported. Hearing loss and specific problems with blood vessels at the back of the eye have also been found in some cases.

Muscle pain is a quite frequent complaint accompanying FSHD, often in the early stages. This may relate to inflammation within the muscles, which seems to occur more in FSHD than other muscular dystrophies.

What are the causes?

Normally, at a particular site on the gene map (region '4q35' at one end of chromosome 4), each of us has many copies of a particular sequence of genetic instruction (DNA). In most cases, FSHD is caused when the number of copies is reduced below a certain level on one of the pair of chromosome 4's. This seems to affect the way that DNA in that region is packed into the chromosome, and may well be triggering the production or assembly of some proteins which would not normally be made in muscle. The effect is to cause damage to the muscle cells.

How is it treated?

There is no one best treatment for this, but different approaches to treatment have been used in different individuals. Research programmes in FSHD are currently mostly aimed at trying to understand these processes and how the genetic fault leads to muscle damage, with the hope that this may eventually lead to treatments which could prevent this.

Inheritance patterns and prenatal diagnosis
Inheritance patterns
Autosomal dominant. This gives a fifty per cent risk for each child of someone proven to have the DNA fault. At least ten per cent of cases, and particularly ones with an early childhood presentation, arise by fresh DNA mutation. Not infrequently, this may arise initially in one of the parents, but without resulting in clinical symptoms in them, and hence mean that further children could also be at risk. However, the unaffected elder brothers or sisters of a severely affected child are very unlikely to carry the same genetic fault or pass it on to their future children.

Prenatal diagnosis
Accurate prenatal testing, performed by Chorionic Villus Sampling, usually at eleven weeks, can be offered at patient request. It is essential that genetic (DNA) tests be performed first on blood samples from the affected parent or child to define the DNA mutation in that family. Blood samples would usually be required from both parents, and in some cases from additional relatives. Techniques to enable pre-implantation genetic diagnosis have now been developed in one or two assisted conception units Worldwide, although this is not yet available for FSHD within the UK.

Medical text written October 2001 by Dr P Lunt. **Last updated April 2007 by Dr P Lunt, Consultant Clinical Geneticist, St Michael's Hospital, Bristol, UK.**

Further online resources
Medical texts in *The Contact a Family Directory* are designed to give a short, clear description of specific conditions and rare disorders. More extensive information on this condition can be found on a range of reliable, validated websites. Further information on these resources can be found in our **Medical Information on the Internet** article on page 21.

Support
FSH MD Support Group
c/o Muscular Dystrophy Campaign, 61 Southwark Street, London SE1 0HL
Tel: 020 8950 7500   Fax: 020 8950 7300   e-mail: fshgroup@hotmail.com
Web: http://www.fsh-group.org
The Group is a Self Help Group, established in 1986. It offers support for affected families and links affected persons where possible. It publishes a newsletter and has information available, details on request. The Group is in touch with over 400 families.
Group details last updated January 2008.

As Facioscapulohumeral MD is a form of muscular dystrophy, advice and information about the condition is also available from the Muscular Dystrophy Group (see entry, Muscular Dystrophy and neuromuscular disorders).

FAMILIAL DYSAUTONOMIA

Background

Familial Dysautonomia (FD) is one example of a group of disorders known as hereditary sensory and autonomic neuropathies (HSAN). The various HSAN disorders are believed to be genetically distinct from each other. Unlike other HSAN, Familial Dysautonomia has been only noted in individuals of Ashkenazi Jewish extraction causing dysfunction of the autonomic and sensory nervous systems. Dysfunction is a result of an incomplete development of the neurons (nerve fibres) of these systems.

For information on Riley-Day syndrome and related dysautonomias see entry, Metabolic diseases.

What are the symptoms?

The most distinctive feature of FD is the absence of overflow tears with emotional crying although it can be normal for a child not to produce tears until seven months of age.

In babies with FD there is a high prevalence of breech presentation births and poor muscle tone (floppy babies).

Other features include:
- a weak or absent suck;
- respiratory congestion due to misdirected swallowing;
- blotching of skin;
- difficulty in maintaining temperature.

Difficulty in feeding is observed in sixty per cent of infants in the neo-natal period. Poor sucking and misdirected swallowing often persist and put the child at risk from aspiration pneumonia which is even more likely to occur if the child also has gastro-oesophageal reflux.

In older children symptoms may include:
- Delay in developmental milestones such as walking and speech;
- Poor balance and unsteady gait;
- Scoliosis (spinal curvature) eighty-five per cent before ten years of age;
- Orthostatic hypotension-extreme drop in blood pressure with change in posture;
- Breath holding until fainting in early years;
- Episodic vomiting;
- Excessive drooling and sweating;
- A smooth tongue and decrease in sense of taste;
- Inappropriate temperature control with very high to very low

temperatures;
- Poor weight gain and growth;
- Frequent lung infections;
- Decreased reaction to pain or no reaction at all;
- Cold puffy hands and feet;
- Extremes of blood pressure;
- Corneal abrasions and dry eyes;
- Gastric dysmotility;
- Dysautonomic 'crisis'.

Dysautonomia crisis is a constellation of symptoms that include nausea, high blood pressure, fast heart rate and a change in personality. It is usually caused by stress and that stress can be either physical, such as an infection, or emotional, such as an upcoming exam. Whatever the catalyst, the child will become nauseated, and may start to retch or vomit. In addition there are usually other symptoms including a marked increase in blood pressure and heart rate, sweating, drooling and blotching of the skin. Irritability and a negative personality change also may accompany these symptoms. Episodes can occur as frequently as daily or some patients will never experience a 'crisis.'

The number and severity of symptoms in children are extremely variable. Patients with FD can be expected to function independently if treatment is begun early and major disabilities avoided. Children with FD are usually of normal intelligence. There has been an increased frequency of learning disabilities however. Early intervention and aggressive therapy in areas of language and learning have been extremely successful in prevention and treatment.

How is it treated?
Treatment of the condition is symptomatic with emphasis on special therapies (feeding, occupational, physical and speech). The absence of overflow tears requires frequent use of topical lubrication. To cope with the labile blood pressures, periodic gastrointestinal problems and dysautonomic crises, special drug management is required. Surgical interventions may be required to protect the child from respiratory problems that result from misdirecting their swallows. As there is a high incidence of spine curvature, surgery may also be needed for this problem. Due to the decreased taste, temperature and pain perception, the child will need particular protection from injury.

Inheritance patterns and prenatal diagnosis
Inheritance patterns
Autosomal recessive. FD has been localised to a gene (IKBKAP) on the long arm of chromosome 9 (9q31).

Prenatal diagnosis

Prenatal diagnosis is available for any couple who are aware that both of them are carriers.

Medical text written January 2002 by Contact a Family. Approved January 2002 by Professor F Axelrod. **Last updated September 2006 by Professor F Axelrod, Professor of Dysautonomia Treatment and Research and Professor of Neurology, New York University School of Medicine, New York, USA.**

Further online resources

Medical texts in *The Contact a Family Directory* are designed to give a short, clear description of specific conditions and rare disorders. More extensive information on this condition can be found on a range of reliable, validated websites. Further information on these resources can be found in our **Medical Information on the Internet** article on page 21.

Support

Dysautonomia Society of Great Britain
PO Box 17679, London NW4 1WS   Tel: 020 8357 0038   Fax: 020 8958 8760
Web: http://www.dsgb.org
The Society is a National Registered Charity No. 285399, established in 1984. It is mainly a fundraising body but it also offers support by telephone and letter. It has information available, details on request. The families of 12 affected children and adults are in membership.
Group details last updated February 2008.

FAMILIAL HYPERLIPIDAEMIAS

Background

Familial hyperlipidaemias are inherited metabolic disorders which include harmful disorders resulting in an excess of cholesterol and/or triglyceride in the blood. Cholesterol is transported round the body in combination with proteins, known as lipoproteins, low density lipoproteins (LDL) and beneficial

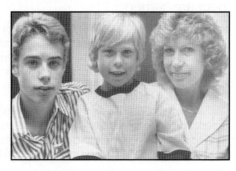

high density lipoproteins (HDL). Triglyceride travels within very low density lipoproteins (VLDL) and chylomicrons.

High levels of cholesterol in the blood may be associated with heart disease and strokes. The most common inherited cause is familial hypercholesterolaemia. High levels of triglycerides without raised cholesterol may be caused by the inherited disorders lipoprotein lipase deficiency and apoC-II deficiency, and can cause the serious condition of acute pancreatitis.

It is believed that approximately three hundred thousand people in Britain are suffering from familial hypercholesterolaemia (FH) and familial combined hyperlipidaemia (FCH).

What are the symptoms?

Familial hypercholesterolaemia (FH) occurs in approximately 1 in 500 people. It is characterised by a high blood LDL level and a greatly increased risk of coronary heart disease at an early age. The risk of heart disease is increased if other family members have had early onset heart disease or if there are other risk factors in the individual such as diabetes or high blood pressure. Xanthomas (fatty deposits) on the tendons of the back of the hand or Achilles tendon, corneal arcus (white ring around the iris) in younger people, and xanthelasmata (yellow deposits round the eye or eyelids) may be present; or the individual or a close relative may have had angina or a heart attack at an early age. Where both parents have the condition, children may inherit a more severe life threatening form known as homozygous FH.

How is it diagnosed?

Diagnosis in affected families can be made at any age after birth by measurement of lipoprotein profile.

How is it treated?

Effective treatment in lowering blood cholesterol is available using a combination of diet, drugs (especially the statin drugs) and lifestyle changes.

In **Familial Combined Hyperlipidaemia** (FCH) where both cholesterol and triglyceride levels are raised, there is an increased risk of early heart disease.

In **Familial Hypertriglyceridaemia**, triglyceride fats are markedly increased in the blood without a major increase in cholesterol. Those affected may have xanthomas as well as an enlarged liver and spleen, and the blood may appear creamy. The most important risk is acute pancreatitis.

Inheritance patterns and prenatal diagnosis

Inheritance patterns

Autosomal dominant in the case of Familial Hypercholesterolaemia, autosomal recessive in the case of Familial Hypertriglyceridaemia.

Prenatal diagnosis

None.

Medical text written November 1991 by Contact a Family. Approved November 1991 by Professor M Patton, Professor of Medical Genetics, St Georges Hospital Medical School, London, UK and Dr J E Wraith, Consultant Paediatrician, Royal Manchester Children's Hospital, Manchester, UK. **Last updated May 2006 by Dr M Sharrard, Consultant Paediatrician with Special Interest in Metabolic disease, Sheffield Children's Hospital, Sheffield, UK and Dr T Gray, Consultant in Chemical Pathology, Northern General Hospital, Sheffield, UK.**

Support

H.E.A.R.T UK – the Cholesterol Charity
7 North Road, Maidenhead SL6 1PE   Tel: 0845 450 5988 (Helpline)   Tel: 01628 777 046
Fax: 01628 628698   e-mail: ask@heartuk.org.uk   Web: http://www.heartuk.org.uk
The group is a National Registered Charity No. 1003904, established in 1984. It offers dietary and lifestyle advice and contact with others affected by high cholesterol, where possible. It publishes a quarterly magazine, 'The Digest' and has a wide range of information, full details on their website. It has approximately 2,000 members.
Group details last updated May 2007.

FAMILIAL SPASTIC PARAPLEGIA

Familial Spastic Paraplegia: Hereditary Spastic Paraplegia; Strumpell disease

Background

Familial Spastic Paraplegia (FSP) describes a group of largely progressive conditions predominantly affecting the legs. As the name suggests there are three main features: the legs become stiff (spasticity); there is a variable amount of weakness (paraplegia) and there is a strong genetic element.

What are the causes?

It is now clear there are a large number of conditions that fall under this grouping and progress has been made in identifying the genetic factors behind some of the more common forms. However, it may be some time before all the genes responsible are found and even longer before the exact molecular and cellular processes that give rise to FSP are understood. It is hoped that further research it will be possible to produce disease modifying and curative treatments.

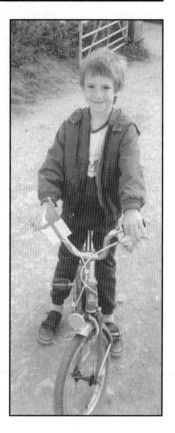

At a clinical level there are two forms of this condition: pure and complicated. The pure form is not associated with additional features, whereas the complicated form is clinically very variable with many different additional features. The pure form is far commoner then the complicated variety. However, it is now established that the situation at a genetic level is even more complicated with several different genes proving responsible for the pure form of FSP.

Inheritance patterns and prenatal diagnosis

Inheritance patterns

A large number of spastic paraplegia genes are now known. At least twenty of these are found on the autosomes (the non sex chromosomes) with three known genes carried on the X chromosome. Although the locations of these genes are known, the actual gene and mutations causing FSP in many cases remain to be identified.

The most common form of inheritance is Autosomal dominant and the commonest gene (spastin found on chromosome 2) for the pure form of FSP is known. However there are many cases of both autosomal recessive and

X-linked inheritance and the genes for some of these are also now known. There will also be families in whom neither the gene nor its location are known so it can be surmised that there are still more genes to be found.

Prenatal diagnosis

Testing for the commoner forms of FSP is being developed but is not yet available. A test for the X-linked condition, adrenomyeloneuropathy is available. This rare condition is a milder adult form of Adrenoleukodystrophy (see entry) but is included by some experts as an X-linked form of FSP.

Medical text written September 2002 by Professor N Wood, Professor of Clinical Neurology and Neurogenetics, Institute of Neurology, London, UK.

Further online resources

Medical texts in *The Contact a Family Directory* are designed to give a short, clear description of specific conditions and rare disorders. More extensive information on this condition can be found on a range of reliable, validated websites. Further information on these resources can be found in our **Medical Information on the Internet** article on page 21.

Support

FSP Group

37 Alexandra Road, Great Wakering, Southend-on-Sea SS3 0HN Tel: 01702 218184 e-mail: FSPgroup@aol.com Web: http://fspgroup.org

The Group is a National Registered Charity No. 1109398, established in 1991. It offers support for families of affected children and adults. It holds an AGM and some regional meetings. The Group has over 200 members.

Group details last updated February 2007.

FANCONI ANAEMIA

Fanconi anaemia: Fanconi's anaemia; Fanconi's anemia (US); Congenital Aplastic anaemia; Congenital Aplastic anemia (US)

Background

This term describes a group of inherited diseases characterised by defects in repairing DNA or protecting it from damage.

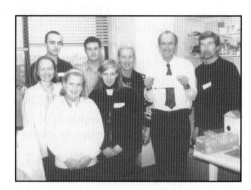

Fanconi's Anaemia Research Team, Guy's Hospital, London with group members

What are the symptoms?

The defects found in Fanconi anaemia result in an abnormal chromosome structure with the following consequences:

- **Congenital birth defects**: these occur in two thirds of affected individuals and may involve one or more body parts. The commonest abnormalities affect the thumb and radial bone of the lower arm. Other areas often affected are the heart, genito-urinary system, other limbs and skin (with abnormal pigmentation);
- **Growth**: short stature is common. Although deficiency of growth and thyroid hormones are seen in Fanconi anaemia, their relevance to poor growth is not clear;
- **Low blood counts**: these often fall with age; many of those with abnormal blood counts during childhood will go on to develop aplastic anaemia (bone marrow failure). This usually occurs by the age of fifteen years and is often severe;
- **Predisposition to cancer**: many types of malignancy are more frequent but the commonest complications are the development of myelodysplasia (pre-leukaemia), acute myeloid leukaemia and head and neck or gynaecological cancers.

How is it treated?

Congenital defects may require surgery. The main indication for treatment is aplastic anaemia. This often responds to administration of the androgenic steroid oxymetholone, although the beneficial effect is not permanent and side effects are common. Bone marrow transplantation can cure blood problems but can also lead to life-threatening complications. The best results have been in children with matched sibling donors who are themselves free of the disease; however, results from matched unrelated donors are improving. Dietary/drug therapy directed towards reducing oxidant levels may also have a role. Gene therapy may be possible in the future.

Inheritance patterns and prenatal diagnosis
Inheritance patterns
Autosomal recessive. Patients can be assigned to 'complementation groups' (called FA-A, -B, -C, -D1, -D2, -E, -F, -G, -I, -J, -L and -M) depending on which of twelve different genes that can cause Fanconi anaemia is affected. The responsible gene for each group is known except for FA-I.
Prenatal diagnosis
Chorionic villus sampling at ten weeks.

Medical text written September 2000 by Dr C G Steward. **Last updated October 2005 by Dr C G Steward, Reader in Stem Cell, Bristol Children's Hospital, Bristol, UK.**

Support
F.A.B. UK
4 Pateley Road, Woodthorpe, Nottingham NG3 5QF
Tel: 0115 926 9634 (Helpline with 24 hour answerphone)
The Group is a Contact Group, established in January 1989. It raises funds for medical and genetic research at Guy's Hospital, London. In addition, it encourages fundraising for F.A.B. UK's Family Comfort Fund. It has information available, details on request. The Group responds to affected families and professional workers nationally and internationally. Advice given on nutrition/diet which supports those with F.A.
Group details last updated September 2007.

FATTY ACID OXIDATION DISORDERS

Background

Fatty acids are one of the body's fuels: oxidation is the process by which they are broken down to release energy. This process has many steps, each catalysed by a different enzyme. Fatty acid oxidation disorders result from deficiency of one of these enzymes:

- Medium-chain acyl-CoA dehydrogenase (MCAD) deficiency;
- Very-long-chain acyl-CoA dehydrogenase (VLCAD) deficiency;
- Short-chain acyl-CoA dehydrogenase (SCAD) deficiency;
- Multiple acyl-CoA dehydrogenase (MAD) deficiency (= Glutaric aciduria type II, GA II);
- Long-chain hydroxyacyl-CoA dehydrogenase (LCHAD) deficiency;
- Trifunctional protein deficiency;
- Carnitine palmitoyl-transferase I (CPT I) deficiency;
- Carnitine palmitoyl-transferase II (CPT II) deficiency;
- Carnitine acylcarnitine translocase deficiency;
- Primary (systemic) carnitine deficiency.

What are the symptoms?

MCAD deficiency is the commonest disorder. Patients with MCAD deficiency are healthy most of the time.

Infections or prolonged fasting, however, can lead to drowsiness and coma or sudden death.

How is it treated?

This can be prevented by avoiding fasting and maintaining a regular intake of sugar during infections - by mouth or intravenously if the child vomits. With this simple management, outcomes are excellent.

Patients with other fatty acid oxidation disorders also need to avoid fasting and to maintain a regular sugar intake during infections. Unfortunately, they can have additional problems, such as muscle problems or heart muscle disease. Treatment usually involves a low fat diet.

Inheritance patterns and prenatal diagnosis

Inheritance patterns

All these disorders show autosomal recessive inheritance.

Prenatal diagnosis

Prenatal diagnosis is available for these disorders.

Medical text written October 2000 by Dr A Morris. **Last reviewed August 2005 by Dr A Morris, Consultant Paediatrician with Special Interest in Metabolic disease, Willink Biochemical Genetics Unit, Royal Manchester Children's Hospital, Manchester, UK.**

Support

While there is no specific support group in the UK for Fatty Acid Oxidation Disorders, support and information is available from a group of families under the umbrella of Climb (see entry, Metabolic diseases). The US FOD Family Support Group http://www.fodsupport.org acts as an international group.
Group details last confirmed January 2008.

The Family Fund helps families of disabled and seriously ill children under the age of 16, giving grants and information related to the care of the child. For more information about this organisation, and other grant-making bodies, call the Contact a Family Helpline.

FETAL ABNORMALITY

Background

For those faced with difficult prenatal test results, information, support and counselling can be vital. Whatever choices need to be made, contact with other parents can be useful. ARC is the specialist organisation providing this support and information.

Support

ARC (Antenatal Results and Choices)

73-75 Charlotte Street, London W1T 4PN   Tel: 020 7631 0285 Helpline
Tel/Fax: 020 7631 0280   e-mail: info@arc-uk.org   Web: http://www.arc-uk.org
ARC is a National Registered Charity No. 299770, founded as SATFA (Support Around Termination for Fetal Abnormality) in 1988 and renamed as ARC in November 1998. ARC provides information and support to parents throughout the antenatal testing process and when an abnormality is diagnosed in their unborn baby. Support is offered through decision making and its aftermath. ARC offers UK-wide support through a network of trained Parent Contacts and an e-mail support group as well as a range of supportive publications including a newsletter.
Group details last confirmed October 2007 .

FETAL ALCOHOL SPECTRUM DISORDER

Background

Fetal Alcohol Spectrum disorder (FASD) ranges from minor individual alcohol-related birth anomalies such as low birth weight to the severe Fetal Alcohol syndrome (FAS).

What are the symptoms?

It is important to note that children with FAS do not grow out of its affects. They may have continuing problems with sleeping and feeding. They often have learning difficulties. Other problems include not being able to understand the link between cause and effect, problems with attention and other behaviour difficulties. Making and keeping friends is often difficult. Learning and behavioural problems tend to persist but can be helped by a stable environment and consistent approach. Children with FAS can be easily overwhelmed in new situations and need constant support.

What are the causes?

FAS occurs when babies are exposed to heavy maternal drinking during pregnancy. Only a small minority of pregnant women with alcohol problems have babies with FAS. The severity of the syndrome appears to relate to the frequency of high doses of alcohol.

Factors which influence whether a baby is affected or not are likely to include maternal polydrug use, poor nutritional status and pattern of drinking.

How is it diagnosed?

Diagnosis is made on the basis of three main areas:

Growth Washington Scale: Children with FAS are small for their age at birth, with weight, length, head circumference, or any combination of these in less than 10th centile (the lowest ten per cent) for their age.

Brain Children with FAS have delayed development and many have learning difficulties.

Facial

Children with FAS have at least two of the following features:

- microcephaly - head circumference below third centile;
- short palpebral fissures (short space between the eyelids) or microphthalmia (small eyes) or both these features;
- poorly developed philtrum, thin upper lip, flattening of cheekbones.

Other features which may occur are congenital heart disease, genito-urinary malformations, squint, cleft palate, bony abnormalities, spina bifida.

Inheritance patterns and prenatal diagnosis

Inheritance patterns

None.

Prenatal diagnosis

Should be monitored if the mother has an identifiable drinking problem.

Medical text written November 1998 by Dr D Cundall, Consultant Community Paediatrician, Leeds Community and Mental Health Trust, Leeds UK. **Last updated October 2003 by Prof Moira Plant, Alcohol & Health Research Trust, University of the West of England, Bristol, UK.**

Further online resources

Medical texts in *The Contact a Family Directory* are designed to give a short, clear description of specific conditions and rare disorders. More extensive information on this condition can be found on a range of reliable, validated websites. Further information on these resources can be found in our **Medical Information on the Internet** article on page 21.

Support

NOFAS-UK

157 Beaufort Park, London NW11 6DA   Tel: 020 8458 5951   Helpline: 08700 333 700
Fax: 020 8209 3296   e-mail: nofas-uk@midlantic.co.uk   Web: http://www.nofas-uk.org
NOFAS-UK (National Organisation for Fetal Alcohol Syndrome-United Kingdom) is a National Registered Charity No. 1101935, established in 2003. It provides information about Fetal Alcohol Spectrum Disorders (FASD) and answers enquiries by phone, letter and e-mail. Where requested it can usually link families on a one to one basis for support. NOFAS-UK has a helpline, holds support group meetings with playgroups for children, family activity days, conferences and training sessions and has a library of resources including the documentary video 'Child for Life' about Fetal Alcohol Syndrome, details on request. It publishes a Family Support Newsletter.
Group details last updated July 2007.

FASawareUK

45 Lakeside Avenue, Billinge, Wigan WN5 7BT   Tel: 01942 223780
e-mail: fasawareuk@blueyonder.co.uk   Web: http://www.fasaware.co.uk
FASawareUK is a National Registered Charity No. 1102118 which aims to educate and raise public and professional awareness of Fetal Alcohol Spectrum Disorder. It provides support to parents and training sessions for professionals. It maintains an online resource containing a wide range of information about the condition, much specifically for professionals, tools for awareness raising and links and signposting on to other sources of help, including other FASD groups around the world.
Group details last updated March 2008.

FETAL ANTI-CONVULSANT SYNDROME

Background

Babies exposed to anti-convulsant (anti-epileptic) drugs taken by the mother during pregnancy have a higher risk of suffering some sort of birth defect, or congenital malformation, than average. This risk is probably about two to three times normal, meaning that five to ten per cent of babies exposed to these drugs may be affected, although some studies have suggested a higher proportion of babies may be at risk.

What are the symptoms?

The risks associated with exposure to more than one anti-convulsant are greater. The type of abnormalities that occur are diverse but include Spina Bifida, Cleft Lip

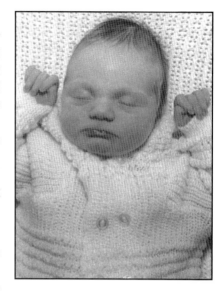

and/or Palate, Upper Limb Abnormalities, Lower Limb Abnormalities (see entries), Congenital Heart disease (see entry, Heart defects) and Kidney problems (see entry, Kidney disease). None of these abnormalities are specific for the condition but the facial features of these children may be distinctive, even though quite subtle, especially as toddlers and especially in association with exposure to Epilim (sodium valproate). The facial appearance becomes more normal with age. In addition, a degree of developmental delay and/or behavioural difficulty in affected children is common but there is very little information about what can be expected as the children grow up through adolescence and into adulthood.

What are the causes?

It is not certain at present if different drugs cause different problems, or whether they all act in the same way. The best information has accumulated on the effects caused by phenytoin (Epanutin), carbamazepine (Tegretol) and sodium valproate. Evidence has been accumulating that sodium valproate carries more risks than the other drugs, both in terms of physical birth defects and learning difficulties. Limb defects are more common after exposure to this drug compared to the other anti-convulsants, and there is also evidence for an increased risk of behavioural problems within the autistic spectrum. There are many newer anti-convulsants being prescribed now and the risks associated with these drugs remains to be fully evaluated. However, early reports suggest that lamotrigine (Lamictal) is relatively safe, though there is no drug that should be regarded as completely safe.

How is it treated?

For those women who need to take anti-convulsant drugs during pregnancy to control epilepsy, it is important to try and take the lowest dose that prevents fits, and if possible take only one drug rather than two or more. It is also important for these women to take folic acid daily around the time of conception and during the early part of pregnancy.

Inheritance patterns and prenatal diagnosis

Inheritance patterns

The precise cause for all these problems is not yet known. Fetal anti-convulsant syndrome(s) is not a "genetic" condition in the usual sense but current opinion is that variations in the way these drugs are metabolised by some pregnant women, and/or their affected children, predisposes the unborn baby to damage. This variation in metabolism probably is genetically determined but there is no test at present to identify which epileptic mothers are at risk. For women who have had one child diagnosed with fetal anticonvulsant syndrome, the risk of having a second affected baby may be as high as forty per cent, assuming the same drug at the same dose through pregnancy.

Prenatal diagnosis

Scanning the baby for spina bifida and other major defects can be specifically requested where a mother has been taking anti-epileptic drugs. In the absence of significant physical defects which can be seen on a prenatal scan there is no guaranteed test to identify those babies affected by exposure to these drugs, especially in relation to learning difficulties.

Medical text written June 1998 by Dr P D Turnpenny. **Last updated December 2005 by Dr P D Turnpenny, Consultant Clinical Geneticist, Royal Devon & Exeter Hospital, Exeter, UK.**

Support

OACS

PO Box 772, Pilling, Preston PR3 6WW   Tel: 01253 790022
e-mail: janet.oacs@btinternet.com   Web: http://www.oacs-uk.co.uk
OACS (Organisation for Anti Convulsant Syndrome) is an National Registered Charity No. 1116497, established in 1999. It provides support, information and signposting on to other relevant support organisations as well as campaigning to raise awareness of the condition. OACS publishes a quarterly newsletter. Regular local group meetings are held in Liverpool, Manchester, Birmingham and London. Enquiries from professionals are welcome. The group is in touch with over 400 families from the UK, Europe and North America.
Group details last confirmed November 2007.

FIBRODYSPLASIA OSSIFICANS PROGRESSIVA

Fibrodysplasia Ossificans Progressiva: Myositis Ossificans Progressiva; MOP; FOP

Background

Fibrodysplasia Ossificans Progressiva (FOP) is a disabling condition which is caused by the formation of bony bars within the muscles of the body. This disorder occurs in all countries in the world and affects about one person in a million. Men and women seem to be equally affected.

What are the symptoms?

Most people affected by FOP have some abnormalities of the fingers or toes. The toes are most commonly involved and are often shortened and deviated. These differences are usually apparent at birth.

This bone formation is usually first noticed in early childhood as a series of hard lumps in the neck or along the spine. These lumps, which may be tender, gradually shrink in size as the affected muscles are replaced by bone. The appearance of bony lumps in muscles is usually spontaneous but can also be provoked by any injury to the muscles. Disability in FOP is physical and very variable in extent; intelligence is unaffected.

Injury to the muscles can often provoke local bone formation. For this reason intramuscular injections should be avoided if possible. Similarly operations on the muscles to remove pieces of bone almost invariably result in increased bone formation. Also, some forms of dental treatment may result in bone formation in the jaw muscles and individuals with MOP should inform their dental practitioner.

What are the causes?

The cause of FOP has been identified as a mutation of the ACVR1 gene on Chromosome 2.

FOP is progressive in that more muscles become involved with increasing age, but the rate of progression is very variable from one person to another. Furthermore, the condition tends to show long periods of inactivity (of up to several years in length).

Certain muscles are never involved in this disease. These include the muscles of the eyes, the face, the tongue, the gullet, the intestines and the muscles of continence (bowel and bladder control). The heart is never involved in this condition. Chest expansion may be reduced in FOP but the diaphragm, which is the single most important breathing muscle is never involved.

How is it treated?

Currently there is no effective treatment for FOP. General health remains good and several people with FOP in Britain are over sixty years old.

Inheritance patterns and prenatal diagnosis

Inheritance patterns

The basic genetic error is thought to occur at the moment of conception. The chance of it happening is very low and is certainly less than 1 in 2,000,000 if both parents are unaffected. For a person with FOP, however, inheritance is autosomal dominant. Genetic advice can be obtained from local or regional genetics centres.

Prenatal diagnosis

None available.

Medical text written March 2004 by Professor J M Connor and abridged by Contact a Family. Approved March 2004 by Professor J M Connor. **Last updated May 2006 by Professor J M Connor, Head of Department and Honorary Consultant, Ferguson-Smith Centre for Clinical Genetics, Glasgow, UK.**

Further online resources

Medical texts in *The Contact a Family Directory* are designed to give a short, clear description of specific conditions and rare disorders. More extensive information on this condition can be found on a range of reliable, validated websites. Further information on these resources can be found in our **Medical Information on the Internet** article on page 21.

Support

FOP UK Support Group
c/o Contact a Family, 209-211 City Road, London EC1V 1JN   Tel: 01772 339296
e-mail: MargaretParkes@btinternet.com
This is a small network, established in 2000 to offer informal support and a listening ear to affected individuals and their families.
Group details last confirmed June 2007.

As Fibrodysplasia Ossificans Progressiva is a neuromuscular disorder information, support and advice is available from the Muscular Dystrophy Campaign (see entry, Muscular Dystrophy and neuromuscular disorders).

FLOATING-HARBOR SYNDROME

Background

The unusual name of this syndrome is derived from the Boston Floating Hospital and the Harbor General Hospital where the first two patients were described.

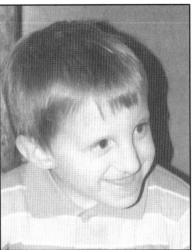

What are the symptoms?

This condition is characterised by an association of three features:

- short stature with delayed bone age;
- language delay usually in the presence of normal motor development;
- characteristic facial features with a prominent nose, deep set eyes and a long, thin upper lip. The ears may be low set and tipped backwards.

Inheritance patterns and prenatal diagnosis

Inheritance patterns

None identified at the present time, all cases have been sporadic

Prenatal diagnosis

None known

Medical text written June 1992 by Dr M Patton, Consultant Clinical Geneticist, St Georges Hospital Medical School, London, UK. **Last updated October 2005 by Dr J Clayton-Smith, Consultant Clinical Geneticist, St Mary's Hospital, Manchester, UK.**

Support

The Floating-Harbour Syndrome Contact Group is currently in abeyance. Families can use Contact a Family's Freephone Helpline for advice, information and, where possible, links to other families. Contact a Family's web-based linking service Making Contact.org can be accessed at http://www.makingcontact.org

FOCAL DERMAL HYPOPLASIA (GOLTZ SYNDROME)

Focal Dermal Hypoplasia: Goltz syndrome; Goltz-Gorlin syndrome

Background

This is an inherited condition that involves many body systems but takes its name from patchy skin abnormalities.

What are the symptoms?

Affected areas of skin are often atrophic (thin) and are characteristically in a linear or line distribution, especially on the limbs. The abnormal areas appear pink or red in colour although they may become less clear and somewhat pigmented with age. Some thinner areas of skin, for instance in the elbows, allow fat from the layers below to protrude forming small yellowish-white lumps. They are not usually sore or itchy and can occur anywhere on the body. In addition, the nails can be brittle and ridged, the teeth can be small or missing and the hair is often sparse and grows slowly. Papillomas (small lumps) can develop around the lips, gums or the side of the nose. The lips themselves are often irregularly formed.

The limbs may also be affected but almost never symmetrically, and the difference between hands and feet can also be remarkably large. Hand (see entry, Upper Limb Abnormalities) and foot (see entry, Upper Limb Abnormalities) anomalies include syndactyly (joined together digits), polydactyly (extra digits) and occasionally missing digits (especially the middle three fingers, giving rise to a 'lobster claw' hand) or the entire hand. The eyes may be involved and there may be a coloboma of the iris (see entry, Coloboma). The abnormalities are again often not the same in each eye. Head circumference can be small. Some children are developmentally delayed, others follow a normal development. Behavioural problems do not specifically occur. The gut may also be involved with malrotation (incorrect turning) of the gut, duodenal atresia (closure) and occasionally exomphalos (protrusion of abdominal contents through the navel) see entry, Abdominal Exstrophies. Congenital heart disease (see entry, Heart Defects) and cleft lip and/or palate (see entry) are also reported but not specific. It must be stressed that the condition is very variable in its presentation and the diagnosis can be difficult to make. There are a few entities like MIDAS that can resemble Focal Dermal Hypoplasia to a great extent.

How is it diagnosed?

There is no definite diagnostic test that can confirm the diagnosis. An X-ray of the long bones can show a characteristic pattern called osteopathia striata which looks like lines of increased density of bone. This occurs in other entities as well however. A skin biopsy (examination of tissue) of the abnormal skin can confirm fatty herniation (protrusion). Most individuals will have a routine chromosome test to check for a small deletion (missing part) of the X chromosome.

Inheritance patterns and prenatal diagnosis

Inheritance patterns

Focal Dermal Hypoplasia is thought to be inherited as an X-linked dominant condition. Males with the affected gene are thought not to survive early pregnancy. The gene has not yet been identified but this inheritance pattern explains why the condition is so patchy in distribution.

Prenatal diagnosis

This is dependent on ultra sound examination in the second trimester (three to six months) of pregnancy. As it is difficult to see skin changes on the ultrasound image, it is not definitive. Limb anomalies can however be picked up. No gene test is currently available.

Medical text written March 2002 by Dr I K Temple, Consultant Clinical Geneticist, Wessex Clinical Genetics Service, Southampton University Hospital Trust, Southampton, UK. **Last updated July 2006 by Professor RCM Hennekam, Professor of Clinical Dysmorphology, Institute of Child Health and Great Ormond Street Hospital for Children, London, UK.**

Further online resources

Medical texts in *The Contact a Family Directory* are designed to give a short, clear description of specific conditions and rare disorders. More extensive information on this condition can be found on a range of reliable, validated websites. Further information on these resources can be found in our **Medical Information on the Internet** article on page 21.

Support

Information, support and advice for features in common with Ectodermal Dysplasia is available from the Ectodermal Dysplasia Society (see entry Ectodermal Dysplasia).

Cross referrals to other entries in The Contact a Family Directory are intended to provide information and advice for these particular features of the disorder. Organisations identified in these entries do not provide support specifically for Focal Dermal Hypoplasia (Goltz syndrome). Families can use Contact a Family's Freephone Helpline for advice, information and, where possible, links to other families. Contact a Family's web-based linking service Making Contact.org can be accessed at http://www.makingcontact.org

FRAGILE X SYNDROME

Background

Fragile X is the most common identifiable form of inherited intellectual disability (see entry, learning disability). It has a prevalence of about 1 in 4,000 males and 1 in 8,000 females.

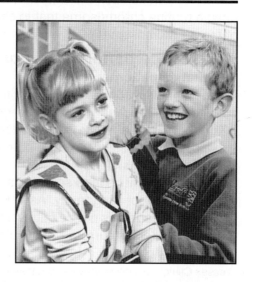

What are the symptoms?

Intellectual disability varies from mild to severe. Girls and women who have a fragile X chromosome are often of normal intelligence. However up to a third have learning problems which are usually mild or moderate but can occasionally be severe.

Other problems experienced by affected individuals include delayed and distorted speech and language development. There can be difficulties with the social use of language, with continuing speech anomalies, repetitive behaviour, attention deficits and overactivity, and autistic-like features, such as poor eye contact, hand flapping, social anxiety, abnormal shyness and an insistence on routine.

Physical features ascribed to fragile X syndrome include a relatively large head, a long face with prominent ears, largish jaw and double-jointedness. However these are rarely obvious in affected individuals. Ten to thirty per cent of people with fragile X syndrome develop epilepsy.

Psychological and behavioural characteristics

Intellectual disability is common in people who carry the Fragile X gene, although abilities do span a wide range. Approximately eighty per cent of males have learning disabilities. These are mostly in the mild to moderate range, but about one-third have severe learning difficulties. Overall, verbal abilities tend to be better than performance abilities, with relative strengths in vocabulary, aspects of simultaneous information processing, and some visual perceptual tasks. Affected individuals are much weaker on tasks of abstract reasoning, sequential processing, visual-spatial abilities and short term memory and numeracy. They tend to have greater difficulty in processing new information than in learning school-related, verbally-based factual material. Even individuals with intelligence in the average or above-average range, females as well as males, show many of these features. There can be accompanying problems with shyness and social anxiety, concentration and freedom from distractibility, difficulties in organising ones thoughts and planning ahead, and maintaining direct eye contact with others. The rate of intellectual development appears to decline with age as individuals approach adolescence. The most notable decline is in the early pubertal years. This is largely attributable to difficulties in processing complex sequences of incoming information.

Language difficulties range from a complete absence of speech through to mild communication problems. Individuals often have characteristic rapid and dysrhythmic speech ('cluttering'). The rate of talking may be fast and fluctuating, with up and down swings of pitch and occasionally garbled and disorganised speech with corrections, frequent shifts of conversation from topic to topic and tangential comments. Speech may not be very fluent. Affected individuals tend to use many incomplete sentences, to repeat themselves when talking and to echo what others say to them. Articulation problems are also common.

Clumsiness and fine motor co-ordination problems occur. However, early motor development is often unremarkable. Oversensitivities to certain sights, sounds, smells, tastes and textures are also frequently witnessed.

Boys with fragile X tend to be overactive and impulsive with marked concentration problems, restlessness, fidgetiness and distractibility. Irritability, tantrums and aggressive outbursts are precipitated by environmental over stimulation, confusing situations or heightened anxiety.

Medication, in particular stimulants such as methylphenidate and dexamphetamine, have been found to be helpful for the attentional deficits in some instances. Overactivity in fragile X syndrome tends to decrease with age, but attention difficulties, restlessness and impulsivity can remain problematic for many adolescents and adults.

Autistic-like behaviours have been reported in individuals who have fragile X syndrome. These include avoidance of eye contact, stereotyped repetitive behaviours such as hand flapping, repetitive speech, resistance to environmental change, and strong preoccupations or fascinations. Only a minority of individuals have 'typical' autism. Most are affectionate and have an interest in relating socially, but have notable difficulties in social interactions and tend to be shy and anxious in social situations. Also, while affected individuals do repeat their own and other people's speech, these repetitions are believed to serve an important communicatory function, since they maintain participation in conversation while the individual is trying to process what is being said. Affected individuals are easily overwhelmed by a variety of sensory stimuli, which they find difficult to cope with. Their poor eye contact and gaze avoidance may therefore be attempts to avoid excessive stimulation. Other features such as hand-biting and hand-flapping are common, and may be provoked by anxiety, excitement and/or frustration. In many instances these features become less evident in adulthood.

Adults with fragile X syndrome often show strengths in domestic daily living skills, relative to their communication and socialisation abilities. Nevertheless, many need a degree of supported living.

Up to one-third of females with fragile X syndrome demonstrate learning and behavioural difficulties that are similar to, but usually less severe than, those seen in affected males. Some twenty-five per cent of females have learning disabilities. However, more subtle problems with learning, behavioural and emotional difficulties are common even in carrier females with a normal IQ. As is the case for affected males, verbal abilities tend to be better than performance skills, and special needs in arithmetic, visuo-spatial abilities and visual and auditory memory are common. The spoken language of carrier females may be high pitched, with repetitions and poor topic maintenance. Difficulties with planning and organising information, sustaining effort, generating problem-solving strategies, and monitoring their own performance are also apparent in many cases, as are difficulties with abstract concepts, information processing, perseverative thinking, attention (with or without overactivity) and impulsivity. Their speech is characterised by the use of tangential language and frequent changes of topic. Extreme shyness, anxiety, social avoidance, withdrawal and poor eye contact are also commonly reported in females with fragile X.

All the above features can be helped substantially by a carefully planned and instituted combination of medical, psychological, educational and social interventions tailored to the individual's particular profile of developmental and behavioural strengths and needs.

What are the causes?
The cause is an abnormal expansion of DNA just above the tip of the X chromosome's long arm, which may be passed from one generation to the next.

How is it diagnosed?
Diagnosis is by blood test usually for the change in the gene using DNA analysis.

Inheritance patterns and prenatal diagnosis
Inheritance patterns
A carrier woman has a fifty per cent chance of passing on the fragile X chromosome to her children. Of these, males are likely to be affected by the syndrome, whilst daughters have a 1 in 3 chance of being clinically affected.

Men can also be unaffected carriers of the fragile X chromosome. In such cases the genetic change is passed to all daughters, but to none of the sons. These daughters will themselves be unaffected but at risk of having affected children. Any sons of carrier males will be completely unaffected as they do not receive their X chromosome from their father.

Prenatal diagnosis

Prenatal diagnosis is possible by chorionic villus sampling or fetal blood sampling. This is likely to give a definitive answer for affected males but cannot always distinguish affected from unaffected carrier females.

Medical text and Psychological and behavioural characteristics text written June 1997 by Dr A Barnicoat, Consultant in Clinical Genetics, Institute of Child Health, London, UK and Professor J Turk. **Last updated December 2005 by Professor J Turk, Professor of Developmental Psychiatry and Consultant Child & Adolescent Psychiatrist, Department of Clinical Developmental Sciences, St. George's Hospital Medical School, London, UK.**

Further online resources

Medical texts in *The Contact a Family Directory* are designed to give a short, clear description of specific conditions and rare disorders. More extensive information on this condition can be found on a range of reliable, validated websites. Further information on these resources can be found in our **Medical Information on the Internet** article on page 21.

Support

Fragile X Society
Rood End House, 6 Stortford Road, Dunmow CM6 1DA   Tel: 01371 875100
e-mail: info@fragilex.org.uk   Web: http://www.fragilex.org.uk
The Society is a National Registered Charity No. 1003981, established in 1990. It offers support, information and advice to affected families and professionals. Family members have the opportunity to participate in research studies and the four family conferences held annually in the UK. It publishes a newsletter three times a year, has a video, helplines on education, epilepsy and benefits and has a wide range of information available, details on request. The Society has over 1,500 members.
Group details last confirmed January 2007.

FREEMAN SHELDON SYNDROME

Freeman Sheldon syndrome: Craniocarpotarsal Dystrophy; Whistling Face syndrome

Background

This condition was first described in 1938 by Freeman and Sheldon.

What are the symptoms?

The features include a lateral deformity of the fingers with contractures at the joints of the fingers, which may resemble the appearance seen in rheumatoid arthritis. There are also facial features such as deep-set eyes and a small pinched mouth. On a few occasions it has been associated with club feet or similar deformities in the feet.

What are the causes?

The underlying cause of the disorder is not known but it is thought to involve the fibrous replacement of muscles.

How is it treated?

Physiotherapy should be used to alleviate the joint contractures. If this is insufficient and the contractures affect the function of the hands, then orthopaedic surgery may be required.

There may be malocclusion of the teeth and orthodontic treatment of this may be required. Opening the mouth fully for dental treatment may be difficult.

Inheritance patterns and prenatal diagnosis

Inheritance patterns

Freeman Sheldon syndrome may be inherited as an autosomal dominant or as an autosomal recessive trait. Abnormalities in one of the muscle protein genes [embryonic myosin MYH3] has been found in some of the dominant families.

Prenatal diagnosis

None available.

Medical text written February 2002 by Contact a Family. Approved February 2002 by Professor M Patton. **Last updated September 2007 by Professor M Patton, Professor of Medical Genetics, St. George's Hospital Medical School, London, UK.**

Further online resources

Medical texts in *The Contact a Family Directory* are designed to give a short, clear description of specific conditions and rare disorders. More extensive information on this condition can be found on a range of reliable, validated websites. Further information on these resources can be found in our **Medical Information on the Internet** article on page 21.

Support

There is no specific support group for Freeman Sheldon syndrome in the United Kingdom. However, STEPS, the support group for Lower Limb Abnormalities (see entry), can provide support and contacts.

There is a United States based support network for Freeman Sheldon syndrome:

Freeman-Sheldon Parent Support Group
e-mail: info@fspsg.org   Web: http://www.fspsg.org
Group details last confirmed September 2007.

"What I liked best was the integration of disabled and non-disabled children in an atmosphere where everyone's abilities were catered for." Feedback from a mother attending a Contact a Family Play Day on art, music and drama.

FRIEDREICH'S ATAXIA

Friedreich's Ataxia: Recessive Spino-Cerebellar Degeneration

Background

Friedreich's Ataxia is a genetic disorder characterised by a progressive degeneration of the spino-cerebellar system due to an abnormality of a gene on chromosome 9 (called Frataxin).

What are the symptoms?

The first sign of the disorder is unsteadiness of gait (ataxia). The onset of the condition is variable but usually occurs between the ages of four and sixteen (but occasionally between eighteen months and thirty years). Although most cases present under the age of twenty-five very rarely it may produce with an ataxia of much later onset. Onsets into the sixth and seventh decades have been found. Therefore it is worth considering even in older patients if some of the other clinical hallmarks are present.

The onset of the condition is insidious and affects co-ordination of the muscles used in speech, the arms and legs. Scoliosis (see entry) may also be a feature of the disorder, as may an enlarged heart
or diabetes.

What are the causes?

The genetic abnormality (mutation) in the majority of patients (ninety-five per cent plus) is an abnormally long repetition of a DNA fragment (expansion) in the Friedreich ataxia genes in both chromosomes 9. This mutation can be readily detected using a variety of molecular methods. However a small percentage (less than five per cent) may just have one expansion in one copy of their gene and the other copy may have a much more subtle abnormality called a point mutation. These latter abnormalities are more difficult to detect and need to be specially requested from the laboratory.

Inheritance patterns and prenatal diagnosis

Inheritance patterns

Autosomal recessive

Prenatal diagnosis

It is now possible to offer, by means of blood tests, carrier detection, prenatal and pre-symptomatic diagnosis in families with an affected child. These tests are only available to those families with an affected member. In such families genetic advice should be sought where a pregnancy is under consideration. Chorionic villus sampling is available at ten to twelve weeks.

Medical text written November 1991 by Contact a Family. Approved November 1991 by Professor M Patton, Professor of Medical Genetics, St Georges Hospital Medical School, London, UK and Dr J E Wraith, Consultant Paediatrician, Royal Manchester Children's Hospital, Manchester, UK. **Last updated November 2005 by Dr P Giunti, Senior Clinical Fellow, University Department of Clinical Neurology, University College, London, UK.**

Further online resources

Medical texts in *The Contact a Family Directory* are designed to give a short, clear description of specific conditions and rare disorders. More extensive information on this condition can be found on a range of reliable, validated websites. Further information on these resources can be found in our **Medical Information on the Internet** article on page 21.

Support

Ataxia UK

Winchester House, 11 Cranmer Road, London SW9 6EJ

Tel: 0845 644 0606 Lo-Call Helpline   Tel: 020 7582 1444 Office   Fax: 020 7582 9444
e-mail: enquiries@ataxia.org.uk   Web: http://www.ataxia.org.uk

Ataxia UK is a National Registered Charity No. 1102391, established in 1964. It supports people affected by Friedreich's, cerebellar and other ataxias. Ataxia UK helps people with ataxia, their carers, families and friends, to live with the condition. It provides information through leaflets, magazines, reports and the website; an information and support helpline; branches, self-help groups and meetings; personal contacts; and welfare grants. It also supports medical and scientific research into causes and potential treatments. Information about this under-diagnosed condition is also available for healthcare and social service professionals.

Group details last confirmed October 2007.

FRONTOTEMPORAL LOBAR DEGENERATION including FRONTOTEMPORAL DEMENTIA

Frontotemporal Lobar degeneration; FTLD; Pick's disease

Background

Frontotemporal Lobar Degeneration (FTLD) is a term for a group of conditions caused by loss of brain cells in the frontal and temporal lobes of the brain. Pick's disease is an older name for the disease and is now mostly used just to mean a particular type of underlying pathology, although some people still use this to mean the clinical syndrome of FTLD.

Anybody can develop FTLD. It affects men and women alike. Although it typically affects people in their fifties and sixties it has been diagnosed in people from the ages of twenty to eighty. The rate of progression varies enormously ranging from a duration of less than two years to well over ten years.

What are the symptoms?

FTLD consists of three syndromes: Frontotemporal Dementia (FTD) or the behavioural variant of FTLD; and two syndromes which present with language problems, Progressive Non-Fluent Aphasia (PNFA) and Semantic Dementia (SD).

Frontotemporal Dementia (FTD) or behavioural variant FTLD

FTD varies in the way it affects individuals. There are however a common core of symptoms. Some or all of these may be present at different stages of the disease. The more common symptoms include:

- personality change:
  - loss of inhibitions, aggression, irritability, impatience, inappropriate behaviour
  - apathy, loss of motivation
  - changes in sexual behaviour
- development of routines and obsessions, hoarding, "childlike" behaviour
- decreased amount of speech
- overeating, obsessional cravings for certain types of food, especially sweet food.

Progressive Non-Fluent Aphasia (PNFA)

In this condition there are progressive difficulties with speech production. This may be the only problem between the ages of two and ten. Reading and writing can become affected as the disease progresses. Patients are usually aware of their speech/language deficit. It is caused by loss of cells in the speech areas of the brain (in most people this is on the left side of the brain). Comprehension of speech is normally unaffected early on but can become a feature later. Similarly, behavioural symptoms can occur as the disease progresses although these are rarely a major problem. This condition is sometimes called Primary Progressive Aphasia (PPA) although this term is also used to mean both PNFA and SD by some doctors.

Semantic Dementia (SD)

SD also presents as a problem with language although it differs from PNFA in being a difficulty with understanding the meaning of words. The first symptom is therefore often difficulty finding the correct words. Speech is still fluent but the person may talk about things in a vague or circumlocutory manner. They often use the wrong word or say 'thing' instead. As the disease progresses there is increased difficulty comprehending what is being said to them. As with PNFA, behavioural symptoms can become a feature later on.

In a small number of patients FTLD overlaps with either Motor Neurone disease (MND) or a disease called Corticobasal Ddegeneration (CBD) see entries. Symptoms of MND can include weakness of the limbs or problems with swallowing. Patients with CBD can get stiffness and/or jerking of one or more of their limbs. Furthermore, some patients with FTLD will later develop symptoms similar to Parkinson's disease such as slowing of movements, tremor and stiffness of the limbs.

What are the causes?

In 1892, Arnold Pick, a German neurologist, described a man who had presented in life with progressive loss of language. After death, the patient's brain was shown to have asymmetric localised atrophy (loss of brain cells) at the front of the brain as opposed to Alzheimer's disease where the atrophy is more general. Brain cells in these areas of atrophy are abnormal and contain abnormal deposition of proteins, either one called tau (which in some cases forms 'Pick bodies') or another one called TDP-43 (also known as ubiquitin-positive, tau-negative inclusions).

How is it treated?

There are currently no known curative treatments for FTLD. However, there are treatments for some of the symptoms such as concurrent depression or behavioural symptoms. Drugs used in Alzheimer's disease (the cholinesterase inhibitors such as donepezil) may worsen behavioural symptoms in some patients. A major international research effort is currently dedicated to understanding FTLD better and ultimately to develop new treatments.

Inheritance patterns and prenatal diagnosis

Inheritance patterns

Between thirty and fifty per cent of all patients with FTLD will have a history of somebody else in their family also suffering from the condition. So far two genes have been found which cause FTLD – one is called tau, and the most recently discovered one is called progranulin.

Prenatal diagnosis

None.

Medical text written October 2001 by Contact a Family. Approved October 2001 by Professor M Rosser, Professor of Clinical Neurology, National Hospital for Neurology and Neurosurgery, London, UK and Medical Adviser to the Pick's Disease Support Group. **Last updated October 2006 by Dr Jonathan Rohrer, Dr Rohani Omar and Dr Jason Warren of the Dementia Research Centre, Institute of Neurology, National Hospital for Neurology and Neurosurgery, London, UK.**

Further online resources

Medical texts in *The Contact a Family Directory* are designed to give a short, clear description of specific conditions and rare disorders. More extensive information on this condition can be found on a range of reliable, validated websites. Further information on these resources can be found in our **Medical Information on the Internet** article on page 21.

Support

Pick's Disease Support Group
3 Fairfield Park, Lyme Regis DT7 3DS   Tel: 01297 445488   e-mail: info@pdsg.org.uk
Web: http://www.pdsg.org.uk
The Group is a National Registered Charity No. 290173 and is under the umbrella of the National Hospital for Neurology and Neurosurgery Development Foundation. It offers regional contacts and an e-mail directory. It publishes a newsletter and has a wide range of information available, details on request. The Group has over 1,000 members.
Group details last confirmed November 2007.

GALACTOSAEMIA

Background

Babies with galactosaemia usually present in the first days and weeks of life with feeding difficulties, vomiting, jaundice, failure to thrive, liver and kidney disease due to their inability to convert galactose, a sugar present in milk, into glucose, the sugar used by the body.

What are the symptoms?

The severity of the illness varies from life threatening to a more chronic problem. If the disorder is not treated promptly there is a risk of death due to liver failure, bleeding or infection.

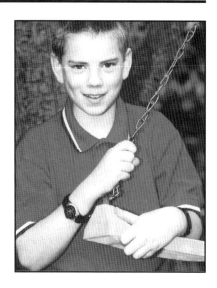

Psychological and behavioural characteristics

The information below has been drawn up by Dr Orlee Udwin of the Society for the Study of Behavioural Phenotypes.

Even with early diagnosis and immediate treatment psychological and learning difficulties are apparent. Intellectual abilities tend to be in the low average or borderline range. Even children with average cognitive abilities have a high prevalence of speech and language problems. These are most marked in the area of expressive language, and include a limited vocabulary, difficulties with word finding, syntax and grammar, articulation disorders, and transpositions of words in sentences. Deficits in verbal recall and problems with abstract reasoning have also been described. In contrast, understanding of language tends to be age appropriate. Some visual-perceptual difficulties have been noted in up to half of the cases, and problems with co-ordination, gait and balance in about one-quarter.

There are reports of progressive neurological disease and a decline in IQ scores in affected individuals with increasing age, though the latter may be due to the use of different cognitive assessments at different ages.

Behavioural and personality characteristics reported to be associated with galactosaemia include lack of confidence and assertiveness, anxiety, social withdrawal and timidity. These can lead to difficulty in obtaining independent employment. Yet some affected adults are reported to cope well with work, marriage and parenthood.

What are the causes?

Children with Galactosaemia cannot make the necessary conversion of galactose, a simple sugar, into glucose. However once galactose is removed from the diet, there is rapid improvement in the clinical symptoms. Babies may have cataracts (see entry) although many of these are minor and resolve with dietary treatment.

How is it treated?

Dietary treatment must be lifelong, but this does not prevent the long-term complications, which occur in the majority of patients. These include damage to the ovaries in most females, speech problems, developmental delay and specific learning difficulties. Growth may be delayed but the final height is normal. The girls may require induction of puberty and counselling about fertility.

Life expectancy of the treated individuals appears normal. However there are increasing reports of neurological complications such as movement disorders and intention tremor with increasing age. The cause of the symptoms is not clear.

Inheritance patterns and prenatal diagnosis

Inheritance patterns

Autosomal recessive

Prenatal diagnosis

Chorionic villus sampling at ten to twelve weeks with amniocentesis at sixteen weeks if necessary

Medical text written October 2002 by Professor J Leonard, Professor of Paediatric Metabolic disease, Institute of Child Health, London, UK. Psychological and behavioural characteristics written by Dr Orlee Udwin of the Society for the Study of Behavioural Phenotypes.

Further online resources

Medical texts in *The Contact a Family Directory* are designed to give a short, clear description of specific conditions and rare disorders. More extensive information on this condition can be found on a range of reliable, validated websites. Further information on these resources can be found in our **Medical Information on the Internet** article on page 21.

Support

Galactosaemia Support Group

31 Cotysmore Road, Sutton Coldfield B75 6BJ   Tel: 0121 378 5143
e-mail: sue@galactosaemia.org   Web: http://www.galactosaemia.org
The Group is a National Registered Charity No. 1020167, established in 1988. It offers help, support and contact with other families. It publishes a newsletter and has information available including lists of lactose free manufactured foods. The Group represents the families of over 200 affected children and adults.
Group details last confirmed April 2007.

As Galactosaemia is a metabolic disease, information and advice are also available from Climb (see entry, Metabolic diseases).

GAUCHER DISEASE

Background

Gaucher disease is a lysosomal storage disorder that is caused by an inherited deficiency of the enzyme glucocerebrosidase.

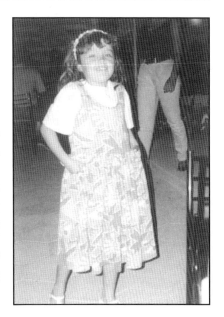

What are the symptoms?

In Type 1 symptoms may appear at any time from infancy to old age. The disease is associated with anaemia, fatigue, bruising and an increased tendency to bleed. An enlarged spleen and liver with abdominal distension may also occur as well as bone pain, fractures and skeletal degeneration. In the neuropathic forms of the condition (Types 2 and 3) involvement of the central nervous system is seen.

Inheritance patterns and prenatal diagnosis

Inheritance patterns

Autosomal recessive inheritance. The most common form (Type 1) affects under 1 in 100,000 of the general population but about 1 in 1,000 of Ashkenazi Jews. Not all these will show symptoms.

Prenatal diagnosis

Chorionic villus sampling at ten to twelve weeks allows the condition to be diagnosed in the early stages of pregnancy.

Medical text written November 1992 by Professor T Cox, Professor of Medicine, University of Cambridge School of Clinical Medicine, Cambridge, UK. **Last reviewed February 2006 by Dr A Velodi, Consultant Paediatrician and Honorary Senior Lecturer, Metabolic Unit, Great Ormond Street Hospital, London, UK.**

Further online resources

Medical texts in *The Contact a Family Directory* are designed to give a short, clear description of specific conditions and rare disorders. More extensive information on this condition can be found on a range of reliable, validated websites. Further information on these resources can be found in our **Medical Information on the Internet** article on page 21.

Support

Gauchers Association

3 Bull Pitch, Dursley GL11 4NG   Tel: 01453 549231   e-mail: ga@gaucher.org.uk
Web: http://www.gaucher.org.uk

The Association is a National Registered Charity No. 1095657, established in 1991. It offers telephone and written support and linking of families where possible. It also has up to date therapy information. It publishes a biannual newsletter and has information available, details on request. The Association has around 250 members.
Group details last confirmed March 2007.

In conjunction with the relationship specialists One Plus One, Contact a Family produces a guide on 'Relationships and caring for a disabled child.'

GENDER IDENTITY DISORDER

Gender Identity disorder: Gender Dysphoria

Background

Gender Identity disorders are rare conditions mainly arising from psychological conflicts within individuals between their physically determined gender and their beliefs and perceptions regarding their personal appraisal of their gender.

A number of causes of Gender Identity disorders have been suggested including genetics, environment, parenting, pre-birth hormonal influences, and exposure early in life to inappropriate sexual material. However, the cause usually remains unidentified and none of the above is necessary.

The two main classifications of Gender Identity disorder are to be found in the International Classification of Diseases, 10th revision (ICD 10) and the Diagnostic and Statistical Manual of Mental Disorders, 4th edition (DSM-IV).

The main diagnostic criteria are:

- Repeatedly expressing a persistent wish to identify with, and be one of, the opposite sex including cross-dressing, preference for cross-sex roles and friends of the opposite sex. In adults and adolescents this often progresses to actions and not just desires;
- Persistent anxieties and feelings that their physical gender is not appropriate for them as individuals, even to the extent of believing they have "been born in the wrong body". In children this is expressed in their feelings, the way they play and behave, the toys and clothes they prefer and certainty that they do not wish to develop the usual adolescent sexual characteristics of their physical gender. In adults this can progress to a desire to take action to alter their physical gender;
- Individuals do not have a specific intersex condition; that is to say, their general physical, including genital, features are appropriate for their genetically determined gender - it is the individuals' overwhelming psychological conviction that they are in fact "made to be" the opposite gender which is characteristic;
- The individual shows major distress in important areas of social interaction, work or other important areas of life as a result of their Gender Identity disorder.

Gender Identity disorders in children

It is very important that difficulties that might be related to Gender Identity disorder in children are identified sensitively and quickly and addressed as early in life as possible in order to minimise undue anxiety, unhappiness and vulnerability to teasing and bullying.

A number of symptoms have been recognised as features of Gender Identity disorders of childhood. However, individually these symptoms are not necessarily indicative of the disorder. In children such symptoms and behaviours may include:

- Behaviours and interests normally associated with the opposite sex;
- A belief that the individual will grow up to be a member of the opposite sex;
- Expressing this wish to be a member of the opposite sex;
- Rejection by, and isolation from, peers because of behaviours and interests more often associated with the opposite sex;
- Anxiety or depression at their isolation and their situation;
- Discomfort with their genitalia and desire for it to be exchanged for that of the opposite sex;
- Discomfort using public lavatories or changing rooms.

As children with Gender Identity disorder become teenagers they may come to:

- Express their desire to live as a member of the opposite sex;
- Dress as a member of the opposite sex;
- Express a desire to alter their genitalia to those of the opposite sex;
- Withdraw from social contact with others;
- Intensely dislike their own genitalia and body shape;
- Be concerned about developing secondary sexual characteristics (e.g. facial hair and voice lowering in biological males; menstruation and breast development in biological females).

They may also suffer continued anxiety or depression at their isolation and their situation leading some to self-harm or even attempt suicide.

Help for an affected individual is available. Counselling for children/teenagers and their families to alleviate stress, resolve conflict and promote understanding may precede reversible hormonal intervention as a teenager approaches adulthood (i.e. to block hormonal production and thus prevent further emotional and physical discomfort). Gender Identity disorders of childhood do not have outcomes that can be easily predicted – but the majority of cases do resolve, and do not necessarily lead to atypical gender identity in adulthood.

Gender Identity disorders in adulthood

Adults with Gender Identity disorder may come to express their concerns by:

- Expressing their desire to live as a member of the opposite sex;
- Dressing as a member of the opposite sex;
- Expressing a desire to alter their genitalia to those of the opposite sex;

- Withdrawal from social contact with others;
- Developing psychological and psychiatric difficulties requiring sometimes intensive and highly expert support and intervention.

Help for affected individuals includes counselling and psychotherapy, and sex reassignment involving surgical intervention and hormone treatment. However, sex reassignment may not be a final answer as there is a possibility that psychological problems will persist. Management, counselling and psychotherapy are unlikely to change the individual's self perception radically. Thus the aim is to help individuals to break out of isolation, become more accepting of their personal predicament and to enable them and their families to be more comfortable with their choices and lifestyles.

Reference: Bradley, S.J. & Zucker, K.J. (1997) Gender identity disorder: a review of the past 10 years. Journal of the American Academy of Child & Adolescent Psychiatry, Vol 36, 872-880.

Medical text written September 2005 by Contact a Family. Approved September 2005 by Professor J Turk, Professor of Developmental Psychiatry and Consultant Child & Adolescent Psychiatrist, Department of Clinical Developmental Sciences, St. George's Hospital Medical School, London, UK.

Further online resources

Medical texts in *The Contact a Family Directory* are designed to give a short, clear description of specific conditions and rare disorders. More extensive information on this condition can be found on a range of reliable, validated websites. Further information on these resources can be found in our **Medical Information on the Internet** article on page 21.

Support

Mermaids

BM Mermaids, London WC1N 3XX

Tel: 07020 935066 Charged at mobile rates (Mon-Sat, 3-7pm, answer machine available)
e-mail: mermaids@freeuk.com   Web: http://www.mermaids.freeuk.com

Mermaids was, established in 1995 and became a National Registered Charity No. 1073991 in 1999. It supports children and teenagers up to the age of 19 who are trying to cope with gender identity issues, also their parents and carers. Mermaids raises awareness about gender issues amongst professionals such as teachers, doctors and social services, and the general public. It campaigns for the recognition of this issue and the increase in professional services. Although for children and teenagers, material on Mermaids' web site will be also be helpful to adults. Mermaids is in touch with over 50 families.

Group details last updated February 2008.

The Gender Identity Research & Education Society (GIRES)

Melverley, The Warren, Ashtead KT21 2SP   Tel: 01372 801554   Fax: 01372 272297
e-mail: admin@gires.org.uk   Web: http://www.gires.org.uk

The Society is a National Registered Charity No. 1068137, established in 1997. GIRES has obtained funding for a national programme to improve the lives of people, including families, who are adversely affected by gender identity and intersex issues. The charity works with the leading international medical and scientific experts in this field. It is engaged in research-based policy and practice development, and provides education for professionals in the medical, legal, employment, teaching, public service and media sectors. It also provides a very wide range of information on its web site and from its office. GIRES has about 350 members, including many from families affected by these issues. Group details last confirmed August 2007.

A donation of £15 a month with Gift Aid would enable ten parents to attend one of our regional workshops each year. A donation form is on page 1088.

GLANZMANN'S THROMBASTHENIA

Background

Glanzmann's thrombasthenia (GT) is a rare genetic bleeding disorder affecting the small cell fragments in the blood called platelets. Platelets are important because after injury they are the first blood components to form the plug which stops bleeding (the haemostatic plug).

What are the symptoms?

Even as a child, easy bruising may be noted and in most cases the diagnosis has been made by the age of five years. The commonest problems are easy bruising, nose bleeds, heavy periods and gum bleeding. Prolonged bleeding has been reported after shedding of deciduous teeth and bleeding is of course prolonged after trauma and surgery.

Not all patients with GT are affected to the same degree. Some patients (Type 1) are severely affected while others (Type 2) are less severely affected. Even within these groups there is considerable variation. The Type 2 patients appear to have a small amount of IIb IIIa (the protein involved in stopping bleeding) on their platelets.

Overall, whilst bleeding after trauma or surgery may be severe, problems from spontaneous bleeding in day to day life are often mild but affected women often need hormonal treatment to reduce or suppress their periods. The oral contraceptive pill may be sufficient.

Many patients, particularly women, become iron deficient as a result of frequent minor blood loss and regular iron supplements may be required.

Pregnancy in women affected by GT can be extremely hazardous, not only for the patient but for the child as well. Advice should be sought from a haematologist.

Drugs such as aspirin and ibuprofen (Nurofen, Cuprofen) which also inhibit platelet function should be avoided. Paracetamol is a useful alternative but there are others; contact your doctor for advice.

Attention to oral hygiene is important to reduce bleeding from gums. Nose bleeds often become less severe after childhood giving the impression that the disorder becomes milder with age.

What are the causes?

In patients with GT a particular protein (called IIb IIIa) is either missing from the platelets or does not work properly. The result is that the platelets cannot stick together adequately to form the haemostatic plug and bleeding is not stopped even from minor injuries. The number of platelets in the blood is normal and specialised tests are required to make the diagnosis.

How is it treated?

Bone marrow transplantation is the only curative form of treatment. However this is generally considered more hazardous than the condition except in exceptional circumstances.

Inheritance patterns and prenatal diagnosis

Inheritance patterns

Inheritance is autosomal recessive. It is equally common in males and females (unlike haemophilia (hemophilia - US)); carriers (the parents and some siblings of patients with GT) are unaffected and it is more common in children whose parents are related.

Prenatal diagnosis

The genes coding for IIb IIIa have been isolated and cloned. Many genetic mutations have already been described. This means that identification of affected pregnancies can be performed at an early stage, but that considerable planning is required and early medical consultation is necessary. Carriers can be identified by testing their platelets or by DNA testing.

Medical text (paediatric) written August 2001 by Dr R F Stevens, Consultant Haematologist/Oncologist, Royal Manchester Children's Hospital, Manchester, UK and (adult) November 2002 by Dr M Laffan. **Last reviewed October 2005 by Dr M Laffan, Reader in Haemostasis and Thrombosis & Honorary Consultant in Haematology, Imperial College School of Medicine, London, UK.**

Further online resources

Medical texts in *The Contact a Family Directory* are designed to give a short, clear description of specific conditions and rare disorders. More extensive information on this condition can be found on a range of reliable, validated websites. Further information on these resources can be found in our **Medical Information on the Internet** article on page 21.

Support

Glanzmann's Thrombasthenia Contact Group

28 Duke Road, Newton, Hyde SK14 4JB   Tel: 0161 368 0219

e-mail: glanzmannsupport@btopenworld.com

This is a Contact Group, established in 1990. It offers contact through telephone and letter with newly diagnosed and affected families. It also has information and advice about problems associated with the condition. The Group is in touch with 35 families and individuals.

Group details last confirmed March 2007.

GLAUCOMA

Background

Glaucoma is an eye disease usually characterised by increased intra-ocular pressure. There are a number of different forms of glaucoma. The condition mainly affects those over the age of forty. However there is a congenital form of the condition which affects babies and children.

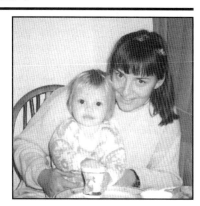

Chronic glaucoma is an insidious condition which may cause restriction of vision. Tests should be performed during routine eye examinations for those over 40, or for people with familial incidence of the condition.

What are the symptoms?

In congenital glaucoma the cornea may look hazy or the eye may enlarge due to increased internal pressure. The first thing a parent may notice is an aversion to light or watering of the eyes in the absence of inflammation.

Acute glaucoma is a painful condition causing blurred vision, haloes round sources of light and is a medical emergency requiring hospital admission.

What are the causes?

In the congenital type of glaucoma the cause of the condition is abnormal development of eye tissue. It is called hydrophthalmia or buphthalmos.

Acute glaucoma is caused when there is a sudden increase of eye pressure.

How is it treated?

In cases of congenital glaucoma, it is necessary to perform a small but delicate operation to allow the eye fluid to circulate, followed by regular monitoring. In most cases early treatment of chronic glaucoma will prevent further deterioration in vision.

Acute glaucoma is a medical emergency requiring hospital admission and usually laser or operative treatment. If treated intensively and without delay, vision subsequently is often little affected.

Inheritance patterns and prenatal diagnosis

Inheritance patterns

A genetic predisposition is recognised in both congenital and chronic glaucoma. Close blood relatives should be examined to exclude a similar condition.

Prenatal diagnosis

No test is yet available. Research is in progress on genetic markers.

Medical text written November 1991 by Contact a Family. Approved November 1991 by Professor M Patton, Professor of Medical Genetics, St Georges Hospital Medical School, London, UK and Dr J E Wraith, Consultant Paediatrician, Royal Manchester Children's Hospital, Manchester, UK. **Last updated February 2005 by Mr R Pitts-Crick, Consultant Ophthalmic Surgeon and President of the International Glaucoma Association, London, UK.**

Further online resources

Medical texts in *The Contact a Family Directory* are designed to give a short, clear description of specific conditions and rare disorders. More extensive information on this condition can be found on a range of reliable, validated websites. Further information on these resources can be found in our **Medical Information on the Internet** article on page 21.

Support

International Glaucoma Association

15 Highpoint Business Village, Henwood, Ashford TN24 8DH

Tel: 01233 648 170 Sightline   Tel: 01233 648 164 Programming Fax: 01233 648179

e-mail: info@iga.org.uk   Web: http://www.glaucoma-association.com

The Association is a National Registered Charity No. 274681, established in 1974. It offers support and reassurance to those with the condition, their relatives and anyone who is concerned. There is a network of support groups. The Association holds meetings and distributes literature as a forum for both professionals and patients to share their knowledge and views on all aspects of the condition. It campaigns for the improved treatment of glaucoma and raises awareness of the need for all three glaucoma tests to be carried out during a routine eye check. It supports much research into glaucoma, both in the UK and abroad. Free information about glaucoma and the work of the charity is available on request. The Association has approximately 10,000 members and friends. Group details last updated February 2008.

GLOBAL DEVELOPMENTAL DELAY (GDD)

Background

Babies are usually born programmed to learn important skills such as speaking, socialising or walking in predictable sequences of stages, with the help of encouragement, teaching and support as they grow up. These skills usually develop in predictable sequences and at predictable times. There are well-established average ages for when these stages of skill development occur, although they are all affected by familial factors (children in some families talk later than in others, walk later, or become dry at night later), racial factors (Black children by and large sit up, crawl and walk earlier than White children do) and social factors (children in homes with lots of books and opportunities to read and where reading is a valued and a frequent pastime will read earlier and better than others).

All the above stages of skill development are known as developmental milestones and there are a number of these within recognised areas of development (developmental domains). A child with Developmental Delay has delayed achievement of one or more developmental milestones in one or more developmental domains. A child with Global Developmental Delay (GDD) is one who is delayed in achieving milestones within most, if not all, of these development domains. The prevalence of GDD is estimated to be 5-10 per cent of the childhood population, and most children with GDD have impairment of all domains.

These domains of development can be summarized as follows:

- Motor skills (milestones in this domain include, gross motor skills such as sitting up or rolling over and fine motor skills such as picking up small objects);
- Speech and language (which also includes babbling, imitating speech, identifying sounds, communicating using non-verbal means such as gesture, facial expression, eye contact and posture, and understanding what others are trying to communicate to you – comprehension or "receptive language");
- Cognitive skills (the ability to learn new things, filter and process information, remember and recall, and to reason);
- Social and emotional skills (interacting with others and development of personal traits and feelings).

Parents will often be the first to worry that their child has delays in one or more developmental domains. However children develop at notoriously different rates and the age at which a particular child reaches a specific developmental milestone can vary substantially. In fact, some children who do not reach developmental milestones on time may catch up later, sometimes with and sometimes without extra support, have no permanent problems and go on to develop normally.

Paediatricians screen routinely for delays and if they suspect GDD they may ask questions regarding the child's progress and evaluate the child with a number of tests, both developmental (checking out what exactly a child is able to do) and medical (usually to try to find a cause for the developmental difficulties.

What are the causes?

The most common causes of GDD are chromosome and genetic abnormalities such as Down syndrome (see entry) and Fragile X syndrome (see entry - Chromosome disorders) or abnormalities with the structure or development of the brain or spinal cord such as Cerebral Palsy or Spina Bifida (see entries). Other causes can include prematurity – being born too early (see entry - Prematurity and sick newborn), infections (such as congenital rubella or meningitis) or metabolic diseases such as having an underdeveloped or underactive thyroid gland (hypothyroidism) (see entry, Metabolic disorders). There are a number of tests that can be done to identify the underlying cause of GDD and sometimes these causes can be treated to cure the developmental delay, or at least to prevent it worsening. However, often the cause is never determined.

How is it treated?

Treatment is tailored to the child's specific needs and, if any, the underlying cause of the GDD. Early assessment, clarification of profile developmental difficulties, strengths and needs, and early commencement of medical, psychological, educational and social interventions as appropriate provide the best chance for improvement, maximizing potential and quality of life, and minimizing the risk of developing further avoidable disabilities.

Inheritance patterns and prenatal diagnosis

Inheritance patterns

These will depend on the underlying cause of the condition. Infections, for example, will never be inherited, although an infected mother can pass on the infection to her unborn child or during the child's delivery. Down syndrome, the most common cause of marked developmental delay, is chromosomal but usually not inherited, the major risk factor being increasing maternal age.

Prenatal diagnosis

This is dependent on the underlying cause of the condition. If there is a strong family history of individuals having Global Developmental Delay, then an expert clinical genetics opinion should be sought for further assessment and testing.

This is dependent on the underlying cause of the condition. If there is a strong family history of individuals having Global Developmental Delay, then an expert clinical genetics opinion should be sought for further assessment and testing.

Medical Text written December 2007, by Contact a Family. Last updated January 2008 by Professor J Turk, Professor of Developmental Psychiatry and Consultant Child & Adolescent Psychiatrist, Department of Clinical Developmental Sciences, St. George's Hospital Medical School, London, UK.

Support

If the underlying cause is known then support can be offered by the relevant condition group. For general developmental delay, also known as general learning (or intellectual) disability, information, support and advice is available from Mencap and Enable (see entry, Learning Disabilities).

BIBIC - British Institute for Brain Injured Children

Knowle Hall, Bridgwater, Somerset TA7 8PJ   Tel: 01278 684060
Fax: 01278 685573   e-mail: info@bibic.org.uk   Web: http://www.bibic.org.uk
BIBIC is a National Registered Charity No1057635. It offers practical help to families caring for children with conditions such as autism, cerebral palsy, Down's syndrome, developmental delay, traumatic and acquired brain injury and specific learning difficulties such as attention deficit hyperactivity disorder, dyslexia and dyspraxia.
Group details last updated January 2008

GLOMERULONEPHRITIS

Background

Glomerulonephritis, inflammation of the glomeruli (small filtering structures in the kidney), is an umbrella name for a range of conditions generally caused by an abnormality of the immune system which is triggered for unknown reasons. Glomerulonephritis is one of the major causes of renal failure, and the main cause of kidney disease in young adults. It is estimated that twenty per cent of those on dialysis have glomerulonephritis.

What are the symptoms?

People with glomerulonephritis may have some or all of the following symptoms: blood in the urine (haematuria), protein in the urine (proteinuria), swelling up due to water and salt retention, progressive or chronic renal failure and high blood pressure (hypertension). Existing treatment consists of careful control of all these symptoms, especially blood pressure.

The identification of the specific form of glomerulonephritis in an individual will depend on a kidney biopsy:

- Minimal change disease, one of the causes of Nephrotic syndrome (see entry) does not lead to renal failure and is common in children;
- Focal and segmental glomerulosclerosis includes Nephrotic syndrome, hypertension and renal failure, and is commoner in young adults;
- Membranous nephropathy is characterised by proteinuria or nephrotic syndrome, renal failure, and is common in middle age;
- IgA Nephropathy is the commonest form of glomerulonephritis and manifests with proteinuria, hypertension and slow renal failure. It mainly affects young adults.
- Acute diffuse glomerulonephritis, which usually follows infection, tends to resolve and is now rare in Western countries. It includes haematuria/proteinuria and hypertension leading to acute nephritis;
- The rare crescentic glomerulonephritis leads to rapid renal failure and is commoner in middle age/older patients.

What are the causes?

The glomerular filters in the kidney take blood under pressure and filter out excess water, waste products and some salts. These filters sometimes become inflamed and enlarged usually due the white blood cells in the body's immune system turning against the body. This causes the inflammation. The underlying mechanism of disease is not well understood and is the subject of much current research. The inflammation can develop at any time and may trigger an occurrence such as an infection in a person with a genetic susceptibility to the disease.

It is unknown why the inflammation of the kidneys gets better in some people once treatment starts while in others the kidneys develop a scarring process and continue to decline.

How is it treated?

A variety of drugs are used to get the balance right and this differs from person to person. In some cases the use of non-specific drugs which affect the immune system (e.g. steroids) may help. In all cases the aim of treatment is to prevent the kidneys completely failing to function. If kidney failure takes place individuals will need dialysis or transplantation.

Inheritance patterns and prenatal diagnosis

Inheritance patterns

None.

Prenatal diagnosis

None.

Medical text written February 2003 by Contact a Family. Approved February 2003 by the Medical Advisor (Consultant Nephrologist) of the National Kidney Research Fund, UK.

Support

As Glomerulonephritis is a kidney disease, information and advice is available from the National Kidney Research Fund (see entry, Kidney disease).

GLYCOGEN STORAGE DISEASES

Background

The term glycogen storage disease (GSD) refers to a number of inherited metabolic conditions where genetic enzyme deficiencies cause excessive accumulation of glycogen within the body. Each type of GSD is most commonly referred to by a number, although the disorders are also referred to by eponyms or according to the enzyme that is deficient.

enzyme deficiency	number	eponym
glucose-6-phosphatase	I	von Gierke disease
α 1,4-glucosidase (acid maltase)	II	Pompe disease
debrancher (amylo-1,6 glucosidase)	III	Cori disease
brancher	IV	Andersen disease
muscle phosphorylase	V	McArdle disease
liver phosphorylase	VI	Hers disease
phosphofructokinase	VII	Tarui disease
phosphorylase b kinase	IX	

What are the symptoms?

Some disorders affect the liver (types I, IV, VI & IX), some the muscles (types V & VII) and some both (type III). Disorders affecting the liver lead to liver enlargement and can be associated with a tendency to a low blood sugar. Those affecting the muscles cause muscle weakness and sometimes kidney disease. Other problems may also arise depending on the particular type of GSD. Type II GSD (Pompe disease, see entry) is both biochemically and clinically very different to the other GSDs.

How is it treated?

Treatment for GSD varies depending on the type. To prevent a low blood sugar, frequent day time feeding and continuous overnight feeding is usually necessary in type I GSD and sometimes in type III GSD. High protein diets may be used in disorders affecting muscle.

The prognosis for most GSD is relatively good although the more severe disorders may be associated with a poorer outcome.

Inheritance patterns and prenatal diagnosis

Inheritance patterns

Autosomal recessive (types I, II, III, IV, V, VII, some IX), & X-linked (some IX).

Prenatal diagnosis

This is available for some types of GSD.

Medical text written May 2000 by Dr J Walter. **Last updated November 2004 by Dr J Walter, Consultant Paediatrician, Willink Biochemical Genetics Unit, Royal Manchester Children's Hospital, Manchester, UK.**

Contact a Family Helpline 0808 808 3555

Further online resources

Medical texts in *The Contact a Family Directory* are designed to give a short, clear description of specific conditions and rare disorders. More extensive information on this condition can be found on a range of reliable, validated websites. Further information on these resources can be found in our **Medical Information on the Internet** article on page 21.

Support

The Association for Glycogen Storage Diseases (UK)
9 Lindop Road, Hale, Altrincham WA15 9DZ   Tel: 0161 980 7303
e-mail: GenSec@agsd.org.uk   Web: http://www.agsd.org.uk
The Association is a National Registered Charity No. 327841, established in 1984. All the Glycogen Storage diseases are individually listed in the Index. It offers support for affected individuals and families and linking families where possible. It can provide information about current treatments and long term prospects for GSD affected people. It publishes 3 newsletters annually, holds an annual Family Conference and AGM, and can provide more detailed information on specific GSD types on request. Workshop reports from the annual Family Conference are available on the Association's website. The Association has almost 200 UK families with an affected child or adult in membership.
Group details last updated October 2007.

Further information, support and advice on Glycogen Storage diseases is available from Climb (see entry, Metabolic diseases) and the Muscular Dystrophy Group (see entry, Muscular Dystrophy and neuromuscular disorders).

GOLDBERG SHPRINZTEN SYNDROME

GOSHS; HSCR cleft palate-mental retardation; Goldberg-Shprinzten megacolon syndrome. OMIM 609460 (not to be confused with Shprintzen Goldberg craniosynostosis syndrome or Shprintzen syndrome – velocardiofacial syndrome. These are different disorders)

Background

Goldberg Shprinzten syndrome (GOSHS) was first described by R Goldberg and R Shprinzten in 1981. Individuals with this condition have learning difficulties and typical facial features. Hirschsprung's disease with or without cleft palate usually alerts the clinician to the diagnosis, but is not an essential feature. Individuals with GOSHS are usually small in height and head size for their age.

GOSHS affects males and females equally. It is a rare condition and has been reported in only a handful of cases worldwide. It is probably under-diagnosed though, as some cases in the past may have been confused with another condition called Mowatt-Wilson syndrome (see entry). The two conditions are genetically separate and are inherited in different ways.

What are the symptoms?

The main features of GOSHS are;

Features present in most individuals:

- Mild - moderate learning disability (see entry). This may cause particular difficulties with expressive speech;
- Typical facial features:
  - highly arched eyebrows;
  - synophrys (eyebrows joined in the middle);
  - hypertelorism (widely spaced eyes);
  - large ears and nose;
  - sparse hair.
- Hirshsprung disease (failure of the nerves in the lower bowel to work correctly, causing constipation or bowel obstruction – see entry);
- Microcephaly (reduced head size - see entry);
- Restricted growth, i.e. height in the lower end of the normal range for age.

Features present in some cases:

- Cleft palate, or problems with palate function. This can lead to:
  - Feeding difficulties and excessive drooling;
  - Speech difficulties including 'nasal' sounding speech;
- Ptosis (drooping eyelids);
- MRI brain scan abnormalities: changes in the grooves of the brain

(polymicrogyria) and other subtle abnormalities can sometimes be seen on high resolution scan;

- Gait and co-ordination problems – e.g. wide based gait;
- Recurrent ear infections leading to hearing difficulties;
- Congenital heart problems (rare).

As children with GOSHS get older, as teens and young adults they may also develop problems with:

- Corneal hypoasthesia (reduced sensation to the surface of the eye). This can cause recurrent eye infections if not monitored;
- Scoliosis or lordosis (increased curvature of the spine);
- Decreased muscle strength – reported in two individuals to date.

In these instances referral to an appropriate specialist, is recommended at an early stage.

What are the causes?

Gene alterations (mutations) in the KIAA1279 gene on chromosome 10.1 are known to cause GOSHS in some patients. Exactly how this gene works is not yet known. Gene alterations in KIAA1279 may interfere with growth and migration of young nerve tissue in a developing fetus. Gene testing for KIAA1279 is available in the Netherlands.

Inheritance patterns and prenatal diagnosis

Inheritance Pattern

Autosomal recessive. Genetic advice and counselling is available for families.

Prenatal diagnosis

This may be possible for some families with an affected child where KIAA1279 gene alterations have been identified.

Medical text written August 2007 by Dr Helen Murphy, Specialist Registrar in Clinical Genetics, c/o Alder Hey Hospital, Liverpool, UK

Further Online Resources

Medical texts in *The Contact a Family Directory* are designed to give a short, clear description of specific conditions and rare disorders. More extensive information on this condition can be found on a range of reliable, validated websites. Further information on these resources can be found in our **Medical Information on the Internet** article on page 21.

Support

There is no support group for Goldberg Shprinzten syndrome. Cross referrals to other entries in the Contact a Family Directory are intended to provide relevant support for these particular features of the disorder. Organisations identified in these entries do not provide support specifically for Goldberg Shprinzten syndrome. Families can use Contact a Family's Freephone Helpline for advice, information and, where possible, links to other families. Contact a Family's web-based linking service MakingContact.org can be accessed at Web: http://www.makingcontact.org

Currently Contact a Family is actively involved in facilitating the formation of a UK support group. If you would like to know more about this, please contact the Rare Disorders Team on Tel: 020 7608 8700 or e-mail: specific-cond@cafamily.org.uk . We look forward to hearing from you.

"I find it helpful to come to these courses not just for information but also as a time to spend with others in similar situations." Parent attending a Contact a Family Wales stress management course

GOLDENHAR SYNDROME

Goldenhar syndrome; Hemi-facial Microsomia; First and Second Branchial Arch syndrome; Facio-Auricular Vertebral Spectrum; Oculo-Auricular Vertebral Dysplasia

Background

The main features of this condition are an unilateral under development of one ear (which may even not be present) associated with under development of the jaw and cheek on the same side of the face. When this is the only problem it is normally referred to as hemi-facial microsomia but when associated with other abnormalities, particularly of the vertebrae (hemi-vertebrae or under developed vertebrae, usually in the neck), it is referred to as Goldenhar syndrome. It is likely however, that these are two ends of the spectrum of the same condition.

What are the symptoms?

The muscles of the affected side of the face are under developed and there are often skin tags or pits in front of the ear, or in a line between the ear and the corner of the mouth. There are often abnormalities of the middle ear and the ear canal may be completely absent and deafness (unilateral) is extremely common.

There are also eye abnormalities including dermoid and notches in the lids, squints and occasionally small eyes. Children with the Goldenhar end of the spectrum may have a variety of heart problems. A variety of kidney abnormalities may also be present. There are a number of other rarer congenital abnormalities that may occur. Most individuals with Goldenhar syndrome are of normal intelligence although learning difficulties can occur in about thirteen per cent of cases. These are usually language problems as a result of deafness. There may also be speech and swallowing problems. Many babies with Goldenhar syndrome have poor weight gain in the first year or two of life.

What are the causes?

No DNA abnormality has been identified. Various environmental causes have been suggested but not proven.

How is it diagnosed?

Diagnosis of Goldenhar syndrome is made clinically and no DNA abnormality has been identified.

How is it treated?

Early identification and treatment of deafness is important and speech therapy is often necessary. Help may be required with managing feeding problems and encouraging weight gain in early infancy. Any associated abnormalities such as the congenital heart problems may need appropriate treatment. Plastic surgeons are now able to improve the growth of the face, particularly the jaw, through the use of bone distraction techniques (this is a device which is able to artificially lengthen the jaw bone). Children with Goldenhar syndrome may also need on-going orthodontic treatment.

Inheritance patterns and prenatal diagnosis

Inheritance patterns

Goldenhar syndrome is almost always a sporadic condition with only a few very rare familial cases.

Prenatal diagnosis

Prenatal scanning may identify the condition in certain cases where facial or skeletal abnormalities are present. Prenatal scanning and genetic advice may be offered for future pregnancies but the risk of having another affected child is very small.

Medical text written November 1999 by Dr J A Hulse, Consultant Paediatrician, Maidstone Hospital, Maidstone, UK. **Last reviewed December 2004 by Professor J M Connor, Head of Department and Honorary Consultant, Ferguson-Smith Centre for Clinical Genetics, Glasgow, UK.**

Further online resources

Medical texts in *The Contact a Family Directory* are designed to give a short, clear description of specific conditions and rare disorders. More extensive information on this condition can be found on a range of reliable, validated websites. Further information on these resources can be found in our **Medical Information on the Internet** article on page 21.

Support

Goldenhar Support Group
18 Nuffield Close, St. John's, Worcester WR2 6JN   Web: http://www.goldenhar.org.uk
The Group is a National Registered Charity No. 1099642, established in 1989. It offers support for individuals and families and linking where possible. It publishes a two-monthly newsletter and has information available, details on request. The Group has around 30 members. To e-mail visit the website.
Group details last updated November 2007.

GORLIN SYNDROME

Gorlin syndrome: Gorlin-Goltz syndrome; Basal Cell Nevus syndrome; NBCCS; Nevoid basal cell carcinoma syndrome

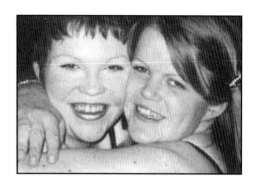

Background

Gorlin syndrome is an inherited predisposition to the development primarily of multiple basal cell carcinomas (localised skin cancers) and the development of multiple cysts within the jaws.

What are the symptoms?

The numbers and age of onset of both can vary greatly from member to member within a family. Harmless inherited abnormalities in bones (such as doubling of the ends of the ribs) are common. There is a tendency to lay down calcium deposits (also harmless) in other parts of the body which are identifiable on x-rays. Although not common, cleft lip and palate, an extra finger, stiff thumbs, stiff great toes and eye problems are also part of the condition. People with Gorlin syndrome are often tall and have large hat sizes.

What are the causes?

Gorlin syndrome is caused by a change in the patched gene which is located on Chromosome 9. Someone with Gorlin syndrome has a usual copy of the gene on one Chromosome 9, but a copy of the altered gene on the other Chromosome 9.

How is it diagnosed?

It may be possible to confirm the diagnosis on the basis of a clinical examination by a doctor with an interest in this condition and x-rays. It is important that people with Gorlin syndrome have regular screening of the skin and jaws so that the localised skin cancers and jaw cysts can be removed before they cause further problems.

How is it treated?

It is strongly recommended that the skin cancers are treated other than by radiotherapy because this can be associated with the appearance of multiple new skin cancers in the treated area. Direct DNA testing of the patched gene is possible to identify the change in the gene.

Inheritance patterns and prenatal diagnosis

Inheritance patterns

Autosomal dominant. Individuals with Gorlin syndrome have a fifty per cent chance of passing on the faulty gene to each of their children. Each child of a person with Gorlin syndrome can inherit either the usual or the changed copy of the gene. There is therefore a fifty per cent chance that a child will inherit the changed gene and so develop features of the condition. In other families, the affected person's condition is caused by a change occurring for the first time in the patched gene (a new mutation). Parents and sibs of such a person would not have the condition but the affected person can pass on the condition to children.

Prenatal diagnosis

When the change in the patched gene has been identified in an affected member, other members of the family may ask to use this information to determine whether or not they have Gorlin syndrome so that appropriate genetic information may be given and surveillance undertaken. It is also possible to use this test early in pregnancy.

Medical text written June 1995 by Dr G Evans, Consultant Clinical Geneticist, St Mary's Hospital, Manchester, UK. **Last updated October 2006 by Professor P Farndon, Consultant Clinical Geneticist, West Midlands Clinical Genetic Service, Birmingham, UK.**

Further online resources

Medical texts in *The Contact a Family Directory* are designed to give a short, clear description of specific conditions and rare disorders. More extensive information on this condition can be found on a range of reliable, validated websites. Further information on these resources can be found in our **Medical Information on the Internet** article on page 21.

Support

Gorlin Syndrome Group
11 Blackberry Way, Penwortham, Preston PR1 9LQ   Tel: 01772 517624
e-mail: info@gorlingroup.co.uk   Web: http://www.gorlingroup.co.uk
The group is a National Registered Charity No. 1096361, established in 1992. It offers contact between affected families where possible. It publishes a periodic newsletter and has information available on the website. Further details on request. The group is in touch with over 300 families.
Group details last confirmed April 2007.

GROUP B STREPTOCOCCUS

Background

The Group B Streptococcus is the commonest cause of infection in babies in the first few days of life. It is an infection that was virtually unknown before the 1960s and is now a worldwide problem affecting between 0.3 to 5 in 1,000 births. A recent UK study demonstrated that the minimum incidence in this country is 0.72 in 1,000 births. The true underlying rate is likely to be considerably higher. The infection may proceed so rapidly that even the most powerful antibiotics do not work. Even with the best treatment available, the death rate following infection is approximately 1 in 10. In addition, another 1 in 5 babies who survive the infection become permanently affected. It is also a recognised but unusual cause of stillbirths and premature onset of labour.

The Group B Streptococcus is related to other Streptococci, some of which are better known. For example, bad sore throats may be caused by a related bacterium, the group A streptococcus (this is known as a 'strep throat'). The Group B Streptococcus bacterium is unusual, however, because it causes infections that most often occur in infants of less than three months of age.

What are the symptoms?

The infection develops most commonly while the baby is still in the womb shortly before birth or hours after birth. The baby is either unwell at birth or rapidly becomes unwell, will not feed and will have difficulty in breathing. A less common form of the infection affects babies from two days after birth up until about three months of age. Infections acquired forty-eight hours after birth are usually complicated by meningitis as well as septicaemia.

What are the causes?

In most cases, the source of the organism is the mother's vagina or gastrointestinal tract. The Group B Streptococcus is a common organism, which resides in the vagina of millions of women. The presence of the Group B Streptococcus in the vagina is normal, unavoidable and does not lead to any illness or medical disorder. As can be appreciated, of all the babies born to mothers who carry the Group B Streptococcus, only a very small minority will develop the infection. There is no known way to identify which babies will become infected and there is no way to eradicate Group B Streptococcus in the mother by using antibiotics, diet or lifestyle change.

How is it treated?

Administering penicillin to the pregnant woman from the onset of labour in those cases where the risk of Group B Streptococcus infection is highest (clindamycin is recommended where the pregnant woman is allergic to penicillin) will prevent the majority of early onset infections. In practice, these means administration of an antibiotic to women with a raised temperature, prolonged rupture of the membranes, pre-term labour, an episode of Group B Streptococcus bladder infection during pregnancy, isolation of GBS from a vaginal or rectal swab during the current pregnancy or a history of a previous child that had a Group B Streptococcus infection. The antibiotic should be given into a vein at the onset of labour and should be continued at regular intervals until the baby delivers.

Inheritance patterns and prenatal diagnosis

Inheritance patterns
Not applicable.

Prenatal diagnosis
A test that establishes whether the mother is a GBS carrier in late pregnancy is now available in the UK, but only privately. Swabs are taken from the anus and vagina at thirty-five to thirty-seven weeks of gestation and are cultured using a special 'enriched broth medium' designed to isolate the GBS. If the swab shows that mother is a GBS carrier, that increases the risk of GBS infection in the baby whereas a negative swab indicates a GBS infection is unlikely.

Medical text written June 2004 by Professor R Feldman, Visiting Professor in Paediatrics, Imperial College, London and Hon. Consultant, Hammersmith Hospital, London, UK.

Support

Group B Strep Support
PO Box 203, Haywards Heath RH16 1GF   Tel: 0870 803 0023   Fax: 0870 803 0024
e-mail: info@gbss.org.uk   Web: http://www.gbss.org.uk
The Group is a National Registered Charity No. 11112065, established in 1996. It offers information by telephone, letter and e-mail and aims to raise awareness of Group B Streptococcus infection in newborn babies and how most of these infections could be prevented. It publishes a twice yearly newsletter to members only and has up to date information available for families, pregnant women and health professionals, current editions of which are available from the website or on request.
Group details last updated July 2007.

GROWTH HORMONE DEFICIENCY

Background

Growth hormone, along with several other hormones controlling growth and general well being, is secreted from the pituitary gland in the base of the brain.

Growth hormone deficiency may occur in isolation or combined with other hormone deficiencies. Growth hormone deficiency may occur spontaneously at a frequency of approximately 1 in 5,000 children and is more common in boys than in girls.

What are the causes?

Growth hormone deficiency and multiple pituitary hormone deficiency may also occur associated with tumours of the brain or as a secondary complication of the treatment of childhood cancer, usually associated with irradiation of the brain.

With the more recent successful outcomes in the treatment of childhood cancer, this is an increasing cause of growth hormone deficiency. It is important that such children be seen by a specialist endocrinologist as the underlying condition can be effectively treated, but the pituitary deficiency may evolve with time.

Inheritance patterns and prenatal diagnosis

Inheritance patterns

This is dependent on the underlying diagnosis. Most cases are not inherited.

Prenatal diagnosis

None.

Medical text written November 1995 by Dr R Stanhope. **Last reviewed July 2006 by Dr R Stanhope, Consultant Paediatric Endocrinologist, Great Ormond Street Hospital, London, UK.**

Support

Growth disorder information, support and advice is available from the Child Growth Foundation (see entry, Restricted Growth).

GUILLAIN-BARRÉ SYNDROME

Guillain-Barré syndrome: GBS; Acute Inflammatory Polyneuropathy

Background

Guillain-Barré syndrome is an acute illness which is caused by inflammation of peripheral nerves leading to loss of sensation, muscle weakness and, in more serious cases, complete paralysis and breathing difficulty.

The disease varies in speed of onset with children reaching their maximal disability over a matter of days or, much more gradually over a period of up to four weeks.

What are the symptoms?

Initial symptoms consist of tingling, numbness, unsteadiness and progressive weakness usually affecting the feet and then the hands and gradually progressing up the limbs. At the height of their illness about a quarter of children remain able to walk but the other three quarters loose their mobility and about sixteen per cent need to be artificially ventilated on an intensive care unit. In almost eighty per cent of children these symptoms follow a recent illness (usually viral). This infection is thought to trigger a faulty response in the immune system.

How is it diagnosed?

The diagnosis of Guillain-Barré syndrome is confirmed with a combination of lumbar puncture, where a high protein content is demonstrated in the cerebrospinal fluid and nerve conduction studies, which show slowing of nerve conduction in the nerve roots and/or peripheral nerves.

How is it treated?

Recovery usually begins in two to three weeks and may be accompanied by pain and tingling in the limbs. Most children are able to walk unaided by six weeks and most are free from symptoms by about three months. A minority do have some residual problems but these children are usually still able to walk unaided. The condition can occur at any age but there appear to be peak ages of onset in childhood at four years and twelve years. In general children make a much better recovery than adults. There is a very small risk of mortality due either to unrecognised respiratory complications or to cardio vascular instability in the most seriously affected children. It is thought that treatment with plasma exchange or intravenous immunoglobulin shortens recovery time in children.

Adults

Treatment with plasma exchange or intravenous immunoglobulin has been shown to shorten recovery time significantly.

Inheritance patterns and prenatal diagnosis
Inheritance patterns
None.
Prenatal diagnosis
Not applicable.

Medical text written December 1996 by Dr S A Robb. Additional material provided June 2000 by Professor R A C Hughes, Professor of Neurology, Division of Clinical Neurosciences, Guy's, King's and St Thomas' School of Medicine, London, UK. **Last reviewed August 2002 by Dr S A Robb, Consultant Paediatric Neurologist, Newcomen Centre, Guy's Hospital, London, UK.**

Further online resources
Medical texts in *The Contact a Family Directory* are designed to give a short, clear description of specific conditions and rare disorders. More extensive information on this condition can be found on a range of reliable, validated websites. Further information on these resources can be found in our **Medical Information on the Internet** article on page 21.

Support
Guillain-Barré Syndrome Support Group
c/o Lincolnshire County Council, Eastgate, Sleaford NG34 7EB   Tel: 01529 304615
Tel: 0800 374803 Helpline   Web: http://www.gbs.org.uk
The Group is a Registered Charity No. 327314, established in 1985. It also covers Chronic Inflammatory Demylenating Polyneuropathy, the chronic form of Guillain-Barré syndrome, and other related illnesses. It offers emotional support including visits from individuals who have personal experience of the condition. The charity provides awareness presentations to health professionals. Membership is available and members receive an annual journal and three newsletters per annum. There is also an annual conference offering members and interested persons the opportunity to hear the latest news on GBS and CIDP.
Group details last updated February 2008.

GUT MOTILITY DISORDERS

Gastro-Oesophageal Reflux; Intractable Vomiting; Intestinal Pseudo-Obstruction; severe constipation

Background

The contents of the gut are moved from mouth to anus in a carefully regulated fashion in order that food may be digested and absorbed and the exhausted waste expelled. The power for movement originates from the muscle coats of the bowel, which are controlled by an intrinsic network of nerves within the gut wall (Enteric Nervous System - ENS). In addition, the function of the ENS and muscles cells is also controlled by the brain via the sympathetic and parasympathetic nerves (extrinsic to the gut), by hormones from endocrine cells and by the immune system. Congenital abnormality or acquired disease may affect any of these components in any part of the bowel to produce dysfunction that results in a gut motility disorder. As a result, such disorders comprise a large group that may vary in their clinical features.

The disorders may be restricted to only part of the gut such as gastro-oesophageal reflux or may diffusely affect the gut and even the urinary bladder as in Hollow Visceral Myopathy. Gastro-oesophageal reflux with a hiatus hernia occurs in 1 in 500 live births and intestinal pseudo-obstruction and very severe constipation in 1 in 4,500. The latter are due to a heterogeneous group of disorders in which developmental abnormality of the enteric nerves and muscle coats occurs. The commonest of these is Hirschsprung's disease (see entry).

What are the symptoms?

Gut motility disorders may present in a variety of ways and these include recurrent vomiting which may be intractable, abdominal distension and recurrent obstruction, severe abdominal pain, severe constipation and/or diarrhoea.

What are the causes?

Some gut motility disorders are now known to be due to genetic abnormality, for example, defects of c-ret and endothelin B receptors (genes known to be involved in the development of the nerves in the gut) in Hirschsprung's disease. Other conditions which may be inherited such as hollow visceral myopathy or congenital absence of argyrophil neurons are extremely rare and relatively few cases are known in the UK.

How is it diagnosed?

Diagnosis of motility disorders requires specialist paediatric gastroenterological and histopathological investigation. Such investigations include tests of co-ordinated gut contraction e.g. manometry. The type of tests used will depend on the part of the gastrointestinal tract most affected.

How is it treated?

Treatment is both pharmacological and surgical and may require nutritional support either enterally or parenterally. Surgery should only be carried out in centres experienced in the field. A register of patients with intestinal pseudo-obstruction is maintained in the Department of Gastroenterology and Histopathology at the Great Ormond Street Hospital for Children in London.

Recently it has become clear that inflammation involving the nerves and the muscles of the gut may underlie motility disorders that occur following infection. Specific treatments for this are now being devised.

Medical text written December 1996 by Professor Peter Milla, Professor of Paediatric Gastroenterology and Nutrition, Great Ormond Street Hospital, London, UK. **Last updated November 2006 by Dr Nikhil Thapar, Clinician Scientist and Honorary Consultant in Paediatric Gastroenterology and Nutrition, Great Ormond Street Hospital, London, UK.**

Support

TummyTrouble
7 Leechon Way, Rochford, Essex, SS4 1TU Tel: 0844 815 1415
e-mail: alex@tummy-trouble.co.uk
TummyTrouble - supporting parents and families of children with gut motility disorders, is a telephone support network covering a range of gut motility disorders established in 1996 as the Gut Motility Disorders Support Network became TummyTrouble in 2007. It has parent volunteers to answer other parents' and family members' enquiries and has medically approved information available, details on request.
Group details last updated February 2008.

HIV INFECTION AND AIDS

Background

Infection with the human immunodeficiency virus results in progressive destruction of the immune system. As a result of this an infected individual becomes susceptible to a number of different infections and is also liable to become wasted and also to develop neurological problems.

The Acquired Immune Deficiency syndrome (AIDS) is a clinical definition. An HIV positive individual is described as having AIDS if they develop one or more of the complications associated with the deteriorating immune system.

What are the symptoms?

The complications of HIV infection and the ways infected children may present are numerous and extremely variable. All the systems of the body may be involved including the gastro-intestinal tract, the lungs and the nervous system. They are also prone to develop recurrent infections and some malignancies.

What are the causes?

HIV can be transmitted by unprotected sexual intercourse, both homosexual and heterosexual, by the administration of contaminated blood products and by contact with infected needles.

HIV infected women can also pass the infection to their unborn children, this may occur while the baby is in utero, at the time of delivery, or transmitted by breast milk.

How is it treated?

Current knowledge now encourages HIV testing during pregnancy. AZT treatment combined with elective caesarean section and bottle-feeding has reduced the chance of a baby being infected from over twenty per cent down to two per cent.

The outlook for children born with the virus has dramatically improved with the introduction of combination retroviral therapy. Three drug combinations have also led to an improved outcome for infected children.

Most children are now well, back at school and leading normal lives apart from taking medication twice a day by mouth. This treatment is relatively new and the long term outcomes and side effects have yet to be assessed.

It is recommended that infected babies and older children with evidence of a damaged immune system are given the antibiotic septrin to prevent them getting PCP. Symptomatic children are given the anti-HIV drug AZT and studies are on going looking at other drugs and combinations of drugs used at various stages of the disease. Children should receive the normal schedule of vaccinations with two exceptions. It is recommended that babies born to infected mothers should not receive BCG and that they should be given the injectable inactivated polio vaccine as opposed to the oral live form. They are also given additional vaccines including one protecting against pneumococcus.

No children with haemophilia (hemophilia - US) have been infected since 1986 when the screening of donated blood for HIV was introduced and the blood products were treated to inactivate the virus.

This is a disease where several members of the same family may be infected. The families face a wide range of problems including social, legal, schooling, employment and bereavement issues. The management of these families is extremely complex and necessitates a team approach involving a range of professionals, voluntary groups and organisations and most importantly the children and their families themselves.

Inheritance patterns and prenatal diagnosis
Inheritance patterns
None; however, the disease may be passed from mother to child by means of vertical transmission.

Prenatal diagnosis
No prenatal diagnostic tests are available although women are now actively encouraged to have an HIV test in pregnancy. Post-natal tests are available for babies born to HIV positive women.

Medical text written November 1995 by Dr J Evans, Paediatric HIV Team, St Mary's Hospital, London UK. **Last reviewed December 2004 by Dr M Sharland, Consultant Paediatrician in Paediatric Infectious diseases and HIV, St George's Hospital, London, UK.**

Support
Children with Aids Charity
Calvert House, 5 Calvert Avenue, London E2 7JP   Tel: 020 7033 8620
Fax: 020 7739 3902   e-mail: info@cwac.org   Web: http://www.cwac.org
Children With Aids Charity is a National Registered Charity No.1027816, established in 1992. It exists to help the youngest of those infected and affected by HIV and AIDS. Its Hardship & Respite Care Project helps alleviate financial stress felt by children and their families enabling them to maintain a better quality of life and a brighter outlook. Its Transport Service ensures children can access treatment and support groups whilst its Education Program tirelessly promotes paediatric HIV and AIDS awareness whilst fighting for a future without prejudice for those living with the virus.
Group details last updated August 2007.

Waverley Care Solas
2/4 Abbeymount, Edinburgh EH8 8EJ   Tel: 0131 661 0982   Fax: 0131 652 1780
e-mail: childcare@waverleycare.org   Web: http://www.waverleycare.org
*Waverley Care Solas is a Scottish Registered Charity No. SC 000765, established in 1991.
It provides a full and confidential range of services for children and families affected by
HIV. Services for children and young people (4-16years) include: support groups; activity
programmes; residentials; and school holiday programmes. Individual counselling is also
available.*
Group details last confirmed September 2006.
*Other organisations providing excellent support and information covering HIV Infection/
AIDS but not specifically geared to children are listed below:*

Positively Women
347-349 City Road, London EC1V 1LR
Tel: 020 7713 0222 Helpline for women living with HIV (Mon-Fri, 10am-4pm)
Tel: 020 7713 0444 (admin)   e-mail: info@positivelywomen.org.uk
Web: http://www.positivelywomen.org.uk
*Positively Women is a National Registered Charity No. 802406, established in 1987. It
is the only national charity working to improve the quality of life of women and families
affected by HIV. All direct services are delivered by HIV positive women, and include:
support, advice and advocacy; helpline; outreach work in hospitals, clinics and prisons;
information service including quarterly newsletter; children and families service;
volunteering opportunities; and complementary therapies.*
Group details last confirmed February 2008.

The Terrence Higgins Trust
314-320 Gray's Inn Road, London WC1X 8DP   Tel: 0845 122 1200 THT Direct Helpline
Tel: 020 7812 1600 Admin   e-mail: info@tht.org.uk   Web: http://www.tht.org.uk
*The Trust is a National Registered Charity No. 288527, established in 1983. It is a national
service and its helpline, THT Direct, offers information, support and advice to anyone living
with, affected by, or concerned about HIV and other sexually transmitted infections. THT
Direct can also refer and signpost callers to relevant services in their area - whether run
by THT or other voluntary or statutory bodies. THT also runs many face-to-face services
through its network of regional centres. These services include advice and information
on welfare benefits, community care, debt, employment, housing and criminalisation to
anyone who is HIV positive, hardship funds, testing, counselling, community support,
support groups and complementary therapies.*
Group details last updated August 2007.

HAEMOCHROMATOSIS

Background

Haemochromatosis (Hemochromatosis - US) is the medical term describing the presence of excess iron in the body. It may be inherited or acquired.

Acquired haemochromatosis usually occurs due to accumulated iron from frequent blood transfusions given to treat haemolytic anaemias. Often these are necessary for children with anaemias, and therefore iron overload can affect this age group. Features include cardiac and liver disease (see entry). This type of haemochromatosis is treated, and indeed prevented, by the use of iron chelation therapy, using a drug such as desferrioxamine which binds iron in the body and allows it to be excreted in the urine. As with genetic haemochromatosis, iron removal may not reverse disease, because of the tissue damage that has already occurred.

Genetic haemochromatosis usually has autosomal recessive inheritance and is the result of excessive absorption of iron from the intestine despite normal or high body iron stores. Over ninety per cent of patients are homozygous for the C282Y mutation in the HFE gene on chromosome 6. Iron accumulates in the liver, pancreas, heart, joints and pituitary. Iron overload only reaches levels where there is tissue damage in the third to fifth decade of life, and therefore children are rarely if ever affected. Moreover, in many people with the genetic condition, iron accumulates only slowly and may not cause the symptoms described below.

What are the symptoms?

In the early stages genetic haemochromatosis may be difficult to recognise as the symptoms are often vague and non-specific. These include fatigue, abdominal pain, and joint aches and pains. The liver function tests may be mildly abnormal. As the disease progresses the skin may take on a tanned appearance (not due to sun exposure) and other more serious features develop including diabetes mellitus (see entry), cirrhosis and heart disease.

How is it diagnosed?

Initial detection of iron overload is by blood tests (transferrin saturation, ferritin). If this is present, mutation analysis for the C282Y mutation identifies those patients with genetic haemochromatosis.

How is it treated?

Early diagnosis and treatment by venesection is important to reduce disease progression. Venesection therapy is the taking of approximately one pint of blood, usually every week, until iron levels return to normal. Subsequently venesection continues at a less frequent rate (three to six monthly) for life to prevent iron accumulation.

Inheritance patterns and prenatal diagnosis

Inheritance patterns

Autosomal recessive

Prenatal diagnosis

Prenatal diagnosis is not currently done. As already mentioned the accumulation of iron takes many years. In children of affected individuals iron studies can be delayed until the late teenage years, and screening by mutation analysis until informed consent can be obtained. The risk to children of an affected individual can be indicated by mutation analysis of the spouse.

Medical text written October 2000 by Dr J S Dooley, Hon. Consultant in Medicine, Royal Free Hospital, London, UK. **Last updated October 2005 by Professor M Worwood, Professor and Clinical Scientist, Director of the Graduate School in Biomedical and Life Sciences, Department of Haematology, School of Medicine, Wales College of Medicine, Cardiff, UK.**

Further online resources

Medical texts in *The Contact a Family Directory* are designed to give a short, clear description of specific conditions and rare disorders. More extensive information on this condition can be found on a range of reliable, validated websites. Further information on these resources can be found in our **Medical Information on the Internet** article on page 21.

Support

Haemochromatosis Society

Hollybush House, Hadley Green Road, Barnet EN5 5PR   Tel/Fax: 020 8449 1363
e-mail: info@haemochromatosis.org.uk   Web: http://www.haemochromatosis.org.uk
The Society is a National Registered Charity No. 1001307, established in 1990. It offers support to individuals and families and contact where possible. It provides a handbook to members, publishes a quarterly newsletter and has information available, details on request.
Group details last confirmed September 2007.

HAEMOLYTIC URAEMIC SYNDROMES

Haemolytic Uraemic syndromes: Hemolytic Uremic syndromes - US

Background

The Haemolytic Uraemic syndromes are a group of disorders which occur throughout the world and are the commonest cause of acute kidney failure in children in North America and Western Europe. They are characterised by a haemolytic anaemia, a low platelet count and kidney failure. The most common form occurs in children and is associated with a diarrhoeal illness. This form of Haemolytic Uraemic syndrome has been termed D+HUS.

What are the symptoms?

Symptoms include pallor, vomiting, a reduction or cessation of urine output and symptoms of neurological involvement. HUS may involve not only the kidneys and central nervous system, but other organs such as the gut, liver, heart and pancreas.

What are the causes?

Most children develop HUS after a preceding illness, usually gastroenteritis. The onset of the breakdown of red blood cells and kidney failure is sudden.

It is now believed that the majority of cases of D+HUS are associated with infection by verocytotoxin producing Escherichia coli (VTEC). These organisms are associated with clinical conditions ranging from mild diarrhoea to haemorrhagic colitis and D+HUS. Food borne transmission of VTEC 0157 has been shown to occur in a large number of outbreaks in various parts of the world. Minced beef and dairy produce are the most commonly implicated foods. Infection has also been associated with the consumption of water, vegetables and fruit juice. Person to person spread and contact with livestock have also been documented as modes of transmission of infection in outbreaks in Europe and North America.

How is it treated?

Despite a wide variety of different treatment modalities, there is a continuing dependence on supportive measures in the treatment of D+HUS. This involves prompt and vigorous control of kidney failure, high blood pressure and chemical imbalance alongside the careful correction of anaemia.

The prognosis for children with D+HUS remains good, but there is an acute fatality and the mortality among HUS cases caused by VTEC 0157 infection is in the range of three to seven per cent. The longer term prognosis following this illness remains more unclear. Follow up studies from different countries have shown between fifteen to forty per cent of survivors having some form of ongoing kidney impairment. In view of the number of patients with longer term problems, albeit in the main generally minor, it is advised that children who have had an episode of this illness be kept under general medical review.

Inheritance patterns and prenatal diagnosis
Inheritance patterns
Not applicable
Prenatal diagnosis
Not applicable

Medical text written June 1998 by Dr M M Fitzpatrick, Consultant Paediatric Nephrologist, St James's University Hospital, Leeds, UK. **Last reviewed October 2004 by Dr R Trompeter, Consultant Paediatric Nephrologist, Great Ormond Street Hospital, London, UK.**

Support
HUSH

PO Box 159, Hayes UB4 8XE   Tel: 0800 731 4679   e-mail: hush@ecoli-uk.com
Web: http://www.ecoli-uk.com

HUSH is a Scottish registered charity (No. SCO 026945), established in 1997 following a large outbreak of E.coli poisoning. It supports families affected by E.coli 0157 and/or Haemolytic Uraemic Syndrome (HUS), and can put affected people in touch with others who have been affected previously. HUSH also raises awareness of the bacterium among members of the public and the medical profession. Information leaflets and posters are available on request. Membership is free and exceeds 290.

Group details last updated August 2007.

HAEMOPHILIA, VON WILLEBRAND DISEASE and other coagulation defects

Background

The conditions covered in this entry are haemophilia A, haemophilia B (Christmas disease), von Willebrand disease (VWD) and some other coagulation defects.

The haemophilias (hemophilias - US) are a group of inheritable blood disorders characterised by various defects in the blood clotting system. The clotting factors present in blood were initially known by Roman numerals, numbered from I to XIII. More recently described factors have been given names and some deficiencies are associated with excessive, rather than reduced, blood coagulation. Factor VIII is deficient in classical haemophilia, also known as haemophilia A. Factor IX is deficient in haemophilia B (also known as Christmas disease). Von Willebrand factor is deficient in VWD and this results in a failure of platelet and vessel wall function with an associated reduction in factor VIII clotting activity.

Haemophilia occurs in about 1 in 10,000 of the population in the UK, with haemophilia A (six thousand patients) being five times as frequent as haemophilia B (one thousand two hundred and fifty patients). Both conditions are sex-linked so that it is almost always males who are affected. VWD occurs equally in males and females and about seven thousand five hundred patients are registered in the UK but the real number of affected people is certainly much greater. These conditions affect all racial groups and occur worldwide.

What are the symptoms?

The haemophilias and VWD may be severe, moderate or mild depending on the functional level of the deficient factor. In the severe form of haemophilia, where factor VIII or factor IX are virtually absent, repeated bleeding into joints and muscles is characteristic and can lead to long term joint damage. These effects are unusual in the milder forms. In VWD, bleeding from the mouth and nose is particularly common and women tend to experience heavy periods but the problem is rarely very severe.

Many other conditions, which are inherited and can give rise to abnormal bleeding, have also been described. These are generally milder than haemophilia and are usually autosomal recessive, only being fully expressed in the homozygous (having two identical forms of the gene, one inherited from each parent) or doubly heterozygous (having two different forms of a particular gene, one inherited from each parent) state. Examples are deficiencies of factors XI, I (fibrinogen), V, VII, X and XIII, all of which are particularly found in communities where consanguinity (blood relationship between parents because of shared ancestry) is common.

Easy bruising and bleeding after injury or surgery can occur in any of the disorders described above unless effective treatment is given.

How is it treated?

Treatment is based at hospitals with a haemophilia centre and there are currently twenty-five Comprehensive Care Centres across the UK, so designated because of the wide range of services they provide. The principle of management is the replacement of the deficient factor by intravenous injection. For those severely affected, regular injection to prevent bleeding (prophylaxis) is well established, especially in children and as a result joint disease has proved to be largely preventable. In the UK, the concentrated clotting factors used for the treatment are now almost exclusively produced artificially (recombinant factors), but concentrates derived from human blood plasma are still often used to treat VWD.

Plasma derived factor concentrates were associated with the transmission of hepatitis and then human immunodeficiency virus (HIV) until 1986 when improved donor selection and viral inactivation techniques were introduced. Over one thousand two hundred people with haemophilia were infected with HIV and the majority have died, although modern treatment has been very effective for those who survive. More than four thousand contracted hepatitis (mostly due to hepatitis C virus) and although some have recovered completely, either spontaneously or through increasingly effective treatment, the majority have evidence of chronic infection and some have developed cirrhosis, liver failure or, more rarely, liver cancer. Plasma derived factor concentrates are now very safe but it is expected that recombinant factor will eventually replace the plasma derived products used for haemophilia care in the developed world.

About six per cent of patients with haemophilia A in the UK have inhibitors (antibodies) to factor VIII and this makes their treatment both difficult and very expensive. The most severely deficient patients are at greatest risk. Inhibitors are rare in haemophilia B, VWD and other inherited coagulation disorders.

For mildly affected patients with haemophilia A and VWD it is often possible to use a hormone called desmopressin (DDAVP) instead of factor VIII concentrate but a recombinant von Willebrand factor is not yet available.

Inheritance patterns and prenatal diagnosis
Inheritance patterns
Haemophilia A and B are sex (X) linked and it is usually possible to determine the causative genetic abnormality but new spontaneous mutations are

not uncommon. Genetic counselling is available at Comprehensive Care Centres and Haemophilia Society publications also give useful information. In VWD there are both autosomal dominant and recessive forms. In many milder affected patients and their families no pattern of inheritance can be demonstrated. For VWD and other coagulation disorders (which are mostly autosomal recessive) genetic counselling is rarely requested or required.

Prenatal diagnosis

Prenatal diagnosis for haemophilia can be performed by a number of techniques from about ten weeks of pregnancy and modern genetics has given parents increasing choice for those who wish to exercise it.

Medical text written April 2002 by Dr Brian Colvin. **Last updated April 2007 by Dr Brian Colvin, Consultant Haematologist, Haemophilia Centre, Royal London Hospital, London, UK.**

Further online resources

Medical texts in *The Contact a Family Directory* are designed to give a short, clear description of specific conditions and rare disorders. More extensive information on this condition can be found on a range of reliable, validated websites. Further information on these resources can be found in our **Medical Information on the Internet** article on page 21.

Support

Haemophilia Society

First Floor, Petersham House, 57a Hatton Garden, London EC1N 8JG

Tel: 0800 018 6068 Helpline   Tel: 020 7831 1020   Fax: 020 7405 4824

e-mail: info@haemophilia.org.uk   Web: http://www.haemophilia.org.uk

The Society is a National Registered Charity No. 288260, established in 1950. It offers information, advice and support to people with bleeding disorders and their families. Details of the bleeding disorders covered, the newsletter HQ and publications can be found on the website or by contacting the helpline.

Group details last confirmed April 2007.

HASHIMOTO'S ENCEPHALITIS

Background

Hashimoto's is a rare, probably autoimmune, encephalitis/encephalopathy usually associated with high levels of thyroid antibodies in the blood.

What are the symptoms?

Often there is a global depression of higher function - drowsiness and sometimes coma. Other features can include amnesia and epileptic seizures.

What are the causes?

The exact cause is unknown - the thyroid antibodies are a marker rather than the cause of the problem. Thyroid function is usually normal.

How is it diagnosed?

It is a diagnosis of exclusion and the differential is wide - from Creutzfeldt-Jakob disease to rare inborn errors of metabolism. Useful tests include Magnetic Resonance Imaging (MRI) of the brain, Electroencephalogram (EEG), Cerebrospinal Fluid (CSF) findings, endocrine and metabolic screens, and viral studies.

How is it treated?

Most patients respond to high dose prednisolone, although improvement may take weeks, even months. Plasma exchange and intravenous immune globulin (IVIg) have been used in some patients.

The prognosis with treatment is generally good. Steroids are often continued for many months.

Inheritance patterns and prenatal diagnosis

Inheritance patterns

None.

Prenatal diagnosis

None.

Medical text written April 2002 by Dr Ian Hart, Senior Lecturer and Consultant Neurologist, University Department of Neurological Science, Walton Centre for Neurology and Neurosurgery, Liverpool, UK.

Support

Support and information for Hashimoto's Encephalitis is provided by the Encephalitis Support Group (see entry, Encephalitis).

HEART and HEART/LUNG TRANSPLANT

Background

In some cases of heart or lung conditions in children there comes a time where treatment with a donor organ is the only remaining option. The need for transplantation presents many difficulties with painful decisions for both the recipient and donor parent.

How is it treated?

Transplantation is the last hope for many children suffering from congenital, viral or genetic heart conditions, of for those with cystic fibrosis and primary pulmonary hypertension

Heart or heart/lung transplantation is not the end of treatment for these children, but the beginning of a new and different course of treatment. But it is also the only hope for such children to enable them to enjoy an extended life with any degree of quality.

Inheritance patterns and prenatal diagnosis

Inheritance patterns

Inheritance patterns of heart and lung conditions vary according to the cause of the underlying problem. The inheritance is autosomal recessive for cystic fibrosis and dominant in some cardiomyopathy conditions.

Prenatal diagnosis

Prenatal diagnosis of heart and lung conditions is sometimes possible:

- certain heart conditions can be detected by fetal ultrasound scanning at sixteen to eighteen weeks;
- cystic fibrosis can be detected in about the 10th week by chorionic villus sampling.

Medical text written May 1997 by Contact a Family. Approved May 1997 by Dr A Reddington, Consultant Paediatric Cardiologist, Royal Brompton Hospital, London, UK. **Last reviewed August 2002 by Dr R Yates, Consultant Fetal and Paediatric Cardiologist, Great Ormond Street Hospital, London, UK.**

Support

Heart Transplant Families Together
PO Box 463, Worthing BN11 9EL   Tel: 01903 606826   Tel: 07852 287713 (mobile)
e-mail: admin@htft.org.uk   Web: http://www.htft.org.uk
The Group is a National Registered Charity No. 1055882, established in 1996 with the help of the Cardiomyopathy Association. It offers support by telephone and linking families where possible. Heart Transplant Families Together supports and promotes the organ donor register and provides links between current development and medical professionals in the transplantation community. It publishes a newsletter and has over 100 members. Group details last updated May 2006.

HEART DEFECTS

OUTLINE OF A NORMAL HEART

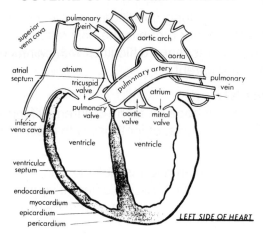

Background

The heart itself is a pump whose function is to supply the body with oxygen by circulating blood throughout the vascular system. Congenital heart anomalies affect about 1 in 125 babies. In approximately half these children surgery may be necessary. Some conditions are minor and do not require treatment. Innocent murmurs come in this category. In ninety per cent of cases the cause of the anomaly is not known.

What are the symptoms?

Some common defects are:

Anomalous Pulmonary Venous Drainage: APVD Some or all pulmonary veins drain into the right side of the circulatory system instead of the left.

Aortic Stenosis A narrowing of the aortic valve opening between the left ventricle and the aorta.

Atrial Septal Defect: ASD A hole between the right and left atrium. There are various types of defect and some may close spontaneously.

Atrioventricular Septal Defect: AVSD A hole between the right and left atrium, a hole between the right and left ventricle and single valve between the atria and the ventricles. This may be partial or complete.

Cardiomyopathy (see entry)
1.   **Dilated Cardiomyopathy** Weak heart muscle usually associated with an enlarged heart.

2.   **Hypertrophic Cardiomyopathy** The heart muscle is thickened and has difficulty in relaxing.

Coarctation of the Aorta A narrowing of the main artery supplying the body.

Double Inlet Ventricle The blood from both atria flows into one ventricle.

Hypoplastic Left Heart syndrome (see entry) The left ventricle is very small and the aortic and mitral valves are narrowed, thickened, or blocked.

Persistent Ductus Arteriosus: PDA The ductus arteriosus which is part of the fetal circulation does not close as it should in the first weeks of life.

Pulmonary Atresia with no Ventricular Septal Defect The pulmonary valve is blocked and the right ventricle may be very small.

Pulmonary Atresia with Ventricular Septal Defect A complete blockage between the heart and pulmonary arteries and hole between ventricles.

Pulmonary Stenosis A narrowing of the pulmonary valve opening.

Transposition of the Great Arteries The aorta and pulmonary artery are transposed so deoxygenated blood is circulated to the body and oxygenated blood back to the lungs.

Tetralogy of Fallot This is a combination of a hole between the two ventricles and narrowing between the right ventricle and pulmonary artery.

Tricuspid Atresia The tricuspid valve situated between the right atrium and ventricle is absent.

Ventricular Septal Defect: VSD A hole between the right and left ventricles which may close spontaneously.

Heart defects may occur with other anomalies in specific syndromes such as **Marfan** or **Down syndromes** (see entries). Occasionally the fetal heart may be damaged by infection: for example German measles, or drugs or medications such as excess alcohol or anti-convulsants.

How is it treated?
Some forms of congenital heart disorder such as myocarditis or cardiomyopathy may require transplantation (see entry, Heart and Heart/Lung Transplant).

Inheritance patterns and prenatal diagnosis
Inheritance patterns
In cases where there is an affected child there is a slightly increased risk that future children may be affected. If two children are affected the future risk increases. In cases of specific syndromes inheritance patterns will depend on the cause of the condition.

Prenatal diagnosis

This is possible for families at higher than average risk, or diabetic mothers, using ultrasound techniques at about sixteen to eighteen weeks. Suspected defects detected during routine ultrasound screening can be referred to a fetal cardiologist for diagnosis.

Medical text written November 1991 by Contact a Family. Approved November 1991 by Professor M Patton, Professor of Medical Genetics, St Georges Hospital Medical School, London, UK and Dr J E Wraith, Consultant Paediatrician, Royal Manchester Children's Hospital, Manchester, UK. **Last updated September 2001 by Dr R Yates, Consultant Paediatric Cardiologist, Great Ormond Street Hospital, London, UK.**

Support

Children's Heart Federation

First Floor, 2-4 Great Eastern Street, London EC2A 3NW   Tel: 0808 808 5000 Helpline
Tel: 020 7422 0630   Fax: 020 7247 2087   e-mail: info@chfed.org.uk
Web: http://www.chfed.org.uk
The Federation is a National Registered Charity No. 800525, established in 1987. The Federation is a national charity which represents 21 regional heart organisations across the U.K. They provide information and support, medical equipment and grants, and campaign to improve the clinical and social care of children with heart conditions.
Group details last updated August 2007.

The Children's Heart Association

26 Elizabeth Drive, Helmshore, Rossendale BB4 4JB   Tel: 01706 221988
e-mail: information@heartchild.info   Web: http://www.heartchild.info
The Association is a National Registered Charity No. 267893, established in 1973. It covers England and Wales and offers support for the families of children with heart disorders (or those who have lost such a child) through a network of branches. It publishes regular newsletters and has information available, details on request.
Group details last confirmed October 2007.

Scottish Association for Children with Heart Disorders (SACHD)

104 Comiston Road, Edinburgh EH10 5QL   Tel: 0131 447 2711
e-mail: secretary@youngheart.info   Web: http://www.youngheart.info
The Association was formerly part of the Association for Children with Heart Disorders. It is a Registered Charity No. SC035499, established in 1973 and registered in 2004. It offers support and understanding in everyday care and welfare to parents and families of children with heart disorders. It publishes a newsletter 'Heartbeat' and has information available, details on request. SACHD is an organisation under the umbrella of the Children's Heart Foundation.
Group details last updated February 2008.

GUCH Patients Association

Saracen's House Business Centre, 25 St Margaret's Green, Ipswich IP4 2BN
Tel: 0800 854759 Helpline e-mail: info@guch.org.uk Web: http://www.guch.org.uk
GUCH PA (Grown up Congenital Heart Patients' Association) is a National Registered Charity No. 1041866, established in 1993. GUCH PA is supported by the British Heart Foundation. It offers support for adolescents and young adults via their helpline and through their website. It aims to raise awareness of the needs of young people with congenital heart disorders. GUCH PA publishes a quarterly newsletter "GUCH News" and has information leaflets available, details on request.
Group details last updated November 2007.

SADS UK

22 Rowhedge, Brentwood CM13 2TS   Tel: 01277 230642   e-mail: info@sadsuk.org
Web: http://www.sadsuk.org
*SADS UK (Sudden Adult Death Trust) is a National Registered Charity No. 1113681,
established in 2000. The trust offers support, information and one to one linking for families
of affected children and affected individuals. It also offers support to bereaved families and
raises awareness about rare arrhythmia conditions such as Cardiomyopathies, Long QT
syndrome, Wolf-Parkinson White syndrome and Brudada syndrome. It provides information
and has medical advisers. SADS UK works closely with SADS America, Canada, Australia
and Europe.*
Group details last updated June 2007.

British Heart Foundation

14 Fitzhardinge Street, London W1H 6DH   Tel: 08450 708070 Heart helpline
Tel: 020 7935 0185   Fax: 020 7486 5820   e-mail: hearthelponline@bhf.org.uk
Web: http://www.bhf.org.uk
*The British Heart Foundation is a National Registered Charity No. 225971, established
in 1961. It funds research into the causes, prevention, diagnosis and treatment of heart
disease. It educates the public, health professionals and heart patients about heart disease
and promotes training in emergency life support skills. It has a wide range of information
available, including publications specifically for children and young people from pre-school
to 18 years old, details on request.*
Group details last updated November 2007.

*The following parent support groups are based around specific regional hospitals carrying
out paediatric cardiac surgery or cover regional parts of the country:*

Heart Link

68 Rockhill Drive, Mountsorrel, Leicester LE12 7DT   Tel: 0500 382152 Helpline
Web: http://www.heartlink-glenfield.org.uk
*The Group is a National Registered Charity No. 513946, established in 1981. It is
organised round the Glenfield Hospital in Leicester and covers Leicestershire, Derbyshire,
Lincolnshire and Nottinghamshire. It offers support, contact and practical help for parents
of affected children. It publishes a newsletter. The Group has over 1,200 members.*
Group details last confirmed September 2007.

Young at Heart

42 Thetford Road, Great Bar, Birmingham B42 2HY   Tel: 0121 357 8200 Information Line
e-mail: youngatheartsue@yahoo.co.uk   Web: http://www.youngatheart.org.uk
*Young at Heart is a National Registered Charity No. 512815, established in 1981. It
supports the families of children being treated at Birmingham Children's Hospital or who
are due to be treated at the hospital. Young at Heart publishes a quarterly newsletter and
has information available, details on request. It supports over 500 families.*
Group details last updated March 2007.

CRY

Unit 7, Epsom Downs Metro Centre, Waterfield, Tadworth KT20 5LR   e-mail: cry@c-r-y.org.uk
Web: http://www.c-r-y.org.uk   Web: http://www.sads.org.uk   Web: http://www.cry-csc.org.uk
*Cardiac Risk in the Young (CRY) is National Registered Charity No. 1050845, established
in 1995. It offers support to bereaved families through a nationwide network of trained
volunteers and holds a bereavement support day. The CRY Surgery Supporters Club
helps young people who have had major surgery to link for mutual support. CRY promotes
diagnostic procedures, offers proactive cardiac screening and raises awareness of the
issues surrounding cardiac risk in the young. It publishes a quarterly newsletter and has a*

wide range of information available, details on request.
Group details last confirmed February 2008.

Wessex Children's Heart Circle
48 South Avenue, Sherborne DT9 6AP   Tel: 01935 816156
e-mail: ange1events@aol.com   Web: http://www.wchc.org.uk
The Group is a National Registered Charity No. 800877, established in 1988. It covers Hampshire, Dorset, the Channel Islands, part of Somerset, Wiltshire, Plymouth area and parts of Cornwall. It offers support and local contact for families of affected children together with financial support where necessary while at the cardio-thoracic unit at Southampton Hospital. It publishes a newsletter and has information available, details on request. The group has over 500 members.
Group details last updated June 2007.

HeartLine Association
Community Link, Surrey Heath House, Knoll Road, Camberley GU15 3HH
Tel: 01276 707636   Fax: 01276 707642   e-mail: admin@heartline.org.uk
Web http://www.heartline.org.uk
The Association is a National Registered Charity No. 295803. It offers support and information on aspects of congenital heart disease in babies and children and parent contact through a nationwide network of groups often centred round a local hospital with a regular paediatric cardiac outpatients clinic. It publishes a quarterly newsletter and has a wide range of information available, details on request. The Association has over 1,400 families in membership.
Group details last confirmed February 2008.

Heartbeat (Northern Ireland)
9 Turloughs Hill, Annalong, Newry BT34 4XD   Tel: 028 4376 8786
e-mail: irwynmckibbin@heartbeatni.org.uk Web: http://www.heartbeatni.co.uk
The group is the support arm of the Northern Ireland Children's Heart Trust which is an organisation recognised by the Inland Revenue as a Charity and which acts as Trustee for Heartbeat. It offers support and parent contact through ward visits and a network of locally based groups. Heart Beat fundraises for equipment for the Clark clinic at the Royal Belfast Hospital for Sick Children. It has a 'Beating Hearts' group for teenagers, publishes a twice-yearly newsletter and has information available, details on request.
Group details last updated September 2005.

ECHO
PO Box 5015, Brighton BN50 9JR   Tel: 01273 248 948
e-mail: admin@echo-evelina.org.uk   Web: http://www.echo-evelina.org.uk
ECHO (Evelina Children's Heart Organisation) is a National Registered Charity No. 287475. It supports families of children born with heart conditions, who are treated at the Evelina Children's Hospital within Guy's and St Thomas' hospitals and their satellite clinics in greater London, Surrey, Kent, Essex, Sussex, Middlesex, Suffolk and Norfolk. It supports it members either by providing contact with other families from it's network of over 550 members or by supplying further information. It also arranges social and fundraising events.
Group details last updated July 2007.

South West Children's Heart Circle
The Hollies, 7 Ryecroft Road, Frampton Cotterell, Bristol BS36 2HJ   Tel: 08701 252307
e-mail: info@heartcircle.org   Web: http://www.heartcircle.org
The Group is a National Registered Charity No. 267323 for the families of all children with heart conditions who live in the South West of England and Wales. It offers support and visiting for families. It publishes an annual newsletter and has information available, details on request. The Group has over 500 families in membership.
Group details last updated June 2006.

HEMIMEGALENCEPHALY

Background

This is a rare brain malformation characterised by the enlargement and malformation of an entire cerebral hemisphere.

What are the symptoms?

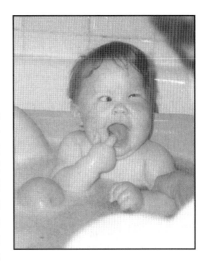

Affected children usually suffer epileptic seizures (see entry, Epilepsy) soon after birth (although these may be delayed until later in infancy) and display learning and psycho-motor difficulties. Later, children will display a hemiplegia (see entry), a weakness down one side. The condition may also be associated with facial enlargement and skin disorders. Other disorders may also involve malformation of one hemisphere, without the enlargement. Such children present with similar clinical features and require a similar course of management. The degree of developmental delay varies from mild to severe.

How is it treated?

Treatments may prevent seizures and improve the quality of life. The first line of treatment for seizures would be medication, although early consideration with regard to surgery should be given. Many children benefit from surgery, namely hemispherectomy, which is disconnection or removal of the abnormal hemisphere. It is unlikely this hemisphere is doing anything except causing seizures, therefore function is unlikely to be compromised over and above what would be inevitable from the malformation (e.g. hemiplegia).

Inheritance patterns and prenatal diagnosis

Inheritance patterns

None

Prenatal diagnosis

Ultra sound scanning may show up the different sizes of the cerebral hemispheres. Prenatal screening and genetic advice may be offered for future pregnancies. Ante-natal MR scan at twenty to twenty-five weeks in specialist units may also give further information.

Medical text written December 2001 by Dr H Cross. **Last updated September 2006 by Dr H Cross, Reader and Honorary Consultant in Paediatric Neurology, Institute of Child Health and Great Ormond Street Hospital, London, UK.**

Further online resources

Medical texts in *The Contact a Family Directory* are designed to give a short, clear description of specific conditions and rare disorders. More extensive information on this condition can be found on a range of reliable, validated websites. Further information on these resources can be found in our **Medical Information on the Internet** article on page 21.

Support

The HME Family Network is no longer operational. Families can use Contact a Family's Freephone Helpline for advice, information and, where possible, links to other families. Contact a Family's web-based linking service Making Contact.org can be accessed at http://www.makingcontact.org

Contact a Family produces Connected four times a year, with contributions from parents, professionals and voluntary organisations. If you would like to contribute to future editions, or would like to order a copy for an annual subscription of £10, Tel: 020 7608 8700

HEMIMELIA

'Hemimelia' literally means 'half limb'. By convention, this series of disorders refer to a deficiency in a skeletal and soft-tissue part which is in the 'distal' (further from the trunk) part of the limb. Usually, at least one of the two paired long bones of the arm (radius/ulna) or leg (tibia/fibula) are deficient.

What are the symptoms?

Fibular hemimelia

This is one of the most common longitudinal limb deficiencies, with an incidence of about 1 in 50,000. The fibular fails to develop in part or whole. The spectrum of abnormality ranges from mild bowing of the leg, to knee joint instability with 'knock knee' appearance, unstable ankle with a reverse "club-foot" appearance, and shortening of the lower leg. Sometimes foot, ligament and thigh bone (femoral) abnormalities are associated. The deformity tends to increase with growth, as there is limited growing potential within the affected bone. Since there is often a significant soft tissue deficiency, severe deformity at the ankle often requires a foot amputation known as a "Symes" amputation. Tibial straightening procedures (osteotomies) and limb lengthening procedures can also be undertaken.

Tibial hemimelia

This is a very rare congenital deficiency, with an incidence of about 1 in 1,000,000, in which the tibia fails to develop in part or in whole. Associated problems may include hip and hand abnormalities. There may be associated ligament absence, and an abnormal end of the thigh bone (femur). Many cases are severe, resulting in amputation at or below the knee which may produce a better quality of life and an ability to walk on the affected leg using a prosthetic.

Radial hemimelia

In this condition, the radius fails to develop normally either in part or in whole, causing the position of the hand to tend to drift to the thumb-side of the wrist. Also known as "radial club hand", the incidence is about 1 in 50,000, and mostly occurs without an obvious cause. A range of severity exists, and may be associated with mild or severe hand abnormalities. This may be associated with other disorders such as TAR syndrome (see entry) that include low platelet count (thrombocytopaenia) or Fanconi anaemia (see entry), a form of anaemia. Rarely cardiac, kidney, and tracheal-gullet anomalies are present. Treatment of moderate and severe deformities involves re-aligning the ulna bone using osteotomies and/or external fixators, and centering the wrist on the remaining ulna. Sometimes an absent thumb will be fashioned from an adjacent finger.

Ulna hemimelia

Much less common than radial hemimelia (1 in 150,000), this condition is also known as "ulnar club hand" in which the ulna bone of the forearm fails to develop in part or in whole. The position of the hand tends to drift to the little-finger-side of the wrist and sometimes fingers may be short or absent too. The radius may be fused to the ulna (synostosis). Rarely, there are associated abnormalities of the femur, fibula or shoulder blade. It may be necessary to undertake re-alignment operations of the lower humerus, the radius or ulna. Function in a synostosis may be improved by changing the angle that the forearm sits in rotation.

Inheritance patterns and prenatal diagnosis

Inheritance patterns

None, except where the abnormality is part of a syndrome such as TAR syndrome which is autosomal recessive.

Prenatal diagnosis

An anomaly ultrasound scan at twenty weeks may show up limb abnormalities.

Medical text written September 2005 by Mr D E Porter, Senior Lecturer & Hon. Consultant in Orthopaedic Surgery, University of Edinburgh, Edinburgh, UK.

Support

Hemimelia Support Group
c/o Contact a Family, 209-211 City Road, London EC1V 1JN
Tel: 0808 808 3555 Freephone Helpline   Tel 020 7608 8700   Fax 020 7608 8701
e-mail: hemimelia@yahoo.co.uk   Web: http://www.hemimelia.org.uk
The Hemimelia Support Group is an international patient and family support network offering a wide range of information on its website about hemimelia and services for affected children and adults. Members have the opportunity to share everyday experiences with others who live with the condition.
Group details last updated October 2007.

HEMIPLEGIA

Background

Childhood hemiplegia is a condition affecting one side of the child's body. It is caused by damage to some part of the brain, which may happen before, during or soon after birth, when it is known as **congenital hemiplegia**; or later, as a result of accident or illness, when it is known as **acquired hemiplegia**. The condition affects approximately one child in a thousand.

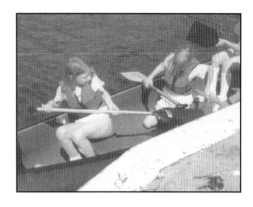

What are the symptoms?

The most obvious result of childhood hemiplegia is weakness or stiffness and lack of control in the affected side of the body. The child may have little use of one hand, may limp or have poor balance. The weakness may often be associated with spasticity (stiffness or tightness of the muscle). Some children with hemiplegia have additional medical problems such as speech difficulties, visual field defects or epilepsy. Many others have less obvious additional difficulties, such as perceptual problems, specific learning difficulties, or emotional and behavioural problems, which may be more frustrating and disabling than their physical problems.

Inheritance patterns and prenatal diagnosis

Inheritance patterns

In general none. However, in one or two very rare instances there may be a genetic factor.

Prenatal diagnosis

None

Medical text written October 1999 by Hemi-Help. Approved October 1999 by Professor Robert Goodman. **Last reviewed January 2004 by Professor Robert Goodman, Professor of Brain and Behaviour, Institute of Psychiatry, London, UK.**

Support

HemiHelp

Camelford House, 89 Albert Embankment, London SE1 7TP

Tel: 0845 123 2372 Helpline (Mon - Fri, 10am - 1pm)   Tel: 0845 120 3713 (Office)

Fax: 0845 120 3723   e-mail: support@hemihelp.org.uk   Web: http://www.hemihelp.org.uk

HemiHelp is a National Registered charity No. 1085349, established in 1991 for children and young people with hemiplegia. It offers information and support by telephone, letter, e-mail and the website and holds regular conferences on topics of interest to parents/ carers and professional workers. It publishes a quarterly newsletter and has a wide range of information available, details on request. HemiHelp has over 3,000 families and professional members.

Group details last confirmed February 2008.

Last year we distributed 98,000 guides for parents caring for a disabled child.

HENOCH SCHONLEIN PURPURA

Background

Henoch Schonlein Purpura (HSP), a non-genetic disorder, is caused by an inflammation of blood vessels (vasculitis). Whilst generally an uncommon condition, most children's doctors will have seen cases each year.

What are the symptoms?

HSP is usually preceded by an infection, often a viral respiratory tract infection, leading on to the many manifestation of this vasculitis: painful, occasionally swollen joints; red/purple skin rash which fails to blanch with pressure (purpura); abdominal pain and kidney inflammation. Generalised abdominal pain may be caused by inflammation and swelling of the wall of the intestines or, more rarely, by a twisting inversion of the lining of the bowel termed acute intussusception.

How is it treated?

Surgery may be necessary to correct acute intussusception. Kidney involvement causes blood (haematuria) and protein (proteinuria) in the urine. Whilst kidney involvement is common, occurring in up to sixty per cent of sufferers, serious kidney damage is very uncommon. Haematuria may persist for months if regular urine testing is performed. Recurrent HSP may recur in association with subsequent infections. However, the prognosis for full recovery is excellent.

Inheritance patterns and prenatal diagnosis

Inheritance patterns

None

Prenatal diagnosis

None

Medical text written October 1996 by Dr A P Windrow Consultant Paediatrician, Kingston Hospital, Kingston upon Thames, UK. **Last updated September 2006 by Dr Graham Smith, Consultant Paediatric Nephrologist, Children's Kidney Centre, University Hospital Wales, Cardiff, UK.**

Support

Henoch Schonlein Purpura Support Group
c/o Contact a Family, 209-211 City Road, London EC1V 1JN
Tel: 01733 204368 (10am - 2pm)   e-mail: hsp.help@klg.myzen.co.uk
This is a small contact group, established in 2003. It offers a listening ear and, where possible, linking for affected adults and families of affected children.
Group details last updated August 2007.

HEREDITARY HAEMORRHAGIC TELANGIECTASIA

Hereditary Haemorrhagic Telangiectasia: HHT; Hereditary Hemorrhagic Telangiectasia - US; Osler-Rendu-Weber; Rendu-Osler-Weber

Background

Hereditary Haemorrhagic Telangiectasia is a genetic disorder that leads to the development of abnormally wide and fragile blood vessels.

What are the symptoms?

Most people affected by HHT experience two problems:

- The fragile blood vessels are prone to bleed, for example, in the nose causing **nose bleeds**, and less frequently in the gut. Generally, this bleeding settles down on its own, but if it leads to anaemia, it may need treatment with iron tablets, or with a blood transfusion if severe;
- The abnormal blood vessels may become visible as **blood spots**, for example on the lips or fingertips.

A few people will have abnormal vessels elsewhere. The lungs are affected in 1 in 5 individuals with HHT and it is important that this is recognised (see below). For other sites, such as the liver and brain, it is not clear that any specific tests or treatment are needed if they are not causing problems already.

About 1 in 5 individuals with HHT develops abnormal vessels in the lungs. These are called pulmonary arteriovenous malformations (PAVMs). These malformations let blood bypass or 'shunt' past the lung airsacs. They are particularly important because individuals who have PAVMs are at risk of having a ministroke or brain abscess even if they feel well. In addition, a few women with PAVMs have complications during pregnancy. It is therefore important to check whether or not PAVMs are present, and if so, arrange for a simple treatment to close them off.

Inheritance patterns and prenatal diagnnosis

Inheritance patterns

Autosomal dominant. The earliest sign of HHT in children is usually nose bleeds, but nose bleeds may not develop until middle age. Because HHT may not become apparent until late in life, we are unable to say that younger members of a family are definitely unaffected. It is sensible for their medical records to include the fact that they have a parent with HHT, and for them to be screened for lung involvement.

Prenatal diagnosis

This is possible in families where a genetic change has been identified.

Medical text written May 2001 by Dr C Shovlin, Senior Lecturer and Honorary Consultant Respiratory Physician, Respiratory Medicine Unit, Hammersmith Hospital, London, UK. **Prenatal diagnosis information last updated November 2005 by Dr M Porteous, Consultant Clinical Geneticist and Reader in Clinical Genetics, Western General Hospital, Edinburgh, UK.**

Further online resources

Medical texts in *The Contact a Family Directory* are designed to give a short, clear description of specific conditions and rare disorders. More extensive information on this condition can be found on a range of reliable, validated websites. Further information on these resources can be found in our **Medical Information on the Internet** article on page 21.

Support

Telangiectasia Self Help Group

39 Sunny Croft, Downley, High Wycombe HP13 5UQ   Tel: 01494 528047
e-mail: info@telangiectasia.co.uk   Web: http://www.telangiectasia.co.uk
The Group was, established in 1985. It offers contact with others affected by the condition where possible. It publishes a periodic newsletter and has information available, details on request. The Group has over 600 members.
Group details last updated November 2005.

Contact a Family offers face-to-face support to over 9,000 families each year.

HEREDITARY MULTIPLE EXOSTOSES

Hereditary Multiple Exostoses: Multiple Hereditary Exostoses; Multiple Osteochondromatosis; Diaphyseal Aclasis

Background

This condition affects the skeleton and is thought to be present in more than one thousand individuals in over five hundred families in the UK.

Affected children and adolescents develop multiple bony spurs with a cap of cartilage (exostoses or osteochondromas) at the end of many bones - especially the long bones of the arms and legs.

What are the symptoms?

Exostoses grow throughout childhood, but usually become fully bony and stop growing at the end of teenage years. When they grow large they are frequently painful and can disturb growth resulting in variable short stature and deformity. Less commonly symptoms occur when exostoses compress adjacent nerves and vessels. Forearm pain, hip, knee and walking problems may occur and flat foot may also exist. Extremely rarely exostoses may become cancerous (less than five per cent of individuals). Rapidly-growing and painful exostoses in late adolescence or adulthood with a cartilage-cap thickness in excess of 10mm are usually those with this potential. Disease severity can range from mild to severe even within families.

How is it treated?

Surgery to remove problematic exostoses is often required during childhood. In childhood, regular review by an orthopaedic surgeon is recommended (perhaps annually or every second year). In adulthood clinical review is tailored to patient need and risk. A specialist exostosis clinic which takes national referrals occurs at the Royal Hospital for Sick Children in Edinburgh every three months. No other specialist exostosis clinic is known to exist in the United Kingdom.

Inheritance patterns and prenatal diagnosis

Inheritance patterns

Autosomal dominant. Up to one third of affected individuals represent 'new cases', in whom neither parent have the condition. Genes responsible for eighty per cent of affected families are EXT1 (chromosome 8q24.1) and EXT2 (chromosome 11p11-13). These genes have been fully identified. Other genes (possibly on chromosomes 1 and 19) may be responsible for the remainder of families.

Prenatal diagnosis

Prenatal or family testing is occasionally available through consultation with a consultant clinical geneticist.

Medical text written May 1998 by Mr D E Porter. **Last updated June 2007 by Mr D E Porter, Senior Lecturer & Hon. Consultant in Orthopaedic Surgery, University of Edinburgh, Edinburgh, UK.**

Further online resources

Medical texts in *The Contact a Family Directory* are designed to give a short, clear description of specific conditions and rare disorders. More extensive information on this condition can be found on a range of reliable, validated websites. Further information on these resources can be found in our **Medical Information on the Internet** article on page 21.

Support

HME Support Group
PO Box 207, Chester le Street DH3 9AR   Tel: 01438 861866
e-mail: support@hmesg.co.uk   Web: http://www.hmesg.co.uk
The Group is a National Registered Charity No. 1091069, established in 1997. It offers support by telephone and letter and linking with other families where possible. It holds regular meetings, has an informative website and produces a newsletter. The Group has over 300 families in membership.
Group details last confirmed September 2007.

HEREDITARY THROMBOPHILIA

Background

Hereditary Thrombophilia is the increased tendency to develop blood clots in veins and arteries. Blood is designed to flow freely round the body and not obstruct blood vessels. At the time of a cut, however, blood thickens and becomes sticky around the injured area forming a semi-solid mass (otherwise known as a blood clot or thrombus). This prevents bleeding and limits blood loss. In thrombophilia, clotting most often occurs within an unbroken vessel at an inappropriate time and place.

Blood clots may form within all blood vessels, but typically occur in the large vessels in the brain, heart, lungs, legs and arms. Clots in the leg or the arm can usually be detected by ultra-sound examination. In addition, clots can be detected by X-ray examination by injecting a substance into the blood to make the clot stand out. A blood clot in the lung is more difficult to diagnose. A radioactive substance may be used to test for a mismatch between the distribution pattern of blood flowing in the vessels and of the air filled spaces in the lungs. Such a mismatch would indicate the presence of a clot.

What are the symptoms?

Clots interfere with normal blood flow by completely or partly obstructing vessels. This leads to a build-up of blood before the clot (in an artery) or behind the clot (in a vein) causing pain and swelling of the tissue around the area. Clots deprive tissues and organs of oxygen and nutrition and may cause permanent damage particularly if the clot obstructs a vital organ, such as in certain parts of the brain. They may grow very quickly and can break apart sending small pieces of the clot (known as emboli) through the blood stream. These emboli can then become lodged in smaller vessels distant from the clot of origin. An emboli lodging within vessels of the lung is known as a pulmonary embolus. By blocking the blood to the lung and depriving the body of oxygen, they may be rapidly life threatening. An emboli lodging in brain vessels can cause a stroke (see entry). These are serious conditions which may be associated with a high risk of disablement. Consequently, thrombotic events may require immediate medical attention and appropriate treatment.

Factor V Leiden

In the most common form of inherited thrombophilia factor V Leiden, the leg may become swollen, painful and red. In some individuals, part of the clot may be dislodged and flow to the lung (pulmonary embolism) which may make breathing difficult. Depending on the size of the blood clot, some individuals may experience severe respiratory difficulty whereas in others breathing problems may be barely noticeable. In very rare cases, a clot might occur in the arm, brain, or liver. Since clots associated with factor V Leiden form in the veins (which take blood to the heart), there is no increased risk of coronary occlusion. However, pregnancy loss and other obstetric complications may occur at an increased rate in women with factor V Leiden.

Factor V Leiden is associated with a change in the factor V gene, otherwise known as factor V Leiden mutation. The factor V gene codes for a coagulant protein. A change (or 'Leiden' mutation) in the factor V gene may lead to an increased tendency to develop an inappropriate blood clot. The first blood clot usually occurs in adulthood (approximately forty-five years) but may occur in premature babies, neonates and pregnant women. The risk of developing a clot is thought to increase with age. Factor V Leiden is associated with both deep and superficial blood clots in the legs (venous thromboses).

What are the causes?

The clotting process (otherwise known as haemostasis) functions as a careful balance between flowing and stopping; and between clotting and dissolving/ reabsorbing clots. The consistency of blood is regulated and maintained by the careful balance of a number of different proteins; some of which are involved in clot formation (coagulation) and some of which are involved in the prevention of clot formation and dissolving of formed clots (anticoagulation or fibrinolysis). Thrombophilia may occur in association with abnormalities in either coagulation or anticoagulation proteins.

Specific genes are known to code for coagulation and anticoagulation proteins. Individuals who inherit changes (or mutations) in these genes may have an increased risk or 'predisposition' to developing thrombophilia compared to the rest of the population. However, in certain individuals there may only be a small increased risk to health. Other people who have inherited a predisposition to thrombophilia will not experience any symptoms and will remain healthy and unaffected. In particular, the predisposition to forming a thrombosis may be of relevance to our lifestyles as for example the increased risk to air travellers.

How is it diagnosed?

Doctors may suspect an inherited predisposition to blood clotting in individuals who have a blocked blood vessel at a young age, or have recurrent thromboses, or have a strong family history of clotting disorders (such as stroke, pulmonary embolism, or deep vein thrombosis). A diagnosis may be made by screening for inherited blood-clotting factors which are known as Factor V Leiden and Prothrombin gene mutation. Screening for these genetic changes should form part of the routine investigations for individuals who present with thromboses.

Inheritance patterns and prenatal diagnosis

Inheritance patterns

Factor V Leiden is inherited as an autosomal dominant trait. However, in some cases, factor V Leiden may be increased as an autosomal recessive trait. This is associated with a greater risk of venous thrombosis.

Prenatal diagnosis

Prenatal testing is not routinely available.

Prothrombin gene mutations

The prothrombin gene is responsible for the production of a protein, which helps the blood to clot. A change (or mutation) in the prothrombin gene may lead to an increased tendency to develop an inappropriate blood clot. Clinically this may manifest in a similar manner to patients with factor V Leiden. Again the risk of thrombosis is heightened in pregnancy. This condition is associated with an increased risk of blood clots in the legs (venous thrombosis) and lungs (pulmonary embolism), but most frequently in the deep veins of the lower extremities. Blood clots may occur in the head (cerebral vein thrombosis). However, clots may also occur in unusual sites, particularly cerebral sinus vein thrombosis.

Inheritance patterns

Prothrombin is inherited as an autosomal recessive trait. Individuals with a mutation in both prothrombin genes, one on each chromosome, are called homozygous and they appear more likely than heterozygotes (one mutated gene and one normal gene) to develop thrombosis.

Prenatal diagnosis

Prenatal testing is not routinely available.

Medical text written February 2002 by Contact a Family. Approved February 2002 by Professor F Cotter, Professor of Experimental Haematology, St Bartholomew's Hospital, London, UK.

Further online resources

Medical texts in *The Contact a Family Directory* are designed to give a short, clear description of specific conditions and rare disorders. More extensive information on this condition can be found on a range of reliable, validated websites. Further information on these resources can be found in our **Medical Information on the Internet** article on page 21.

Support

There is no specific support organisation for Hereditary Thrombophilia but Stroke support organisations (see entry) can provide help if Hereditary Thrombophilia disorders lead to stroke. Families can use Contact a Family's Freephone Helpline for advice, information and, where possible, links to other families.

HERPES VIRUS INFECTION

Background

Herpes Simplex virus infection usually occurs on the face causing small blisters which are called 'cold sores'.

The virus can infect any area of skin, but as it is passed on by direct skin-to-skin contact with friction, it occurs mostly on the face, hands (where it causes Herpetic Whitlows) or, once a person is sexually active, on the genital or anal areas where it is called Genital Herpes Simplex. Cold sores are extremely common: by the age of twelve years, one quarter of children have contracted the virus, mostly without having any noticeable symptoms.

What are the symptoms?

A first infection can include fever and ulcers inside the mouth and throat. When that is over, some Herpes Simplex virus remains in the nearest ganglion (nerve junction) and can occasionally reactivate. This may be in response to illness, tiredness, or sunlight/UV light directly on the skin. The symptoms usually reappear at the same place or nearby. For example, when the virus has been caught on the face, reappearing cold sores are usually on the lips or nose. Very rarely it will reactivate in one eye which can be serious as, without treatment, it can cause corneal ulceration with possible scarring leading to impaired vision.

How is it diagnosed?

A GP can diagnose the condition by carrying out a Fluorescein Stain. Very rarely, and seriously, a facial infection will reactivate in the brain causing severe headache, and altered consciousness (see entry, Encephalitis).

How is it treated?

Herpes Simplex sores on the skin will get better without treatment. However, during the first infection, antiviral tablets may be given to speed up healing. Repeat outbreaks are usually treated symptomatically with an ointment containing lignocaine to relieve itchiness or soreness and a lubricant cream to prevent the skin at the edge of the scab from drying and cracking.

Inheritance patterns and prenatal diagnosis

Inheritance patterns

Not applicable.

Prenatal diagnosis

Not applicable.

Medical text written October 2003 by the Herpes Viruses Association. Approved October 2003 by Dr G Kinghorn, Clinical Director of Genito-Urinary Medicine, Royal Hallamshire Hospital, Sheffield, UK.

Further online resources

Medical texts in *The Contact a Family Directory* are designed to give a short, clear description of specific conditions and rare disorders. More extensive information on this condition can be found on a range of reliable, validated websites. Further information on these resources can be found in our **Medical Information on the Internet** article on page 21.

Support

Herpes Viruses Association
41 North Road, London N7 9DP   Tel: 0845 123 2305 Helpline
Tel: 020 7607 9661 Main office and membership   e-mail: info@herpes.org.uk
Web: http://www.herpes.org.uk
The Association is a National Registered Charity No. 291657, established in 1985. The patient-run association offers support and information by telephone and website to people with herpes viruses. Members receive leaflets, quarterly journals and invitations to seminars, workshops and get-togethers. A local contact scheme operates nationally. Professionals can order posters and hand-outs, details on request. The Association has approximately 1,300 members.
Group details last updated February 2008.

HIRSCHSPRUNG'S DISEASE

Hirschsprung's disease: Hirschsprung disease; Aganglionosis

Background

Hirschsprung's disease (HD) affects 1 in 4,500 live births throughout the world. In the United Kingdom this equates to about one hundred and fifty to two hundred new cases of HD each year.

HD affects the nerves of the large intestine (colon). The main function of the colon is to conserve water and salt, to store faecal material (stool), and to regulate its release from the body. Normally, special nerve cells (ganglion cells) control the pushing movement of muscles in the colon and push stool to the anus where it is expelled from the body.

What are the symptoms?

In most patients, HD presents during the first few days of life. The major symptoms of HD in a newborn baby are delayed first bowel movement (meconium stools), abdominal distension, chronic constipation, and reluctance to feed. Babies with HD may grow and develop more slowly than other babies (failure to thrive). Older children may experience constipation alternating with bouts of diarrhoea, vomiting, pain and anaemia (a shortage of red blood cells) due to blood being lost in the stool, so-called enterocolitis. When HD becomes apparent during adolescence and adulthood (acquired HD), constipation and anaemia are characteristic symptoms. Acquired HD may be associated with diseases such as Parkinson's disease, scleroderma (see entries), intestinal pseudo-obstruction, Chagas disease and drug induced or idiopathic (cause unknown) constipation.

The length of colon affected can vary from child to child. Short segment HD involves up to a third of the large intestine and long segment HD involves more than one third, often the whole colon. Seventy per cent of individuals have short segment HD. The severity of the symptoms is not always consistent with the length of the intestinal segment involved but children with the whole colon involved tend to have more severe symptoms.

What are the causes?

In HD, ganglion cells can be missing (aganglionosis) from any part of the colon. As a result the colon becomes narrowed and unable to function. Stool will then build up behind the narrowed segment and that part of the colon becomes chronically distended, giving rise to the name 'megacolon.' Usually, a ring of muscles just inside the body (internal anal sphincter) automatically relaxes to allow stool to pass from the body. In HD the internal anal sphincter becomes permanently contracted and so stool either passes through with great difficulty or not at all.

How is it diagnosed?

Currently, HD diagnosis is confirmed with a rectal biopsy. This involves taking a small biopsy from the wall of the last part of the large bowel (rectum) to confirm the absence of ganglion nerves.

How is it treated?

If HD is not treated, stool can fill the large intestine causing problems such as infection, bursting of the colon and sometimes death. Individuals diagnosed with HD, therefore, require immediate surgery. A number of procedures have been developed and vary depending upon on the extent of the involvement of the colon, the age of the patient, the severity of the symptoms and presence of enterocolitis. In the majority, surgery essentially involves removal of the aganglionic segment and rejoining of the remaining bowel. This is effective in relieving the obstruction caused by HD and most children with HD may lead near normal lives thereafter. Drug therapy is not effective.

Inheritance patterns and prenatal diagnosis

Inheritance patterns

HD develops in children before they are born and is due to genetic factors. It is not caused by anything the mother did while pregnant. HD is a familiar disease, but is not inherited as a simple Mendelian trait.

Prenatal diagnosis

None at present.

Medical text written January 2003 by Contact a Family. Approved January 2003 by Professor P Milla, Professor of Paediatric Gastroenteritis and Nutrition, Great Ormond Street Hospital, London, UK. **Last updated November 2006 by Dr Nikhil Thapar, Clinician Scientist and Honorary Consultant in Paediatric Gastroenterology and Nutrition, Great Ormond Street Hospital, London, UK.**

Support

Support for families of children with Hirschsprung's disease can be obtained from Tummy Trouble (see entry, Gut Motility disorders).

HISTIOCYTOSIS

Background

Histiocytoses are diseases affecting white blood cells known as histiocytes, which are part of the immune system and, in health, are important in preventing infections. There are several types of histiocyte and therefore several diseases caused by these cells and known as histiocytoses.

Langerhans Cell Histiocytosis (LCH) is a disease in which cells called Langerhans dendritic cells, accumulate with other immune cells in many parts of the body and cause damage by the release of chemicals. In health, Langerhans cells form a network in the skin and take up foreign materials such as bacteria or viruses that break through the skin surface. The Langerhans cells then move to lymph nodes to start a protective immune response. In the disease, the skin, bone and pituitary gland are commonly affected but the disease may also involve the lungs, intestines, liver, spleen, bone marrow and brain. The disease is found in children and adults but tends to be most severe in very young children.

Haemophagocytic Lymphohistiocytosis (HLH) affects histiocytes called macrophages. Affected children have fever, enlargement of the liver and spleen, a fall in the number of normal blood cells, abnormalities of blood clotting and accumulation of macrophages and other white blood cells within affected tissues, typically the bone marrow, liver, spleen and lymph nodes.

Rosai-Dorfman disease, also called **Sinus-Histiocytosis with Massive Lymphadenopathy**, presents with swelling of lymph nodes (typically in the neck), and there may be general ill health with fever and changes in the blood count. The disease is generally self-limiting, but, on occasion, treatment with corticosteroids, cytotoxic drugs, surgery or radiotherapy may be used.

In **Malignant Histiocytosis** some subtypes of acute myeloid leukaemia affect cells of monocyte/macrophage lineage. Other malignant disorders of histiocytes are extremely rare.

What are the symptoms?

Langerhans Cell Histiocytosis (LCH) is very variable, ranging from single skin or bone lesions, which may not require treatment, to a severe illness involving many organs. The pituitary gland is commonly affected and this results in failure to concentrate the urine so that patients drink and excrete large volumes, producing diabetes insipidus (not sugar diabetes, or diabetes mellitus), and they may not grow because of a lack of growth hormone. Other symptoms are very variable because of the large number of organs that may be affected.

What are the causes?

The cause of Langerhans Cell Histiocytosis (LCH) is unknown.

Haemophagocytic Lymphohistiocytosis (HLH) occurs in primary and secondary forms and secondary HLH typically occurs in people receiving treatment that reduces the function of the body's immune system (immune suppressive therapy), or children born with inherited abnormalities of immunity.

How is it treated?

In time Langerhans Cell Histiocytosis (LCH) may burn itself out, but there may be long-standing problems due to damage caused by the disease process. Not all patients require specific treatment but, when this is indicated, they usually receive corticosteroids (Prednisolone) or cytotoxic drugs.

Haemophagocytic Lymphohistiocytosis (HLH) is often triggered by viral or other infection and improvement generally follows treatment for the precipitating infection and removal of immune suppression, if this is possible. Primary HLH is a genetic disorder which usually presents in very young children with no other known immune abnormality. This group of children usually require drug treatment with corticosteroids, cytotoxic chemotherapy, or the immune suppressive drugs antithymocyte globulin and Cyclosporin. Children with a definite family history (familial HLH) generally receive a bone marrow transplant once the disease is adequately controlled and this is often also necessary for other children with primary HLH who do not have a definite family history.

Medical text written December 1997 by Dr David Webb Consultant Paediatric Haematologist/Oncologist, Great Ormond Street Hospital, London, UK. **Last updated September 2006 by Professor Peter Beverley, Institute for Vaccine Research, Newbury, UK.**

Further online resources

Medical texts in *The Contact a Family Directory* are designed to give a short, clear description of specific conditions and rare disorders. More extensive information on this condition can be found on a range of reliable, validated websites. Further information on these resources can be found in our **Medical Information on the Internet** article on page 21.

Support

Histiocytosis Research Trust

18 Western Road, Wylde Green, Sutton Coldfield B73 5SP   Tel: 0121 355 5137
e-mail: info@hrtrust.org   Web: http://www.hrtrust.org
The Trust is a National Registered Charity, No. 1004546 formally, established in 1991. It has strong links with international organisations and three trustees are members of the UK Children's Cancer Study Group. The Trust operates a 'Circle of Friends' for mutual support through information, newsletters, family days and road shows led by Histiocytosis experts. Funding from the Trust supports the UK & Ireland epidemiology research project at Newcastle University and a project by a team of research scientists at the Univerity of Lausanne in Switzerland. The Trust is in touch with well over 100 families around the UK and overseas.
Group details last confirmed October 2007.

HOLOPROSENCEPHALY

Holoprosencephaly: HPE

Background

Holoprosencephaly is a series of brain malformations in which there is incomplete development of the cerebrum. Its effects on the child range from severe and lethal to mild and almost undetectable.

In the most severe form, alobar HPE, the cerebrum is a single U-shaped mass rather than being divided into right and left hemispheres. Death most often occurs before, during or soon after birth. Among liveborn children with alobar HPE, half will have died by four months of age, but survival for several years has been noted in a number of children.

What are the symptoms?

In the most severe form, alobar HPE, those who survive have profound learning disabilities, but they usually acquire some basic developmental skills such as visual tracking, responding to sound, smiling, and evidence of memory. Most children with alobar HPE will have seizures requiring anticonvulsant medication. Muscle spasticity and periods of marked irritability are present to some degree in all, and various medications may be helpful. Episodes of irregular breathing and pulse rate and highly variable body temperature control can be particularly troublesome. Endocrine problems due to pituitary gland malfunction may require medication. Feeding is a major problem, and tube or gastrostomy feeding is often recommended. Constipation is a common problem but can be managed successfully.

In the less severe forms, semilobar and lobar HPE, there is more complete development of the brain into right and left hemispheres. In general, survival is longer than with the alobar type, with many affected children living into adulthood, although early death is also common. Some degree of learning disability is the rule and is often severe. These more severely affected children will have many of the same problems found with alobar HPE. With the mildest forms of lobar HPE, the child may have minimal disability and a normal lifespan.

Associated malformation of the face is often present, most commonly with the alobar type of HPE. Cyclopia, median cleft lip and/or single nostril are markers of the severe end of the spectrum. Absent sense of smell and single maxillary central incisor tooth may be the only facial features at the mild end of the spectrum.

Inheritance patterns and prenatal diagnosis

Inheritance patterns

HPE has many different causes. In most instances it is only one feature of a multiple malformation or chromosomal anomaly syndrome (particularly trisomy 13, Patau syndrome).

When it is an isolated malformation or accompanied only by face malformation it may be caused by an abnormal dominant gene (several different dominant genes have now been identified, but more remain to be discovered). It has also occurred among the offspring of mothers with insulin-dependent diabetes mellitus or severe alcohol abuse.

Prenatal diagnosis

Prenatal detection of alobar HPE is possible by targeted ultrasound examination. The milder forms of HPE may not be evident by prenatal ultrasound examination.

Medical text written May 1998 by Dr M Barr Jr, University of Michigan, USA. **Last reviewed March 2006 by Dr A Habel, Consultant Paediatrician, Great Ormond Street Hospital, London, UK and Dr M Lees, Consultant Geneticist, Institute of Child Health, London, UK.**

Further online resources

Medical texts in *The Contact a Family Directory* are designed to give a short, clear description of specific conditions and rare disorders. More extensive information on this condition can be found on a range of reliable, validated websites. Further information on these resources can be found in our **Medical Information on the Internet** article on page 21.

Support

The support group covering Holoprosencephaly is currently in abeyance. This medical description is retained for information purposes. Families can use Contact a Family's Freephone Helpline for advice, information and, where possible, links to other families. Contact a Family's web-based linking service Making Contact.org can be accessed at http://www.makingcontact.org

HOLT-ORAM SYNDROME

Background

Holt-Oram syndrome is the name given to the association of heart defect and upper limb abnormality first described by Dr Mary Holt and Dr Samuel Oram in 1960. Since then over a hundred cases have been reported worldwide.

What are the symptoms?

Heart defects

Most commonly this is an Atrial Septal Defect (ASD) or Ventricular Septal Defect (VSD) but other congenital heart defects can occur. Conduction disturbances are often seen on electrocardiography (ECG) and may be the only sign of the condition.

Upper limb

Abnormalities affect both arms but not necessarily in the same way. The thumb is usually abnormal (triphalangeal, like a finger), absent or underdeveloped. The forearms may be short or absent. The shoulders are usually narrow and sloping. The mildest abnormalities are abnormal bending of the fifth finger and limited rotation of the joints of the forearms which allow palm of hands to face up. The most severe involve absence of all or part of the upper limb.

The lower limbs are not involved and no other abnormalities are seen in the Holt-Oram syndrome.

Inheritance patterns and prenatal diagnosis

Inheritance patterns

The Holt-Oram syndrome is inherited by autosomal dominant inheritance. Where a child is born to an affected parent there is a 50/50 chance of that child having the syndrome. Because the severity is very variable a mildly affected parent may have a severely affected child. The causative gene has been identified (TBX5) enabling molecular genetic diagnosis.

Prenatal diagnosis

In families where the specific gene mutation has been identified, genetic prenatal diagnosis may be available by Chorionic Villus Sampling.

Medical text written May 1995 by Dr R Newbury-Ecob. **Last updated December 2005 by Dr R Newbury-Ecob, Consultant in Clinical Genetics, Clinical Genetics Service, St Michael's Hospital, Bristol, UK.**

Further online resources

Medical texts in *The Contact a Family Directory* are designed to give a short, clear description of specific conditions and rare disorders. More extensive information on this condition can be found on a range of reliable, validated websites. Further information on these resources can be found in our **Medical Information on the Internet** article on page 21.

Support

There is currently no effective support group covering Holt-Oram syndrome. This medical description is retained for information purposes. Families can use Contact a Family's Freephone Helpline for advice, information and, where possible, links to other families. Support specifically for the upper limb abnormalities of Holt-Oram Syndrome is available from Reach (see entry, Upper Limb Abnormalities.) Contact a Family's web-based linking service Making Contact.org can be accessed at http://www.makingcontact.org

"The money's made a lot of difference: it's eased the pressure on my husband. We were relying on him to do overtime to see us through, but now he's able to spend more time with my daughter who has cerebral palsy, and my little boy." A parent who received specialist benefits advice from our helpline.

HUGHES SYNDROME

Hughes syndrome: Antiphospholipid syndrome

Background

Antiphospholipid syndrome (APS), also known as Hughes syndrome, was first described by Dr Graham Hughes in 1983. The features of the clinical picture may include migraine, memory loss, vein and artery thrombosis, multiple sclerosis (see entry) and recurrent miscarriage. Because one of the main features includes thrombosis (blood clotting), the name 'sticky blood syndrome' has often been used as a shorthand to describe this condition. APS affects individuals from all ethnic backgrounds. Although individuals of all ages may be affected, most show features of APS before forty-five years.

What are the symptoms?

The increased tendency to form blood clots in individuals with APS may have a devastating effect on any part of the body including the legs, arms, chest, head and a number of 'internal' organs such as the kidney and liver. Commonly, blood clots develop in the veins of the legs (deep vein thrombosis) causing pain and swelling, usually starting in the calf. Clotting in the leg may happen once or several times. Clots may also occur in the lung (pulmonary embolus). Clotting in arteries can result in strokes (see entry) or heart attacks.

The brain appears to be particularly sensitive to the clotting. In fact, in many patients, headaches precede clotting for many years. Also, individuals may develop slight speech disturbance, suggestive of a mini-stroke or epilepsy. Other forms of brain abnormality include movement disorders such as chorea (St Vitus Dance) and more commonly, fits. Epilepsy (see entry) in all its forms, from petit mal (absences) through to grand mat (fits), are important features of Hughes syndrome.

Women affected with APS may experience spontaneous pregnancy losses due to complications in the blood supply to the unborn baby in the womb. If clotting occurs in the placenta, the baby's blood supply is cut-off leading to miscarriage, possibly late in pregnancy. Many women with a history of recurrent miscarriages have no other features of APS. In fact, many women may never develop any medical problems outside pregnancy. In some patients, therefore, the only manifestation of APS is recurrent miscarriage. In other women, headaches or speech or visual/neurological disturbances may be the primary feature.

The manifestations of APS are very variable and a number of other clinical features have been described including 'blotchiness' of the skin (livedo reticularis) such as blue knees or purplish vein coloration on the back of the wrists. Another feature is a low platelet count or 'thrombocytopenia.'

APS is an autoimmune syndrome. The function of the immune system is to keep the body healthy by producing antibodies to fight germs and viral infections from the environment. Occasionally, however, certain types of antibodies mistakenly attack the body's own healthy tissues. One such type, Antiphospholipid antibodies, target body fats known as phospholipids. Phospholipids are important 'membranes' in platelets and blood vessels.

Some patients with APS are also affected with Lupus (see entry), another disorder of the immune system causing fatigue, rashes, joint pain and in some patient's potentially life-threatening kidney and brain disease. It is a relatively common condition which particularly affects women. Lupus and Antiphospholipid syndrome are related. In both, there is an over-production of antibodies. However, most individuals with APS do not go on to develop more generalised Lupus.

How is it diagnosed?

There are two very positive features of recognizing APS. Firstly, that the cause 'sticky blood' can be detected by simple blood tests, and secondly that the disease is treatable.

Most laboratories and clinics use two main tests:
- 'Anticardiolipin' (aCL);
- The somewhat confusingly named 'lupus anticoagulant' which although a more complicated clotting test, is far less reliable.

As these tests give different results, individuals may be offered both tests to confirm a diagnosis of APS. Because antibody levels can fluctuate, and even disappear, the blood tests for APS need to be repeated at least six weeks from the first time of testing to make sure that they are still positive.

A diagnosis of APS depends upon an individual's past medical history, medical examination and the results of specific tests. Although many people have not heard of APS, Professor Hughes predicts that 'sticky blood' will be the most common autoimmune disease of the 21st century, more prevalent than Multiple Sclerosis, Lupus and Rheumatoid Arthritis. The good news, however, is that this condition is treatable and patients show incredible improvement once they are taking the right medication.

How is it treated?

Any decision about treatment at a particular time (such as pregnancy) depends upon the individual's previous medical history, as well as laboratory and clinical criteria. Anti-clotting (anticoagulation) treatment is available to prevent the symptoms of APS. This works through the action of thinning the blood. The three drugs most commonly used for this purpose in the treatment of APS are aspirin, warfarin (Coumadin) and heparin. For most patients long term low-dose aspirin (75-100 mg daily) is sufficient. For those with more severe clotting problems, warfarin is mandatory.

Inheritance patterns and prenatal diagnosis

Inheritance patterns

None.

Prenatal diagnosis

None available.

Medical text written December 2001 by Contact a Family. Approved December 2001 by Dr G Hughes. **Last updated March 2006 by Professor G Hughes, Consultant Rheumatologist, London Lupus Centre, London Bridge Hospital, London, UK.**

Further online resources

Medical texts in *The Contact a Family Directory* are designed to give a short, clear description of specific conditions and rare disorders. More extensive information on this condition can be found on a range of reliable, validated websites. Further information on these resources can be found in our **Medical Information on the Internet** article on page 21.

Support

Hughes Syndrome Foundation

Louise Coote Lupus Unit, Gassiot House, St Thomas' Hospital, London SE1 7EH

Tel: 020 7188 8217   e-mail: hsf@btconnect.com   Web: http://www.hughes-syndrome.org

The Foundation is a National Registered Charity No. 1089077, established in 2001. It offers a network of support groups, information and education to the medical profession and supports research into the condition. It publishes a newsletter three times a year and has information available, details on request. The Foundation receives over 1,500 enquiries a year.

Group details last updated March 2007.

HUNTINGTON'S DISEASE

Huntington's disease: Huntington's Chorea

Background

Huntington's disease (HD) is a neurodegenerative disorder, characteristically affecting the basal ganglia but also affecting other areas of the central nervous system. Onset is usually in the fourth or fifth decade, but HD can occur more rarely in childhood or extreme old age.

Juvenile Huntington's disease

The age of onset of HD is very variable: in around five per cent of cases onset can be under the age of twenty years and in very rare cases the onset can be under the age of ten years. Given that juvenile HD (JHD) is defined by the age of onset, it follows that at any one time a number of people who started with HD under the age of twenty years will now be over twenty years old.

What are the symptoms?

The clinical features of Huntington's disease (HD) can be thought of as a triad of emotional, cognitive and motor disturbances. Early in the disease, manifestations can include subtle changes in co-ordination, minor involuntary movements, difficulty thinking through problems, and often, a depressive and irritable mood. In the middle stage, the involuntary movement disorder, known as chorea may become prominent, and difficulty with voluntary motor activities will be more evident. Speech becomes more difficult to understand, and there can be difficulties in swallowing safely. As cognitive and movement problems increase, the patient will be unable to work. Patients in the late stage may have chorea but quite often have slow voluntary movements. They may become unable to speak and bedridden and will require total care. The cognitive impairment is selective so, despite their difficulties with speech, patients may still be able to understand conversations, although their ability to make decisions will be very impaired. The duration of the disease is variable with an average of fifteen years frequently quoted.

In general, young people with juvenile HD (JHD) are likely to present with difficulties at school and perhaps some clumsiness. The earliest features of JHD are not very specific so parents may experience a delay between being concerned about a young person and a genetic test being performed; this may lead to frustration.

The neurological features of JHD differ from that seen with the more classical onset. Slowness of movement, called bradykinesia, rather than chorea is likely to occur; as the disease progresses, there may be slurred speech, dystonic movements (which result in the limbs adopting unusual postures) and muscle cramps. Epilepsy is more likely to occur in JHD than in the more usual form.

As with the adult form of HD the intellectual problems are selective which may manifest itself as behavioural problems.

How is it diagnosed?

A genetic test can answer the question as to whether or not the gene for Huntington's disease (HD) is present but the decision about whether or not the condition has started remains a matter of judgement. As the early features of juvenile HD (JHD) are often non-specific, doctors may wait for clearer neurological signs before doing the test.

How is it treated?

There is no cure for Huntington's disease (HD) at present, though much research is underway. None the less it is possible to find out whether one has the responsible mutation (or genetic change) which causes the disease. This predicts with great accuracy whether someone will develop the disease or not. The knowledge that one has the gene for HD can create significant difficulties with insurance, employment and relationships, even before the disease manifests itself, and it is important to seek expert advice from a clinical genetics centre about such tests.

Inheritance patterns and prenatal diagnosis

Inheritance patterns

It is inherited as an autosomal dominant so that each child of an affected parent has a fifty per cent risk of inheriting the disease.

Prenatal diagnosis

Where a parent has had a predictive test showing gene carrier status the fetus may be tested for the presence of the gene.

Where the parent does not want a predictive test for himself/herself exclusion testing on the fetus may be possible. This will either give the fetus a low risk status or the same risk status as the parent. Further details can be obtained from regional genetic centres

Medical text written November 1996 by Dr S Simpson. **Last updated September 2005 by Dr S Simpson, Associate Specialist/ Senior Lecturer in Clinical Genetics Clinical Genetics, Grampian University Hospitals, Aberdeen, UK. Additional material on Juvenile Huntington's disease written July 2005 by Dr D O Quarrell, Consultant in Clinical Genetics, Centre for Human Genetics, Sheffield, UK.**

Further online resources

Medical texts in *The Contact a Family Directory* are designed to give a short, clear description of specific conditions and rare disorders. More extensive information on this condition can be found on a range of reliable, validated websites. Further information on these resources can be found in our **Medical Information on the Internet** article on page 21.

Support

Huntington's Disease Association

Downstream Building, 1 London Bridge, London SE1 9BG   Tel: 020 7022 1950
Fax: 020 7022 1953   e-mail: info@hda.org.uk   Web: http://www.hda.org.uk
The Association is a National Registered Charity No.296453, established in 1971. It offers Regional Care Advisers, branches and support groups throughout England and Wales together with care, advice and support. It publishes a twice-yearly newsletter and has a wide range of information available, details on request. The Association has over 8,500 members.
Group details last confirmed January 2007.

Scottish Huntington's Association

Thistle House, 61 Main Road, Elderslie, Johnstone PA5 9BA   Tel: 01505 322245
Fax: 01505 382980   e-mail: sha-admin@hdscotland.org   Web: http://www.hdscotland.org
The Association is a Scottish Registered Charity No. SCO10985, established in 1989. It offers a network of local self-help groups together with support and information for families and professionals. The Association has a national youth project manager, youth adviser and a dedicated website section for children and young people. It publishes a bi-annual newsletter and has information available, details on request.
Group details last confirmed August 2007.

Huntington's Disease Association of Northern Ireland

c/o Contact a Family, 209-211 City Road, London EC1V 1JN
Tel: 028 9022 1950   e-mail: s.mckay1@ntlworld.com
The Association is a support network, established in 1976 working with the Northern Ireland Regional Genetic Centre. It offers support, information and care for families. It also promotes research and knowledge about the condition. It has information available, details on request. The Association responds to the needs of approximately 180 families.
Group details last confirmed February 2008.

HYDRANENCEPHALY

Background

Hydranencephaly is a condition that usually arises in mid/late pregnancy when a major reduction of blood supply to the brain results in loss of most of both cerebral hemispheres. The more primitive parts of the brain (brain stem, thalamus and cerebellum) are preserved so that usually the vital functions of breathing, heart function and temperature regulation are possible. The head mainly contains fluid-filled cavities with occasional small islands of the cerebral cortex remaining, particularly at the back of the head. A related condition of multiple cavities with more surviving brain is referred to as multicystic encephalomalacia.

What are the symptoms?

The head may be abnormally small, of normal size, or large. Sometimes there may be an excessive rate of head growth and it may be appropriate to insert a shunt system for hydrocephalus (see entry) to prevent the development of a very large head. Babies with hydranencephaly normally show no visual behaviour or other developmental progress. The life span is usually limited to weeks or months but is sometimes longer. Those who are most severely affected may die at birth.

This description is of the severe or true hydranencephaly. Some babies have more surviving brain tissue and may therefore have some developmental progress and a longer life span.

What are the causes?

Despite the severity of the damage, there is often no clear event in the pregnancy to account for it. There may be a reduction in fetal movements but the mother is often quite unaware of any problem. Recognised causes of this condition include intrauterine death of a twin, or blood loss from the baby by a number of possible mechanisms. A number of acute illnesses/injuries to the mother in pregnancy have been reported in the medical literature in a small number of instances but this is uncommon. Ultrasound late in pregnancy can show the abnormality but may only be perestablished in high-risk situations. Sometimes a similar situation may occur as a result of severe damage during or immediately after birth but the acute brain illness is then obvious.

Sometimes the birth is slow and it may be mistakenly thought that the damage occurred at birth.

Despite the severity of the brain defect, the baby may apparently behave normally at birth with spontaneous limb movements, crying and sucking. Others are unwell with spasticity and feeding and temperature regulation problems.

Epileptic seizures (see entry, Epilepsy) are quite common and may not respond to treatment.

How is it diagnosed?

The diagnosis is made by ultrasound of the head. In severe cases, the EEG shows no activity.

Inheritance patterns and prenatal diagnosis

Inheritance patterns

This is regarded as an acquired disorder and not genetic. A small number of families have had more than one baby with the disorder. It occurs equally in boys and girls. Counselling is therefore directed to looking for obstetric factors which might be identifiable and remediable. However, this is in the main a sporadic disorder with a low risk of recurrence.

Prenatal diagnosis

Late ultrasound in utero may find the abnormality.

Medical text written May 2003 by Professor B Neville, Professor of Paediatric Neurology, Institute of Child Health, London, UK.

Further online resources

Medical texts in *The Contact a Family Directory* are designed to give a short, clear description of specific conditions and rare disorders. More extensive information on this condition can be found on a range of reliable, validated websites. Further information on these resources can be found in our **Medical Information on the Internet** article on page 21.

Support

There is no UK support group for Hydranencephaly. There is an International Hydranencephaly Support Group with a UK contact person. Families can use Contact a Family's Freephone Helpline for advice, information, access to the UK contact person for Hydranencephaly and, where possible, links to other families. Contact a Family's web-based linking service Making Contact.org can be accessed at http://www.makingcontact.org

Cross referrals to other entries in the Contact a Family Directory are intended to provide relevant support for these particular features of the disorder. Organisations identified in these entries do not provide support specifically for Hydranencephaly.

HYDROCEPHALUS

Background

Hydrocephalus is commonly, but inaccurately, known as 'water on the brain.' A watery fluid known as Cerebro Spinal Fluid (CSF) flows through narrow passageways in the brain from one ventricle to the next, out over the inside of the brain and down the spinal cord. CSF is continuously absorbed into the blood stream and the amount of pressure is kept within a narrow range. If the flow of fluid is obstructed at any point, it accumulates in the ventricles causing them to enlarge and compress surrounding brain tissue. In babies - but not older children or adults - the head will enlarge.

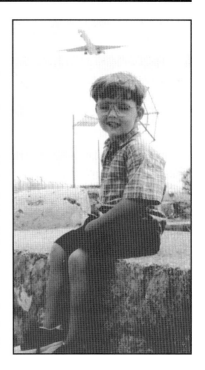

What are the symptoms?

Symptoms caused by raised pressure usually improve, but other signs of brain damage may remain. These can include subtle learning difficulties.

Shunts can become blocked leading to headache, nausea, photophobia, inertia and irritability. Chronic infection may cause gradual deterioration in overall performance. Medical advice should be sought in cases of mental or physical deterioration in those with shunts, or if a shunt blockage is suspected.

What are the causes?

The most common causes of hydrocephalus in children are infections such as Meningitis or Toxoplasmosis, premature birth, head injury, or a brain tumour. In adults, hydrocephalus can be caused by meningitis, trauma or brain tumour, or blockage of the brain pathways (aqueduct stenosis) of unknown cause. Other forms of hydrocephalus in adults include 'Normal Pressure Hydrocephalus' (see entry) which is suggested by deterioration in mental performance including memory, walking difficulties, and sometimes incontinence. Once diagnosis is confirmed, the treatment is shunting, preferably using an adjustable valve.

How is it treated?

Treatment may be by insertion of a 'shunt' to redirect the excess CSF or, in some cases, by a third ventriculostomy. This will entail a hole being made in the floor of the 3rd ventricle to allow CSF flow.

Inheritance patterns and prenatal diagnosis

Inheritance patterns

Genetically related (inherited) hydrocephalus is very rare, and is usually X-linked: only boys are affected. It is usually accompanied by abduction of the thumbs. Diagnosis is determined by genetic tests.

Spina Bifida is genetically determined and the risk is higher in families who already have a member with this or a similar condition. Almost all people with spina bifida have hydrocephalus, though this might not require treatment .

Prenatal diagnosis

Often, but not always, seen prenatally on ordinary ultrasound. Fetal Anomaly Scanning is recommended in suspected cases.

Medical text written July 1994 by the Association of Spina Bifida and Hydrocephalus. Approved by Dr C.R.Birch, Consultant Physician and Medical Director, Grantham and District Hospital, Grantham, UK. **Last updated June 2003 by Dr R Bayston, ASBAH and Senior Lecturer, University of Nottingham Medical School, Nottingham, UK.**

Further online resources

Medical texts in *The Contact a Family Directory* are designed to give a short, clear description of specific conditions and rare disorders. More extensive information on this condition can be found on a range of reliable, validated websites. Further information on these resources can be found in our **Medical Information on the Internet** article on page 21.

Support

Support and advice about Hydrocephalus are available from ASBAH (Association for Spina Bifida and Hydrocephalus), see entry, Spina Bifida.

HYPEREKPLEXIA

Hyperekplexia: Startle disease

Background

Hyperekplexia means excessive startle. An affected adult will startle easily at a sudden sound or unexpected touch or bump and may fall and be injured. The fall will be stiff and fast. This excessive startle will be much improved if the individual takes daily clonazepam. Although doctors may have some concerns about addiction, benzodiazepine drugs do not appear to be a significant risk in this condition.

What are the symptoms?

If an unborn baby is affected, this may first be noticed by the mother as abnormal intrauterine movements. When an affected baby is born he or she is often stiff. For those unfamiliar with hyperekplexia, this feature may easily be misdiagnosed as spastic cerebral palsy. When a baby startles, there may be a tendency for severe nonepileptic convulsions with increased stiffness and fast quivering. Even a bath may bring this on. Such convulsions are potentially dangerous because they induce a severe syncope with lack of oxygen to the brain. Individuals with hyperekplexia are of normal intelligence and may live as fulfilling and productive lives as other people.

What are the causes?

The underlying basis for the hyperekplexia is a mutation or change in the gene involved in the action of a neurotransmitter called glycine. Glycine is called an inhibitory transmitter because it damps down the action of nerve cells particularly in the spinal cord and brain stem. When glycine receptors are impaired, the nerve cells are too easily excited. When strychnine poisoning was more prevalent something very similar would happen, since strychnine targets these same glycine receptors. So much so, that scientists call the receptors involved in hyperekplexia strychnine-sensitive glycine receptors. It is now possible for mutations in the genes controlling these receptors to be detected, admittedly in only a few laboratories.

How is it diagnosed?

Diagnosis of hyperekplexia is carried out by a nose tap test. Tapping the tip of the nose of an unaffected baby will elicit no response, but in hyperekplexia there is an obvious startle response which is repeated each time the nose is tapped.

Hyperekplexia is often misdiagnosed as epilepsy (see entry). Accurate recognition of hyperekplexia in a newborn is important to avoid an incorrect diagnosis of epilepsy with consequent treatment with anticonvulsants. Secondly, so that children with hyperekplexia are monitored and treated so that abnormal startle reactions do not lead to convulsions and falls. Thirdly, in some families to identify those at risk in any subsequent pregnancy.

How is it treated?

There are two effective treatments for hyperekplexia. First, if the baby is flexed, that is made to curl up by pressing the head towards the knees, the convulsion will stop. Secondly, if the doctor starts the baby on clonazepam the excessive startle will diminish and the condition will improve as the baby grows older. Some develop minor complications such as a hernia.

Inheritance patterns and prenatal diagnosis

Inheritance patterns

Hyperekplexia is usually inherited as an autosomal dominant trait. Affected families are advised to seek genetic counselling. In some cases, hyperekplexia occurs sporadically.

Prenatal diagnosis

Possible in some cases.

Medical text written February 2002 by Professor J B P Stephenson, Honorary Professor of Paediatrics in Neurology, University of Glasgow, Glasgow, UK.

Further online resources

Medical texts in The Contact a Family Directory are designed to give a short, clear description of specific conditions and rare disorders. More extensive information on this condition can be found on a range of reliable, validated websites. Further information on these resources can be found in our **Medical Information on the Internet** article on page 21.

Support

Hyperekplexia Contact Group

216 Westcott Crescent, London W7 1NU   Tel: 020 8578 0456 (7.30-10pm)

This is a small contact group. It offers support by telephone and letter. It has information available, details on request, please send SAE.

Group details last confirmed September 2007.

HYPERMOBILITY SYNDROME

Background

The term hypermobility means 'more movement' and describes the over flexibility of the joints. Hypermobility syndrome (HMS) is an inherited condition in which the protein, collagen, which makes up the supporting tissues and gives the body its intrinsic toughness, is more flexible than usual. A person's joints are lax because they have inherited looser and more brittle connective tissue, particularly their ligaments, tendons, joints and muscles. This makes the joints more mobile, sometimes unstable, thus more prone to injury. Some children may have more severe problems that may lead to subluxations (excessive movement of the joint) or dislocations. The degree of difference and hence tendency towards painful symptoms, varies from individual to individual, even in the same family.

HMS is a composite term bringing together all the various difficulties that may arise in people with hypermobile or lax joints. It is probably more correct to refer to the Hypermobility syndromes (in the plural) as a family of genetically based conditions which differ not only in the particular protein affected, but also in the degree of difference of formation. At one end of the spectrum are the diseases with potentially serious complications such as Marfan syndrome or Ehlers-Danlos syndrome Vascular Type (formally EDS IV) see entries. At the other end, are what is now called, on good evidence, the Benign Joint Hypermobility syndrome (BJHS) or Ehlers-Danlos Hypermobile Type (formerly EDS III). These may cause troublesome and persistent problems but do not affect the vital organs and thus do not pose a serious threat to life. Because joints do not look arthritic, the problem is often overlooked by health professionals.

What are the symptoms?

Although some people with Benign Joint Hypermobility syndrome (BJHS) have little or no trouble, in others, pain can be a recurring or, in some, even a constant, problem. This renders them prone to the effects of injury and over-use resulting in acute (short-term) pain on prolonged and unaccustomed exercise. More chronic day-in day-out pain is also seen and may require a variety of measures, which can vary from one person to another in order to control it.

About seven to ten per cent of the population of school age children has been found to have loose joints and occasional pain in the joints and muscles, especially after exercise or at night. Most children with HMS complain of joint pains in the evening or sometime after exercise. These mostly occur in the knees, ankles or non specifically in the legs. Sometimes the joints may appear to be swollen. Swelling should be treated as with any injury: RICE (rest, ice, compression, and elevation). Young children generally do not like ice, but it can be used with older children. If the joint pain persists, a doctor should be consulted.

Children with HMS often wake up in the night complaining of pain in the legs. For the majority, symptoms will improve as they grow older as their supporting muscles and ligaments get tighter and this is why this used to be called 'Growing Pains' which we now feel does not exist.

How is it treated?

Others may need to have physiotherapy, occupational therapy, podiatry and pain management through psychology, to help strengthen specific muscles that stabilise joints and cope with their pain. It is important that children continue to exercise and do sport to build up their strength and muscles.

Inheritance patterns and prenatal diagnosis

Inheritance patterns

As in most of the Heritable Disorders of Connective Tissue the pattern of inheritance for the Benign Joint Hypermobility syndrome is autosomal dominant. This means that fifty per cent of the offspring may carry the gene for the condition. In the BJHS this does not imply that they will inherit any particular set of symptoms, since many affected people have no ill effects at all. It used to be thought that Hypermobility simply represented the upper end of the normal distribution of joint laxity. This view has been challenged as increasing evidence emerges to suggest that it is also a genetic connective tissue disorder, (albeit a relatively mild one) in its own right.

Prenatal diagnosis

If a genetic form of Hypermobility is known to affect members of a family, referral for genetic advice or counselling should be sought.

Medical text written October 2001 by Professor Rodney Grahame. **Last updated October 2006 by Professor Rodney Grahame, Emeritus Professor Rheumatology, University College London, London, UK and Dr Nathan Hasson, Paediatric Rheumatologist, Great Ormond Street Hospital, London, UK.**

Support

Hypermobility Syndrome Association
12 Greenacres, Hadleigh, Benfleet, Essex SS7 2JB
Tel: 0845 3454465 (Mon-Fri & first Sat of month, 9am-1pm)
e-mail: info@hypermobility.org   Web: http://www.hypermobility.org
The Association is a National Registered Charity No. 1011063, established in 1992. It offers support and information together with contact opportunities where possible. It promotes knowledge and understanding within the medical community and the public at large, gives life-style information and holds yearly residential weekends for member families. It publishes a newsletter and has information available, details on request. The Association has over 700 members.
Group details last updated October 2007.

HYPOCHONDROPLASIA

Hypochondroplasia: HCH; Hypochondrodysplasia

Background

Hypochondroplasia is a rare inherited skeletal dysplasia (condition of abnormal bone growth or development) causing short stature due to short limbs. HCH affects both males and females. Where the only feature in an individual is short stature, medical intervention may not be sought. As a result, the incidence of HCH is uncertain. It is thought that its incidence could be 1 in 15,000 to 1 in 40,000 live births.

What are the symptoms?

To a lesser or greater degree, the features of HCH may include:

- Short stature with an adult height in the range of 128 -151 cm (4 feet, 2 inches to 4 feet 11 inches);
- Disproportionate arms and legs with short, broad hands and feet;
- Macrocephaly (an enlarged head);
- Limitation of elbow movement;
- Lordosis (exaggerated curvature at the lower end of the spine);
- Increased joint mobility;
- Learning problems (it has not yet been determined whether this is in fact a feature of HCH).

What are the causes?

About seventy per cent of people with HCH have an identifiable mutation in the FGFR3 gene on chromosome 4p16.3. The remaining thirty per cent will either have a so far unrecognised mutation in the FGFR3 gene or a mutation in other as yet unidentified genes.

How is it diagnosed?

It is not easy to diagnose HCH in very young children and may be even be missed in adults. Diagnosis is made by identifying the features known to appear in HCH together with radiological (x-ray) findings. DNA based testing can confirm the FGFR3 gene mutation but cannot be used to eliminate the diagnosis.

How is it treated?

HCH is not a curable condition and treatment will be symptomatic for specific features. Surgical limb lengthening can be considered but is a drawn out and painful process. Human growth hormone therapy has been given to some children with HCH but has shown mixed results. A range of support for families, based on perception of the effect of being of short stature at school and in the wider community, is available. Families can obtain information about aids to ameliorate difficulties in access and operation of equipment from local and national statutory and support organisations.

Inheritance patterns and prenatal diagnosis
Inheritance patterns
Autosomal dominant.
Prenatal diagnosis
Chorionic Villus sampling or amniocentesis is available if a parent has HCH and a mutation in the FGFR3 gene has been identified. Where the mutation has not been identified ultrasound scanning is the only method of prenatal testing. Families where HCH has been diagnosed should seek genetic counselling.

Medical text written September 2004 by Contact a Family. Approved September 2004 by Dr M Wright, Consultant Clinical Geneticist, Institute of Medical Genetics, International Centre for Life, Newcastle upon Tyne, UK.

Further online resources
Medical texts in *The Contact a Family Directory* are designed to give a short, clear description of specific conditions and rare disorders. More extensive information on this condition can be found on a range of reliable, validated websites. Further information on these resources can be found in our **Medical Information on the Internet** article on page 21.

Support
As Hypochondroplasia is a condition of restricted growth, support and advice is available from the Restricted Growth Association (see entry, Restricted Growth).

HYPOMELANOSIS OF ITO

Hypomelanosis (Pigmentary Mosaicism): Hypomelanosis of Ito; Incontinentia Pigmenti Achromians; Ito syndrome; Pigmentary Mosaicism

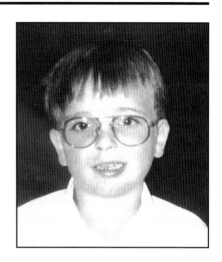

Background

The condition was first described by Dr M Ito in 1951 and confirmed to have wider systemic associations by Dr T Hamada in 1967. Hypomelanosis of Ito is a group of disorders with the common feature of increased and/or decreased pigmentation in a characteristic formation with swirling patterns around the trunk and linear patterns down the legs and arms. Dermatologists call this pattern Blaschko's Lines.

Very few epidemiological data exist on this condition but it appears to be the third most common neurocutaneous disorder (after Neurofibromatosis type 1 and Tuberous Sclerosis, see entries) and is diagnosed in 1 in 8,000 - 10,000 unselected patients in a paediatric hospital.

What are the symptoms?

Associated abnormalities are thought to occur in approximately seventy per cent of patients with cutaneous lesions. These include:

- Neurological problems (the most common) with:
    - Learning difficulties (see entry, Learning Disability)
    - Seizures
    - Hemimegalencephaly (asymmetric enlarged brain) see entry
- Visual problems (see entry, Vision disorders in childhood):
    - Retinal pigment abnormalities
    - Myopia
    - Night blindness
    - Detached retina
- Orthopaedic problems:
    - Scoliosis, see entry
    - Hemihypertrophy (asymmetry of growth on either side of the body)
- Precocious puberty (see entry, Premature Sexual Maturation)
- Cardiac abnormalities (see entry, Heart defects).

What are the causes?

It is now known that this pattern occurs when there are two populations of cells in the skin which vary because of a chromosome problem in one set of cells or a gene change. When skin cells are cultured, an abnormal chromosome pattern is found in one population of cells in about one third of affected individuals. The typical skin manifestations usually present in the first year of life with up to fifty-four per cent being noticeable at birth.

Inheritance patterns and prenatal diagnosis

Inheritance patterns

This is not an inherited disorder since the error occurs after conception in one population of cells. Reports in older literature of familial cases are unconvincing. It is believed to be due to chromosomal mosaicism and sporadic gene changes. The specific gene(s) involved has not been confirmed. Pigmentary mosaicism should be differentiated from the X-linked condition of Incontinentia Pigmenti where the areas of increased pigment are preceded by blistering skin lesions.

Prenatal diagnosis

This condition is not recurrent. Management in future pregnancies should be routine, although detailed scanning may provide added reassurance.

Medical text written October 1999 by Professor Dian Donnai, Consultant Clinical Geneticist, St Mary's Hospital, Manchester, UK. **Last updated October 2006 by Dr Wayne Lam, Consultant Clinical Geneticist, Western General Hospital, Edinburgh, UK.**

Support

HITS (UK) Family Support Group
99 Great Cambridge Road, London N17 7LN   Tel: 01803 401018
Tel: 020 8352 1824 Helpline (Tuesdays 7-9pm)   Fax: 020 8352 1824
Web: http://www.e-fervour.com/hits   e-mail: tgrant@hitsuk.freeserve.co.uk
The Group was originally, established in 1991 and was re-established in 1999. It offers support by telephone, letter, e-mail, internet chatroom, monthly live chats and an annual Ito family day (usually in London). It also offers links with other similarly affected families where possible. It publishes two newsletters a year with additional information available on request.
Group details last updated January 2007.

HYPOPLASTIC LEFT HEART SYNDROME

Background

Hypoplastic Left Heart syndrome (HLHS) is a complex congenital heart condition that occurs in 1 in 5,000 children. Currently two hundred diagnoses are made annually in the United Kingdom and Ireland.

What are the symptoms?

The syndrome is a collection of malformations on the left side of the heart:

- Mitral Atresia/Stenosis;
- Hypoplastic Left Ventricle;
- Aortic Atresia/Stenosis;
- Hypoplastic Aorta.

How is it diagnosed?

Currently fifty per cent of cases are diagnosed antenatally. Early detection gives parents the opportunity to explore treatment options - palliative surgery at birth, comfort care or termination of pregnancy.

In cases were the diagnosis is made after birth parents have less time to make a treatment choice as the baby is often critically ill. They have the options to offer comfort care or palliative surgical treatment.

How is it treated?

Transplantation of the heart in infants is not an option commonly offered in the UK as there are not enough donor hearts available to make this a viable option.

Surgical treatment is presently offered in a limited number of paediatric cardiac centres in the UK. The complexity of the surgery requires a dedicated, experienced team approach, this often means that families choosing the surgical path for their child will have to travel to receive treatment.

Palliative Surgery is offered as a three stage procedure:

1. The Norwood procedure is offered within the first week of life, with babies being maintained on Prostaglandin therapy until surgery is possible. The children are hospitalized for many weeks after this stage of surgery. This operation holds the highest risks. The cardiac team will quote an individual risk for each child as the complexity of the condition may vary.

2. Cavopulmonary Shunt or Hemi Fontan procedure is offered between three to nine months of age. This operation holds lower risk than stage one and the children are usually in hospital for a shorter period of time.

3. The Fontan Procedure is offered from three years upwards. Children are often hospitalized for some weeks following surgery because of the dramatic change in circulation. Post third stage the children generally have a great

563

deal more energy.

The overall survival of all the children starting down the surgical treatment path is that sixty per cent will still be alive at five years of age.

A majority of children recover well from surgery and lead happy full lives. Their exercise tolerance is reduced but they still enjoy normal childhood games. Indications are that they are broadly within the normal educational range of their peers. It is difficult to predict the future for children with HLHS. The indications from experience in the US is that the children will need a heart transplant in their late teens or early twenty's. Presently the oldest child in the UK is only ten years old.

Medical text written February 2002 by Left Heart Matters. Approved February 2002 by Dr O Stumper, Consultant Paediatric Cardiologist, Birmingham Children's Hospital, Birmingham, UK.

Further online resources

Medical texts in *The Contact a Family Directory* are designed to give a short, clear description of specific conditions and rare disorders. More extensive information on this condition can be found on a range of reliable, validated websites. Further information on these resources can be found in our **Medical Information on the Internet** article on page 21.

Support

Little Heart Matters

11 Greenfield Crescent, Edgbaston, Birmingham B15 3AU   Tel: 0845 330 9801
Tel: 0121 455 8982   Fax: 0845 330 9802   e-mail: info@lhm.org.uk
Web: http://www.lhm.org.uk
Little Heart Matters, formerly Left Heart Matters, is a National Registered Charity No. 1058735, established in 1996. It provides support for families affected by any single ventricle heart condition such as Hypoplastic Left Heart Syndrome, Tricuspid Atresia, Complex Pulmonary Atresia and Double Inlet single ventricle conditions. It offers support by telephone, e-mail and letter and linking families where possible. It publishes a bi-monthly newsletter and has information available, details on request. Please send SAE. The organisation has over 700 families and 150 professionals in membership.
Group details last confirmed June 2007.

HYPOSPADIAS

Background

In Hypospadias, the urethral opening, normally situated at the tip of the glans penis, is located somewhere on the under side of the penis, in mild cases on the glans itself and in more severe cases at some point along the penile shaft.

Hypospadias is one of the most common congenital deformities, affecting approximately 1 in 200 new born boys.

What are the symptoms?

The foreskin is also almost always affected, being imperfectly formed beneath, and this deformity may be more obvious than the hypospadias itself In a proportion of cases, there is also a downward bend on the shaft of the penis (chordee) which becomes exaggerated during penile erections and as a general rule the more severe the hypospadias the greater the chance of significant chordee. The position of the urethral opening may result in a downwardly deflected urinary stream, a problem for boys once they are toilet trained, while chordee may cause difficulties with sexual intercourse during adult life.

In the most severe cases, which are fortunately rare, the gender of the child may not be certain in which event further investigation will be required.

What are the causes?

Except in a small number of cases where there is a positive family history, the cause is unknown.

How is it treated?

Surgical repair is always merited in the event of a misdirected urinary stream or of chordee and may also be advisable for cosmetic reasons in patients without these complications. Although many forms of hypospadias repair have been devised, in practice only about half a dozen are currently commonly performed, some in a single-stage and others as two-stage procedures.

As a rule, the repair is undertaken some time between twelve months and two years of age or after toilet-training, between three and four years of age. Although repair is usually successful, there is an appreciable (fifteen to thirty per cent) rate of complications requiring further surgery. Because the foreskin may be needed for the repair, the child should not be circumcised. After treatment, most boys will appear almost normal and should not have any long-term problems.

Occasionally, following several unsuccessful attempts at repair, there may be insufficient penile skin remaining to achieve a satisfactory result. Tissue grafts may be taken from other areas such as the lining of the mouth or the skin behind the ear and used to replace the deficient skin on the penis.

Inheritance patterns and prenatal diagnosis
Inheritance patterns
Possibly familial
Prenatal diagnosis
None

Medical text written June 2001 by Mr A M K Rickwood, Consultant Urological Surgeon, Alder Hey Children's Hospital, Liverpool, UK. **Last updated March 2006 by Miss H F McAndrew, Consultant Paediatric Urologist, Alder Hey Children's Hospital, Liverpool, UK.**

Support
Hypospadias Support Group
20 Barnack Close, Padgate, Warrington WA1 4JH   Tel: 01925 496510
e-mail: support@hypospadias.co.uk   Web: http://www.hypospadias.co.uk
This is a small support group, established in 1999. It offers support by telephone and letter. It has information available, details on request. The group is in touch with over 200 families.
Group details last confirmed October 2006.

HYPOTHALAMIC HAMARTOMA

Background

Hypothalamic hamartoma (HH) describes a benign brain tumour located close to or within the hypothalamus. This part of the brain produces the hormones that control body processes such as thirst, hunger, sex hormone regulation and the release of hormones from the thyroid and adrenal glands.

What are the symptoms?

HH is associated with a number of features including difficult epilepsy, particularly gelastic (laughing) seizures, behavioural problems and precocious (early) puberty. The range and severity of these features varies widely between individuals.

Gelastic seizures are a rare type of seizure characterised by highly distinctive episodes of laughter. Seizures are both unpredictable and unprovoked, lasting for between five to sixty seconds, and occurring frequently. Because the seizures resemble natural laughter, parents and doctors initially may not recognize the child's behaviour as a seizure, thus delaying a diagnosis of HH.

In later childhood, the laughing seizures become longer and more severe, taking on less natural sounds and the pattern of seizure may change. Gelastic seizures may progress to complex partial seizures, tonic, atonic or generalized tonic-clonic seizures. In a generalized tonic-clonic (also known as a grand mal) seizure, individuals usually cry out, lose consciousness and fall to the floor. Their muscles stiffen (tonic phase) and then their arms and legs will jerk and twitch (clonic phase). The development of seizures associated with HH varies widely between individuals.

Later in development a child with HH may start to show outbursts of aggression and rage (often referred to as hypothalamic rage) and poor social adjustment. Increasing problems with learning often occurs. Some HH children display signs of autism. The frequency of the seizures and the subsequent disruption to the brain often makes deterioration of the child's mental state unavoidable.

Individuals with HH may show precocious puberty (see entry, Premature Sexual Maturation). This is the onset of puberty with the development of secondary sex characteristics before the age of eight years in girls and nine years in boys. Girls may begin their periods before nine years of age. Early onset of puberty is associated with a number of problems. Although an early growth spurt can initially cause tall stature, rapid bone maturation causes growth to cease too early resulting in short adult stature. The early appearance of breasts or periods in girls and increased libido in boys may cause emotional distress for both children and parents.

How is it treated?

In most individuals, surgery to remove the hypothalamic hamartoma is extremely difficult. Furthermore, seizures resulting from HH are notoriously difficult to control with medical treatment.

Inheritance patterns and prenatal diagnosis

Inheritance patterns

Some people with HH are affected by an extremely rare genetic disorder, Pallister Hall syndrome. In most other cases, HH occurs sporadically.

Prenatal diagnosis

Although little is known about the origin of hamartomas, some research suggests that hypothalamic hamartomas develop during the sixth or seventh week of gestation. Diagnosis of a hypothalamic hamartoma might be possible on antenatal ultrasound, but this would need to be confirmed using magnetic resonance imaging (MRI).

Medical text written July 2003 by Contact a Family. Approved July 2003 by Dr T McShane, Consultant Paediatric Neurologist, John Radcliffe Hospital, Oxford, UK.

Support

HHUGS UK

c/o Contact a Family, 209-211 City Road, London EC1V 1JN   Tel: 01494 728564
e-mail: hhugsuk@hotmail.com   Web: http://www.hhugs.com

HHUGS UK (Hypothalamic Hamartoma Uncontrolled Gelastic Seizures) is a National Registered Charity No. 1098698 providing support by letter, telephone and e-mail. Families will be linked where possible and if requested. The group has information and access to medical advice and is in touch with over 20 families.

Group details last confirmed October 2006.

HYPOTONIA

Background

Hypotonia literally means low muscle tone. Therefore, this is not a diagnosis of a particular condition but simply refers to low muscle tone that can be caused by a variety of conditions. In addition, its severity can vary significantly from mild to severe hypotonia depending on the underlying cause.

What are the symptoms?

Hypotonic infants appear floppy. Head control may be poor causing the head to fall forwards, backwards and/or sideways in the sitting position. This is also reflected in head lag when pulling the child to sitting from lying down. Often children with hypotonia have good arm and leg movements but the range of movements at the hips, elbows and knees is excessive. Poor sucking and chewing may also be present in some hypotonic children depending on the underlying condition.

In a significant number of cases hypotonia is merely a reflection of increased joint laxity and the term 'benign hypermobility syndrome' is often used in these cases. The joint laxity and associated hypotonia tends to improve with time in the majority of children.

What are the causes?

In some children the hypotonia might be the manifestation of an underlying more complex condition, such as the chromosomal disorder Prader-Willi syndrome (see entry). In other children it might be a sign related to a form of Cerebral Palsy (see entry) in which hypotonia is associated with reduced or abnormal movements. In other cases a neuromuscular disorder, i.e. a condition affecting muscles or the way muscles are activated by nerves, has to be suspected such as Spinal Muscular Atrophy (see entry) or a congenital myopathy. The long term prognosis in these latter cases is usually more severe compared to those cases with Benign Hypermobility syndrome especially if the breathing and feeding muscles are significantly affected.

The underlying problem is therefore significantly different in different children and this does affect the long term prognosis.

How is it diagnosed?

In some cases the doctors involved might decide to do specific tests to rule out individual conditions; in other instances the clinical examination will be sufficient to rule out serious conditions, and it should be noticed that the majority of children with hypotonia do not have a severe underlying problem.

Inheritance patterns and prenatal diagnosis

Inheritance patterns

Depends on the underlying condition.

Prenatal diagnosis

Depends on the underlying condition.

Medical text written October 2002 by Professor F Muntoni. **Last updated September 2007 by Professor F Muntoni, Professor and Consultant in Paediatric Neurology, Imperial College of Science, Technology and Medicine, Hammersmith Hospital, Neuromuscular Centre, London, UK.**

Support

UK Congenital Hypotonia Network

Flat 1, Frognal Court, 158 Finchley Road, London NW3 5HL

e-mail: nbrownlaco@hotmail.com   Web: http://freespace.virgin.net/bch.hypotonia

The UK Congenital Hypotonia Network is an informal parent support group providing support and information to families. There are over 50 families in touch with the network. Initial contact is by e-mail or by phone to the Contact a Family Freephone Helpline 0808 808 3555.

Group details last confirmed August 2007.

ICHTHYOSIS

Background

Ichthyosis is the term used to describe persistent scaling of the skin due to an abnormality of the outermost part of the skin, the epidermis.

What are the symptoms?

It occurs as a result of a number of different genetic disorders. Some of these conditions primarily affect the skin such as: **Ichthyosis Vulgaris; X-linked Ichthyosis; Non-Bullous Ichthyosiform Erythroderma; Lamellar Ichthyosis; Bullous Ichthyosiform Erythroderma and Harlequin Ichthyosis** others are multisystem disorders and these include: **Netherton syndrome** (see entry); **Sjögren Larsson syndrome; Refsum disease; Trichothiodystrophies; Neutral Lipid Storage disease; KID syndrome and Conradi-Hunermann syndrome** (see entry) , as well as a number of other more rare disorders.

This is a large mixed group of conditions all having in common scaling of the skin, which can vary in severity from mild scaling in ichthyosis vulgaris to the severe large dark plate-like scales of lamellar ichthyosis. In some, the skin is inflamed and red as well as scaly (non-bullous ichthyosiform erythroderma and Netherton syndrome, in others it may blister (bullous ichthyosiform erythroderma).

What are the causes?

The cause of inherited ichthyosis may be due to an abnormal protein in the skin (one of the keratins) or due to an abnormality of lipids, which act as a 'cement' in the skin. In some of the disorders the basic abnormality is recognised, but in others it is unknown. Hopefully, through research, we will understand more about these disorders with the development of more specific treatments and better prenatal diagnosis by molecular genetic testing.

Inheritance patterns and prenatal diagnosis

Inheritance patterns

This depends on which form of Ichthyosis is involved. The underlying genetic mutations have now been discovered for most forms of Ichthyosis; these can be mutations in lipids, proteins, enzymes or transport molecules.

Prenatal diagnosis

For a few of the conditions prenatal diagnosis may be available, but for most this is not possible yet.

Medical text written December 1997 by Professor J Harper, Consultant In Paediatric Dermatology, Great Ormond Street Hospital, London UK. **Last updated July 2003 by Dr D Paige, Consultant in Dermatology, Royal London Hospital, London, UK.**

Further online resources

Medical texts in *The Contact a Family Directory* are designed to give a short, clear description of specific conditions and rare disorders. More extensive information on this condition can be found on a range of reliable, validated websites. Further information on these resources can be found in our **Medical Information on the Internet** article on page 21.

Support

Ichthyosis Support Group
PO Box 7913, Reading RG6 4ZQ   Tel: 0845 602 9202   e-mail: isg@ichthyosis.org.uk
Web: http://www.ichthyosis.org.uk
The Group is a National Registered Charity No. 1084783, established in 1997. It offers support by telephone and letter and linking families where possible. It publishes a newsletter and has information available, details on request. The Group has over 400 members.
Group details last confirmed August 2007.

It is not known how many children live without a diagnosis of their condition or disorder. Contact a Family produce a guide 'About Diagnosis', call the helpline for a copy.

IMMUNE (IDIOPATHIC) THROMBOCYTOPENIC PURPURA

Background

Childhood Immune (Idiopathic) Thrombocytopenic Purpura (ITP) is a disorder that affects around 4 in 100,000 children every year. Its basis is a dramatic and often sudden reduction in the number of circulating platelets - small blood cells that have an essential role in the prevention of bleeding.

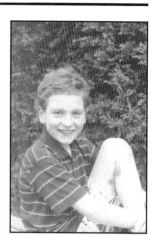

What are the symptoms?

It comes to light by the occurrence of abnormal bruising, small pin-point bleeds into the skin, and occasionally nosebleeds or other abnormal blood loss. It often follows a viral infection.

What are the causes?

The platelets are removed by the body's immune system - they are inappropriately regarded as foreign tissue. ITP is thus a type of auto (self) immune disorder.

How is it treated?

In most children (ninety per cent) ITP is a trivial and rapidly self-correcting condition (acute ITP), and nearly all cases eventually spontaneously resolve within six months. The risk of serious bleeding in childhood ITP is very small, and usually no treatment is necessary other than avoidance of Aspirin or Ibuprofen, which increase the risk of bleeding. Treatment, if required, is aimed at suppressing the immune system to stop the inappropriate destruction of platelets, and so reduce the risk of serious internal bleeding. This is usually achieved by either a short course of steroid drugs (by mouth or, occasionally, by intravenous drip) which suppress the immune system, or an intravenous injection of large amounts of human, soluble antibody protein from blood donors (intravenous immunoglobulin) which interfere with the destruction of platelets by the immune system.

In a few children, ITP runs a more prolonged course (chronic ITP). These children will usually be investigated further, including having a bone marrow test. They are also more likely to require treatment. Some children, with persistent and troublesome ITP associated with bleeding, may be treated by removal of the spleen - the site of inappropriate platelet destruction.

Inheritance patterns and prenatal diagnosis
Inheritance patterns
None
Prenatal diagnosis
Not applicable

Medical text written 1996 by Professor Sir John S Lilleyman, Mark Ridgewell Professor, Barts and the London NHS Trust, London, UK. **Last updated January 2005 by Dr S Ball, Consultant Paediatric Haematologist, St George's Hospital Medical School, London, UK.**

Support
The ITP Support Association
'Synehurste', Kimbolton Road, Bolnhurst , Bedford MK44 2EW   Tel/Fax: 0870 777 0559
e-mail: shirley@itpsupport.org.uk   Web: http://www.itpsupport.org.uk
The ITP Support Association is a National Registered Charity No. 1064480, established in 1995. It offers support by a helpline, patient/parent contact network, access to an ITP Nurse, and Annual Convention. It funds ITP Research, a National ITP database and ITP Seminars for health professionals. The Association has been in touch with approximately 3,000 affected families and ITP Societies in the USA, Israel and Holland and has around 1,600 members.
Group details last updated September 2007.

INCONTINENTIA PIGMENTI

Incontinentia Pigmenti: Bloch-Sulzberger syndrome

Background

Incontinentia Pigmenti (IP) is a rare inherited ectodermal dysplasia (see separate entry) affecting the skin, hair, teeth and central nervous system. The disorder is almost always lethal in males due to miscarriage or still birth. This results in IP affecting females almost exclusively. IP is found in all populations but is more common in caucasian people.

What are the symptoms?

The hallmark features of IP appear on the skin:

- In the first months of life, abnormal redness of the skin followed by lines of blisters in all areas except the face;
- As the blisters heal, warty areas occur on the skin of the hands and feet. In most cases these clear by six months of age;
- Hyperpigmented (excessive brown pigmentation) streaks or whorls occurring mainly on the trunk but which fade in adolescence. These give IP its name;
- From adolescence into adulthood, pale hairless streaks or patches.

Other features of IP include:

- Absent, small or misshapen teeth;
- Alopecia (baldness) or coarse, wiry dull hair;
- Ridging or pitting of the nails;
- Excessive formation of blood vessels in the retina of the eye.

Occasionally, seizures and learning disability occur. Life expectancy is normal.

What are the causes?

IP is caused by mutations in the NEMO gene on the X chromosome also known as the IKBKG gene.

How is it diagnosed?

IP is diagnosed by the characteristic clinical signs of the disorder and a skin biopsy can provide confirmation. In about eighty per cent of people mutations can be identified in the NEMO gene for which tests are available. Tests can be used to confirm a diagnosis or carrier status.

How is it treated?

In the early months of life, management aims to reduce the risk of infection of the blisters which can be treated by topical (locally applied) medications and discomfort relieving baths. However, such treatment does not shorten the period in which blisters occur.

Pigmented areas can be treated with skin camouflage (see "Visible Difference" in section, Procedures and Management), cosmetics or obscuring clothes. These areas fade over time. In the case of scalp alopecia, a dermatologist can prescribe wigs from a hospital medical appliance department or a prescription can be used for a reduction of the cost of a wig from a commercial retailer.

Numerous eye abnormalities in IP have been reported but the majority of them result from retinal vascular defects of the retinal blood vessels. These abnormalities, which can lead to retinal detachment, represent the major cause of severe visual defects in IP. The mechanisms causing the changes in blood vessels are not fully understood. The natural history of retinal disease in IP is also unknown and optimal treatment of the retinal problems is not clear at present. There are reports of successful treatment of proliferative retinopathy (overgrowth in the retinal blood vessels) with cryotherapy (freezing treatments) and laser.

An ocular examination should be performed as soon as possible after birth and IP patients should be followed carefully by an ophthalmologist. Parents may be advised of the possibility of retinal detachment and the need to have any apparent changes checked promptly. A study from Sweden of 30 patients with IP recommended eye screening for all newly diagnosed infants with IP and the female offspring of affected women. The following scheme was suggested: ocular examination as soon as possible after birth, monthly until three to four months, three monthly until one year of age, and then bi-annually until three years of age.

Our knowledge of the natural history of the retinal changes in IP is not complete and the duration of screening remains unclear and therefore ophthalmology review should perhaps be continued on an annual basis throughout childhood. An ocular assessment can be arranged by referral to the local ophthalmology department from a GP, clinical geneticist, paediatrician/neonatologist or dermatologist.

Continued evaluation by a dentist should take place and referral to a speech therapist for help with speech and feeding should be part of the management/treatment process.

Inheritance patterns and prenatal diagnosis
Inheritance patterns
X-linked dominant.
Prenatal diagnosis
This is available for families already known to be affected.

Medical text written October 2005 by Contact a Family. Approved October 2005 by Dr H Stewart, Consultant Clinical Geneticist and Lead Clinician, Churchill Hospital, Oxford, UK. Additional ophthalmic information written March 2006 by Mr C. E. Willoughby, Consultant Ophthalmic Surgeon, Royal Victoria Hospital, Belfast, UK and Senior Lecturer in Ophthalmology, Queen's University, Belfast, UK.

Further online resources

Medical texts in *The Contact a Family Directory* are designed to give a short, clear description of specific conditions and rare disorders. More extensive information on this condition can be found on a range of reliable, validated websites. Further information on these resources can be found in our **Medical Information on the Internet** article on page 21.

Support

Support for Incontinentia Pigmenti is available from the Ectodermal Dysplasia Society (see entry, Ectodermal Dysplasia). Contact a Family's web-based linking service Making Contact.org can be accessed at http://www.makingcontact.org

IRRITABLE BOWEL SYNDROME

Background

Irritable Bowel syndrome (IBS) is a painful and disabling abdominal illness, characterised by frequent attacks of abdominal pain or discomfort associated with disturbances in defecation which might be either constipation, diarrhoea or a combination of the two.

What are the symptoms?

Sufferers also frequently complain of a variety of other symptoms, especially fatigue, breathlessness, headaches, indigestion, backache, anxiety and depression. Symptoms are commonly brought on by life changes, and difficult life situations, but they may also be triggered by food.

What are the causes?

It is one aspect of a spectrum of medically unexplained illnesses that are perhaps best regarded as visceral responses to unresolved emotional tension. As such there is a strong overlap with other illnesses such as Chronic Fatigue syndrome, Fibromyalgia syndrome, Functional Dyspepsia and many others.

Sometimes the illness appears to be instigated by an attack of gastroenteritis, but this association is more likely if a person is anxious or depressed at the time of the acute illness. Physiological studies show enhanced gastrointestinal motility and sensitivity in some patients.

How is it treated?

Symptoms may be alleviated with antispasmodics, such as Colofac and Spasmonal, and with bowel regulators, such as Imodium and Fybogel.

Severe and chronic illness is often unresponsive to such treatments, but may show improvement and resolution with more holistic therapies, such as psychotherapy, hypnotherapy and complementary therapies. For most people, IBS is a fairly benign condition that tends to recur at times of change, but for some it is profoundly disabling, ruling their lives and confining them to their homes.

Medical text last written January 2003 by Professor N W Read, Consultant Physician and Psychotherapist, Chairman of Trustees for the IBS Network.

Further online resources

Medical texts in *The Contact a Family Directory* are designed to give a short, clear description of specific conditions and rare disorders. More extensive information on this condition can be found on a range of reliable, validated websites. Further information on these resources can be found in our **Medical Information on the Internet** article on page 21.

Contact a Family Helpline 0808 808 3555

Support

The Gut Trust

Unit 5, 53 Mowbray Street, Sheffield S3 8EN

Tel: 0114 272 3253 Helpline (Mon-Fri, 6-8pm; Sat, 10am-noon)

Tel: 0114 272 3253 General enquiries only (Mon-Fri, 10am-3pm)

Fax: 0114 201 1112

e-mail: info@theguttrust.org.uk

Web: http://www.theguttrust.org

The Gut Trust is a National Registered Charity No. 1057563, established in 1996. It offers advice, information and support to those with IBS, carers and professionals. It has a network of local self-help groups and a Junior Network, and provides information for the media. The network also has a unique self management programme. It aims to raise public awareness of IBS and the issues surrounding the condition. It publishes a quarterly journal 'Gut Reaction'. It runs a befrienders and penpals service, an e-mail discussion group and has information and details of other sources of help available (details on request). The Network has around 3,000 members.

Group details last updated October 2007.

"Families from ethnic minority groups and families with pre-school children reported the highest levels of unmet need [for community equipment services]." Extract from a study conducted by the Social Policy Research Unit in 2003 - 'The Community Equipment Needs of Disabled Children and Their Families'

ISODICENTRIC 15

Isodicentric 15: idic (15)

Background

Isodicentric 15 is a rare chromosomal disorder (see the Chromosome Abnormalities section in Patterns of Inheritance). Individuals with idic (15) have an extra chromosome made up of some material from the 15th pair of chromosomes. This means that there are forty-seven chromosomes (or occasionally forty-eight or forty-nine) in these cells rather than 46. The extra piece of chromosome 15 has been duplicated end-to-end like a mirror image and is referred to as an 'isodicentric 15', an 'inverted duplication 15', or a 'supernumerary marker.'

What are the symptoms?

There are two main types of idic (15). Type 1 has the more obvious features and contains one, or more usually two, extra copies of the so-called Prader-Willi-Angelman critical region (PWACR) on Chromosome 15. This region may be deleted in patients with Prader-Willi or Angelman syndrome. Except in very rare circumstances, people with idic (15) do not have Prader-Willi or Angelman syndrome. It is the presence of this extra genetic material that is thought to account for the symptoms seen in individuals with this disorder. Those with Type 2 do not have extra copies of the PWACR. Type 2 is not usually associated with any problems but, unlike Type 1, it is often passed down through a family.

The features associated with Type 1 idic (15) are 'non-specific', in other words, they tend not to form an easily recognisable pattern (syndrome), and they are seen in a range of other disorders. The most common features are:

Hypotonia (reduced muscle tone), see entry. This is usually present at birth but usually decreases with age. Babies may appear 'floppy' and have difficulty sucking. Motor milestones (rolling over, sitting up and walking) may be delayed. Most individuals are able to walk independently.

Seizures (see entry, Epilepsy). Many, but not all, affected children and adults have seizures at some point in their lives. These may be occasional or frequent, short or prolonged.

Developmental delay (see entry, Learning Disability). Learning difficulties vary in severity but are often moderate to severe.

Autistic behaviours (see entry, Autism Spectrum disorders) are also associated with idic (15) including hand flapping, poor eye contact, repetitive or poorly developed speech and a need for 'sameness' in environment or daily routine. Although individuals do not appear unusual, many share similar facial characteristics including a flattened nasal bridge giving a 'button' nose, skin folds, called 'epicanthi' at the inner corners of the eyes, downward slanting eyes and full lips.

How is it diagnosed?

Distinguishing between the two types of idic (15) is important and is not easily done on a routine chromosome test. Laboratories will need to use additional techniques, either FISH (fluorescent in situ hybridisation) or DNA analysis, to show whether extra copies of the PWACR are present.

Inheritance patterns and prenatal diagnosis

Inheritance patterns

Type 1 idic (15) is clinically important and almost always occurs sporadically. In other words, no other family member, brother or sister, is usually affected. However, Type 2 idic (15) can be inherited. Genetic advice and counselling should be sought.

Prenatal diagnosis

This is rarely carried out specifically to look for idic (15), however, the diagnosis may be made for the first time by examination of chorionic villus samples (CVS) or amniotic fluid taken for Down syndrome screening. If the idic (15) anomaly is identified, expert advice should be sought.

Medical text last updated October 2002 written by Contact a Family and approved by Dr N Dennis, Senior Lecturer in Clinical Genetics and Hon. Consultant Clinical Geneticist, Princess Anne Hospital, Southampton, UK.

Support

As Isodicentric 15 is a Chromosome Abnormality, information, support and advice is available from Unique – the Rare Chromosome Support Group (see entry, Chromosome Disorders).

IVEMARK SYNDROME

Ivemark syndrome: Right Atrial Isomerism

Background

Ivemark syndrome is the association of congenital absence of the spleen with abnormalities predominantly of the cardiovascular system.

What are the symptoms?

The common clinical presentation is with cyanosis (blueness). Other symptoms include shortness of breath, loss of energy and cardiac failure due to the severe heart abnormalities. The cardiac abnormalities include: Pulmonary Stenosis, Total Anomalous Pulmonary Venous Drainage (TAPVD), Transposition of the great vessels, Double Outlet Right Ventricle and Atrioventricular Canal Defects. Other abnormalities include: mirror imaging of the lungs (isomerism) with both resembling a normal right lung, midline liver and varying degrees of malrotation and malfixation of the bowel.

What are the causes?

The exact cause of Ivemark syndrome is not known. To date it affects more males than females.

Inheritance patterns and prenatal diagnosis

Inheritance patterns

Not clear but probable autosomal recessive inheritance.

Prenatal diagnosis

No genetic prenatal diagnosis. Ivemark syndrome may be detected prenatally when associated with severe cardiac abnormalities seen on ultra sound scanning.

Medical text written December 1996 by Professor A Redington, Professor of Congenital Heart Disease, Great Ormond Street Hospital, London UK. **Last updated October 2001 by Dr R Yates, Consultant Paediatric Cardiologist, Great Ormond Street Hospital, London, UK.**

Further online resources

Medical texts in *The Contact a Family Directory* are designed to give a short, clear description of specific conditions and rare disorders. More extensive information on this condition can be found on a range of reliable, validated websites. Further information on these resources can be found in our **Medical Information on the Internet** article on page 21.

Support

Ivemark Syndrome Association
18 French Road, Poole, Dorset BH17 7HB Tel/Fax: 01202 699 824
e-mail: ingrid@imgladki.freeserve.co.uk
The Association is a small support group started in 1996. It offers support by telephone and letter and linking families where possible. It has information available, details on request.
Group details last updated June 2007

JACOBSEN SYNDROME

Background

Jacobsen syndrome was first described in 1973 by a Danish geneticist, Dr Petrea Jacobsen. It is a rare chromosomal condition which affects about 1 in 100,000 births.

What are the symptoms?

Jacobsen syndrome is associated with a recognisable pattern of features. The children are usually of a pleasant disposition with a characteristic face, somewhat more pear shaped than normal. However, there is also some developmental delay which basically means learning difficulties (see entry, Learning Disability) varying from mild to more severe; speech and language (see entry) may also be slow to develop and growth may be slower. However, heart problems such as an enlarged left heart syndrome (see entry, Heart Defects) can be more debilitating, sometimes requiring surgery. Blood disorders, mainly in the form of easy bruising and prolonged bleeding due to low numbers of platelets (thrombocytopenia - reduction in the number of platelets present in the blood and refered to as Paris-Trousseau syndrome) are common. Gastrointestinal problems including a narrowing of the outlet from the stomach to the small intestine (pyloric stenosis) and frequent respiratory problems also are seen. Individuals with Jacobsen syndrome may show some or all of these features although there is great variability in the number and severity of symptoms.

The life expectancy for individuals with Jacobsen syndrome currently remains unknown but is increasing as we understand more about the symptoms and how to manage them. The two most common causes of illness and death are congenital heart defects and bleeding. The improved outcomes in children with most forms of congenital heart disease, however, suggests that the outcomes for children with Jacobsen syndrome with congenital heart defects are also likely to continue to improve.

What are the causes?

It is caused by the loss of a small portion of a chromosome at conception. A chromosome is made up of DNA code in a thread-like structure present in the nucleus of most cells in the body. The DNA code in turn carry genes which are the all important instructions about how each cell in the body should divide, grow and die. Genes are 'strung' along chromosomes rather like beads are strung along a necklace. In each cell, there are twenty-three pairs of chromosomes. The body needs a full compliment of chromosomes for normal health and development. Sperm and ova ('egg cells') carry one representative of each chromosome and at fertilisation fuse to create a baby with the full number of chromosomes shared equally from both parents. In

Jacobsen syndrome a small piece of the 11th chromosome is missing (or deleted) and this causes a range of clinical features in individuals with this condition. The features are related to the genes that are absent from the small piece of chromosome 11 that is missing. The reason for the loss of the piece of chromosome is not fully understood. Jacobsen syndrome occurs more frequently in females than males.

Inheritance patterns and prenatal diagnosis

Inheritance patterns

Jacobsen syndrome occurs sporadically. For this reason, it is unusual for any other member of the family, brother or sister, to be affected.

Prenatal diagnosis

None available.

Medical text written September 2003 by Contact a Family. Approved September 2003 by Professor F Cotter, Professor of Experimental Haematology, St Bartholomew's Hospital, London, UK.

Further online resources

Medical texts in *The Contact a Family Directory* are designed to give a short, clear description of specific conditions and rare disorders. More extensive information on this condition can be found on a range of reliable, validated websites. Further information on these resources can be found in our **Medical Information on the Internet** article on page 21.

Support

Support for families of children with Jacobsen syndrome can be obtained from Unique – the Rare Chromosome Support Group (see entry, Chromosome Disorders).

JOUBERT SYNDROME

Background

Joubert syndrome is a rare neurological condition characterised by developmental delay, floppiness (see entry, Hypotonia), lack of muscle control (ataxia) and difficulty controlling horizontal eye movements (oculomotor apraxia). Other symptoms include abnormal breathing patterns (hyperpnea), kidney abnormalities and a characteristic facial appearance. Individuals with Joubert syndrome may show some or all of these features and, in addition, may be differently affected by the severity of symptoms.

What are the symptoms?

Hypotonia is particularly evident in the neonatal period and during infancy. Children may be moderately or severely affected and may lack head control, have difficulties rolling over, sitting, standing and walking. Unsteadiness (ataxia) and balance problems may also be present. Joubert syndrome also affects breathing and abnormal breathing commonly occurs during the neonatal period. This may, however, improve with age. Sadly, some infants die within the first three years from breathing problems.

Individuals with Joubert syndrome have abnormal eye movements including a squint (see entry, Vision Disorders in Childhood) with or without retinal degeneration (see entry, Vision Disorders in Childhood), and with or without congenital blindness (see entry, Vision Disorders in Childhood). Young infants with Joubert syndrome often have a characteristic appearance and have a large head, prominent forehead, high rounded eyebrows, broad nasal ridge, mild epicanthus (fold of skin on the upper eyelid), upturned nose with evident nostrils, open mouth and protruding tongue. This appearance becomes less pronounced as the child grows.

Cognitive and physical development is delayed in Joubert syndrome. Moderate to severe learning difficulties are common. Language may be delayed making it difficult for children to make themselves understood. Some children with Joubert syndrome are hyperactive, aggressive and difficult to manage whilst others are pleasant, friendly, easy to guide and socially adaptable.

What are the causes?

Joubert syndrome is caused by changes in a gene on chromosome 9. These changes affect development of certain parts of the brain including the cerebellar vermis and brain stem. The cerebellar vermis is responsible for controlling posture, co-ordinating head and eye movements and fine-tuning muscles. The brain stem is responsible for maintaining the body's involuntary functions such as heartbeat, breathing, and thermoregulation. The cerebellar vermis and brain stem are underdeveloped or absent in individuals with Joubert syndrome. Such changes may be identified on an MRI scan of the brain.

How is it treated?

Treatment for Joubert syndrome is symptomatic and supportive. Infant stimulation, physical, occupational, and speech therapy may have beneficial effects.

Inheritance patterns and prenatal diagnosis

Inheritance patterns

Joubert syndrome is inherited as an autosomal recessive trait.

Prenatal diagnosis

Features of Joubert syndrome may be visualised by ultrasound scan by eighteen to twenty weeks.

Medical text written May 2003 by Contact a Family. Approved May 2003 by Professor M Patton, Professor of Medical Genetics, St George's Hospital Medical School, London, UK.

Further online resources

Medical texts in *The Contact a Family Directory* are designed to give a short, clear description of specific conditions and rare disorders. More extensive information on this condition can be found on a range of reliable, validated websites. Further information on these resources can be found in our **Medical Information on the Internet** article on page 21.

Support

Cross referrals to other entries in the Contact a Family Directory are intended to provide relevant support for these particular features of the disorder. Organisations identified in these entries do not provide support specifically for Joubert syndrome.

Joubert Syndrome in the UK
c/o Contact a Family, 209-211 City Road, London EC1V 1JN
Tel: 0808 808 3555 e-mail: saidid@aol.com Web: http://www.jsuk.btik.com
JSUK is a small web based network of families whose children have Joubert Syndrome. (Information about the use of online groups is available in our 'Medical Information on the Internet: Seeking Quality' article on page 21.) The group was founded in 2007 and all contact should initially be by email or via their website. They have medical information available, details on request. The group can also provide support for other related condition: Meckel-Gruber Syndrome, COACH Syndrome, Senior-Løken Syndrome, Dekaban-Arima syndrome and Varadi-Papp syndrome.
Group details last updated March 2008

KABUKI SYNDROME

Kabuki syndrome: Kabuki Make-Up syndrome

Background

Kabuki syndrome is a pattern of physical and developmental problems which was first noted in children in Japan. The doctors who first wrote about this condition felt that the facial features of the affected children looked like the characters in a type of Japanese theatre called Kabuki theatre, hence they named the condition Kabuki syndrome. The syndrome has now been identified worldwide.

What are the symptoms?

Children and adults with Kabuki syndrome have a distinctive facial appearance with long eye openings which may slant upwards. The eyebrows are usually arched. The ears may appear prominent and the corners of the mouth tend to turn downwards. There is a little indentation below the lower lip.

Some children with Kabuki syndrome are loose jointed and almost all have rather prominent finger pads. Other physical features including heart, kidney and bowel problems have been found in some, but certainly not all, of the children.

Most children with Kabuki syndrome grow slowly even though many have been of normal size at birth. Some children have a head size which is below the normal range.

Some children are susceptible to infections when young, especially ear infections. In some girls early breast development may be noted.

Kabuki syndrome is associated with the presence of learning disability, typically in the mild to moderate range. That said, the degree of learning disability varies considerably, and some individuals may be of normal general intelligence.

Oromotor co-ordination may be impaired and feeding difficulties may occur in children with or without cleft palates. Some speech articulation errors can resolve over time but other anomalies persist.

Early speech and language delay is very common and some language-related difficulties usually persist. These are evident even in cases of apparently age-appropriate general cognitive functioning, and are not necessarily only a result of structural anomalies of the mouth and throat. Other areas of language understanding and expression may be affected.

Psychological and behavioural characteristics

The syndrome has not been closely linked to a distinctive pattern or profile of behaviours. Many children may be very expressive and sociable, whereas others may display 'autistic-like' difficulties in their social communication, interactions with their peers, repetitive behaviours, and sensory interests.

How is it treated?

There is relatively little information about the long term outcome for individuals with Kabuki syndrome. It seems that this may vary widely. That said, life expectancy may be normal if potential medical complications, such as heart or kidney defects, are treated in childhood.

Children with Kabuki syndrome usually learn at a slower rate than normal but they do have the ability to continue learning and make progress. Help can be given to encourage a child's progress and special education can help them achieve their own potential.

Inheritance patterns and prenatal diagnosis

Inheritance patterns

Sporadic incidence but there may be an underlying genetic cause. The cause of Kabuki syndrome is not yet known but it is most likely to be due to a tiny piece of one chromosome missing.

Prenatal diagnosis

None.

Medical text written October 1999 by Professor Dian Donnai. **Last updated May 2004 by Professor Dian Donnai, Consultant Clinical Geneticist, St Mary's Hospital, Manchester, UK. Psychological and behavioural characteristics information last updated March 2004 by Dr O Udwin, Consultant Clinical Child Psychologist, West London Mental Health NHS Trust, London, UK and Dr A Kuczynski, Child Clinical Psychologist, South London & Maudsley NHS Trust, London, UK.**

Support

The Kabuki syndrome Support Group is currently in abeyance. Families can use Contact a Family's Freephone Helpline for advice, information and, where possible, links to other families. Contact a Family's web-based linking service Making Contact.org can be accessed at http://www.makingcontact.org

KAWASAKI DISEASE

Kawasaki disease: Mucocutaneous Lymph Node syndrome

Background

Kawasaki disease is an acute illness predominantly affecting young children that was first described in 1967 by Dr Kawasaki in Japan.

What are the symptoms?

Affected children develop a high fever lasting longer than five days together with redness of the eyes, the inside of the mouth and the lips. There may also be a skin rash, swollen glands, and redness and swelling of the hands and feet. Children with Kawasaki disease often have joint pains or arthritis (see entry, Arthritis - Juvenile Idiopathic) and have characteristic miserableness. Later in the illness there may be peeling of the skin around the finger nails or elsewhere on the hands and feet. Some children do not develop all of these typical features and various other rarer symptoms occur in others. These include aseptic meningitis (see entry), liver dysfunction (see entry), hydrops of the gall bladder, diarrhoea, otitis media (see entry, Deafness), uveitis (see entry), pneumonitis erythema and induration (hardness) at the site of BCG vaccination, together with atypical or incomplete presentations of the classical features of Kawasaki disease.

How is it diagnosed?

Abnormal blood tests usually include a rise in the level of white blood cells (neutrophil count), raised markers of inflammation in the blood known as CRP (C-reactive protein) and ESR (erythrocyte sedimentation rate), and a raised level of platelets (a type of cell that is involved in making blood clots), the latter occurring during the second week of the illness.

There is no specific test for Kawasaki disease and the cause of the condition is not known for certain. For this reason Kawasaki disease may be confused with other conditions that have similar symptoms including scarlet fever, measles and other viral infections, mycoplasma, leptospirosis, Lyme disease, toxoplasmosis, Rickettsial disease, Stevens-Johnson syndrome, drug reactions, mercury poisoning, juvenile chronic arthritis, and Still's disease.

Although most affected children recover completely by two weeks after the onset of fever, in up to twenty-five per cent of cases the illness results in damage to the coronary arteries supplying blood to the heart muscle. This damage is seen as widening of the coronary arteries (known as aneurysms). Up to half of these aneurysms will spontaneously resolve but there is a risk of heart attacks and death. The heart attacks are caused by blood clots that develop in the damaged blood vessels, starving the heart of its blood supply.

How is it treated?

Treatment early in the disease with gamma globulin (IVIG), significantly reduces the risk of coronary aneurysms (by up to five times) and often leads to rapid resolution of all symptoms. If possible IVIG should be administered within ten to twelve days of onset of symptoms, though most experts will still use it later than this if symptoms of Kawasaki disease are present.

Although most children who suffer from Kawasaki disease make a full recovery, those who have had injury to their coronary arteries and have developed coronary artery aneurysms may suffer long term consequences of the disease. There is a small risk of narrowing of the coronary arteries developing months or even years after the acute illness, which can result in angina or heart attack. Death occurs in less than two per cent of patients with aneurysms during childhood and adolescence as a result of heart attacks. Most of these heart attacks occur in the first few months. Long term follow up of the severely affected children is often required, and they may be treated with drugs, such as Aspirin, to reduce the risk of clots forming within the damaged coronary arteries. Some authors have suggested that unrecognized Kawasaki disease may account for 1 in 10 of the sudden deaths from heart attacks that occur in young adults. Occasionally the disease may recur in the same child (up to three per cent of cases).

Inheritance patterns and prenatal diagnosis

Inheritance patterns

None.

Prenatal diagnosis

Not applicable.

Medical text written May 1996 by Professor M Levin, Professor of Paediatrics, St Mary's Hospital Medical School, London, UK. **Last reviewed April 2007 by Dr A J Pollard, Reader in Paediatric Infection and Immunity, University of Oxford, Oxford, UK.**

Support

Kawasaki Support Group

13 Norwood Grove, Potters Green, Coventry CV2 2FR   Tel: 024 7661 2178
e-mail: kssg1sue@hotmail.com
This support group was established in 1994. It offers support by telephone and letter and has an area family linking service. It publishes an occasional newsletter and has information available, details on request. The Group has over 1,200 members.
Group details last confirmed September 2007.

KERATOCONUS

Background

Keratoconus is a rare eye condition which results in blurred vision. The incidence of Keratoconus (conical or cone-shaped cornea) varies between 1 in 3,000 and 1 in 10,000. It usually affects both eyes, although one eye is normally affected before the other.

Keratoconus rarely appears in an individual until puberty or beyond. Although it is uncertain how far Keratoconus will develop in an individual, the condition does not cause blindness. With the current treatment available most people should be able to lead a normal lifestyle when they have the condition.

What are the causes?

The cornea is the major focussing surface of the eye. In Keratoconus, the cornea becomes stretched and thin near its centre, and the thinned part of the cornea bulges making the vision more short-sighted and irregular. As a result the vision is distorted. The stretching of the cornea tends to progress but the rate varies. Sometimes one eye may be badly affected while the other eye may show very little sign of the condition.

How is it treated?

The first line of treatment is usually with rigid contact lenses although some people with early Keratoconus may be able to wear spectacles or soft contact lenses. However, good vision may be difficult to maintain at times as the condition progresses and contact lens tolerance varies.

There is a small risk of infection when wearing contact lenses and the risk becomes much greater if the lenses are not kept clean. It is, therefore, important to strictly follow the hygiene instructions given when the lenses are fitted. Contact lenses do not, unfortunately, slow down the rate of progression of the cone, but they do give good vision during that period which could not otherwise be achieved. Drops, ointment, dietary changes and eye exercises also don't help but the condition does eventually stabilise, although it may take many years before that happens.

In about ten to twenty per cent of Keratoconus patients the cornea may become extremely steep, thin and irregular or the vision cannot be improved sufficiently with contact lenses. The cornea may then need to be replaced surgically with a corneal transplant or graft. Visual recovery after a transplant takes a long time - sometimes as long as eighteen months - to settle down and there is a strong possibility that the eye will still need to be fitted with a contact lens afterwards in order to see properly. Surgery is therefore not a shortcut to perfect vision nor a way of avoiding contact lens wear.

There is also a risk of the transplant rejecting afterwards although over ninety per cent of corneal transplants that are done for Keratoconus are successful. If affected individuals feel that this is a possibility they should discuss this with their contact lens practitioner or attend their hospital's Accident and Emergency (Casualty) Department.

Inheritance patterns and prenatal diagnosis

Inheritance patterns

The inheritance mode has not been established but Keratoconus is known to be familial.

Prenatal diagnosis

Not applicable.

Medical text written July 2004 by Mrs L Speedwell, Senior Optometrist, Great Ormond Street Hospital, London, UK.

Further online resources

Medical texts in *The Contact a Family Directory* are designed to give a short, clear description of specific conditions and rare disorders. More extensive information on this condition can be found on a range of reliable, validated websites. Further information on these resources can be found in our **Medical Information on the Internet** article on page 21.

Support

UK Keratoconus Self Help and Support Group
P O Box 26251, London W3 9WQ   Tel: 020 8993 4759
e-mail: chair@keratoconus-group.org.uk   Web: http://www.keratoconus-group.org.uk
The Group provides information and support for people with Keratoconus in the UK. It organises regular meetings for members, often with guest speakers, produces a regular newsletter, raises money for research and works to raise awareness of Keratoconus.
Group details last updated August 2007.

KIDNEY DISEASE

Each kidney contains about one million nephrons, or filtering units, which continuously filter the blood to remove waste products and excess fluid from the body. Kidney disease can result in two different sorts of problems:

- Kidney failure occurs when the function of the filtering unit is reduced, and waste products start to accumulate in the body. In acute kidney (renal) failure there is a sudden loss of kidney function, whereas in chronic kidney failure the decline in kidney function is more gradual;
- Nephrotic syndrome (see entry) describes the situation when the filters allow lots of protein (mostly albumin) to leak into the urine, resulting in low levels of proteins in the blood.

Causes of kidney failure in children include:

- Abnormalities in the development of the kidneys or urinary tract. These may be inherited, or occur in children with no family history of kidney disease. The terms dysplasia or hypoplasia are used to describe a failure of the kidneys to develop or grow properly;
- Vesico-ureteric reflux describes a condition in which urine can flow back up into the kidneys as a child empties their bladder. This can cause scarring to the kidneys, particularly if the urine is infected.

In cystic kidney disease fluid filled sacs, or cysts, develop in the kidney, interfering with normal kidney function. The commonest form is **adult polycystic disease** (see entry, Polycystic Kidney disease), which is inherited as an autosomal dominant. It is a common cause of kidney failure in adults, but cysts rarely cause problems in childhood. In **autosomal recessive polycystic kidney disease** cysts can develop before birth, leading to kidney failure in infants and children. The condition may be associated with liver problems.

Glomerulonephritis (see entry) describes inflammation of the glomeruli, or filters of the kidney. Often the cause or trigger is unknown. In haemolytic uraemic syndrome (see entry) damage to the kidneys often follows infection with a bacterium called Escherichia coli.

Diabetes and Kidney disease. It is estimated that at least one third of individuals with diabetes develop some form of kidney disease although this does not lead to dialysis or transplantation in all cases. Diabetes affects approximately two point three per cent of the population in the UK.

Individuals with diabetic renal disease may develop other complications of diabetes such as poor vision, arterial disease in the limbs which may be severe enough to cause gangrene, heart disease and impaired function of the nerves to the limbs and sometimes the internal organs. These complications may affect decisions on how to treat chronic renal failure if it develops.

Diabetic nephropathy is one of the major complications of diabetes mellitus in which there is damage to the glomeruli, the structures which filter blood so that waste products can be eliminated.

In many individuals affected by diabetic nephropathy, the onset of kidney disease is asymptomatic until it is well advanced. At this stage symptoms of chronic renal failure such as nausea, vomiting, loss of appetite and itching develop. In the silent phase of diabetic nephropathy the condition may be detected by finding excess protein in the urine. The finding is an important warning that diabetic nephropathy is likely to develop in twelve to fifteen years. It is important to have regular screening for microalbuminuria.

Nephrotic syndrome in children is usually caused by a condition known as minimal change disease, so called because there is little abnormal to see if you look at a kidney biopsy from an affected child under the microscope. It is associated with leakage of protein into the urine, but does not affect the other functions of the kidney, and so does not cause kidney failure. It usually responds to treatment with steroids.

Treatment of kidney problems in children involves a team, which includes nephrologists, dieticians, nurses, and pharmacists, all with specialised knowledge of the needs of children with kidney disease. If the kidneys fail their function can be replaced by dialysis or kidney transplantation. Haemodialysis involves using a dialysis machine and an artificial kidney to filter the blood. In peritoneal dialysis a soft tube is placed through the skin over the abdomen into the lining of the tummy. Fluid is cycled in and out of the tummy. This allows waste products to pass across the lining of the peritoneum into the fluid, and be removed every time the fluid is drained out.

Inheritance patterns

In the **adult type** of **polycystic disease** inheritance is autosomal dominant or by a new mutation.

Infantile polycystic disease inheritance is autosomal recessive.

Juvenile nephrophthisis inheritance is autosomal recessive.

Prenatal diagnosis

Infantile polycystic disease can be detected by ultrasound scanning. The adult autosomal dominant disorder may be diagnosed by DNA analysis and chorionic villus sampling if there is an appropriate family history.

Medical text written October 2000 by Dr J Bradley. Additional material on Diabetes and Kidney disease written February 2003 by Contact a Family. Approved February 2003 by the Medical Advisory Board (Consultant Nephrologist) of the National Kidney Research Fund, UK. **Last reviewed May 2005 by Dr J Bradley, Consultant Nephrologist, Director of Renal Medicine, Addenbrooke's Hospital, Cambridge, UK.**

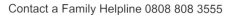
Contact a Family Helpline 0808 808 3555

Support

British Kidney Patient Association

Bordon GU35 9JZ   Tel: 01420 472021/2   Fax: 01420 475831
Web: http://www.britishkidney-pa.co.uk
The Association is a National Registered Charity No. 270288 and is concerned with the welfare of individual kidney patients and their families. The organisation is closely associated with the major renal units throughout the UK. Where necessary, it offers financial support to cover the expenses incurred as the result of the kidney condition and the costs of hospital visiting. It has a wide range of information available, details on request. Membership is available to all renal patients throughout the UK.
Group details last confirmed November 2007.

National Kidney Federation

6 Stanley Street, Worksop S81 7HX   Tel: 0845 601 0209 Helpline   Tel: 01909 487795
Fax: 01909 481723   e-mail: nkf@kidney.org.uk   Web: http://www.kidney.org.uk
The Federation is a National Registered Charity No. 1106735, established in 1978. It has over 70 member Associations and aims to present a national voice to Government on behalf of kidney patients. It offers practical help and contact through member groups located at regional hospitals. It attempts to help families deal with the stress of life-long care, promotes organ donation and campaigns for improved renal services. Patient Support services include a quarterly magazine 'Kidney Life', Patient Helpline, Advocacy Services, website, annual patients conference and a vast range of patient information leaflets available, details on request.
Group details last updated August 2007.

Kidney Research UK

King's Chambers, Priestgate, Peterborough PE1 1FG   Tel: 0845 300 1499 Helpline
Fax: 01733 704699   e-mail: kidneyhealth@kidneyresearchuk.org
Web: http://www.kidneyresearchuk.org
Kidney Research UK, formerly the National Kidney Research Fund, is National Registered Charity No. 252892, established in 1967. It publishes a quarterly newsletter 'PURE' and has a wide range of patients' information booklets. Its services are free, confidential and provided by professional staff.
Group details last updated May 2007.

KLINEFELTER SYNDROME

Klinefelter syndrome: XXY syndrome (sometimes includes XXXY and, until recently, XXXXY)

Background

Klinefelter syndrome was first described in a paper of 1942 by Dr Harry Klinefelter and colleagues. It occurs only in males and is due to a chromosomal abnormality. A chromosome is a rod-like structure present in the nucleus of all body cells, with the exception of the red blood cells, and which stores genetic information. Normally humans have twenty-three pairs of chromosomes, the unfertilised ova and each sperm carrying a set of twenty-three chromosomes. On fertilisation the chromosomes combine to give a total of forty-six (twenty-three pairs). A normal female has an XX pair and a normal male an XY pair.

What are the symptoms?

There is an enormous variation in the expression of this condition. The commonest symptom is infertility. Some men are entirely normal and the diagnosis is only made for an incidental reason. It is important to give an open diagnosis to such children and not just paint a picture of the 'full blown' condition which is described below. It may be that just some of the features are present, such as tall stature or delayed puberty.

The syndrome is characterised by small testes, sterility and scant body hair. Breast development may appear after puberty in twenty-five per cent of those affected. In some cases intellectual difficulties, especially in verbal skills,may be experienced. Additionally psychological problems with self image may be experienced by adolescent boys and adult men.

Other chromosome abnormalities involving more than two X chromosomes in males may lead to learning difficulties.

Psychological and behavioural characteristics

The information below has been drawn up by Dr A Kuczynski, Child Clinical Psychologist, South London & Maudsley NHS Trust, London, UK and Dr O Udwin, Consultant Clinical Child Psychologist, West London Mental Health NHS Trust, London, UK. It has also been approved by the Society for the Study of Behavioural Phenotypes.

As pointed out above, many individuals with the syndrome may be relatively unaffected. Current knowledge may emphasise the more obvious problems in some cases of the syndrome, rather than those who develop comparatively normally.

That said, it is thought that affected individuals are more susceptible to learning problems than the general population, especially in the areas of early speech delay, persistent language difficulties, and difficulties in reading and writing.

Children with the syndrome have been described as relatively placid and compliant. The combination of learning difficulties and abnormal development of sexual characteristics can contribute to low self-esteem and individuals may experience social difficulties in adolescence and adulthood, varying from withdrawal to aggression.

What are the causes?

The male affected by Klinefelter syndrome has two X chromosomes, as well as one Y, resulting in the formation XXY. A mosaic form also occurs where only a percentage of body cells contain XXY while the remainder carry XY. The extent of the affect will depend upon the proportion of XXY to XY throughout the body.

Inheritance patterns and prenatal diagnosis

Inheritance patterns

A sporadic event. However, there is an increased risk in the children of older mothers.

Prenatal diagnosis

Chorionic villus sampling at ten to twelve weeks or amniocentesis at about sixteen weeks is available to older mothers.

Medical text written November 1991 by Contact a Family. Approved by Professor M Patton, Professor of Medical Genetics, St Georges Hospital Medical School, London, UK and Dr J E Wraith, Consultant Paediatrician, Royal Manchester Children's Hospital, Manchester, UK. **Last updated September 2005 by Dr R Stanhope, Consultant Paediatric Endocrinologist, Great Ormond Street Hospital, London, UK. Psychological and behavioural characteristics last updated March 2004 by Dr A Kuczynski, Child Clinical Psychologist, South London & Maudsley NHS Trust, London, UK and Dr O Udwin, Consultant Clinical Child Psychologist, West London Mental Health NHS Trust, London, UK.**

Further online resources

Medical texts in *The Contact a Family Directory* are designed to give a short, clear description of specific conditions and rare disorders. More extensive information on this condition can be found on a range of reliable, validated websites. Further information on these resources can be found in our **Medical Information on the Internet** article on page 21.

K

Support

Klinefelter's Syndrome Association

56 Little Yeldham Road, Little Yeldham, Halstead CO9 4QT   Tel: 0845 230 0047
e-mail: suavecook@aol.com   Web: http://www.ksa-uk.co.uk
The Association is a National Registered Charity No.1058319, established in 1990. It offers support for adults and families by telephone and letter and linking families where possible. It holds an annual conference, publishes a quarterly newsletter and has information available, details on request. The Association has over 160 members.
Group details last updated August 2005.

Klinefelter Organisation

PO Box 9969, Colchester CO1 9FQ   Tel: 01206 870430   e-mail: ko.info@talk21.com
Web: http://www.klinefelter.org.uk
The Organisation is a self help group for all those who are affected by Klinefelters syndrome, including parents and partners, established in 1997, the Klinefelter Organisation offers support and links to other affected individuals where possible. It holds regional meetings and publishes 'The Link' newsletter quarterly and a range of factsheets on request. The organisation is in touch with over 100 affected individuals.
Group details last updated October 2007.

KLIPPEL-FEIL SYNDROME

Background

Klippel-Feil syndrome is a rare disorder caused by failure of the division of the bones in the cervical (neck) section of the spinal column during embryonic development.

Three types of Klippel-Feil syndrome have been described and these depend upon the number of vertebrae joined together and whereabouts in the spine they are joined.

Type I involves fusion of the bones in the neck and the upper part of the back.

Type II is the commonest type of Klippel-Feil syndrome and involves the whole spine from the neck down to the low back. Commonly, two or three bones are joined together, but there may also be some abnormally shaped vertebrae such as hemi-vertebrae (this means the absence of half a bone).

Type III involves almost the whole of the spine from the neck down to the lower back.

What are the symptoms?

Common signs are short neck, impaired movement of the head and neck especially from side to side and a low hairline at the back of the neck. The extent to which individuals are affected by these features can vary widely, ranging from mild cosmetic concerns to more severe impairment.

Other features associated with Klippel-Feil syndrome include: Scoliosis (see entry); spina bifida occulta, an extremely mild form of spina bifida (see entry); one shoulder blade higher than the other (sprengel deformity of the shoulder); kidney (see entry) and urinary tract problems; cleft palate (see entry); fusion of two or more ribs; problems with movements including when one side of the body is moved, the other side wanting to do exactly the same (otherwise known as mirror movements); and hearing problems (see entry, Deafness).

When individuals with Klippel-Feil syndrome are examined specific X-ray findings are seen. Typically, these involve at least two of the seven bones in the neck (otherwise known as the cervical vertebrae) being joined together or fused. Fusion or anomalies of vertebrae in the thoracic (chest area) or lower back may also be seen in Klippel-Feil syndrome.

Klippel-Feil syndrome is associated with conditions including MURCS Association and Wildervanck syndrome.

Only females are affected with MURCS Association. In this condition the Klippel-Feil anomaly is associated with kidney abnormality and underdevelopment of the female reproductive organs, the uterus, fallopian tubes and vagina. The problems may range from very mild, in which all the organs are present but the uterus may be slightly small or an unusual shape, to more severe when the uterus and tubes may be completely absent. Sometimes there may actually be a double uterus and vagina.

Wildervanck syndrome is also more likely to be found in females than males. The Klippel-Feil anomaly is associated with deafness and with eye problems so that the eyes tend to look inwards. This specific eye problem associated with Wildervanck syndrome is known as Duane Retraction syndrome (see entry).

How is it treated?

Complications associated with Klippel-Feil syndrome do not normally develop before the age of twenty-five years and may be treated surgically. Individuals with Klippel-Feil syndrome usually have a normal lifespan. Activities that can injure the neck should be avoided.

Inheritance patterns and prenatal diagnosis

Inheritance patterns

Most cases of Klippel-Feil occur sporadically. In these cases, no other family members are affected. In a few families, Klippel-Feil syndrome is inherited as an autosomal dominant or an autosomal recessive trait.

Prenatal diagnosis

Some of the features of Klippel-Feil syndrome may be identified by ultrasound examination.

Medical text written October 2002 by Contact a Family. Approved October 2002 by Dr K Metcalfe, Consultant Clinical Geneticist, St Mary's Hospital, Manchester, UK.

Further online resources

Medical texts in *The Contact a Family Directory* are designed to give a short, clear description of specific conditions and rare disorders. More extensive information on this condition can be found on a range of reliable, validated websites. Further information on these resources can be found in our **Medical Information on the Internet** article on page 21.

Support

There is no support group for Klippel-Feil syndrome. Cross referrals to other entries in The Contact a Family Directory are intended to provide relevant support for these particular features of the disorder. Organisations identified in these entries do not provide support specifically for Klippel-Feil syndrome. Families can use Contact a Family's Freephone Helpline for advice, information and, where possible, links to other families. Contact a Family's web-based linking service Making Contact.org can be accessed at http://www.makingcontact.org

KLIPPEL-TRENAUNAY SYNDROME

Background

Klippel-Trenaunay syndrome is a rare congenital disorder of blood vessel abnormalities resulting in port wine stains which are present at birth on a limb along with enlargement of that limb.

What are the symptoms?

Less common effects include more complex blood vessel malformations involving the lymphatic system, enlargement of one side of the body, pain from bleeding in the tissues or thrombophlebitis, risk of infection especially if the leg is affected and rectal bleeding where there is pelvic involvement.

How is it treated?

Medical care in Klippel-Trenaunay syndrome requires multidisciplinary management involving orthopaedic care in relation to leg length inequality, compression bandages, laser treatment for the port wine stain, surgical intervention and psycho-social support.

There is a significant degree of variation and medical care needs to be tailored to the individual needs.

Inheritance patterns and prenatal diagnosis

Inheritance patterns

The cause of Klippel-Trenaunay syndrome is unknown

Prenatal diagnosis

None

Medical text written October 1998 by Dr J Harper. **Last updated November 2004 by Professor J Harper, Consultant in Paediatric Dermatology, Great Ormond Street Hospital, London, UK.**

Further online resources

Medical texts in *The Contact a Family Directory* are designed to give a short, clear description of specific conditions and rare disorders. More extensive information on this condition can be found on a range of reliable, validated websites. Further information on these resources can be found in our **Medical Information on the Internet** article on page 21.

Support

Support for individuals and families with Klippel-Trenaunay syndrome is available from the Proteus Family Network (see entry, Proteus syndrome).

KRABBE DISEASE

Background

Krabbe disease is a rare genetic, degenerative disorder of the nervous system. It is one of a group of genetic disorders called the leukodystrophies. The term leukodystrophy comes from the Greek word 'leuko', meaning white, and referring to the 'white matter' of the nervous system. This is a fatty cover which acts as an insulator around nerve fibres of the brain. The word 'dystrophy' means imperfect growth or development. In Krabbe disease the growth of the white matter (otherwise known as myelin sheath) is affected.

What are the symptoms?

Krabbe disease is a very variable condition and the extent to which individuals are affected by their symptoms also varies. The onset of Krabbe disease usually occurs between three to six months. Features include loss of developmental skills, unexplained fevers, irritability, myoclonic seizures (sudden shock-like contractions of the limbs), blindness, spasticity (stiffness of the limbs) paralysis and weight loss. There are three stages of the disorder. Stage I is characterised by general irritability, stiffness, arrest of motor and mental development, and episodes of high temperature without the presence of an infection. During Stage II infants may have severe arching of the back and have myoclonic-like jerks of arms and legs, hypertonic fits, bouts of fever and regression of learned skills. In Stage III infants are severely impaired with no voluntary movement. Sadly, the average age of death is between thirteen months to two years, although this may be earlier due to infections and respiratory failure.

In addition to the infantile form of Krabbe disease, there are also juvenile and adult forms. Although older infants and juveniles with the disorder regress at an unpredictable rate, all will become severely incapacitated. Some adolescents and adults have symptoms confined to weakness, without intellectual deterioration, others become bedridden and continue to deteriorate mentally and physically. Adults may present with loss in manual dexterity, burning paraesthesia (numbness or tingling) in extremities, weakness and dementia. It is nearly impossible to predict the life expectancy of a newly diagnosed older infantile, juvenile, adolescent or adult patient.

What are the causes?

Each nerve in the body is surrounded by myelin sheath. This transmits the electrical impulses to every other nerve in the body. Myelin sheath is a made up of a number of chemicals and Krabbe disease is caused by reduced activity of an enzyme known as galactocerebrosidease (GALC). This enzyme is coded for by a gene on chromosome 14.

How is it diagnosed?

Although a characteristic feature of Krabbe disease may be identified by 'globoid cells' in brain tissue, diagnosis of this disease is confirmed by a blood test which measures the activity of an enzyme known as galactocerebrosidase (GALC). Mutation analysis of the galactocerebrosidase gene may also be carried out to diagnose this disease.

How is it treated?

Although there is no specific cure for Krabbe disease, recently the results of umbilical cord blood transplantation from unaffected donors has been reviewed. Neonatal transplant of umbilical cord blood significantly modifies a severe disease when given to newborn infants who are known to carry two copies of the causal gene; however there are long term risks from the procedure and the appearance of Krabbe disease is not prevented by this treatment. Marrow transplantation may have a role in late onset or adult forms of the condition where it may prevent further progression of the established disease.

Treatment of infants who are diagnosed when significant symptoms are evident is limited to supportive care to control irritability and spasticity. Some symptoms, however, can be treated and physical therapy can help muscle tone.

Inheritance patterns and prenatal diagnosis

Inheritance patterns

Krabbe disease is inherited as an autosomal recessive trait; because of this, the disorder may appear suddenly with no prior history in the family.

Prenatal diagnosis

Where requested, enzymatic and genetic tests can be used to carry out prenatal diagnosis in specialised laboratories.

Medical text written April 2002 by Contact a Family. Approved April 2002 by Professor T Cox. **Last updated March 2007 by Professor T Cox, Professor of Medicine, University of Cambridge School of Clinical Medicine, Cambridge, UK.**

Further online resources

Medical texts in *The Contact a Family Directory* are designed to give a short, clear description of specific conditions and rare disorders. More extensive information on this condition can be found on a range of reliable, validated websites. Further information on these resources can be found in our **Medical Information on the Internet** article on page 21.

Support

While there is no specific support group for families of children in the UK for this condition, information is available from Climb (see entry, Metabolic diseases) and support is available from a group of families under the umbrella of Climb.

Support for the dementia aspects of Krabbe disease in adults can be obtained from the Alzheimer's Society (see entry, Alzheimer's disease). There is no specific support organisation in the UK for adults with metabolic diseases.

"When I visit the hospitals with mum, I can take a step back and take more in." Parent talking about support from her mother. Contact a Family publishes a 'Grandparents' guide recounting grandparents' experiences and detailing information and support available.

LANDAU-KLEFFNER SYNDROME

Background

Landau-Kleffner Syndrome (LKS) is a rare type of childhood epilepsy, in which children develop normally for at least the first two to three years and then show loss of skills, particularly of language (acquired aphasia) which is usually gradual, but may fluctuate and include sudden loss of language following a seizure.

What are the symptoms?

Although characteristically the children lose language understanding (auditory agnosia) which limits speech, a wide range of additional impairments are seen. These include problems with social communication such as seen in Autism Spectrum disorders (see entry), some global reduction in learning abilities, and in more than half, difficulties with co-ordination of walking, feeding and hand function. The lack of response to speech, and even to familiar sounds in some cases, may suggest hearing loss but audiological testing is normal. Many of the children have behaviour problems including impulsivity, hyperactivity, distractibility and challenging behaviour.

Three quarters have epileptic seizures. These are commonly partial motor seizures, or accompanied by loss of responsiveness but a significant minority do not have obvious seizures. All, however, show epileptic discharges on electroencephalogram (EEG) in the central region of the brain with a characteristic increase in the rate of discharges in sleep which are often continuous (non-convulsive status). Magnetic resonance imaging (MRI) scans are usually normal.

This situation of loss of skills associated with a high rate of subclinical epileptiform activity (resembling epilepsy but not detectable by the usual clinical tests) is an example of an epileptic encephalopathy (brain disease) in which it is assumed that the epileptic activity stops normal functioning of that part of the brain. It is, however, a poorly understood phenomenon.

How is it treated?

Treatment with routine antiepilepsy drugs is usually quite effective in seizure control but much less so for the encephalopathy. Corticosteroid drugs are more effective and help more than half of those treated, but have significant side effects.

Occasionally there is a dramatic spontaneous or drug induced total recovery but more commonly problems continue and some long term impairments persist. Occasionally surgical treatment by multiple subpial transactions (severing horizontal connections controlling electrical changes in the brain; this surgical intervention was developed after research showed that the normal structural organisation of the brain relied on vertical connections) is used. Such treatment requires the accurate identification of the source of seizure activity using a range of neurophysiological techniques which may include a methohexitol suppression test and magnetoencephalography. The aim of the methohexitol suppression test is to suppress all the electrical activity in the brain and then to see in which area of the brain the abnormal electrical activity returns first. This area may be the one that is primarily responsible for the problem. Magnetoencephalography is a noninvasive technique that detects and records the magnetic field associated with electrical activity in the brain.

In those children with multiple communication and behavioural impairments, major educational, medical and care support may be required. The active phase of the condition usually burns out in the early part of the second decade, but may leave the child with long term disability.

In addition to the above clinical presentation there are 'variants' with a younger age of onset, and some with abnormal MRI scans which may require different management. There is as yet no evidence to regard the more common presentations of autism in the first two years of life as an early type of LKS.

Inheritance patterns and prenatal diagnosis
Inheritance patterns
None are known
Prenatal diagnosis
None

Medical text written November 2004 by Professor B Neville, Professor of Paediatric Neurology, Institute of Child Health, London, UK.

Further online resources
Medical texts in *The Contact a Family Directory* are designed to give a short, clear description of specific conditions and rare disorders. More extensive information on this condition can be found on a range of reliable, validated websites. Further information on these resources can be found in our **Medical Information on the Internet** article on page 21.

Support
F.O.L.K.S. (Friends of Landau-Kleffner Syndrome)
3 Stone Buildings (Ground Floor), Lincoln's Inn, London WC2A 3XL   Tel: 0870 847 0707
e-mail: info@friendsoflks.com   Web: http://www.friendsoflks.com
The Group is a National Registered Charity No. 1059499, established in 1989. It offers support for families and information about treatment and education for affected children. It also offers contact and linking with others where possible. It publishes a regular newsletter and has information available, details on request. Please send SAE. The Group has over 200 families and interested professional workers in membership.
Group details last confirmed May 2007.

LANGER-GIEDION SYNDROME

Langer-Giedion syndrome: Trichorhinophalangeal syndrome Type II

Background

Langer-Giedion syndrome (LGS) is named after the two doctors who undertook the main research into the condition in the 1960s. It is a very rare condition and diagnosis is usually made at birth or in early childhood

What are the symptoms?

The features associated with this condition include mild to moderate learning difficulties, short stature, unique facial features, small head (microcephaly) and skeletal abnormalities including bony growths projecting from the surfaces of bones. These may include benign bony growths on various bones of the body or cone-shaped extensions on the growing ends (epiphyses) of certain bones, particularly in the hands, and specific craniofacial features. Typically individuals with LGS have fine scalp hair, ears which may be large or prominent, broad eyebrows, deep-set eyes, bulbous nose, long narrow upper lip and missing teeth.

Other features associated with this condition may include loose-wrinkled skin and joint laxity or floppiness, hearing loss (see entry, Deafness) and delayed speech (see entry, Speech and Language Impairment). Individuals with LGS may show a susceptibility to infections during the first years of life, especially chest infection. Individuals may show some or all of these features and, in addition, may be differently affected by the severity of their symptoms. The outlook for children with LGS depends greatly on the severity of the features.

What are the causes?

LGS is caused by a small deletion of chromosomal material. A chromosome is a thread-like structure which is present in the nucleus of all body cells. The chromosomes carry the genes which are the instructions about how to make a new baby from a sperm and an egg. Genes are 'strung' along chromosomes rather like beads are strung along a necklace. In LGS a small piece of the 8th chromosome is missing (or deleted) comprising a number of genes. The loss of these genes is responsible for some of the overall characteristics of LGS.

Inheritance patterns and prenatal diagnosis

Inheritance patterns

Most cases of LGS occur sporadically which means that the loss of genetic material is often not present in the parent and usually other family members are not affected. This issue should be discussed with a clinical geneticist.

Prenatal diagnosis

Chorionic villus sampling (CVS) or amniocentesis may be available for a family if the missing part of the chromosome is large enough to be seen with these techniques. A local genetics centre would be able to offer information on this.

Medical text written October 2002 by Contact a Family. Approved October 2002 by Dr O Quarrell, Consultant in Clinical Genetics, Centre for Human Genetics, Sheffield, UK.

Further online resources

Medical texts in *The Contact a Family Directory* are designed to give a short, clear description of specific conditions and rare disorders. More extensive information on this condition can be found on a range of reliable, validated websites. Further information on these resources can be found in our **Medical Information on the Internet** article on page 21.

Support

There is a US based support group, Trichorhinophalangeal Syndrome Association, which offers an e-mail group at http://health.groups.yahoo.com/group/TRPSA (information about the use of online groups is available in our 'Medical Information on the Internet: Seeking Quality' article). This service is moderated. The Association is also in the process of developing and extending the support which they provide to include an annual family meeting, newsletter and website. If you do not have internet access please telephone our free phone helpline on 0808 808 3555.
Group details last updated February 2007.

There is no support group for Langer-Giedion syndrome in the UK. Cross referrals to other entries in The Contact a Family Directory are intended to provide relevant support for these particular features of the disorder. Organisations identified in these entries do not provide support specifically for Langer-Giedion syndrome. Families can use Contact a Family's Freephone Helpline for advice, information and, where possible, links to other families. Contact a Family's web-based linking service Making Contact.org can be accessed at http://www.makingcontact.org

LARSEN SYNDROME

Background

Larsen syndrome was first described in 1950 by an orthopaedic surgeon, Joseph Larsen. He noticed that a number of his patients shared common features including multiple dislocations of the major joints (wrists, elbows, hips and knees), deformities of the feet and an unusual facial appearance characterised by a flat nasal bridge, wide-spaced eyes, and a prominent forehead.

What are the symptoms?

The wide range of features associated with Larsen syndrome include abnormalities of the growth centres and length of the bones. This leads to short stature, Scoliosis (see entry), short stubby fingers, broad thumbs, short metacarpals (the bones between the wrist and the base of the fingers) and foot deformities. Individuals may also have abnormalities of the cervical spine (the seven bones of the top end of the backbone that form the neck) leading to cervical kyphosis (forward curving of the spine); the thoraco-lumbar spine (the twelve bones below the cervical spine together with the five bones of the lower back) leading to spina-bifida (see entry) and scoliosis; cleft lip and/or palate (see entry); tracheomalacia (softening of the cartilages in the trachea); difficulties in swallowing and breathing; and poorly developed kidneys (see entry, Kidney disease), ureters and urinary bladder. Mixed hearing loss (see entry, Deafness) has been reported.

There is variation in the severity of the syndrome. A rare lethal form has been described but is likely to be a different disorder.

What are the causes?

Larsen syndrome is thought to be caused by a generalised embryonic connective tissue disorder during gestation. It is categorised as one of a number of connective tissue disorders including Ehlers-Danlos syndrome, Brittle Bone Disease/Osteogenesis Imperfecta and Marfan syndrome (see entries).

How is it treated?

Treatment of Larsen syndrome varies according to an individual's specific features. Joint abnormalities may require prolonged orthopaedic treatment including special exercises, casting, braces, or surgery. Abnormal spinal segmentations may be treated either by use of a brace or surgical procedure. Early diagnosis of cervical kyphosis followed by operative stabilisation may help to avoid neurological side effects. Surgery of the inner ear bones may be possible and may be treated with hearing aids. Cleft palate or cleft lip may be managed with speech therapy or surgical procedures. Respiratory problems can be treated with chest physiotherapy, tracheotomy (opening made in the front of the neck so that air can be drawn in), and the assistance of a ventilator. Given the wide range of features associated with Larsen syndrome, a number of different specialists may be involved in the management of the condition.

Inheritance patterns and prenatal diagnosis
Inheritance patterns

Larsen syndrome may be inherited as either an autosomal dominant trait or an autosomal recessive trait. More commonly, it is inherited as an autosomal recessive trait. Changes (or mutations) in a gene on chromosome 3 are thought to be responsible for the dominant form of Larsen syndrome. Changes in genes on either chromosome 1 or chromosome 6 are thought to be associated with the autosomal recessive form of Larsen syndrome.

It is not possible to categorise, on the basis of clinical features alone, the inheritance pattern of Larsen syndrome in an individual case, either as an autosomal dominant trait or an autosomal recessive trait. However, features such as syndactyly, cleft palate, genital anomalies and severe short stature and milder 'flat face' appearance are more commonly associated with the recessive form of the condition. The variability of the effects of this condition make genetic counselling for Larsen's syndrome complex.

Prenatal diagnosis

Ultrasonographic diagnosis may be possible prenatally for features such as dislocations of specific parts of the body. Confirmation of a diagnosis of Larsen syndrome after birth is important for genetic counselling.

Medical text written October 2003 by Contact a Family. Approved October 2003 by Professor M Patton, Professor of Medical Genetics, St George's Hospital Medical School, London, UK.

Further online resources

Medical texts in *The Contact a Family Directory* are designed to give a short, clear description of specific conditions and rare disorders. More extensive information on this condition can be found on a range of reliable, validated websites. Further information on these resources can be found in our **Medical Information on the Internet** article on page 21.

Support

There is no support group for Larsen Syndrome. Cross referrals to other entries in the Contact a Family Directory are intended to provide relevant support for these particular features of the disorder. Organisations identified in these entries do not provide support specifically for Larsen Syndrome . Families can use Contact a Family's Freephone Helpline for advice, information and, where possible, links to other families. Contact a Family's web-based linking service Making Contact.org can be accessed at http://www.makingcontact.org

LEARNING DISABILITY

Learning Disability: Intellectual Disability

Background

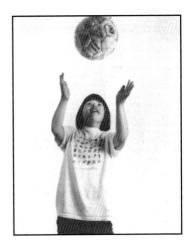

Learning disability (formerly known as mental handicap) and referred to increasingly as intellectual disability covers a wide range of intellectual impairments.

Mild learning disability (roughly equivalent to an IQ of fifty to seventy) is analogous to the educational term 'moderate learning difficulties'. It is usually caused by a combination of restricted learning and social opportunities plus a high rate of low-average intellectual ability and learning disability in close relatives.

Moderate-to-profound learning disability (roughly equivalent to an IQ below fifty) is analogous to the educational term 'severe learning difficulties'. It usually has a specific biological cause. However there are exceptions either way.

What are the symptoms?

Generally someone is considered to have a learning disability when they function at a level of intellectual ability which is significantly lower than their chronological age. This is usually considered to be equivalent to having an IQ of seventy or less and occurs in approximately two to three per cent of the population. Increased difficulties in acquiring basic independence, self-care and life skills, and increased dependence on others are common. Specialist educational input is usually required. This is increasingly possible within mainstream school settings, though sometimes specialist school placement still proves to be most beneficial.

What are the causes?

Learning disability may occur in isolation, in association with other sensory or physical handicaps, or as part of a recognisable genetic syndrome. Emotional and behavioural difficulties are common in individuals who have a learning disability, for a variety of biological, psychological and social reasons. Assessment and management of such difficulties can be problematic and may require a specialist multi-disciplinary team involving professionals from health, education and social services as well as the private and voluntary sector.

The cause of learning disability is often undetermined (see Undiagnosed Children). However there are five main areas in which intellectual impairment can occur:

- chromosomal and genetic abnormalities such as Down syndrome and Fragile X syndrome (see entries);
- infections such as toxoplasmosis (see entry) and congenital rubella (see entry, Rubella);
- toxins such as alcohol (see Fetal Alcohol Spectrum disorder) and certain medications (see Fetal Anti-convulsant disorder);
- injury or physical trauma such as road traffic accidents (see Brain Injuries);
- socio-environmental factors such as profound neglect.

How is it treated?

Broadly, important components of management include:

- breaking the news of the child's disabilities to parents as soon, professionally and supportively as possible;
- counselling on promotion of development;
- dealing with associated disabilities and any emotional and behaviour issues;
- advising on appropriate education;
- genetic and lifestyle counselling as appropriate;
- providing social and emotional support to individual and family members.

Once diagnosed, likely challenges and progress of children with intellectual disability will depend more especially on:

- the severity of the intellectual impairment;
- associated physical, sensory, emotional and behavioural issues;
- quality of care and education received;
- cause of the intellectual disability.

Inheritance patterns and prenatal diagnosis

Inheritance patterns

These will depend upon the fundamental underlying cause of the condition. This is often unknown. Genetic counselling is important and is available through regional genetic centres. Genetic counselling appointments can be arranged through general practitioners or hospital specialists.

Prenatal diagnosis

This is dependent upon the underlying condition and may include 'chorionic villus sampling' (testing a small piece of material from near the placenta), ultrasound scanning, amniocentesis, fetal blood sampling and fetoscopy (examining the developing baby through a small telescope).

Early identification, evaluation and remedial input are essential to maximising the abilities and progress of individuals with learning disability.

Medical text written May 2001 by Professor J Turk. **Last updated November 2005 by Professor J Turk, Professor of Developmental Psychiatry and Consultant Child & Adolescent Psychiatrist, Department of Clinical Developmental Sciences, St. George's Hospital Medical School, London, UK.**

Support

Mencap (The Royal Mencap Society)
123 Golden Lane, London EC1Y 0RT   Tel: 020 7454 0454   Fax: 020 7608 3254
Tel: 0808 808 1111 Helpline (England)   Tel: 0808 8000 300 Helpline (Wales)
Tel: 0845 7636227 Advice line (Northern Ireland)   Tel: 0808 808 8181 Text
e-mail: help@mencap.org.uk   Web: http://www.mencap.org.uk
Web: http://www.askmencap.info
Mencap is a National Registered Charity No. 222377, established in 1946. It works with children and adults with learning disabilities in England, Wales and Northern Ireland. It offers information, advice and support through a network of Community Support Teams and affiliated groups. It campaigns and influences at a national and local level and provides housing, residential and domiciliary support. It also provides employment via the Pathway Employment services and leisure opportunities via Gateway Clubs. It publishes a national newspaper 'Viewpoint' and has a wide range of information available, details on request or via the website. Mencap has over 1,200 affiliated groups.
Group details last updated June 2006.

ENABLE Scotland
6th Floor, 7 Buchanan Street, Glasgow G1 3HL
Tel: 0141 226 4541 Information Service (Mon-Fri, 1pm-4pm)
Fax: 0141 204 4398   e-mail: info@enable.org.uk   Web: http://www.enable.org.uk
ENABLE Scotland is a Scottish charity No. SCO09024, established in 1954. It campaigns locally and nationally and provides information and legal advice. A network of local groups offers support and contact between families. In different parts of Scotland, its local services can provide vocational training and job support, after-school care, family-based short breaks for children, supported living and day services for adults. It publishes a quarterly newsletter 'Newslink' and has a wide range of information available, details on request. Members can join nationally or through a network of local branches. It has over 4,000 members.
Group details last updated May 2007.

LEBER'S CONGENITAL AMAUROSIS

Background

Leber's Congenital Amaurosis (LCA) is not a single specific disorder. It is the term used for a group of conditions that have in common abnormality of retinal receptors that results in severe vision impairment from birth. Many older publications do not differentiate between retinal conditions that are now given a more specific diagnostic label.

What are the symptoms?

At an early age it may not be possible to differentiate LCA from syndromic disorders where the child may have disability due to a systemic disorder that affects other organs than the eyes. Caution therefore is advised before attaching this diagnostic label in a very young child especially if there are developmental concerns too marked to be explained by vision impairment.

It is difficult to assess residual vision from behaviour in a very young child. Many who are severely visually impaired will develop some useful vision in the first six months. However, over childhood this may gradually be lost. In LCA, it is uncommon to achieve even navigational vision and older children rarely retain sufficient vision to read print.

In more severely visually impaired children who have no vision or only light perception in common with other individuals blind from birth, eye poking behaviour may develop resulting in Keratoconus (see entry) - the cornea becoming thinned and conical in shape, in the lens becoming cataractous, and in the fat around the eye shrinking leading to a sunken eye appearance.

What are the causes?

Within the LCA group genetic testing can now, in some cases, identify which of more than six distinct genes has an error, but as yet this does not alter management.

How is it diagnosed?

Electrodiagnostic testing is essential in the differential diagnosis. All types of LCA have poor function of both the rod and cone receptors in the retina. The ERG (electroretinogram) will be unrecordable or very small and eye movements will be roving or jerky (see entry, Nystagmus).

A few children initially given the diagnostic label of LCA will later have a revised diagnosis if problems become apparent apart from the eyes. Some of these children will even develop moderate visual function. Other features which may lead to a modified diagnosis include: kidney problems - Senior-Loken syndrome and Joubert syndrome (see entry); heart problems - Alström syndrome (see entry); and panting breathing pattern in infancy and later head shaking when using vision to track - Joubert syndrome (see entry).

LCA is a completely different condition from Leber's Hereditary Optic Neuropathy (see entry) - the only connection being a description by the same doctor.

How is it treated?

A few children may see slightly better with hypermetropic (thick) glasses. However, there is considerable variation as this is not one disorder.

Gene therapy, with the goal of at least stabilising any residual vision, may be a possibility in the not too distant future for the small number of children with the RPE65 genotype.

Inheritance patterns and prenatal diagnosis

Inheritance patterns

Inheritance is autosomal recessive.

Prenatal diagnosis

None.

Medical text written January 1999 by Miss Isabelle Russell-Eggitt FRCS FRCOphth. **Last updated September 2004 by Miss Isabelle Russell-Eggitt FRCS FRCOphth, Consultant Ophthalmic Surgeon, Great Ormond Street Hospital for Children, London, UK.**

Further online resources

Medical texts in *The Contact a Family Directory* are designed to give a short, clear description of specific conditions and rare disorders. More extensive information on this condition can be found on a range of reliable, validated websites. Further information on these resources can be found in our **Medical Information on the Internet** article on page 21.

Support

There is no support group for Leber's Congenital Amaurosis. Cross referrals to other entries in the Contact a Family Directory are intended to provide relevant support for those particular features of the disorder. Organisations identified in those entries do not provide support specifically for Leber's Congenital Amaurosis. Families can use Contact a Family's Freephone Helpline for advice, information and, where possible, links to other families. Contact a Family's web-based linking service Making Contact.org can be accessed at http://www.makingcontact.org

LEBER'S HEREDITARY OPTIC NEUROPATHY

*Leber's Hereditary Optic Neuropathy:
Leber's Optic Atrophy: LHON*

Background

This is a rare inherited condition which involves the optic nerves with either complete or partial loss of central vision. This disorder is unrelated to Leber's Congenital Amaurosis (see entry) - the only connection being that they were described by the same doctor.

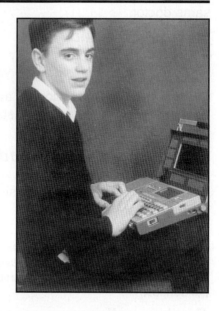

The optic nerve is the 'information cable' joining the eye, the 'camera', to the brain. If damage occurs to the retina or the optic nerve then some of the 'wires' in the optic nerve will die. The 'finest wires' that allow us to see fine detail are lost in LHON. The nerve health can be assessed by looking into the eye. A healthy nerve looks pink and one that has been damaged pale and is called 'atrophic'. However, early in LHON the nerve can look abnormally pink and slightly swollen.

What are the symptoms?

Normally males lose their eyesight between the ages of fifteen to forty-five, but visual loss may occur in young children or later in life. Often vision is lost in one eye a few months before the other. There may be spontaneous marked improvement in vision several months or even years after abrupt severe vision loss. This observation makes it difficult to assess efficacy of any treatments.

There is loss of central vision and diminished colour vision. Children will have difficulty with reading and fine detail tasks especially with low contrast and small detail work.

Very rarely individuals have other problems including mild neurological symptoms and cardiac conduction defects with irregularity of heart beat.

What are the causes?

The genetic defect causing LHON is in the mitochondria, small bodies inside cells that generate their energy.

Several studies have shown increased risk of vision loss in smokers, in heavy alcohol drinkers and in those with diets deficient in natural antioxidants (substances that inhibit oxidation or reactions promoted by oxygen).

How is it treated?

There may be spontaneous marked improvement in vision several months or even years after abrupt severe vision loss. This observation makes it difficult to assess efficacy of any treatments.

The value of vitamin supplementation to a normal diet is not of proven value. There is some evidence of a possible benefit of drugs including steroids and Idebenone in acute disease.

Inheritance patterns and prenatal diagnosis

Inheritance patterns

This disorder is due to a mutation in the DNA of the mitochondria passed by a mother to her child. LHON may be passed on by mothers who have no symptoms, as females are often mildly affected or unaffected. Males do not pass on LHON to their child.

Genetic testing in one of UK's national reference laboratories, Web: http://www.lwh.nhs.uk/genetics/molecular/services.html is available for adults who may be asymptomatic but who have a close relative with LHON and who wish to know if they are at risk of developing symptoms and their risk of passing on the genetic defect.

Genetic testing is only advised for children with visual loss in whom a diagnosis of LHON is being considered on clinical signs. The mutation (spelling mistake in the DNA) can be detected in about ninety per cent of cases thought clinically to have LHON. The majority have one of the following mutations: 11778, 3460, 14484. Whilst symptomatic individuals with 14484 generally have better vision outcome there is much variation even within each group.

Many individuals with these genetic defects, especially females, may have normal vision throughout life. At the moment there is no way of predicting which people carrying a LHON gene will actually go on to lose their eyesight, or how badly their eyesight will be affected.

Prenatal diagnosis

None.

Medical text written October 2004 by Miss Isabelle Russell-Eggitt FRCS FRCOphth, Consultant Ophthalmic Surgeon, Great Ormond Street Hospital for Children, London, UK.

Further online resources

Medical texts in *The Contact a Family Directory* are designed to give a short, clear description of specific conditions and rare disorders. More extensive information on this condition can be found on a range of reliable, validated websites. Further information on these resources can be found in our **Medical Information on the Internet** article on page 21.

Support

There is currently no effective support group covering Leber's Hereditary Optic Neuropathy. This medical description is retained for information purposes. Families can use Contact a Family's Freephone Helpline for advice, information and, where possible, links to other families. Contact a Family's web-based linking service Making Contact.org can be accessed at http://www.makingcontact.org

---

"One of the main ways in which young disabled people might use direct payments is to purchase personal assistance." From a study undertaken by the Joseph Rowntree Foundation in 2003 examining the issues related to 16 and 17 year olds managing direct payments and what information and services exist.

LEIGH SYNDROME

Leigh syndrome: Leigh's disease; Leigh's Encephalopathy

Background

This is a progressive disease affecting the brain. The clinical course is very variable.

Most patients have problems by the age of two years, deteriorate rapidly and die within a year or two. Other patients have a step-wise downhill course starting later in childhood: these patients may deteriorate suddenly and then show partial recovery, followed by periods in which their condition is stable.

What are the symptoms?

Common problems in young children include poor weight gain and floppiness. Later there may be problems with movement (such as stiffness or tremor), loss of vision, abnormal eye movements, difficulty swallowing or abnormal breathing patterns.

How is it diagnosed?

Diagnosis of Leigh syndrome is difficult. Scans usually show changes in parts of the brain called the brainstem and basal ganglia. There also tends to be a high level of a chemical called lactic acid in the fluid round the brain (CSF). A muscle biopsy can help to identify the underlying biochemical abnormality.

How is it treated?

In the vast majority of patients, there is no effective treatment.

Inheritance patterns and prenatal diagnosis

Inheritance patterns

Leigh syndrome is caused by defects in the cell's pathway for producing energy. This process occurs in parts of the cell called mitochondria. The defect can involve several different steps in the pathway (e.g. pyruvate dehydrogenase or the mitochondrial respiratory chain). The pattern of inheritance depends on which step is affected: most cases are autosomal recessive but a few are X-linked or show 'maternal inheritance' (due to mtDNA mutations).

Prenatal diagnosis

This is available in some cases of Leigh syndrome but it is not possible in all cases.

Medical text written November 2000 by Dr A Morris. **Last updated August 2005 by Dr A Morris, Consultant Paediatrician with Special Interest in Metabolic disease, Willink Biochemical Genetics Unit, Royal Manchester Children's Hospital, Manchester, UK.**

Further online resources

Medical texts in *The Contact a Family Directory* are designed to give a short, clear description of specific conditions and rare disorders. More extensive information on this condition can be found on a range of reliable, validated websites. Further information on these resources can be found in our **Medical Information on the Internet** article on page 21.

Support

While there is no specific support group in the UK for Leigh syndrome, information is available from Climb (see entry, Metabolic diseases) and support is also available from a group of families under the umbrella of Climb.

Is your child affected by a condition for which there is no support group? If you would like to speak to other affected families, Contact a Family may be able to organise a telephone conference. Tel: 020 7608 8700 for details.

LENNOX-GASTAUT SYNDROME

Background

Lennox-Gastaut syndrome is the name given to a group of severe epilepsies which occur in childhood. It sometimes follows the onset of seizures in the first year of life, which may include infantile spasms (see entry, West syndrome).

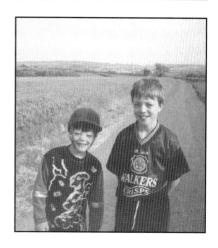

The onset, which is usually under the age of five years, may be quite acute, with multiple seizures and loss of skills, or initially as infrequent seizures. Although originally described as having a characteristic EEG (electroencephalogram) pattern of slow spike-wave, the main clinical features of this condition are of a child developing several types of seizures with slowing or regression in development.

What are the symptoms?

The seizures include tonic (generalised stiffening) myoclonic (fast jerks), atypical absences (loss of responsiveness which may not be complete), partial (stiffening and jerking of one body segment) and generalised (stiffening and jerking of the whole body) tonic clonic attacks. Very commonly the seizures also include episodes of non-convulsive status epilepticus in which the child lapses into a groggy state and may have difficulty with communication, feeding and walking. There are more children and young adults with multiple seizure types and regression than those who fit the above EEG definition and from the families' point of view it is reasonable to include all within the group.

Most children have learning difficulties which may vary both in extent and from time to time. A range of psychological problems, including attention deficit, and autistic features are common.

How is it treated?

This condition is often resistant to drug treatment and may pose long term problems with variable and unpredictable levels of functioning. A small number of children show a milder and self-limiting pattern. The condition may occur in a child with normal or slow early development. Occasionally surgical treatment may be possible if there is removable area of brain damage responsible for the seizures or if drop attacks are the main seizure type.

Inheritance patterns and prenatal diagnosis

Inheritance patterns

None has been found

Prenatal diagnosis

None

Medical text written December 1996 by Professor B Neville. **Last updated January 2003 by Professor B Neville, Professor of Childhood Epilepsy, Institute of Child Health, London, UK.**

Further online resources

Medical texts in *The Contact a Family Directory* are designed to give a short, clear description of specific conditions and rare disorders. More extensive information on this condition can be found on a range of reliable, validated websites. Further information on these resources can be found in our **Medical Information on the Internet** article on page 21.

Support

Lennox-Gastaut Support Group

9 South View, Burrough on the Hill, Melton Mowbray LE14 2JJ   Tel: 01664 454305

e-mail: andrew.gibson15@btopenworld.com

The Lennox-Gastaut Support Group offers support and information by telephone and letter and linking families where possible. It has information available, details on request. The group is in contact with over 200 families and health care professionals.

Group details last confirmed November 2007.

LESCH NYHAN SYNDROME

Lesch Nyhan syndrome: Hypoxanthine Guanine Phosphoribosyl Transferase deficiency; HPRT deficiency

Background

Lesch Nyhan syndrome was first described in 1964. It is a very rare genetic metabolic disorder usually occurring in boys but carried by females. A few affected females have also been reported. It is caused by virtually complete deficiency of the enzyme Hypoxanthine Guanine Phosphoribosyl Transferase (HPRT) which is important in purine metabolism. Cases have been described where HPRT deficiency was incomplete and associated with no obvious neurological or behavioural abnormalities.

What are the symptoms?

Infants with Lesch-Nyhan syndrome appear normal at birth; motor delay and low muscle tone become apparent within the first few months. Dystonia (see entry) and choreoathetosis (involuntary jerky movement of the body) usually develop towards the end of the first year. Dystonia is a disorder of muscle tone producing typical contractile spasms or fixed postures in the limbs or trunk, which interfere with purposeful movements and speech development. The condition may be misdiagnosed as cerebral palsy (see entry). Feeding difficulties and hiatus hernia are common. About half the children have seizures. There may be testicular damage causing small size and delayed puberty.

Intellectual development is impaire. Most affected individuals have moderate or severe learning difficulties, although some have low average intellectual abilities and attain age appropriate reading skills.

A build up of uric acid in the blood and urine results in kidney damage and production of kidney stones. Some infants have severe kidney problems and may present in kidney failure.

Compulsive self-injurious behaviour (see An introduction to behavioural phenotypes) is reported in eighty-five per cent of cases. It usually starts in the second year though can be as late as ten years. Biting of the lips, inside the mouth and tongue or of the fingers is common. Marked dystonic spasm with arching of the back and neck that may cause spinal cord damage is also common. This behaviour fluctuates and may be associated with aggressive outbursts towards carers and anxiety and depression in boys. Restraints such as arm splints and neck support may be required and requested.

What are the causes?

Affected males inherit the gene mutation (change) that results in HPRT deficiency from females who show no symptoms of disease, or as a result of a new mutation.

The full spectrum of disease associated with HPRT deficiency is now recognised as ranging from isolated hyperuricaemia (excess uric acid in the blood) resulting in gout to hyperuricaemia associated with profound neurobehavioral dysfunction. In recognition of the careful early clinical description the full spectrum of clinical abnormalities associated with HPRT deficiency have been designated Lesch Nyhan disease (LND). Patients who lack the full clinical manifestations as a result of partial HPRT deficiency are designated LND variants in which case patients may only have kidney problems and gout as a result of the high level of uric acid in the blood though some also have mild neurological problems.

How is it diagnosed?

Diagnosis should be carried out in a specialist centre as it depends on a careful examination of HPRT activity in the blood. Uric acid levels will usually be raised in blood and urine but levels may be misleading causing missed diagnosis.

How is it treated?

Allopurinol is a drug used to reduce uric acid production but the dose must be carefully monitored as too much can produce xanthine, which is more insoluble than uric acid and will cause kidney damage and stones.

The effectiveness of medication in treating the self-injurious behaviour has been variable. Behaviour modification techniques can be helpful in some cases. Stress reduction is generally viewed as a useful and effective method of intervention. The mechanism of the neurological impairments is not fully understood and there are as yet no effective treatments for these neurological complications. Life expectancy is reduced. In many cases death occurs in the twenties or thirties but some men are living beyond forty.

Inheritance patterns and prenatal diagnosis

Inheritance patterns

X-linked recessive. Up to four boys will be born annually in the UK and one third of cases will be new mutations. Carrier detection is not perfect, only eighty-five per cent can be identified positively using DNA probes. However, genetic counselling and investigation is important for the wider family. In 2004 a database of three hundred and two mutations associated with both full and partial phenotypes was described.

Prenatal diagnosis

Detection of HPRT deficiency is possible in the first twelve weeks of pregnancy using chorionic biopsy material

Medical text written May 2002 by Dr G T McCarthy. **Last updated February 2006 by Dr G T McCarthy FRCP FRCPCH, Honorary Consultant Neuropaediatrician, Chailey Heritage Clinical Services, Lewes, UK.**

Further online resources

Medical texts in *The Contact a Family Directory* are designed to give a short, clear description of specific conditions and rare disorders. More extensive information on this condition can be found on a range of reliable, validated websites. Further information on these resources can be found in our **Medical Information on the Internet** article on page 21.

Support

As Lesch Nyhan syndrome is a purine metabolic disorder, support and information can be obtained from PUMPA (see entry, Purine and Pyrimidine Metabolic diseases). Support is also available from a group of families under the umbrella of Climb (see entry, Metabolic diseases).

A donation of £500 would pay for a workshop for local parents. A donation form is on page 1088

LEUKAEMIA and other allied blood disorders

Background

Leukaemia (see also Cancer) is a group of potentially life-threatening malignant diseases affecting the production of blood cells. Blood cells are derived from haemopoietic ('blood forming') stem cells which are found in the bone marrow (a spongy tissue found in nearly all bones in children and in the spine, pelvis, ribs, skull and upper ends of arm and leg bones in adults).

There are three main types of blood cell: white cells; platelets (which assist in blood clotting); and red cells (which carry oxygen). The white cells include granulocytes (neutrophils, eosinophils and basophils), monocytes and lymphocytes. The most common type is the neutrophil which is needed to fight bacterial infection. Lymphocytes are divided into B cells which are involved in producing antibodies and T cells which are involved in the immune response.

Leukaemia (Leukemia - US) can be classified into two main groups depending on whether myeloid cells (neutrophils, basophils, eosinophils and monocytes) or lymphoid cells (lymphocytes) are chiefly affected. The other key distinction is between acute leukaemia in which primitive cells accumulate in the marrow and which is rapid in onset and, if untreated, in progression; and *chronic leukaemia* in which there is an increase in mature neutrophils or lymphocytes in the blood and which is slower in onset and usually slower to progress, even if untreated. There are thus four main types of leukaemia: acute myeloid; acute lymphoblastic; chronic myeloid; and chronic lymphocytic. The most common form of leukaemia in children is acute lymphoblastic leukaemia, whereas the most common form in older adults is chronic lymphocytic leukaemia.

Acute Lymphoblastic Leukaemia (ALL)

This mainly affects children, with a peak age of onset at four years; about eighty-five per cent of childhood leukaemia is of this type. Children may complain of bone or joint pains, may be anaemic (pale and easily tired), may have repeated, persistent infections and may have excessive bruising or bleeding problems or they may be non-specifically unwell. The lymph glands (nodes) in the neck, armpits and groins may be enlarged. The disease may also cause neurological problems, such as headaches, difficulties with vision because of meningeal disease, or it may cause testicular enlargement. Diagnosis is by full blood count followed by bone marrow examination, which shows accumulation of primitive cells (lymphoblasts), and reduction in normal blood forming cells. Treatment is by chemotherapy. The cure rate in children is high (about seventy-five to eighty per cent). A minority of children may require a stem cell transplant. From 2003 to 2009 a large scale clinical study, UKALL 2003, is being carried out in the UK; some children are not eligible for this study, but it is likely that most parents will be asked to consider enrolling their child in this trial. Adults receive similar, but more intensive, treatment than children but the outlook is less good. Stem cell transplantation is recommended more frequently, even in first remission. Teenagers have been found to fare better when they are given childhood type treatment rather than that given to adults.

Acute Myeloid Leukaemia (AML)

This is rare in childhood (accounting for about fifteen per cent of cases) and uncommon in young adult life; most patients are diagnosed in later life. It may arise with no preceding illness or follow other bone marrow diseases or cancer therapy (secondary AML). Patients may be anaemic (pale and easily tired), may have repeated, persistent infections with fevers and may have excessive bruising or bleeding problems. Diagnosis is by full blood count followed by bone marrow examination which shows an accumulation of primitive cells (myeloblasts). Treatment is by repeated courses of intensive chemotherapy. Some patients may require a stem cell transplant. If a patient's age or general health limits treatment, they may be given treatment aimed at controlling symptoms, rather than attempting cure.

Chronic Lymphocytic Leukaemia (CLL)

This mainly occurs in older adults (over forty years of age); it is not seen in children. It is often diagnosed by chance when a full blood count is done for another reason, e.g. routine screen. Patients may be anaemic (pale and easily tired), may have repeated, persistent infections and may have excessive bruising or bleeding. There may be enlargement of the lymph nodes, for example in the neck and/or spleen. Diagnosis is by full blood count usually followed by bone marrow examination and immunological characterisation of the leukaemic cells. Patients with early stage CLL do not require any treatment. Treatment for most patients, when it becomes necessary, is by chemotherapy, usually initially in tablet form as an outpatient.

Chronic Myeloid Leukaemia (CML)

This mainly occurs in adults (peak age forty to fifty years). It may be diagnosed as a chance finding on full blood count done for another reason. Patients may be anaemic (pale and easily tired), have abdominal discomfort due to an enlarged spleen, fevers, sweating and loss of weight. Diagnosis is by full blood count followed by bone marrow examination. There are typically three phases to CML: a chronic phase which may last some years during which the disease can be easily controlled with mild chemotherapy; an accelerated phase lasting some months during which the symptoms are more marked and the disease progresses more rapidly; and finally a blast phase or crisis lasting weeks to months in which the condition has transformed to acute leukaemia. Treatment for most patients, in the chronic phase, is by chemotherapy by mouth or injections of Interferon. A relatively new drug, called Gleevec (Imatinib Mesylate, STI-571), has shown promise in the treatment of CML. It has recently received a full license in the UK. Younger patients may be recommended to have a stem cell transplant (particularly if they have a tissue matching brother or sister) which is the only curative treatment for the disease.

Related disorders

Other allied disorders are lymphomas (tumours of the lymph glands) (see entry). There are two main types, Hodgkin's Lymphoma and Non-Hodgkin's Lymphoma. Both involve the lymph nodes and may also involve other tissues. Multiple Myeloma is the excessive production of one particular type of lymphoid cell, plasma cells, in the bone marrow which is often associated with bone problems. Aplastic Anaemia is a condition where the bone marrow is empty and fails to produce adequate numbers of blood cells - Acquired Aplastic Anaemia (see entry); Congenital Aplastic Anaemia (see entry, Fanconi Anaemia).

Inheritance patterns and prenatal diagnosis

Inheritance patterns

The majority of cases of leukaemia are not hereditary. Identical twins of children with ALL show a significant excess chance of developing ALL. Down syndrome (see entry) is associated with an incidence of acute leukaemia, about twenty times higher than is seen in the general population. There is evidence that a small minority of cases of CLL and of AML may be familial.

Prenatal diagnosis

Not applicable.

Medical text written November 2001 by Ken Campbell, Leukaemia Research Fund. Approved November 2001 by Professor Victor Hoffbrand, Emeritus Professor of Haematology, Royal Free and University College Medical School, London, UK. **Last updated August 2006 by Ken Campbell MSc (Clinical Oncology), Leukaemia Research Fund, London UK.**

Support

Leukaemia CARE

One Birch Court, Blackpole East, Worcester WR3 8SG
Tel. 0800 169 6680 CARE Line (24hr, 365 days a year)   Tel: 01905 755977
Fax: 01905 755166   e-mail: info@leukaemiaCARE.org.uk
Web: http://www.leukaemiacare.org.uk
Leukaemia CARE is a National Registered Charity No. 259483, established in 1969. It provides a freephone CARE Line 24/7 for patients and their families to enable people to discuss their feelings, concerns and emotions. In some cases it is able to offer financial assistance and also has a holiday programme. CARE Teams operate throughout the UK and do their best to offer local support for Patients and their families. The organisation publishes a newsletter twice per year and has a wide range of information available, details on request. The charity is also involved in patient advocacy. There are over 10,000 members.
Group details last updated October 2007.

Leukaemia Research Fund

43 Great Ormond Street, London WC1N 3JJ   Tel: 020 7405 0101   Fax: 020 7242 1488
e-mail: info@lrf.org.uk   Web: http://www.lrf.org.uk
The Fund is a National Registered Charity No. 216032, established in 1960. It is the only charity in the UK devoted/dedicated exclusively to researching blood cancers and disorders including leukaemia, Hodgkin's and other lymphomas, and myeloma. It offers patient information booklets and general advice on treatment. It has a wide range of information available, details on request.
Group details last updated May 2007.

Leukaemia Society (UK)

PO Box 68314, London N22 8XG   Tel/Fax: 020 8374 4821
e-mail: info@leukaemiasociety.org   Web: http://www.leukaemiasociety.org
The Society is a National Registered Charity No. 1040984, established in 1994. It offers support to affected children and adults, their families and carers and has a special interest in bone marrow transplantation. It runs mobile bone marrow donor recruitment clinics and its visiting officer can arrange visits when treatment takes place a long distance from the patient's home.
Group details last updated August 2007.

The following organisations also provide support and information to families caring for children with leukaemia. Their details appear in the Cancer entry:

- Christian Lewis Trust
- CLIC Sargent
- Teenage Cancer Trust
- Children's Cancer and Leukaemia Group

Other organisations providing excellent support and information covering all types of cancers and leukaemias but not specially geared to children are listed below. Their details appear in the Cancers entry:

- CancerBACUP
- Macmillan Cancer Support

Additionally there are a number of very supportive local self help groups around the country. If you want to contact one of these and have been unable to do so through the organisations in this directory please get in touch with Contact a Family.

LI-FRAUMENI SYNDROME

Background

Li-Fraumeni syndrome (LFS) was first identified in 1969 by Dr Fred Li and Dr Joe Fraumeni. The syndrome is a rare heritable condition which predisposes many members of a family to a wide range of cancers (see entry).

What are the symptoms?

Many individuals with LFS are first affected in childhood and a hallmark of the syndrome is onset of cancer, particularly a cancer called a sarcoma, before the age of forty-five. Less than four hundred families world-wide have been diagnosed with LFS.

The types of cancers affecting individuals with LFS include sarcomas (soft tissue tumours), osteosarcomas (bone cancer), brain tumours (see entry), breast cancer, adrenocortical carcinomas (adrenal gland cancer) and leukaemia (see entry). However, cancers of other organs can also occur.

Due to the wide range of types of cancer involved with LFS, clinics offer an "SOS" system whereby any symptom that lasts longer than three weeks should be discussed with the specialist cancer genetics clinic. This enables families to allow everyday symptoms that affect the general population to subside but, at the same time, to follow up any symptoms that could be significant as part of the syndrome. In particular, any lump in a part of the body that persists for longer than three weeks should be checked. As there may be interaction with irradiation in this syndrome, it is recommended that, if possible, the investigations and treatment use modalities that avoid radiation e.g. MRI or ultrasound and surgery respectively. Sometimes, this is not possible as the best test/treatment may involve x-rays and, in this instance, it is better to make a diagnosis and give the treatment.

What are the causes?

In three quarters of families with LFS, the cause is a mutation of the tumour suppressor gene TP53 on chromosome 17 at p13.1. Tumour suppressor genes restrain cell growth and mutations in these genes allow the uncontrolled division of cells and the formation of tumours. Children in families known to have LFS need to have annual checks, (some centres offer ultrasound of the tummy) and breast screening from the early twenties. Magnetic Resonance Imaging (MRI) of the breasts in women is being studied and may be offered annually from the age of twenty-five to sixty years.

How is it diagnosed?

Diagnosis of LFS is made if three criteria are met:
1.   A sarcoma is found in a person under forty-five years of age;

2.   This person has a first degree relative diagnosed with any cancer when younger than forty-five years;

3.   Another first or second degree relative of the person is diagnosed with any cancer when younger than forty-five years or a sarcoma diagnosed at any age.

Li-Fraumeni Like syndrome (LFL) shares some, but not all of the features listed for LFS. LFL can be diagnosed in an individual if there is a sarcoma at any age with two tumours in first/second degree relatives (or two tumours in one individual - this counts as two individuals) of the following:

1.   breast cancer at under fifty;

2.   or sarcoma at any age;

3.   or brain tumour/leukaemia/adrenocortical carcinoma/melanoma/germ cell tumour/stomach cancer/prostate cancer at under sixty.

Alternatively, another definition of LFL is a childhood tumour diagnosed at less than twenty years with two other tumours in the family, (sarcoma/breast cancer/brain tumour/leukaemia/adrenocortical tumour at any age and another relative with cancer at less than sixty years).

How is it treated?

Treatment in LFS is determined by the type of cancer involved and may include surgery, chemotherapy or radiotherapy. However, radiotherapy and screening using x-rays should be avoided if possible. Urgent TP53 mutation screening is indicated for young onset breast cancer at under thirty in individuals in families with LFL or for breast cancer usually at under forty for those in a family known to be affected by classical LFS. This screening will help to determine if surgery rather than radiotherapy should be used in the breast cancer treatment.

Inheritance patterns and prenatal diagnosis

Inheritance patterns

In LFS inheritance is autosomal dominant. Families known to be at risk should seek genetic advice.

Prenatal diagnosis

This is possible by chorionic villus sampling (CVS) or amniocentesis if the mutation is identified in a family but requires careful genetic counselling.

Medical text written October 2004 by Contact a Family. Approved October 2004 by Dr R Eeles, Reader in Clinical Cancer Genetics and Hon. Consultant in Cancer Genetics and Clinical Oncology, Institute of Cancer Research, Royal Marsden NHS Trust, Sutton, UK.

Further online resources

Medical texts in *The Contact a Family Directory* are designed to give a short, clear description of specific conditions and rare disorders. More extensive information on this condition can be found on a range of reliable, validated websites. Further information on these resources can be found in our **Medical Information on the Internet** article on page 21.

Support

There is no support group for Li-Fraumeni syndrome. Cross referrals to other entries in The Contact a Family Directory are intended to provide relevant support for these particular features of the disorder. Organisations identified in these entries do not provide support specifically for Li-Fraumeni syndrome. Families can use Contact a Family's Freephone Helpline for advice, information and, where possible, links to other families. Contact a Family's web-based linking service Making Contact.org can be accessed at http://www.makingcontact.org

Contact a Family receives funding from the Revenue to help families with tax credit problems. Call the Contact a Family Helpline if you would like more information about tax credits and a copy of a free guide.

LIVER DISEASE

Background

There are about one hundred different liver diseases and conditions which may occur. Some are genetic, some viral, but for many they occur for no apparent reason and are often life-threatening, serious conditions. Some of these diseases and conditions are confined to adults or are very uncommon in childhood.

What are the symptoms?

The signs and symptoms of liver disease can be non-specific but may include:

- Jaundice;
- Nausea;
- Yellow urine;
- Pale-coloured stools;
- Change of sleep patterns;
- Vomiting of blood or blood in the stools;
- Abdominal swelling caused by a large liver, large spleen or excess fluid in the abdomen;
- Lethargy, tiredness or general loss of stamina.

Genetic liver diseases

There are many liver diseases which may be passed from parents to their babies. Sometimes the parents actually have the condition; in other cases one or both may be carriers of the gene although well themselves.

Improved understanding of genetics has given great hope for the future for parents of children with inherited metabolic liver disorders. Advances in technology, therapy and treatment show great promise for gene therapy in the future.

Alpha-1 antitrypsin deficiency

The alpha-1 antitrypsin deficiency gene is as common as cystic fibrosis, affecting about 1 in 2,500 people. It is the most common genetic cause of liver disease in children and the most common genetic condition for which liver transplantation is carried out in children.

An Alpha-1 antitrypsin deficiency is usually diagnosed while testing a baby for jaundice shortly after birth or at family screening.

Most babies with Alpha-1 antitrypsin deficiency lose their jaundice but a small number may require liver transplantation in the first five years of life. The outcome of children diagnosed after family screening is usually good, but as adults they may develop liver disease or lung disease. Smoking and alcohol are best avoided as they can make lung and liver damage worse. Antenatal screening is available.

Inheritance patterns
Autosomal recessive disorder.

Prenatal diagnosis
Chorionic villus sampling between eleven to fourteen weeks of gestation for genotype analysis is practised in some units.

Wilson's disease

Wilson's disease is an inherited condition and affects 1 in 30,000 to 50,000 people. The defect lies in lack of copper excretion from the liver. The excess copper can build up in the liver and/or brain causing liver damage and/or neurological problems. Between half to two-thirds of those with Wilson's disease show symptoms before the age of fifteen years. The symptoms are usually non specific, like abdominal pain, bone pains, haemolytic anaemia (hemolytic anemia - US), gallstones, deterioration of handwriting, abnormal movements or speech problems.

Rarely the condition presents as acute liver failure with involvement of the central nervous system. When this happens, there is nearly one hundred per cent death unless the patient receives a liver transplant. The patient presenting with chronic symptoms or diagnosed during family screening needs life-long treatment with drugs called copper chelators (Penicillamine, Trientine, Zinc or Tetrathiomolybdate). It is best to avoid foods like seafood, chocolates or nuts which are rich in copper. The outlook is good. It is important to screen all the young members of the family once a case is diagnosed in the family.

Inheritance patterns
Autosomal recessive.

Prenatal diagnosis
Prenatal diagnosis is possible.

Crigler-Najjar syndrome type 1

Crigler-Najjar syndrome type 1 is a genetic condition in which the liver cannot process bilirubin. The condition is usually suspected shortly after birth when the baby fails to clear jaundice. Treatment includes exchange blood transfusion or phototherapy as failure to reduce the bilirubin levels can cause brain damage. The long term treatment for this condition is phototherapy in which the child has to lay under lights for many hours a day. In school age children this may increase to about fifteen hours a day so interfering considerably with schooling and daily life. In these circumstances liver transplantation, either whole liver replacement or partial (auxiliary) liver transplantation, is the treatment of choice. A mild variant of the condition called type 2 is less serious and jaundice responds to drugs like Phenobarbitone.

Inheritance patterns

Autosomal recessive.

Prenatal diagnosis

Prenatal diagnosis is possible. Analysis of amniotic fluid or chorionic villus sampling (CVS) has been used to establish the diagnosis in the fetus.

Tyrosinaemia type I

Tyrosinaemia is a relatively rare genetic liver disease in which a defect in a particular enzyme in a metabolic pathway leads to liver failure. A new drug (NTBC) plus dietary restriction, gives a good outlook for children with this disorder but some patients do require liver transplantation.

Inheritance patterns

Autosomal recessive.

Prenatal diagnosis

Prenatal diagnosis is possible by the measurement of succinylacetone in the amniotic fluid or by measuring fuamryl acetoacetate hydrolase levels (the missing enzyme responsible for this condition) in the cultured amniocytes or chorionic villus cells.

Viral infections

A number of viruses can affect the liver and cause either acute self-limiting liver disease called acute viral hepatitis or chronic disease of variable severity called chronic viral hepatitis. Common viral infections of the liver are:

Hepatitis A

The hepatitis A virus is spread via the hands of infected people, especially when preparing food, or by contaminated food. There is no specific treatment for hepatitis A as it is generally a mild disease and nearly all children recover completely without any lasting effects. The infection is not very common in developed countries. An effective vaccine is available and before visiting Asia, Africa or Southern America immunisation against the virus is recommended.

Hepatitis B and C

Hepatitis B and C are serious viral diseases which affect the liver and are blood borne. Both viruses may cause acute illness. However, in the majority of children these viruses become chronic with liver damage only becoming apparent in adulthood. The common way of spreading or acquiring the infection are babies born to hepatitis B or C positive mothers, sharing of toothbrushes or razors amongst family members, or intravenous drug abuse. Current treatments of both viruses are not very successful but research is underway into more effective medicines.

There is an effective vaccine available for hepatitis B, but unfortunately in the

UK it is only available for those at high risk unlike the rest of the developed world where this vaccine is part of the universal immunisation programme. However, all pregnant women are now routinely offered a test for hepatitis B.

Neonatal conditions

Biliary Atresia

Biliary atresia is unique to babies, affecting about 1 in 16,000 live births. In this condition, bile ducts within and outside the liver are progressively damaged by inflammation, and become blocked. The condition is suspected in babies who fail to clear the jaundice after two weeks of age and also have pale or white stools. Special tests are required to establish the diagnosis and an early referral to one of the liver specialist centres in the country is recommended, as the outcome of the surgery depends on the expertise of the surgeon and time of the operation. Corrective surgery, called a Kasai-portoenterostomy, seeks to establish bile drainage by using a loop of bowel. This is a complicated procedure and is carried out at three specialist centres in England. The cause of biliary atresia is not very clear and despite corrective surgery a large number of children still need liver transplantation.

Neonatal Hepatitis

This group includes most babies with prolonged neonatal jaundice who tend to have coloured stools and after detailed tests are not found to have any definitive cause of jaundice. Most of these babies lose jaundice after a few months and are not left with any long term damage. Vitamin and nutritional supplements are required while the baby is jaundiced.

Neonatal Haemochromatosis

Neonatal haemochromatosis is a condition in which iron builds up in all body tissues but particularly the liver, causing hepatitis which progresses so rapidly that the baby often dies within a few days of birth or in many cases is stillborn. Liver transplantation is required. It is not the same gene as haemochromatosis in adults. Recently usage of intravenous immunoglobulins in the antenatal period has been shown to reduce the severity of liver disease in the newborn baby.

Inheritance patterns
Not yet established but there is a very high recurrence in the affected families.

Prenatal diagnosis
Not available, but close follow up of pregnancies at risk may identify an affected fetus in the third trimester. Abnormalities described are placental or fetal oedema.

Other childhood liver diseases
The following list is not exhaustive but gives examples of other liver conditions

which may appear in childhood:

Progressive Familial Intrahepatic Cholestasis (PFIC)

A group of disorders where jaundice and itching are the main symptoms. This usually starts in the first few months of life. The defect usually lies in the transport of bile acids from liver cells to the biliary tree. All the conditions have a genetic basis. It is usual to treat the symptoms but if this fails, then liver transplantation has been successful.

Inheritance patterns

Autosomal recessive.

Prenatal diagnosis

Not available. However antenatal diagnosis is available for families with an affected sibling.

Alagille syndrome

This is a rare multisystem disease affecting liver, heart, kidneys with typical facial features (triangular facial expression, deep-set eyes, prominent forehead). The presentation is variable from life threatening heart disease to very mild facial features. The liver disease severity is also variable, from minimal symptoms of itching and jaundice, to the need for liver transplantation in the first few years of life. A genetic defect has been identified but antenatal diagnosis is not routinely available.

Inheritance patterns

Autosomal dominant with variable penetrance.

Prenatal diagnosis

Prenatal diagnosis is possible.

Choledochal cyst

A disorder of the bile ducts, usually presents as abdominal pain, jaundice or recurrent fever. Diagnosis is usually by ultrasound of the liver. The treatment is surgery with good outcome.

Hepatoblastoma

Hepatoblastoma is a liver tumour of childhood. When chemotherapy is combined with surgery the outlook is very good. In a small number of patients where it is not possible to remove the tumour after chemotherapy, liver transplantation is needed.

Autoimmune Hepatitis

A rare liver disease of childhood usually presents in teenage but may also affect young children. Mostly non specific symptoms of malaise, lethargy or jaundice. There is usually a family history of autoimmune conditions like thyroiditis, diabetes or arthritis. The diagnosis is based on the presence of autoantibodies in blood with high immunoglobulins and liver biopsy showing variable degree of inflammation. The treatment is immunosuppression with Prednisolone and

Azathioprine. The prognosis is good, but treatment is long term.

Budd Chiari syndrome

A very rare liver disease, either seen as a complication after chemotherapy or a result of thrombotic tendency that causes blockage of veins in the liver. Can present as acute liver failure. If supportive treatment fails, then liver transplantation may be necessary.

Galactosaemia

Galactosaemia (see entry) is a metabolic condition affecting the liver due to absence of an enzyme that metabolises the milk sugar, galactose. The usual presentation is neonatal jaundice with vomiting or septicaemia. The symptoms resolve once galactose is eliminated from the diet.

Inheritance patterns

Autosomal recessive.

Treatment

Treatment of childhood liver disease will depend upon the actual condition. Through greater knowledge of the biochemical and molecular activities of the liver there have been spectacular advances in treatments available. Not only has this improved the outcome for young people, but their quality of life is also better. Liver transplantation has revolutionised the management of liver disease with long term survivals of more than eighty-five per cent.

Medical written July 2001 by Dr Anil Dhawan. **Last updated October 2006 by Professor Anil Dhawan, Consultant Paediatric Hepatologist, Paediatric Liver Centre, King's College Hospital, London, UK.**

Further online resources

Medical texts in *The Contact a Family Directory* are designed to give a short, clear description of specific conditions and rare disorders. More extensive information on this condition can be found on a range of reliable, validated websites. Further information on these resources can be found in our **Medical Information on the Internet** article on page 21.

Support

Children's Liver Disease Foundation
36 Great Charles Street, Birmingham B3 3JY   Tel: 0121 212 3839   Fax: 0121 212 4300
e-mail: info@childliverdisease.org   Web: http://www.childliverdisease.org
The Foundation is a National Registered Charity No. 1067331, established in 1980. It fights childhood liver disease through providing pioneering research, effective education and giving professional, caring emotional support to families and young people with a liver disease. It aims to develop its programmes of activities to provide an authoritative and effective voice in its support, in every respect, of young people, families and healthcare professionals. It publishes a magazine 'Delivery' and has a wide range of information available, details on request. The Foundation represents over 5,000 families. Each year approximately 1,000 children are diagnosed with some form of liver disease.
Group details last confirmed September 2007.

British Liver Trust
2 Southampton Road, Ringwood BH24 1HY   Tel: 0800 652 7330 Helpline
Tel: 0870 770 8028   Fax: 01425 481335   e-mail: info@britishlivertrust.org.uk
Web: http://www.britishlivertrust.org.uk
The Trust is a National Registered Charity No. 298858, established in 1988. It offers
support for adults affected by liver disease and their carers. It also promotes and funds
liver disease research. It has a wide range of information available on the website.
Group details last updated August 2007.

Where the cause of the liver disorder is a metabolic disease, further information and
support is available from Climb (see entry, Metabolic diseases).

In 2006 Contact a Family and other
charities launched a major new
campaign to get rights and justice for
every disabled child. To find out more
visit www.edcm.org.uk

LONG QT SYNDROME

Long QT syndrome: Romano-Ward syndrome; Jervell-Lange-Nielson syndrome

Background

Long QT syndrome is an unusual condition which is poorly recognised. An individual with Long QT may develop rhythm abnormalities of their heart. These often occur in response to exercise, stress, fear or sudden noise.

What are the symptoms?

The abnormal rhythm is fast and does not allow the heart to pump out blood as well as it should, so the person may faint during an attack. As a result of this, a mis-diagnosis of epilepsy is often made. The attacks can be life threatening.

What are the causes?

Long QT syndrome results from an abnormality of the cells of the muscle of the heart.

How is it diagnosed?

The condition can sometimes be diagnosed by recording an ECG, which shows a characteristic prolongation of an interval between the onset of excitation and the finish of recovery of the heart beat. This is the QT interval. In some people the QT interval is greatly prolonged and is easy to recognise. In others it is only marginally prolonged. This can lead to difficulties in recognition.

How is it treated?

Ninety-five per cent of affected individuals respond extremely well to beta block drugs. The few who do not, often respond to implantation of a pacemaker or implantable defibrillator.

Inheritance patterns and prenatal diagnosis

Inheritance patterns

The condition is congenital and may be inherited. Many children with this condition develop it as a result of a spontaneous mutation in their DNA. There are now over seven different recognised genetic defects and it would appear that all behave slightly differently. One of the mutations is associated with sensory neural deafness and is inherited in a recessive form. The others appear to be inherited in a dominant fashion with incomplete penetrance. Genetic testing for some of these is now available.

Prenatal diagnosis

At present there is no prenatal diagnosis.

Medical text written January 2000 by Dr Jan Till. **Last updated January 2005 by Dr Jan Till, Consultant Paediatric Electrophysiologist, Royal Brompton and Harefields Hospitals, London, UK.**

Further online resources

Medical texts in *The Contact a Family Directory* are designed to give a short, clear description of specific conditions and rare disorders. More extensive information on this condition can be found on a range of reliable, validated websites. Further information on these resources can be found in our **Medical Information on the Internet** article on page 21.

Support

Further support for young people with Long QT syndrome, including linking to other affected young people, is available from CRY - Cardiac Risk in the Young (see entry, Heart Defects).

Support and linking for affected families and support for bereaved families of adults and children who have died as a result of Long QT syndrome is provided by the Sudden Adult Death Trust (SADS UK) (see entry, Heart Defects).

LOWE SYNDROME

Lowe syndrome: Oculo-Cerebro-Renal syndrome

Background

Lowe syndrome was first described by Doctors Lowe, Terrey, and MacLachlan in 1952. It is a rare, inherited, progressive, metabolic disease affecting the eyes, brain and kidneys. Lowe syndrome affects boys of all ethnic groups. The majority of female carriers of the syndrome show the characteristic ophthalmic findings in the lens of each eye. The incidence of Lowe syndrome is thought to be a few per one hundred thousand births but currently there is no accurate data.

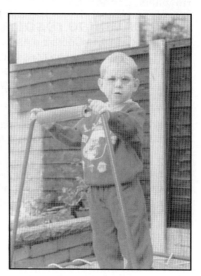

What are the symptoms?

Features of Lowe syndrome include:

- Congenital (present at birth) glaucoma (see entry);
- Nystagmus (see entry);
- Opacity of the cornea, the transparent covering of the iris and pupil, due to overgrowth of scar tissue in about half of affected people;
- Renal tubular dysfunction which may lead to kidney failure;
- Learning disability (see entry) ranging from mild to severe;
- Behavioural problems;
- Seizures, affecting about half of the children diagnosed with the syndrome (see entry, Epilepsy).

What are the causes?

The cause of Lowe syndrome has been identified as mutation of the OCRL1 gene on the X chromosome. Recently, mutations in the same gene have also been found to cause a different syndrome, Dent disease. Patients with Dent disease have similar kidney problems to patients with Lowe syndrome but do not have the other features found in Lowe syndrome. The exact relationship between Lowe syndrome and Dent disease remains to be worked out.

How is it diagnosed?

Reduction of a specific enzyme is known to be involved in Lowe syndrome so diagnosis is made by demonstrating the loss of function of this enzyme and can be carried out by a laboratory test. At present, carrier status can be determined clinically by family history and/or, in most cases, upon careful examination of the lenses of the eye for minor, but nonetheless characteristic, abnormalities. Direct detection of the carrier state can be accomplished in some families by testing the DNA itself. The enzyme test in skin samples is not useful for determining the carrier state.

How is it treated?

Treatment of many of the features of Lowe syndrome is symptomatic and may include surgical intervention for cataracts. Speech therapists and nurses specialising in feeding problems can often help. Medication may be needed if children have seizures. Although the use of human growth hormone has been used successfully, careful consideration is needed to balance its use against drawbacks. The renal tubular dysfunction, which causes loss of phosphate, acidosis, short stature, and renal rickets, may be treated by phosphate and bicarbonate replacement therapy.

Inheritance patterns and prenatal diagnosis

Inheritance patterns

X-linked or sporadic (with no other affected family members).

Prenatal diagnosis

Available by direct enzyme testing by chorionic villus sampling (CVS) or amniocentesis. In some families, direct testing of the DNA may also be useful for prenatal testing. Prenatal testing should be discussed with the geneticist prior to pregnancy.

Medical text written October 2005 by Contact a Family. Approved October 2005 by Dr A Norden, Consultant in Chemical Pathology, Addenbrooke's Hospital, Cambridge, UK.

Further online resources

Medical texts in *The Contact a Family Directory* are designed to give a short, clear description of specific conditions and rare disorders. More extensive information on this condition can be found on a range of reliable, validated websites. Further information on these resources can be found in our **Medical Information on the Internet** article on page 21.

Support

Lowe Syndrome Association

29 Gleneagles Drive, Penwortham, Preston PRI 0JT   Tel: 01772 745070
e-mail: info@lowesyndrome.org (International Lowe Syndrome Association)
Web: http://www.lowesyndrome.org (International Lowe Syndrome Association)
The Association is part of the International Lowe Syndrome Association based in the USA and was established in 1982. It offers mutual support to affected families and aims to raise public awareness. It publishes a tri-annual newsletter 'On the Beam' and has information available, details on request. Worldwide there are around 515 members (about 253 affected families and 100 professionals). There are about 50 known cases in the UK.
Group details last confirmed February 2008.

L

Lowe Syndrome Trust
77 West Heath Road, London NW3 7TH   Tel: 020 8458 6791
e-mail: lowetrust@homechoice.co.uk   Web: http://www.lowetrust.com
The Lowe Syndrome Trust is a National Registered Charity No. 1081241, established in 2000. The Trusts works to fund medical research into Lowe Syndrome. It has a wide range of information on its web site.
Group details last confirmed October 2006.

As Lowe syndrome is a metabolic, disease support and advice are also available from Climb (see entry, Metabolic diseases).

Genetic counselling involves giving information to individuals and families about genetic conditions and the way these are inherited. For more information, and a copy of the factsheet 'About Diagnosis', call the Contact a Family Helpline.

LOWER LIMB ABNORMALITIES

Background

Common lower limb disorders, such as femoral torsion (abnormal twisting of the femur), tibial torsion (twisting of the bone between the knee and the ankle) which can cause intoeing (feet turning inwards), and foot disorders such as metatarsus adductus (curving of the foot) and flat feet, rarely need complex treatment. Observation and waiting to see how the child grows is often all that is required.

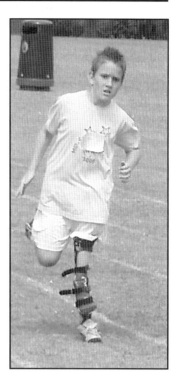

Leg Length discrepancy and Lower Limb Reduction defects

A difference in limb length can occur before or after birth and cover a wide spectrum of conditions which affect the bones in the leg, most commonly involving shortened and/or absent bones. These can range from the mild such as a slightly shortened femur or a missing toe, to severe such as a complete absence of the femur (thigh bone), no hip joint or an abnormal knee joint.

Conditions affecting the thighbone:

- Congenital (present at birth) short femur;
- Proximal Focal Femoral Deficiency (PFFD).

Conditions affecting the lower leg:

- Congenital short tibia (shin bone) with Fibular hemimelia (absent or hypoplastic (underdeveloped) calf bone);
- Congenital Dysplasia (abnormal development) or absence of the tibia with intact fibula (Tibial hemimelia);
- Congenital Tibia Recurvatum (bending backwards of the shin bone) or bowing of the back part of the tibia which frequently corrects itself.

These are called length defects and, in addition, there are a range of abnormal musculature and joints with missing ligaments associated with them. They include Congenital pseudarthrosis (false joint) of the tibia which is quite often associated with Neurofibromatosis (see entry).

Some limb reduction defects result in a failure of growth causing a complete absence of the limb beyond a certain level. Except for very minor conditions such as toe loss, these are defects requiring prosthetic (artificial) replacement and can sometimes be associated with amniotic band syndrome.

What are the symptoms?

Limb length discrepancies of less than 2cm are commonplace and rarely cause a problem. Greater differences cause problems with posture and, if left untreated, may lead to problems with the back, knee or hip in later life.

How is it treated?

Treatment options include:

- surgical limb equalisation techniques;
- orthotic support (the use of external help such as braces);
- prosthetic replacement;
- amputation with prosthetic replacement.

Inheritance patterns and prenatal diagnosis

Inheritance patterns

These are variable and dependent upon the causes of the condition.

Prenatal diagnosis

Some conditions occurring before birth can be detected by prenatal ultrasound scan.

Medical text written June 2005 by steps. Approved July 2005 by Mr J A Fernandes, Consultant Paediatric Orthopaedic Surgeon, Sheffield Children's NHS Trust, Sheffield, UK.

Support

Steps

Warrington Lane, Lymm WA13 0SA   Tel: 0871 717 0044 Helpline (Mon-Fri, 9.30am-4pm) Fax: 01925 750270   e-mail: steps@itl.net   Web: http://www.steps-charity.org.uk

Steps is a National Registered Charity No. 1094343, established in 1980. It supports individuals and families with lower limb conditions, such as clubfoot (congenital talipes equinovarus, see entry), congenital dislocation and developmental dysplasia of the hip (see entry) and lower limb reduction defects. It can offer support and contacts for other conditions with musculoskeletal problems such as amputation caused by meningitis (see entry) or trauma, Blounts disease, Congenital Pseudarthrosis, Congenital Tibial Bowing, Freeman Sheldon syndrome (see entry), Larsen syndrome (see entry), Sacral Agenesis (see entry) or Vertical Talus. It publishes a regular newsletter and has information available, details on request. Steps has over 4,000 members.

Group details last confirmed September 2007.

LUNG DISEASES

Background

Normal breathing draws air into the lungs so that they can extract and absorb oxygen. Damage, which has many causes, limits the extraction of oxygen from the air and the elimination of waste carbon dioxide.

The respiratory syncytial (RS) virus is a major cause of chest infections in young babies. This virus is most common in children less than six months of age, often appearing as a winter epidemic. The damage caused by infection of the lung at this early age can lead to continuing lung problems in later life.

Lung diseases include alpha-one anti-trypsin deficiency, aspergillosis, bronchial asthma, bronchiectasis, chronic bronchitis, chronic obstructive pulmonary disease (COPD), emphysema, fibrosing alveolitis, pulmonary fibrosis and occupational lung diseases.

Inheritance patterns and prenatal diagnosis

Inheritance patterns

Vary according to the particular lung condition.

Prenatal diagnosis

Not applicable.

Other disorders involving the lungs

Other disorders in the Contact a Family Directory having lung involvement to a major or lesser degree include:

Asthma (see entry). This is a complex condition that affects the airways – the small tubes that carry air in and out of the lungs. The usual symptoms are coughing, wheezing, breathlessness or a tight feeling in the chest.

Broncho Pulmonary Dysplasia (see entry). This is a condition found in a small number of premature infants who have needed respiratory support from a ventilator. It is more common the more immature the baby and is more likely to occur in babies who have required ventilation because of lung immaturity or in association with infections.

Cystic Fibrosis (see entry). While the lungs of people with Cystic Fibrosis are normal at birth, thick mucus collects in the lungs blocking some airways and resulting in damage caused by the infection.

Familial Dysautonomia (see entry). This is one of the hereditary sensory and autonomic neuropathies (HSAN) with many features which include respiratory congestion due to misdirected swallowing and frequent lung infections.

Hereditary Haemorrhagic Telangiectasia (see entry). About 1 in 5 people with Hereditary Haemorrhagic Telangiectasia develop abnormal vessels in the lungs called pulmonary arteriovenous malformations (PAVMs). These malformations let blood bypass or 'shunt' past the lung air sacs.

Hereditary Thrombophilia (see entry). This is a disorder in which blood clots develop in the large vessels of major body organs including the lungs. By blocking the blood to the lung and depriving the body of oxygen, they may be rapidly life threatening.

Ivemark syndrome (see entry). One of the features of Ivemark syndrome is mirror imaging of the lungs (isomerism) with both resembling a normal right lung.

Marfan syndrome (see entry). In Marfan syndrome features include pneumothorax (collapse of lung due to air leaking from the lungs into the chest cavity), bronchiectasis (a chronic inflammatory or degenerative condition of one or more bronchi or bronchioles marked by dilatation and loss of elasticity of the walls) and emphysema (over-dissention and destruction of the air spaces in the lungs leading to chronic shortness of breath).

Primary Pulmonary Hypertension (see entry). This is the term used when no cause is found. The term pulmonary hypertension is used when it is associated with other conditions such as severe sleep apnoea, emphysema, pulmonary emboli, some congenital heart defects, left heart failure and autoimmune disorders. In Primary Pulmonary Hypertension (PPH) blood pressure in the lungs rises far above normal levels leading to the heart having a lowered ability to pump enough blood back to the lungs to collect oxygen to send round the body.

Prune Belly syndrome (see entry). Underdevelopment of the lungs is one of the possible complications of Prune Belly syndrome.

Pulmonary Hypertension of the Newborn (see entry). This is a rare disorder of the lungs which occurs at birth or shortly thereafter. The symptoms include cyanosis (blue cast of the skin due to deficient oxygenation of the blood), respiratory distress, tachypnea (increased rate of respiration), and minimal retractions (movement of an organ) during the first day of life.

Sarcoidosis (see entry). This is a multisystem disorder of unknown cause which can affect any organ of the body but most commonly attacks the lungs. It takes the form of cells which cluster together in tiny nodules, or sarcoid granulomas. The word sarcoid comes from the Greek meaning "flesh like".

Tuberculosis (see entry). Tuberculosis (or 'TB') is an infection caught from other people, as with a cold or 'flu. It most often occurs in the lungs and lymph glands but can affect any part of the body.

Medical text written June 2005 by Contact a Family. Approved June 2005 by Dr A Jaffe, Consultant and Honorary Senior Lecturer in Respiratory Research, Great Ormond Street Hospital for Children and Institute of Child Health, London, UK.

Support

Breathe Easy

British Lung Foundation, 73-75 Goswell Road, London EC1V 7ER

Tel: 0845 850 5020 Helpline (Mon-Fri, 10am-6pm)   Tel: 020 7688 5555

Fax: 020 77688 5556   e-mail: enquiries@blf-uk.org   Web: http://www.lunguk.org

The British Lung Foundation provides information, advice, support, friendship and possible contacts to anyone affected by lung disease. The Helpline is staffed by specialist respiratory nurses and welfare benefits advisers who are able to provide advice and information on a wide range of issues affecting people living with a lung condition, including children's lung conditions. There is also a network of support groups, Breathe Easy groups, and a pen-pal scheme.

Group details last updated July 2007.

A donation of £4,000 would pay for the production and distribution of one issue of our magazine 'Connected'. A donation form is on page 1088

LUPUS

Background

Lupus is a chronic inflammatory autoimmune disease of unknown origin which affects many organs and tissues in the body. It is characterised by flares and remissions and is adversely affected by sunlight and possibly ultraviolet light B (UV-B) emitted by some fluorescent lights. The condition is nine times as common in females as in males, more common in black, Chinese, or Asian people than Caucasians, and usually presents between fifteen to fifty years, though children can be affected.

What are the symptoms?

There are several types of lupus:

Discoid Lupus which affects the skin causing a rash and lesions usually on the face and upper part of the body.

Systemic Lupus Erythematosus (SLE) is a more severe form which can affect any body system or organ, notably the joints, kidneys, brain, heart and lungs. It may be life threatening. However, early diagnosis and control of the disease is possible so that many affected individuals can lead relatively normal lives with a normal life expectancy. The disease is characterised by a variety of antibodies which can be detected in the blood. A strongly positive anti-nuclear antibody or antibodies in DNA are particular features of SLE.

Children may be affected by the condition though incidence is very small before the age of 5. Children often present with fever, joint pains, rash in the mouth and recurrent infections. It is important for their prognosis that diagnosis is made early.

Characteristics of the condition include fever, fatigue, joint pains, photosensitivity, central nervous system disorders, pericarditis, pleurisy, kidney problems and mouth ulcers. Other symptoms include hair loss, skin rashes, loss of appetite and miscarriages. However the condition is very variable and may present with only one or two of the symptoms.

Neonatal Lupus is a rare form of the disease due to the transmission of certain types of antibodies from mother to fetus. It causes abnormalities in the child's heart beat and skin rashes. Pregnancy clinics are held at several London hospitals.

What are the causes?

The disease is of unknown origin. **Drug Induced Lupus** is caused by a reversible adverse reaction to a small number of different drugs.

Inheritance patterns and prenatal diagnosis

Inheritance patterns

A genetic predisposition to develop the disease is present. Thus the concordance rate (presence of a trait in twins) for identical twins is twenty-five per cent but among non-identical twins it is two to three per cent. However, it is rare for children of affected mothers to develop the disease - around 1 in 100 cases.

Prenatal diagnosis

None

Medical text written June 1995 by Professor D A Isenberg. **Last updated November 2005 by Professor D A Isenberg, ARC Diamond Jubilee Professor of Rheumatology, University College London, London, UK.**

Further online resources

Medical texts in *The Contact a Family Directory* are designed to give a short, clear description of specific conditions and rare disorders. More extensive information on this condition can be found on a range of reliable, validated websites. Further information on these resources can be found in our **Medical Information on the Internet** article on page 21.

Support

Lupus UK

St James House, Eastern Road, Romford RM1 3NH   Tel: 01708 731251
Fax: 01708 731252   e-mail: headoffice@lupusuk.org.uk
Web: http://www.lupusuk.org.uk
The Group is a National Registered Charity No. 1051610, established in 1995. It offers support and contact with others through regional groups and individual contacts. It publishes a newsletter 'News & Views' three times a year and has a wide range of information available, details on request. The Group has over 8,000 members.
Group details last updated August 2007.

LYMPHOEDEMA

Background

Lymphoedema (Lymphedema - US) is a chronic condition which results in swelling usually of one of more limbs. The lymphatic vessels fail to drain the tissues of excess fluid (lymph) and transport it to the nearest lymph glands and ultimately back to the blood circulation. Lymphoedema arises as a result of failure of this system.

What are the symptoms?

Painless, swelling (oedema) of one foot or ankle is the most common sign of the condition. Recurrent infections of the affected (swollen) part may also develop as a result of lymph drainage failure.

What are the causes?

Secondary Lymphoedema describes swelling which arises from damage to lymph conducting pathways due to an acknowledged cause, e.g. cancer treatment, accidental injury or infection. Primary Lymphoedema is due to swelling which arises from a weakness in the lymph conducting pathways determined at birth. In such circumstances the condition usually develops for no obvious reason.

Inheritance patterns and prenatal diagnosis

Inheritance patterns

Lymphoedema occurring at, or soon after, birth is called congenital lymphoedema. It may be due to a fault in development before birth (not inherited and usually one limb affected) or to a genetic fault (often inherited). Milroy disease is congenital familial lymphoedema due to changes (mutations) in a gene called vascular endothelial growth factor receptor 3 (VEGFR3). The onset of most forms of primary Lymphoedema however are delayed in onset until after puberty. The gene for one such type, associated with distichiasis (double row of eyelashes), is lymphoedema-distichiasis syndrome. This condition is due to gene mutations in the FOXC2 gene.

Both Milroy disease and lymphoedema distichiasis syndrome are dominantly inherited. This means that there is a 1 in 2 chance that an affected individual will pass the altered gene to their child. In many cases the underlying cause of lymphoedema is not clear and further genes may soon be discovered.

Prenatal diagnosis

In Milroy disease, oedema of the feet may be detected in the third trimester by ultrasound.

Medical text written October 1994 by Dr P Mortimer. **Last updated February 2005 by Professor P Mortimer, Professor of Dermatological Medicine, St George's Hospital, London, UK.**

Contact a Family Helpline 0808 808 3555

L

Further online resources

Medical texts in *The Contact a Family Directory* are designed to give a short, clear description of specific conditions and rare disorders. More extensive information on this condition can be found on a range of reliable, validated websites. Further information on these resources can be found in our **Medical Information on the Internet** article on page 21.

Support

Lymphoedema Support Network

St Luke's Crypt, Sydney Street, London SW3 6NH

Tel: 020 7351 4480 Information and Support   Tel: 020 7351 0990   Fax: 020 7349 9809

e-mail: adminlsn@lymphoedema.freeserve.co.uk   Web: http://www.lymphoedema.org/lsn

The LSN is a National Registered Charity No. 1018749, established in 1991. The network provides information and support to people with lymphoedema. It runs a telephone helpline, produces a quarterly newsletter and a wide range of factsheets, and maintains a website. It works to raise awareness of lymphoedema and campaigns for better national standards of care.

Group details last updated January 2007.

LYMPHOMA

Background

Hodgkin's Lymphoma (HL) and **Non-Hodgkin's Lymphoma (NHL)** are both lymphomas, a form of cancer which affects the lymphatic system (a network of glands throughout the body). The lymphatic glands produce a clear fluid known as lymph which circulates round the body and contains lymphocytes (particular white blood cells). Lymphocytes are part of the normal defence system of the body. Lymphomas are potentially life threatening.

What are the symptoms?

Hodgkin's Lymphoma most commonly presents with painless swelling of the lymph glands which continues for some weeks or months. The first glands to be affected are often in the neck or in the area above the collar bone. Sometimes glands in the axilla (armpit) or groin may be affected. Where glands in the chest are affected, a troublesome cough or breathlessness may be apparent.

In **Non-Hodgkin's Lymphoma** there is an enlargement of a group of lymph glands somewhere in the body: for example, in the neck, throat, chest or abdomen. Initially the swelling is painless. Where glands in the chest become very enlarged, difficulty in breathing and a puffy face and neck may develop.

How is it treated?

With present treatment the prognosis for children with Lymphoma is good. These conditions are uncommon in children of any age and very rarely develop in children under three years of age.

Inheritance patterns and prenatal diagnosis

Inheritance patterns

None.

Prenatal diagnosis

None.

Medical text written November 1991 by Contact a Family. Approved November 1991 by Professor M Patton, Professor of Medical Genetics, St Georges Hospital Medical School, London, UK and Dr J E Wraith, Consultant Paediatrician, Royal Manchester Children's Hospital, Manchester, UK. Last updated May 2000 by Dr Paul Revell. **Last reviewed April 2005 by Dr Paul Revell, Consultant Haematologist, Staffordshire General Hospital, Stafford, UK.**

Further online resources

Medical texts in *The Contact a Family Directory* are designed to give a short, clear description of specific conditions and rare disorders. More extensive information on this condition can be found on a range of reliable, validated websites. Further information on these resources can be found in our **Medical Information on the Internet** article on page 21.

Support

Lymphoma Association
PO Box 386, Aylesbury HP20 2GA
Tel: 0808 808 5555 Helpline (Mon-Thur, 9am-6pm; Fri, 9am-5pm)
Tel: 01296 619400 Admin   Fax: 01296 619414   e-mail: information@lymphoma.org.uk
Web: http://www.lymphoma.org.uk
Web: http://www.lifesite.info *Lymphoma Association Information for Young Adults*
The Association is a National Registered Charity No. 1068395, established in 1986. It offers emotional support and telephone links to other families with experience where possible. It publishes a quarterly newsletter and has a wide range of information available, details on request. The lifesite.info website hosts a chat room and message board. The Association has over 2,000 members.
Group details last confirmed June 2007.

The following organisation also provides support and information. Details appear in the Cancer entry:
● CLIC Sargent.

The following organisations also provide support and information. Their details appear in the 'Leukaemia and other allied blood disorders' entry:
● Leukaemia Care;
● Leukaemia Research Fund.

Other organisations providing excellent support and information covering all types of cancers and leukaemias but not specially geared to children are listed below. Their details appear in the Cancer entry:
● Cancerbackup;
● Macmillan Cancer Support.

M-CMTC SYNDROME

M-CMTC syndrome: Macrocephaly – Cutis Marmorata Telangiectasia Congenita syndrome

Background

The main characteristic of the M-CMTC syndrome is cutis marmorata telangiectasia congenita, a marbled appearance of the skin which is present at birth and is due to malformation of the underlying blood vessels.

What are the symptoms?

In addition to a marbled appearance of the skin, individuals with this condition may have other, more discrete pink/red birth marks (see entry, Vascular Birthmarks), particularly over the upper lip. Other distinctive features include a large head size and webbing between the second and third toes and sometimes between the fingers. Sometimes extra fingers or toes may be present. Whilst cutis marmorata telangiectasia congenita can occur as an isolated finding, only individuals with the other, additional features can be said to have the M-CMTC syndrome.

Cutis Marmorata Telangiectasia Congenita syndrome (CMTCS) can appear in isolation or with other features which are not part of the M-CMTC syndrome. In some cases this is felt to be part of the Klippel Trenaunay syndrome/Sturge-Weber syndrome spectrum (see entries).

Babies with M-CMTC syndrome often have a high birth weight and the pregnancy may have been complicated by the presence of excess amniotic fluid or premature delivery. It is common for children with this condition to have low muscle tone and as a consequence there may be initial difficulties with feeding.

Although large at birth, children with M-CMTC syndrome usually have normal growth in later childhood. It is also common to have one side of the body which is slightly larger than the other (hemihypertrophy). The head size continues to be large, and occasionally surgery will be recommended to drain fluid from the brain. An MRI scan may reveal characteristic appearances. In many children, although the head is larger than average, growth stabilises and no treatment is needed. The marbled appearance of the skin tends to get less obvious with time.

There are other, rarer complications of M-CMTC syndrome which include heart problems, seizures, internal blood vessel malformations and developmental abnormalities of the brain. These are not present in every patient.

Children with M-CMTC syndrome are often slow to learn to sit and walk because they have low muscle tone and very mobile joints. Many children with M-CMTC learn at a slower rate than normal but the condition is extremely variable, and whilst some children will need a lot of extra help, others will be very mildly affected.

Very occasionally a child with M-CMTC will be born with a life threatening complication. The majority of children, however, have good general health. The condition is much more difficult to recognise in adulthood but some adults with this condition have been described.

Inheritance patterns and prenatal diagnosis

Inheritance patterns

To date, about 80 individuals with M-CMTC syndrome have been reported worldwide, although the condition is being recognised more frequently and is probably relatively common. Those individuals with milder features are probably underreported. M-CMTC is sporadic, and usually affects only one member of a family. The cause of the condition is so far unknown.

Prenatal diagnosis

No specific tests available. Ultrasound scan abnormalities including increased amniotic fluid, large head size and signs of increased fluid around the baby have been observed in some affected pregnancies.

Medical text written February 2002 by Dr Jill Clayton-Smith. **Last updated September 2007 by Dr Jill Clayton-Smith, Consultant Clinical Geneticist, St. Mary's Hospital, Manchester, UK.**

Further online resources

Medical texts in *The Contact a Family Directory* are designed to give a short, clear description of specific conditions and rare disorders. More extensive information on this condition can be found on a range of reliable, validated websites. Further information on these resources can be found in our **Medical Information on the Internet** article on page 21.

Support

M-CMTC Network
c/o Contact a Family, 209-211 City Road, London EC1V 1JN
Tel: 0808 808 3555 Freephone Helpline   e-mail: keith@macrocephaly-cmtc.com
Web: http://www.Macrocephaly-cmtc.com
The Network provides support by linking families of affected children around the UK and internationally. The Network has further information on the syndrome.
Group details last confirmed September 2007.

MACULAR DISEASE

Age Related Macular Degeneration

Macular Degeneration is a disorder leading to the loss of central vision (the ability to see straight ahead). It is the most common cause of vision loss in people over sixty. By the age of seventy-five, it is thought that nearly fifteen per cent of people are affected. Macular degeneration does not lead to total blindness as it only affects central vision and not peripheral vision.

Macular Degeneration occurs when there is damage to the cells of the macula (the central part of the retina). Light enters the eye through the pupil and is focused on the retina. The retina sends the messages it receives to the brain. In the centre of the retina is an area called the macula. The function of the macula is to allow people to see straight ahead. When there is damage to the cells of the macula, this ability is impaired and people cannot see the fine detail that is required for reading, writing and colour perception.

Normally, both eyes are affected by Macular Degeneration but a diagnosis may be delayed by only one eye being affected before the other and the loss of central vision not being so obvious.

There are two main types of Macular Degeneration: 'wet' and 'dry'. They can be detected by an optometrist but are not perceived as wetness or dryness by an affected individual. In wet Macular Degeneration, there is a build up of fluid under the retina. It is the resulting scarring that leads to a rapid deterioration of central vision. Dry Macular Degeneration progresses over a longer period of time and results from the cells of the macula gradually ceasing to act.

The first signs of loss of central vision can include :
- distorted or blurred objects;
- shape and size distortion of objects;
- undulating or fuzzy straight lines;
- light sensitivity;
- perception of non-existent lights and shapes.

Whilst there is no cure or reliable therapy for dry Macular Degeneration, there are approved treatments for some people with wet Macular Degeneration. These may involve various types of laser, one of which, used in photodynamic therapy (PDT), combines the injection of Visudyne with cold laser treatment. Others include surgical operations on the macula and injections into the eye of substances which can halt the progress of scar formation.

The effects of Macular Degeneration have a major impact on the life of the affected individual who cannot drive or continue to carry out ordinary every day tasks. For younger people with Macular Degeneration who are of working age, the impact on their ability to work is very profound.

Optometrists, GPs and ophthalmic specialists can advise on ways to maximise the visual abilities of affected people. Among the ways of doing this is effective use of peripheral vision and use of vision aids such as magnifiers.

Inheritance patterns
Macular Degeneration may occur in certain families, but the inheritance pattern is variable and at present usually unpredictable.
Prenatal diagnosis
None.

Macular Dystrophy
The term Macular Dystrophy describes the appearance of the macula (central part of the retina) and it occurs in a number of eye conditions. Some Macular Dystrophies are congenital (exist at birth) but many develop in childhood or early adulthood. Often the cause is unknown (Idiopathic) but examples of inherited Macular Dystrophy include Best disease, Stargardt Macular Dystrophy (see entry), Bull's Eye Dystrophy and cone dystrophies. Each condition is rare.

The macular dystrophies can be divided into three main types:
- affecting only the macula;
- affecting the macula and other parts of the retina;
- conditions in which the macular dystrophy is a part of a syndrome/ condition.

Sometimes problems can be picked up during a pre-school or school screening programme. When a parent (or in an older child, the child him/ herself) becomes aware of sight difficulties, a number of examinations and tests can be performed by an ophthalmologist to identify the problem. The ophthalmologist can check the way the eye reacts to bright light and can look at the optic nerve and the retina. Macular Dystrophy can be diagnosed if the ophthalmologist sees that the macula is pale with small specks of black, brown or red. A test called Electroretinogram (ERG) can be performed but this is not easy to carry out on a young child due to the need for sticky patches to be placed round the eyes with wires leading to a machine recording electrical signals made by the eyes.

In the macular dystrophies, the child's vision will be blurred (especially the central vision), the child will have photophobia (dislike bright light) and they will have poor colour vision. However, when young, the child will not realise that their vision is poor but this becomes apparent to the child as they grow older.

Some activities will be unaffected; peripheral vision is good so that the child will be able to run around safely but activities needing good central vision will be affected. Height changes, such as at kerbs will cause confusion and may result in falls. Similar problems will result in difficulties in games at home or at school.

There is no cure for the macular dystrophies so treatment is symptomatic. Encouragement to wear visual aids such as spectacles, contact lens or a low vision aid (LVA) is important. Shielding from bright lights with a brimmed hat will help. Teachers should be advised on classroom methods to help children with macular dystrophies and there is computer software that can be used to good effect. Advice gained from the experience of parents and children previously diagnosed is very helpful.

Inheritance patterns
This will depend on the specific form of Macular Dystrophy. For example Best disease, Butterfly-Shaped Dystrophy, and Bull's Eye Dystrophy are autosomal dominant.

Prenatal diagnosis
This may be possible in cases where there is a previous child in the family. Genetic advice should be sought.

Medical text written December 2004 by Contact a Family. Approved December 2004 by Mr T ffytch, Consultant Ophthalmic Surgeon, London Clinic, London, UK.

Further online resources
Medical texts in *The Contact a Family Directory* are designed to give a short, clear description of specific conditions and rare disorders. More extensive information on this condition can be found on a range of reliable, validated websites. Further information on these resources can be found in our **Medical Information on the Internet** article on page 21.

Support
Macular Disease Society
PO Box 1870, Andover SP10 9AD   Tel: 0845 241 2041 Helpline
e-mail: info@maculardisease.org   Web: http://www.maculardisease.org
The Society is a National Registered Charity No. 1001198, established in 1987. It is a membership society for people with any form of macular degeneration which has led to loss of central vision. The Society's aim is to build confidence and independence for those with central vision impairment. It provides information and practical support, especially at the time of diagnosis. Services provided are a freephone helpline, counselling, magazine and professional journal in print and on tape, national network of self support groups, conferences, leaflets and information and patient support in eye clinics. The Society also sponsors research and works with the RNIB and others to lobby for new treatments and facilities.
Group details last confirmed October 2007.

MAJEWSKI OSTEODYSPLASTIC PRIMORDIAL DWARFISM TYPE II

Background

Majewski Osteodysplastic Primordial Dwarfism Type II (MOPD II) is a form of Primordial Dwarfism which is the name given to a group of disorders where growth delay happens in the earliest development of the human embryo. In many other disorders of short stature (see entry, Restricted Growth) a baby is born with average length and a diagnosis of a specific disorder may be made by observation of other characteristics at birth or short stature may become apparent at a later stage. Babies with one of the primordial dwarfism disorders are affected by intrauterine growth retardation (growth delay in the womb) which leads to very much smaller than average size at birth. Other conditions coming under the heading of Primordial Dwarfism include Silver-Russell syndrome (see entry) and Seckel syndrome.

What are the symptoms?

The features include:

- Low birth weight at full-term delivery, typically just over 1kg (2.3lbs) and with a length of less than 40.6cm (16");
- Microcephaly (small head) see entry – usually average at birth but becoming smaller in proportion as the child grows;
- Conspicuous nose;
- Dental anomalies;
- Scoliosis (sideways curvature of the spine) see entry and kyphosis (outward curvature of the chest area of the spine) in later childhood;
- Disproportionate development of the forearm;
- Dislocation of the hip at birth in some children (see entry, Congenital Dislocation and Developmental Dysplasia of the Hip) and bowing of the knees laterally with age which may lead to dislocation;
- Sparse and fine hair in some children;
- In adulthood, a typical height of less than 1m (39");
- Precocious Puberty (see entry, Premature Sexual Maturation) in some girls;
- Farsightedness in some children with MOPD II (see entry, Vision Disorders in Childhood);
- Renal anomalies (see entry, Kidney disease) are found in some children;
- Aneurisms (small out pouching of the blood vessels in the head) which lead to a predisposition to stroke-like episodes (see entry, Stroke) have been seen in a number of children in the form of Moya Moya disease (see entry).

What are the causes?

MOPD II is a very rare inherited disorder; it is thought that it affects about 1 in 3 million people. The disorder occurs in people of both sexes and all ethnic groups. The cause of MOPD II is not known.

How is it diagnosed?

Diagnosis is made by observation of known characteristics, x-ray, history and elimination of other test findings. Aneurisms can be diagnosed by a cerebral angiography (a test in which a dye is injected into the arteries of the brain to show up faults).

How is it treated?

There is no cure for MOPD II and treatment is symptomatic. Many children with MOPD II have feeding problems and can benefit from help such as frequent feeding with small amounts and in some cases with naso-gastric feeding (through a tube to the stomach). Monitoring is required of:

- the eyes for the development of farsightedness;
- the kidneys for renal anomalies;
- the cerebral vascular system for any indication such as Moya Moya syndrome and the possibility of stroke.

Inheritance patterns and prenatal diagnosis

Inheritance patterns

Although the genes involved in MOPD II have not yet been identified or the mode of inheritance described, it has been suggested that the disorder is autosomal recessive.

Prenatal diagnosis

None.

Medical text written August 2006 by Contact a Family. **Last updated October 2006 by Professor J Hall, Professor Emerita of Pediatrics and Medical Genetics, Department of Pediatrics, British Columbia Children's Hospital, Vancouver, Canada.**

Further online resources

Medical texts in *The Contact a Family Directory* are designed to give a short, clear description of specific conditions and rare disorders. More extensive information on this condition can be found on a range of reliable, validated websites. Further information on these resources can be found in our **Medical Information on the Internet** article on page 21.

Support

There is no support group for Majewski Osteodysplastic Primordial Dwarfism Type II. Cross referrals to other entries in the Contact a Family Directory are intended to provide relevant support for those particular features of the disorder. Organisations identified in those entries do not provide support specifically for Majewski Osteodysplastic Primordial Dwarfism Type II. Families can use Contact a Family's Freephone Helpline for advice, information and, where possible, links to other families. Contact a Family's web-based linking service Making Contact.org can be accessed at http://www.makingcontact.org

MALIGNANT HYPERTHERMIA

Background

When first identified Malignant Hyperthermia (MH) was known as malignant hyperpyrexia. First described in Australia, MH is an inherited condition in which susceptible patients can develop a potentially fatal reaction to certain anaesthetic agents.

What are the causes?

The condition is thought to be due to a loss of the normal control of calcium homeostasis in skeletal muscle when exposed to these agents. This results in marked metabolic stimulation which in turn produces the clinical signs of an MH reaction, one of which is a rapid rise in temperature, hence its name.

How is it diagnosed?

The clinical diagnosis needs to be confirmed by laboratory testing of living muscle tissue, a muscle biopsy. If the test is positive the patient is provided with full information about MH and the family is offered screening based on the autosomal dominant pattern of inheritance, that is parents, siblings and children of the patient in the first instance. About forty per cent of families carry one of the 22 RYR1 diagnostic mutations associated with MH. Genetic testing using DNA from blood samples has recently become available as a preliminary screen for suitable familes but this will still need to be coordinated through a MH centre.

Patients known to be susceptible to MH or who have a family history of MH must inform any anaesthetist treating them about their condition in order to provide safe alternative anaesthesia. Advice can be obtained from the MH centre.

The condition does not affect the general health of the patient and previous uneventful general anaesthesia does not exclude MH.

How is it treated?

Originally, mortality was seventy to eighty per cent but this is now significantly reduced to two to three per cent due to the improved monitoring facilities in the operating theatre and the availability of Dantrolene, the only specific treatment, enabling the reaction to be detected much earlier and successfully treated.

Referral Centre

The UK MH referral centre and National MH register is:

The MH Investigation Unit, Academic Department of Anaesthesia,
Clinical Sciences Building, St James's University Hospital, Leeds LS9 7TF
Tel: 0113 2065274   Tel: 07947 609601 Hotline for medical emergencies only
Fax: 0113 2064140   Web: http://www.leeds.ac.uk/medicine/LeedsMH.html

There is also a European MH Group (EMHG) composed of 23 MH centres throughout Europe. For further information please contact the Secretary of the EMHG, Dr P J Halsall, at the St James University Hospital address, above.

Medical text written October 2000 by Dr J Halsall. **Last updated May 2004 by Dr J Halsall, Honorary Research Fellow (Anaesthetics) and Associate Specialist in Anaesthesia, MH Investigation Unit, Clinical Sciences Building, St James's University Hospital, Leeds, UK.**

Further online resources

Medical texts in *The Contact a Family Directory* are designed to give a short, clear description of specific conditions and rare disorders. More extensive information on this condition can be found on a range of reliable, validated websites. Further information on these resources can be found in our **Medical Information on the Internet** article on page 21.

Support

British Malignant Hyperthermia Association
11 Gorse Close, Newthorpe, Nottingham NG16 2BZ Tel: 01773 717901
e-mail: helpline@bmha.co.uk   Web: http://www.bmha.co.uk
The Association is a National Registered Charity No. 1007739, established in 1983. It has close links with the MH Investigation Unit in Leeds. Two doctors from the MH Unit sit on the BMHA Management Committee. It offers medical and medico-social support to affected individuals and families together with medical updates with regard to safe drugs, screening procedures, research, etc. It provides medical emergency discs and warning cards for those susceptible and family members. It publishes a newsletter and has information available, details on request. The Association has around 400 members.
Group details last confirmed February 2008.

MARFAN SYNDROME

Background

A person with Marfan syndrome will usually be characteristically tall and slim, with lax joints.

What are the symptoms?

Complications may arise, but it is important to note that the range of complications caused by Marfan syndrome, and their severity, varies considerably between individuals. These complications may include:

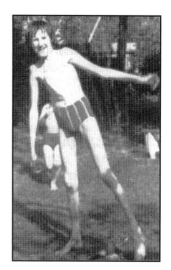

Cardiovascular

Aortic aneurysm, aortic dissection (tears in the wall of the aorta), and mitral valve prolapse sometimes requiring surgical repair. For this reason, each person suspected of this diagnosis should have an echocardiogram (a harmless ultrasound picture of the heart and big blood vessels)

Skeletal

Scoliosis (curvature in the upper thoracic spine) or kyphosis (forward bending curvature in the spine) and, possibly, loose painful joints.

Eyes

Myopia (shortsightedness), dislocation of the ocular lens, retinal detachment, glaucoma.

Lungs

Pneumothorax (collapse of lung due to air leaking from the lungs into the chest cavity), bronchiectasis and emphysema.

Each family has different manifestations.

What are the causes?

This heritable disorder of connective tissue is due to a mutation in the gene for fibrillin, located on chromosome 15. Fibrillin is an important protein component of blood vessel walls, eyes, tendons and ligaments, and lung.

How is it diagnosed?

Marfan syndrome is diagnosed when classical signs of weakness in at least two systems (heart, eyes, skeleton) are found. Diagnosis is made on the basis of family history, physical examination including slit lamp examination for possible dislocated lens, and echocardiogram. Linkage to the gene on chromosome 15 may be studied if affected family members in two generations are available.

Inheritance patterns and prenatal diagnosis
Inheritance patterns
Autosomal dominant inheritance, with one affected parent in seventy-five per cent of cases. In twenty-five per cent of cases the condition occurs as the result of a new spontaneous mutation in the causative gene on chromosome 15.

Prenatal diagnosis
For those who wish to seek prenatal diagnosis, this may be performed by linkage if a large family with other affected members is available for study, or by mutation identification, if the mutation has been identified in the affected parent. Prenatal diagnosis should be discussed with a geneticist prior to pregnancy.

Medical text written November 1991 by Contact a Family. Approved November 1991 by Professor M Patton, Professor of Medical Genetics, St Georges Hospital Medical School, London, UK and Dr J E Wraith, Consultant Paediatrician, Royal Manchester Children's Hospital, Manchester, UK. **Last updated July 2002 by Dr M Briggs, Occupational Health Physician, Hove, UK.**

Further online resources
Medical texts in *The Contact a Family Directory* are designed to give a short, clear description of specific conditions and rare disorders. More extensive information on this condition can be found on a range of reliable, validated websites. Further information on these resources can be found in our **Medical Information on the Internet** article on page 21.

Support
Marfan Association UK
Rochester House, 5 Aldershot Road, Fleet GU51 3NG   Tel: 01252 810472
Fax: 01252 810473   e-mail: marfan@tinyonline.co.uk
Web: http://www.marfan-association.org.uk
The Association is a National Registered Charity No. 802727, established in 1984. It offers support, advice and encouragement for patients and their families, undertakes meetings for patients and the many medical specialists associated with the care of a patient with Marfan syndrome, and actively undertakes and participates in Marfan research. It publishes a twice-yearly magazine "In Touch" and has a wide range of information available, details on request. The Association represents over 1,600 affected families.
Group details last updated February 2008.

Further support for young people with Marfan syndrome is available from CRY - Cardiac Risk in the Young (see entry, Heart Defects).

MARINESCO-SJÖGREN SYNDROME

Marinesco-Garland syndrome: Marinesco-Sjögren-Garland syndrome; Torsten Sjögren; cataract-oligophrenia; hereditary oligophrenic cerebellolental degeneration

Background

Marinesco Sjögren Syndrome (MSS) is a rare disorder with the major features of developmental delay, muscle weakness, early onset cataracts (see entry) and congenital cerebellar ataxia (see entry). Short stature and hypergonadotrophic hypogonadism (underactive sexual organs causing a lack of development at puberty) are common.

Currently over 200 cases of MSS have been reported. It occurs in all ethnic groups but is more common in isolated populations.

What are the symptoms?

Cerebellar Ataxia causes a lack of co-ordination as seen in other conditions (e.g Friedreich's Ataxia, Ataxia telangiectasia - see entries). There are other conditions that resemble MSS.

A child with MSS will have delays in reaching the motor milestones (e.g sitting without support and crawling) and ataxia will become very evident by the time the child is able to sit up. Growth is often poor and pubertal development may not occur due to hypogonadism. Mental retardation can be mild or severe or the child may have no intellectual impairment at all.

Although many adults with MSS are severely disabled, life span seems to be near normal and some individuals will be able to walk with assistance. Other adults have had slowly progressive muscle weakness and use wheelchairs.

How is it diagnosed?

MSS presents at birth because babies are hypotonic (muscle weakness). Although the cataracts are not usually present at birth they can develop quite rapidly in childhood. The diagnosis is usually based on the symptoms observed but eye examinations to confirm cataracts and a MRI of the brain to show a frequently small cerebellum can be helpful. Recently, about 2/3 of the patients with MSS have been found to have mutations in the SIL1 gene.

How is it treated?

MSS is usually treated based on each symptom. This can involve removal of the cataracts through surgery, physical therapy and special education to help visual and motor problems. Hormone replacement therapy is also available if there is hypogonadism.

Inheritance patterns and prenatal diagnosis

Inheritance patterns

Autosomal recessive trait

Prenatal diagnosis

May be available using genetic molecular techniques from laboratories offering custom prenatal testing for families with an affected family member.

Medical Text written February 2007 by Contact a Family. **Last updated August 2007 by Dr William R. Wilcox, Medical Genetics Institute, Cedars-Sinai Medical Center, USA** Group details

Further Online Resources

Medical texts in *The Contact a Family Directory* are designed to give a short, clear description of specific conditions and rare disorders. More extensive information on this condition can be found on a range of reliable, validated websites. Further information on these resources can be found in our **Medical Information on the Internet** article on page 21.

Support

Marinesco-Sjögren Syndrome

There is an online support group for this condition,
Web: http://www.marinesco-sjogren.org e-mail: mss@marinesco-sjogren.org (information about the use of online groups is available in our 'Medical Information on the Internet: Seeking Quality' article on page 21). This group is moderated and refers affected adults, children and their families to relevant and trusted sources of information. It also puts families in touch with one another. Their website has information on this condition endorsed by medical professionals. If you do not have internet access, please telephone our freephone helpline on 0808 808 3555.
Group details last updated August 2007.

MASTOCYTOSIS

Cutaneous mastocytosis; systemic mastocytosis

Background

Mastocytosis is a disorder found in both children and adults, which results from too many mast cells in the body. Found in the skin, stomach lining, intestine and connective tissue (cartilage and tendons) they play an important role in helping your immune system to fight disease and infection. There are several types of mastocytosis recognized in the skin (cutaneous) while those that appear in internal organs are called systemic. Urticaria Pigmentosa (UP) is the most common cutaneous mastocytosis pattern and involves small pink or brown marks on the skin. The condition is usually more unsightly than harmful with some patients even improving naturally. Researchers first described Urticaria Pigmentosa in 1869. Systemic mastocytosis was first reported in the scientific literature in 1933. The true incidence of both types is unknown but it is a rare condition affecting one person in every 500,000.

What are the symptoms?

Mastocytosis is linked to a genetic change in a protein called "kit" on the mast cell which results in too many of them accumulating. Increased numbers of mast cells show as pink or dark marks that may itch.

Too many mast cells in your body result in:

- Skin lesions – these can be pink or brown in colour and vary in size and location depending on the type of cutaneous mastocytosis;
- Itching – this can be quite uncomfortable for patients but often improves with time and can be helped by treatment, wearing loose clothing and keeping cool;
- Swelling – in some types of mastocytosis lesions can swell or blister when rubbed. For some children this may happen less as they grow older and often disappears in adult life;
- Allergies – histamine is the main chemical released during an allergic response. If a mastocytosis patient develops an allergy too much histamine can be released, occasionally causing individuals to collapse;
- Abdominal symptoms – more likely to happen with systemic mastocytosis they can include acid indigestion, cramps, diarrhoea and occasionally ulcers;
- Wheezing – very unusual with cutaneous mastocytosis but possible with systemic disease;
- Bone problems – osteoporosis is a recognized complication of systemic mastocytosis and should be checked for with DEXA scans;

- Anaemia – regular blood checks should be made about once a year if the disease is systemic.

How is it diagnosed?

Diagnosis for mastocytosis can be confirmed by skin biopsy, blood tests and scans of the internal organs or bones. A bone marrow biopsy is the best test for systemic mastocytosis.

How is it treated?

There is no cure for mastocytosis but treatments can relieve the symptoms. Antihistamines can be taken to relieve itching and to treat indigestion. Steroid creams and moisturizers can be used to treat the skin although the use of strong steroid cream use is often limited by the need to avoid thinning of the skin. Better treatments may become available in the future as understanding of the genetic basis of the condition advances.

For most individuals with the condition, mastocytosis will often be no more than an inconvenience requiring no specific treatments or visits to specialists. If symptoms indicate the systemic disease may be developing it is sensible to have investigations and check ups with someone who understands the disease.

Inheritance patterns and prenatal diagnosis

Inheritance patterns

While research is being done into the genetic basis for the condition it does not appear to run in families.

Prenatal diagnosis

Not available.

Medical text written February 2008 by Contact a Family. Approved February 2008 by Dr Clive Grattan, Consultant Dermatologist, St.Johns Institute of Dermatology, St.Thomas's Hospital, London, UK.

Support

UK Mastocytosis Support Group
c/o Contact a Family, 209-211 City Road, London EC1V 1JN Tel: 01506 431908
e-mail: winegums@blueyonder.co.uk Web: http://www.ukmasto.co.uk
The UK Mastocytosis Support Group was established in 2004. The Group provide understanding support and up to date information for adults and parents affected by Mastocytosis and Mast Cell Related Conditions. It is a private e-mail group with additional phone support. It has meetings within the UK for group members and medical professionals. Ultimately the Group aims to become a registered charity.
Group details last updated February 2008.

McCUNE-ALBRIGHT SYNDROME

McCune-Albright syndrome: Albright syndrome

Background

McCune-Albright syndrome is a rare genetic disorder affecting the bones and skin pigmentation. It is also associated with endocrine problems, notably premature sexual development (see entry, Premature Sexual Maturation). In its classic form, McCune-Albright syndrome involves at least two of these features. Life expectancy is near normal.

What are the symptoms?

The hallmark feature of McCune-Albright syndrome is premature puberty in females. Early development of breasts and pubic hair and an increased rate of growth are common. Menstrual periods may begin in early childhood and early menstrual bleeding is caused by estrogens - chemicals secreted into the bloodstream as a result of the formation of ovarian cysts. The cysts and irregular menstrual bleeding may continue into adolescence and adulthood. Many adult women with McCune-Albright syndrome do not have affected fertility.

Less commonly early sexual development occurs in males, involving the development of testes, pubic and underarm hair and increased growth rate.

The spectrum of features has broadened to include problems associated with the heart and liver. Individuals can be differently affected by the range and severity of features. Some children may be affected by bone disease in early infancy and have a range of hormonal problems; others may be entirely healthy.

Many individuals with McCune-Albright syndrome have thyroid gland abnormalities including goitre (generalised enlargement) and irregular masses called nodules and cysts. Some individuals show an excessive secretion of pituitary growth hormone which causes the coarsening of facial features, enlargement of hands and feet and arthritis. Less commonly, some affected individuals may have the features of Cushing syndrome/disease (see entry).

Individuals with McCune-Albright syndrome also have Polyostotic Fibrous Dysplasia (abnormal fibrous tissue growth in many bones). The severity of the bone disease is very variable and any bone in the body may be affected. When the Polyostotic Fibrous Dysplasia occurs in weight-bearing bones, such as the femur (upper leg bone), limping, bowing, pain and sometimes fractures may result. If the bones that form the upper jaw and skull are affected, deafness or blindness can result from 'pinched nerves' and facial asymmetry. Some children are affected minimally and in others severe bone disease has a permanent effect upon mobility and physical appearance. Hypersecretion from the parathyroid glands (with elevated parathyroid hormone levels and raised serum calcium) may make the bone disease more severe.

Most children with McCune-Albright have café-au-lait spots (irregular, flat areas of increased skin pigment so called because in children with light complexions, they are the colour of coffee with milk). These may be extensive and usually have irregular margins. They are different from the café-au-lait spots seen in Neurofibromatosis. In dark skinned children, these spots may be difficult to see. The skin pigmentation is not present at birth, but usually from about a month to six weeks of age. The pigmentation does not become more extensive with time.

Inheritance patterns and prenatal diagnosis

Inheritance patterns

McCune-Albright syndrome is caused by somatic mutations (or changes) in the GNAS1 gene that take place after conception. As these mutations do not take place in the germ cells (egg and sperm), McCune-Albright syndrome is not inherited but sporadic with no other family member, brother or sister likely to be affected.

Prenatal diagnosis

It may sometimes be possible to perform prenatal diagnosis by chorionic villus sampling (CVS) or amniocentesis during pregnancy. Genetic counselling may be helpful for individuals and families affected by this condition.

Medical text written July 2004 by Contact a Family. Approved July 2004 by Dr R Stanhope, Consultant Paediatric Endocrinologist, Great Ormond Street Hospital, London, UK.

Support

There is no support group for McCune-Albright syndrome. Cross referrals to other entries in the Contact a Family Directory are intended to provide relevant support for these particular features of the disorder. Organisations identified in these entries do not provide support specifically for McCune-Albright syndrome. Families can use Contact a Family's Freephone Helpline for advice, information and, where possible, links to other families. Contact a Family's web-based linking service Making Contact.org can be accessed at http://www.makingcontact.org

MELNICK-NEEDLES SYNDROME

Melnick-Needles: Melnick-Needles Osteodysplasty

Background

This rare genetic syndrome is best described in females, with a small number of severely affected males also reported.

What are the symptoms?

The condition in females is characterised by thickening or sclerosis of a number of bones in the body. This leads to deformity in the bones, especially in the skull, pelvis and long bones of the arms and legs, in addition to short stature. Secondary osteoarthritis may occur. Other features may vary in the child but may include scoliosis (see entry), kyphosis (forward curvature), small rib cage with the ribs distorted in shape and short thumbs and big toes. Ear and chest infections are common. Obstructive lesions of the ureters are common and deafness (see entry) and cardiac abnormalities have occasionally been described. Mental development is not affected.

Inheritance patterns and prenatal diagnosis

Inheritance patterns

Most cases are sporadic and a gene resident on the X chromosome has been shown to be mutated in the disorder.

Prenatal diagnosis

Prenatal diagnosis has not been described.

Medical text written November 1995 by Dr M Patton, Consultant Clinical Geneticist, St George's Hospital, London, UK. **Last updated January 2003 by Professor Stephen Robertson, CHRF Professor of Paediatric Genetics, Dunedin School of Medicine, University of Otago, Dunedin, New Zealand.**

Further online resources

Medical texts in *The Contact a Family Directory* are designed to give a short, clear description of specific conditions and rare disorders. More extensive information on this condition can be found on a range of reliable, validated websites. Further information on these resources can be found in our **Medical Information on the Internet** article on page 21.

Support

MNS Support Group
4 Kinver Lane, Bexhill on Sea TN40 2ST   Tel: 01424 217790
e-mail: gill@melnickneedlesyndrome.com   Web: http://www.melnickneedlesyndrome.com
The Group was, established in 1994. It offers support by telephone and letter. It has information available, details on request. The Group is in touch with over 12 families.
Group details last confirmed October 2006.

MELORHEOSTOSIS

Background

Melorheostosis was first described in 1922 by Léri and Joanny as "Hyperostose en Coulée" or "Hyperostosis (flowing overgrowth of bone) resembling dripping candle wax". Melorheostosis is a rare and progressive disease characterised by hyperostosis of cortical (outer layer) bone. Melorheostosis affects both bone and soft tissue (muscle and tendons) growth and development. The age of diagnosis varies widely but it commonly starts in childhood. Melorheostosis is somewhat more common in individuals who have an otherwise benign disorder of bone known as osteopoikilosis ('spotty bones').

What are the symptoms?

While the disorder is not life threatening, it often results in severe pain, limitation of movement, malformed and immobilized muscles, limbs or tendons.

The symptoms can include;

- Irregular bone growth including cortical thickening and 'candle wax' appearance;
- Limb length inequalities;
- Joint swelling and fusion;
- Soft tissue abnormalities including tendon and ligament shortening, absent or abnormal muscles, calcification, contractures resulting in malformed or immobilized joints;
- Range of motion limitations;
- Pain and stiffness;
- Sensitivity to cold;
- Hyper-pigmentation of skin;
- Vascular abnormalities.

What are the causes?

The cause is currently unknown. It is believed the LEMD3 gene (a gene critical to bone formation and the cause of osteopoikilosis) may play a role in melorheostosis but its exact role has not yet been clarified. Researchers are investigating the role of LEMD3 and other related proteins which may eventually lead to identifying the cause and the introduction of effective treatments.

How is it diagnosed?

Melorheostosis is usually diagnosed through X-ray which often shows the characteristic pattern of thickened bone lesions that resemble dripping candle wax.

How is it treated?

Treatment options may include surgery, physical and occupational therapy, hydrotherapy, and medications to alter the bone remodelling process. However most cases do not require surgical intervention.

In many cases of melorheostosis pain management is required. These medications although helpful in the early stages of the chronic progression, can be less so for the severely affected. In extremely rare cases where the pain is unbearable patients have even undergone amputation.

Inheritance patterns and prenatal diagnosis

Inheritance patterns

Melorheostosis is somewhat more common in individuals who have osteopoikilosis, an unusual benign disorder characterized by a spotty appearance to the ends of the bones. This is associated with mutations in the LEMD3 gene but does not usually have clinical consequences. Melorheostosis itself affects the tissues in a segmental fashion and does not follow a Mendelian pattern of inheritance. Most cases occur sporadically in the general population (but somewhat more commonly against the background of osteopoikilosis in the family) and the genetic/biochemical cause is not known for certain.

Prenatal diagnosis

The condition cannot be predicted prenatally.

Medical text written August 2007 by Contact a Family. Approved August 2007 by Prof Paul Wordsworth, Professor of Clinical Rheumatology (Oxford University) and Honorary Consultant Rheumatologist (Nuffield Orthopaedic Centre).

Further Online Resources

Medical texts in *The Contact a Family Directory* are designed to give a short, clear description of specific conditions and rare disorders. More extensive information on this condition can be found on a range of reliable, validated websites. Further information on these resources can be found in our **Medical Information on the Internet** article on page 21.

Support

Melorheostosis Association UK

1 Greengate, Cardale Park, Harrogate, HG3 1GY

Tel: 01423 709993 Web: http://www.melo.eu.com

The Melorheostosis Association UK began in 2004 by an affected adult. The Group have been successful in fundraising and are now funding a research post in Oxford. They have a panel of medical advisers and close links with the US group.

Group details last updated August 2007.

MÉNIÈRE'S DISEASE

Background

Ménière's disease (MD) is a disease of the inner ear. The inner ear is composed of the organ of balance (semicircular canals) and the organ of hearing (the cochlea). In MD these organs are damaged causing a triad of symptoms which include vertigo (dizziness, illusion of movement), noises in the ear - tinnitus (see entry) and hearing loss (see entry, Deafness). The severity and frequency of symptoms varies between people and with time in the individual person. MD affects mainly white people and affects both sexes equally. It can occur at all ages, including childhood, but its onset is most frequent in the twenty to forty age group.

What are the symptoms?

MD is a long-term progressive illness which tends to follow a series of stages. In the early stage, episodes (or 'attacks') of vertigo occur unexpectedly and these may be associated with nausea and vomiting. There may also be some hearing loss, a sensation of fullness and discomfort in the affected ear and tinnitus. MD usually affects one ear, but fifteen per cent of people have both ears affected at the start of symptoms. Initially episodes tend to be intermittent varying in frequency from daily to every few months and can last from a few minutes to several hours. Periods of remission vary from days to months or even years, making MD an unpredictable disease. Hearing and sensation return to normal during these times.

In the intermediate stage, episodes of vertigo continue but may be less severe. Attacks may be preceded or be followed by a period of imbalance and movement induced giddiness. Furthermore, permanent hearing loss develops and continues to fluctuate with the vertigo. As attacks increase, tinnitus fluctuates and becomes more prominent. Remissions are variable.

In the later stages and as the disease progresses, up to fifty per cent of individuals develop symptoms in both ears. Hearing loss increases and may be severe. As there is permanent damage to the balance organ in the ear, significant general balance problems are common, especially in the dark. Often the episodes of vertigo diminish or stop.

Different symptoms of MD may be more pronounced in specific situations. For example, individuals may experience hearing loss when attending meetings, balance problems when trying to decorate at home, or tinnitus when trying to get to sleep. Additionally, individuals may not be able to identify a main symptom of their disease or experience the fluctuation of many changing symptoms early in the illness.

Anxiety and depression may be associated with MD and professional assistance is available for coping psychologically and physically with self-management and lifestyle adjustment to MD.

What are the causes?

For many individuals with MD, the cause of their disease currently remains unknown. A number of factors are, however, known to be involved in the development of the disease. These include an increased pressure of the fluid in the endolymphatic sac in the inner ear; a genetic predisposition; allergic factors damaging the inner ear; some specific viral infections; vascular factors (there is an association between migraine and MD); metabolic factors and other unknown factors. The relationship between these factors and the progression of MD currently remains unclear.

How is it diagnosed?

As yet, there is no specific test that, on its own, is reliable in diagnosing MD. Vertigo and dizziness are associated with a number of other diseases and consequently misdiagnosis may be frequent in individuals with MD. Occasionally patients with anaemia (anemia - US), hypothyroidism (see entry), diabetes mellitus (see entry), autoimmune disease, and syphilis may have symptoms similar to MD.

How is it treated?

Treatment for the 'ear related symptoms' of MD is focused on the control of symptoms. These are medical (drugs) and surgical treatments for control of the vertigo. Masking devices and retraining therapy can help tinnitus and appropriate hearing aids can be valuable.

Inheritance patterns and prenatal diagnosis

Inheritance patterns

In some cases, MD is familial.

Prenatal diagnosis

None available.

Medical text written June 2002 by Contact a Family. Approved June 2002 by Dr G Osborne, Medical Adviser to the Ménière's Society, UK.

Further online resources

Medical texts in *The Contact a Family Directory* are designed to give a short, clear description of specific conditions and rare disorders. More extensive information on this condition can be found on a range of reliable, validated websites. Further information on these resources can be found in our **Medical Information on the Internet** article on page 21.

Support

Ménière's Society
The Rookery, Surrey Hills Business Park, Wotton, Dorking RH5 6QT
Tel: 0845 120 2975 Helpline   Tel: 01306 876883 Admin   Fax: 01306 876057 & minicom
e-mail: info@menieres.org.uk   Web: http://www.menieres.orgo.uk
The Ménière's Society is a National Registered Charity No. 297246, established in 1984.
It offers support to affected individuals, including a small number of children and young
people, and their carers and links members where possible. It also promotes and funds
research. It publishes a quarterly magazine 'SPIN' and has information available, details on
request. The Society has over 5,500 members.
Group details last confirmed April 2007.

"What brilliant news to hear that you've found another family and that they want contact with us. You may not think it but you've done so much for us." Parent.

MENINGITIS

Background

Meningitis is a condition in which inflammation of the meninges (lining) of the brain and spinal cord occurs due to a bacterial, viral or, rarely, fungal infection. The bacterial form is life threatening. Fungal meningitis also tends to be severe while the viral form is usually less so.

Prevention in the form of safe and effective vaccines against some forms of meningitis are now available. A primary course of conjugate Hib, meningococcal C and pneumococcal vaccines is given between eight and sixteen weeks of age. Boosters are given at twelve and thirteen months. Mumps vaccine is part of the MMR vaccine, the first of two doses being given at thirteen months old. BCG vaccine against tuberculosis is offered to all children and babies who are felt to be at higher risk.

What are the symptoms?

Complications of meningitis include deafness (which may be total), brain damage, cerebral palsy, epilepsy and changes in eyesight. Behavioural changes such as subsequent temper tantrums, aggression and mood swings may also cause problems. Meningococcal disease, which involves blood poisoning, may cause the loss of fingers, toes and sometimes even part of a limb.

What are the causes?

Bacterial meningitis can be caused by many different bacteria including meningococcus, Haemophilus influenzae type b (Hib), pneumococcus, leptospirosis (including Weil's disease), tuberculosis, listeria, streptococcus and E.coli. The organisms affecting the newborn baby are often different from those affecting the older child or adult and the outcome is more serious.

Viral meningitis is commonly caused by the coxsackie and ECHO viruses. Some viruses cause a combination of meningitis and encephalitis (see entry) i.e. meningoencephalitis. Mumps meningoencephalitis was common, but no longer so, because of the widespread use of the MMR vaccine.

Children and adults with particular diseases, such as those of the immune system, including HIV infection, may be more susceptible to some forms of bacterial or fungal meningitis.

Inheritance patterns and prenatal diagnosis

Inheritance patterns

Usually none. Very rarely a tendency to meningococcal disease may run in families. Tests are available to check on this, where appropriate.

Prenatal diagnosis
None.

Medical text written February 2001 by Dr D Elliman and Dr H Bedford. **Last updated October 2006 by Dr D Elliman, Consultant in Community Child health, Islington Primary Care Trust, London, UK and Great Ormond Street hospital, London, UK and immunisation Co-ordinator, Islington Primary Care Trust and Dr h Bedford, Senior lecturer, Centre for Paediatric Epidemiology and Biostatistics, institute of Child health, London, UK.**

Further information can be found by referring to the Immunisation page and the Health Promotion, England Web: http://www.immunisation.org.uk

Support
Meningitis Trust
Fern House, Bath Road, Stroud GL5 3TJ
Tel: 0800 028 1828 Freephone Nurse-lead Helpline (24 hours)
Tel: 01453 768003 Minicom   Fax: 01453 768001   e-mail: info@meningitis-trust.org
Web: http://www.meningitis-trust.org
Web: http://www.inmed.co.uk (for health professionals)
Web: http://www.meningitis-schools.org (resources for teachers of children 14-16 years)
The Trust is a National Registered Charity No. 803016, established in 1986. It aims to ensure that affected people receiving quality care and support for life and is working towards the eradication of menintitis and meningococcal septicaemia (blood poisoning). It offers a range of services to affected people, professionals and the general public. The Trust provides professional counselling, home visiting and financial grants. It raises awareness of Meningitis throught education, training and research.
Group details last confirmed September 2007.

Meningitis Research Foundation
Midland Way, Thornbury, Bristol BS35 2BS   Tel: 080 8800 3344 (24-hour helpline)
Tel: 01454 281811   Fax: 01454 281094   e-mail: info@meningitis.org
 Web: http://www.meningitis.org
The Foundation is a National Registered Charity No. 328205, established in 1989. It offers information, befriending and support for people affected by Meningitis and funds scientific research into the prevention, detection and treatment of meningitis and septicaemia, the blood poisoning form of Meningitis. It publishes a quarterly newsletter 'Microscope' and has a wide range of information available, details on request. The Foundation has 5,000 members in the UK and Republic of Ireland.
Group details last confirmed March 2007.

MENTAL HEALTH

Background

Mental health and mental health problems are not exact terms. But the components of mental health can broadly be said to include the following: the ability to develop socially, emotionally and intellectually; the ability to initiate and sustain mutually satisfying relationships; the ability to empathise with others; and the ability to learn from periods of emotional difficulty and distress, and to develop because of them. Defined in this way mental health, rather than physical health, is something of an ideal state.

Mental health problems are difficulties which arise in these areas, and are likely to have their roots in constitutional, environmental or social factors, or a combination of these. Such problems cover a wide spectrum of emotional and behavioural difficulties which vary significantly in their severity and duration. At one end of the spectrum, mental health problems in children may be relieved by the love and support of families and other carers without the need for intervention from a mental health professional. At the other end of the spectrum, mental or psychiatric disorders suggest the existence of a clinically recognisable set of symptoms or behaviour in accordance with the standards set out in the World Health Organisation's International Classification of diseases (ICD10) which means that children are likely to need specialist help.

Doctors have become more aware recently of a number of situations that leave children vulnerable and many of them with mental health problems. Children who have a parent with a mental health problem are one such group. If a parent has a major psychiatric illness, they may experience disruptions of carer and place. Each admission of the parent may mean they go to grandparents or into foster care unless there is a partner to keep them. Parents with their own troubled backgrounds including abuse and neglect may have personality disorder and often children in these families receive inconsistent and unpredictable parenting that leaves them troubled. Depressed parents can be emotionally preoccupied, unavailable to their child and often these children have considerable difficulties. Parents may also be using a range of substances, alcohol, cocaine, heroin that at times leave them unable to function as parents, the child may be ignored or left, in the overwhelming need to obtain their substance and there may be little money left for the practical care of the child.

What are the causes?

Doctors are also more aware that some groups of children are more vulnerable to mental health problems. Asylum seekers enter the country and some have children with them, other young people come in as unaccompanied minors. Often they have witnessed horrendous events and may have been subjected to many traumatic and abusive experiences. They can be fearful, suspicious, with depression, despair and post traumatic stress disorder. Some children in the population are abused or neglected or both. Physical, sexual and emotional abuse, emotional neglect and physical neglect go on and the children are often left troubled and damaged. They have problems with relationships and trust, they find concentration and learning difficult and their self-esteem is very low. These children may still live in their family or may be in foster care or be 'looked after' children. Often they are depressed, anxious and aggressive. Children who are bullied in school can also become anxious and depressed.

When parents divorce, which is now very common, children are often transiently troubled but then settle. However, some remain distressed and if there was domestic violence then the child with ongoing contact can become more disturbed over time. Many of these children can be seen as suffering psychosocial problems but the mental health sequelae are significant and sometimes the problems can be such as to mimic the disorders such as ADHD, Aspergers or psychotic episodes. These disorders therefore need careful diagnosis to ensure the appropriate intervention.

Mental health services

Perhaps the biggest change in recent years has been the recognition of the needs of children, particularly in the area of emotional health and psychological wellbeing.

The National Service Framework (NSF) for services for children included an NSF for Child Mental Health and this led to a great many changes. A mapping exercise of all services for Child, Adolescent and Family Mental Health revealed massive under-provision and Government set aside considerable sums of money. It was recognised that the workforce was quite inadequate and expansion has been greatly encouraged. Priority areas were highlighted and these included services for looked after children, children whose parents had mental health problems, were in prison or were using excessive alcohol or illegal substances. Refugees and asylum-seeking families were also seen to have considerable mental health problems. Also new areas of need were highlighted, these included children and adolescents with learning difficulties who had in addition mental health problems and similarly, children with chronic physical illness or sensory deprivation.

Gaps were recognised and slowly attempts are being made to fill them. When young people reach sixteen years, many are no longer eligible for CAMHS services but adult services do not feel capable of assisting. Transition services are being developed to bridge the gap and also to help where conditions such as Attention Deficit Hyperactivity disorder (see entry), Asperger syndrome (see entry, Autism Spectrum disorders including Asperger syndrome), and Obsessive Compulsive disorder (see entry) are seen as mental health problems in CAMHS but not in adult mental health services. There are now specialist substance abuse services for adolescents and early intervention in psychosis teams that treat fourteen year olds and over.

The legal context has also changed with the Children and Adoption Act 2002 and the Children Act 2004. This latter act sets in train Children's Trusts bringing all the services together (Virtual Trusts) to plan a comprehensive service for each locality to try and ensure prevention and early intervention as well as the best use of the resources available.

Finally, and maybe most significantly, the voice and experience of the users, children, young people and their families, is at the core of all developments and the evaluation of the services so that their perspective can make a central contribution to the next phase of moves to improve the mental health of our children, young people and their families.

Medical text written February 1997 by Dr J Trowell. **Last updated November 2005 by Professor J Trowell, Consultant Child and Adolescent Psychiatrist, Director of the Child and Adolescent Mental Health Services Research Team, University of Worcester, Worcester, UK.**

Support

YoungMinds
48-50 St John Street, London EC1M 4DG   Tel: 0800 018 2138 freephone Parents' Information Service (Mon & Fri, 10am-1pm; Tues & Thurs, 1-4pm; Wed, 1-4pm & 6-8pm)
Tel: 020 7336 8445 Office   e-mail: enquiries@youngminds.org.uk
Web: http://www.youngminds.org.uk
YoungMinds is a National Registered Charity No. 1016968, established in 1989 which is committed to improving the mental health of all children. Services include the Parents' Information Service, a free confidential telephone helpline offering information and advice to any adult with concerns about the mental health of a child or young person. YoungMinds also offers consultancy, seminars and training, leaflets and booklets for young people, parents and professionals and publishes 'YoungMinds Magazine' every two months.
Group details last confirmed October 2006.

Mind
15-19 Broadway, London E15 4BQ
Tel: 0845 766 0163 Infoline (Mon-Fri, 9.15am - 5.15pm, voice and text)
Tel: 020 8519 2122   Fax: 020 8522 1725   e-mail: info@mind.org.uk
Web: http://www.mind.org.uk
Mind is a National Registered Charity No. 219830, established in 1946. It has taken the lead in promoting mental health throughout England and Wales, and working for a better life for everyone with experience of mental distress. It offers mental health services through a network of local Mind associations including: Sheltered homes; Drop-in centres; Counselling; Advocacy; and Employment schemes. It publishes a bi-monthly magazine 'OpenMind' and has a wide range of information available, details on request.
Group details last confirmed September 2007.

Scottish Association for Mental Health
Cumbrae House, 15 Carlton Court, Glasgow G5 9JP
Tel: 0141 568 7000 SAMH Information Service (Mon-Fri, 2.00-4.30pm)
Fax: 0141 568 7001   e-mail: enquire@samh.org.uk   Web: http://www.samh.org.uk
The Association is a Scottish Registered Charity No. SC008897, established in 1923. It offers a range of community based services throughout Scotland. It monitors government policy and campaigns with and on behalf of people with mental health problems. It also promotes positive mental health through training, education and publicity. It has a wide range of information available, details on request. The Association has an information service for mental health service users, their families and carers. Legal and benefits advice is given free of charge.
Group details last confirmed September 2007.

The Contact a Family Website had over 1.7 million visits during 2007.

METABOLIC DISEASES

Background

Metabolic diseases are a group of more than one thousand inherited disorders in which there is genetic fault in metabolism (the body's chemistry).

What are the symptoms?

The effect of the defect on the patients is very varied and not always predictable. Many defects cause severe illness and death whilst others seem to cause no problems.

What are the causes?

Metabolism is a very complex process that occurs in small steps, each one being regulated by an enzyme (complex protein). Some involve anabolism (the build-up of essential components of the body) and others involve catabolism (the break down of essential components of the body). As a consequence of a genetic defect the enzyme may be completely missing or have worked inefficiently. The enzymes are usually grouped in pathways and if there is a blockage then the compound accumulates before the block and the substance that is normally formed will be reduced.

How is it treated?

For some metabolic diseases there is life-long treatment with diet, medicines, enzyme replacement therapy or with organ transplantation. Gene and stem cell therapy give hope for the future.

Inheritance patterns and prenatal diagnosis

Inheritance patterns

These depend on which chromosome the gene is to be found and the type of defect. Most are recessive but some are X-linked or dominant and a few are sporadic. Genetic counselling should always be sought.

Prenatal diagnosis

Prenatal diagnosis is often available but is dependent on the precise metabolic disease and several other factors.

Medical text written November 1991 by Contact a Family. Approved November 1991 by Professor M Patton, Professor of Medical Genetics, St Georges Hospital Medical School, London, UK and Dr J E Wraith, Consultant Paediatrician, Royal Manchester Children's Hospital, Manchester, UK. **Last updated November 2004 by Professor J Leonard, Professor of Paediatric Metabolic Disease, Institute of Child Health, London, UK.**

Further online resources

Medical texts in *The Contact a Family Directory* are designed to give a short, clear description of specific conditions and rare disorders. More extensive information on this condition can be found on a range of reliable, validated websites. Further information on these resources can be found in our **Medical Information on the Internet** article on page 21.

Support

Climb National Information and Advice Centre for Metabolic Diseases
176 Nantwich Road, Crewe CW2 6BG
Tel: 0800 652 3181 Freephone Family Service Helpline Tel: 0845 241 2173
Fax: 0845 241 2174   e-mail: info.svcs@climb.org.uk Web: http://www.climb.org.uk
Climb is a National Registered Charity No 1089588, established in 1981. Offering information and support on over 700 metabolic diseases. For a full list of conditions please take a look at their website or contact CLIMB directly. Climb offers information and advice to families and professionals on metabolic diseases. Long term support and advice for families is also offered even from the pre-diagnosis stage. Climb publishes newsletters throughout the year and a magazine three times a year which has a wide range of factual information, services and contacts. Climb also funds research into Metabolic diseases, makes small grants to family members in need, provides a national network of befrienders, support groups, family contacts and friends of Climb. Climb has internet message forums available to families/individuals for specific disease groups. Climb conferences and meetings are arranged regularly in various venues across the UK.
Group details last updated February 2008.

MICROCEPHALY

Background

In Microcephaly there is sub-optimal growth of the brain which causes it to be smaller than usual.

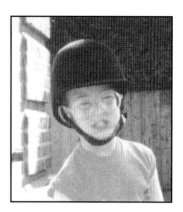

What are the symptoms?

Children and adults who are affected by microcephaly have variable neurological impairments, from very mild learning difficulties (see entry, Learning Disability) to much more severe problems including feeding difficulties, profound learning disability, epilepsy (see entry) and spasticity (see entry, Cerebral Palsy).

What are the causes?

Microcephaly may be caused by many different conditions that may be genetic or entirely non-genetic in origin. For example, genetic causes include different chromosome disorders, different single gene abnormalities and specific genetic syndromes. Non-genetic causes include infections contracted by the baby in the womb (intrauterine infections), reduction in blood supply to the developing fetal brain during pregnancy and some post-natal infections or traumas.

Intrauterine infections which can cause Microcephaly include Cytomegalovirus (CMV), Toxoplasmosis (see entries) and Rubella (see entry).

Rare syndromes which cause disturbed brain development and Microcephaly, usually with other physical disabilities, include Cornelia De Lange syndrome, Rubinstein Taybi syndrome (see entries) and Seckel syndrome.

How is it diagnosed?

At or after birth, Microcephaly is detected by measuring the head circumference. Detailed brain imaging, such as a magnetic resonance scan, may demonstrate an alteration in brain structure, for example, a decrease in the number and complexity of the folds on the surface of the brain (see entry, Cortical Malformations). However, quite frequently, the brain scan appearance simply confirms reduction in overall size of the brain that is otherwise normally formed.

Inheritance patterns and prenatal diagnosis

Inheritance patterns

Complexity arises because different inheritance patterns of genetic Microcephaly are possible. It is known that faults in the function of many different genes may cause genetic Microcephaly. In autosomal dominant Microcephaly, there is one affected parent who has a fifty per cent chance of transmitting the gene fault to each child they may have. In autosomal recessive Microcephaly, both parents are unaffected but both carry a single, recessive Microcephaly gene. It is only when both parents transmit this gene to their child (twenty-five per cent risk of this happening) that the child will be affected by Microcephaly. In X-chromosome linked Microcephaly, an unaffected mother who carries an X-chromosome linked Microcephaly gene has a twenty-five per cent chance of having a son who is affected by Microcephaly. Of these three different inheritance mechanisms, autosomal recessive Microcephaly is probably the most common and this condition is most often characterized by Microcephaly that is present at birth and learning disability that is non-progressive.

Prenatal diagnosis

It is unusual for genetic Microcephaly to be diagnosed by ultrasound scan in early pregnancy but a reduction in fetal brain growth may be discovered by scans undertaken during in the last few months of pregnancy. A number of Microcephaly genes have been discovered but it is rare for any of these to be detected in an affected child. The most common gene defects are found in the ASPM gene, also called MCPH5, and laboratory diagnostic DNA tests for this condition are being introduced at present.

Medical text written May 2002 by Dr J Tolmie. **Last updated August 2006 by Dr J Tolmie, Consultant Clinical Geneticist, Ferguson-Smith Centre for Clinical Genetics, Glasgow, UK.**

Further online resources

Medical texts in *The Contact a Family Directory* are designed to give a short, clear description of specific conditions and rare disorders. More extensive information on this condition can be found on a range of reliable, validated websites. Further information on these resources can be found in our **Medical Information on the Internet** article on page 21.

Support

Microcephaly Support Group

PO Box 519, Pinner HA5 9DR   Tel: 01638 552689   e-mail: gill@microcephaly.org.uk
Web: http://www.microcephaly.co.uk
This is a small parent support group re-established in 2002. The group offers support and information by letter, telephone and email. It publishes a regular newsletter 'Connections' and is in touch with approximately 300 families.
Group details last updated January 2007.

MIGRAINE

Background

Migraine is the name given to recurrent headaches that are not secondary to any other medical problem.

What are the symptoms?

They are usually one-sided, often with throbbing or pounding pain, associated with nausea, and sensitivity to light, and sound and head movement. Movement of the head makes the symptoms worse. Migraine usually comes at intervals with complete freedom between attacks. About twenty per cent of patients have visual or other disturbances known as the migraine aura. In the UK, fifteen per cent of the population suffer migraine, with about six per cent of children affected. The condition is much more prevalent in women with over eighteen per cent of women reporting migraine in the last year, compared to eight per cent of men.

The headache in childhood may also be severe and the abdominal symptoms which include sickness, vomiting and stomach aches are often pronounced. Some children have prominent associated dizziness.

What are the causes?

Precipitants can include missed meals, dehydration, lack of sleep, stress, fatigue, exertion, particularly relaxation after stress, weekends and holidays, intense strenuous exercise, bright lights, excitement, change of sleep pattern, dietary and hormone factors.

Migraine is now much better understood, and considered to be a disorder involving brain areas involved in the processing and control of pain, other sensory input, and the blood vessels of the head. It is now considered that changes in brain chemistry cause the well-recognised blood vessel changes.

How is it diagnosed?

If migraine is suspected in adults and children and attacks do not respond to simple pain killers, the diagnosis should be confirmed by a medical practitioner who can advise on specific management strategies. Most patients with migraine will have a family history of the problem.

Inheritance patterns and prenatal diagnosis

Inheritance patterns

Only the rare condition familial hemiplegic migraine has an autosomal dominant pattern of inheritance. There is undoubtedly a familial link but whether migraine is a learned response or a true genetic condition is the subject of debate.

No specific pattern of inheritance has been identified for the more typical types of migraine, and although a genetic component may be present, environmental factors are also important.

Prenatal diagnosis

None.

Medical text written November 1991 by Contact a Family. Approved November 1991 by Professor M Patton, Professor of Medical Genetics, St Georges Hospital Medical School, London, UK and Dr J E Wraith, Consultant Paediatrician, Royal Manchester Children's Hospital, Manchester, UK. **Last updated February 2006 by Dr A MacGregor, Director of Clinical Research, The City of London Migraine Clinic, London, UK.**

Support

The Migraine Trust

2nd Floor, 55-56 Russell Square, London WC1B 4HP   Tel: 020 7436 1336
Fax: 020 7436 2880   e-mail: info@ migrainetrust.org   Web: http://www.migrainetrust.org
The Trust is a National Registered Charity No. 1081300, established in 1965. It publishes 'Migraine News' and has a helpline with a wide range of information available. It also raises funds to support research and hosts an International Symposium every two years. The Trust's web site carries extensive information on the management and incidence of Migraine which, it is estimated, affects one in six people in the UK.
Group details last confirmed March 2007.

Migraine Action Association

6 Oakley Hay Lodge, Great Fold Road, Corby NN18 9AS   Tel: 01536 461333
Fax: 01536 461444   e-mail: info@migraine.org.uk   Web: http://www.migraine.org.uk
The Association is a National Registered Charity No. 207783, established in 1958. It produces a quarterly newsletter, a range of publications and has a website for children, Web: http://www.migraine4kids.org.uk. The Association also has information specifically regarding abdominal migraine. It has over 10,000 members.
Group details last updated March 2007.

MITOCHONDRIAL CYTOPATHIES and related disorders

Background

Mitochondrial Cytopathies are a group of disorders which may present at any age and are extremely variable in presentation and outlook.

What are the symptoms?

One of the characteristic features of these conditions is the very variable clinical presentation and outlook for each individual patient. Mitochondrial cytopathies can involve either one tissue alone, such as muscle, or several different tissues. In addition, the outlook for each individual patient will depend upon the organs involved and the severity of the defect.

What are the causes?

These conditions are all caused by abnormal function of the mitochondria. Mitochondria are the powerhouses of the cell and convert food into energy in the form of adenosine triphosphate. Any failure of this process causes a lack of energy in the cells and this will severely impair the working of organs such as the brain, heart or skeletal muscle.

How is it treated?

Energy production in mitochondria is an extremely complicated process and this may go wrong at several different sites. For most patients there is no cure, but supportive care to prevent complications is very important. Some patients respond to certain vitamins including Ubiquinone.

Inheritance patterns and prenatal diagnosis

Inheritance patterns

This is particularly complicated for Mitochondrial Cytopathies because the mitochondria is synthesised with the products of two genomes. Most proteins that make up the mitochondria are encoded by the nucleus and then transported to the mitochondria. However, the mitochondria also contain their own DNA which produces thirteen key proteins. The mitochondrial DNA abnormalities are only transmitted by the mother. Thus, the inheritance pattern of mitochondrial disease will depend upon whether the nuclear or mitochondrial DNA is affected.

Prenatal diagnosis

There have been only a few reports of successful prenatal diagnosis. This can only be attempted if the genetic or biochemical defect is identified. This is not available for the majority of patients and is still at a very early stage. Genetic counselling for these disorders is still difficult, but guidance is possible.

In the UK there has been recent funding (April 2007) of Specialist

Commissioning for Rare Mitochondrial Disorders of Adults and Children. This funding allows specialist biochemical and genetic testing, as well specialist clinics, in three centres - Newcastle, London and Oxford.

Medical text written December 1996 by Professor D M Turnbull. **Last updated June 2007 by Professor D M Turnbull, Professor of Neurology, Mitochondrial Research Group, School of Neurology, Neurobiology and Psychiatry, University of Newcastle, Newcastle upon Tyne, UK.**

Further online resources

Medical texts in *The Contact a Family Directory* are designed to give a short, clear description of specific conditions and rare disorders. More extensive information on this condition can be found on a range of reliable, validated websites. Further information on these resources can be found in our **Medical Information on the Internet** article on page 21.

Support

Information on support for children with Mitochondrial Cytopathies can be obtained from Climb (see entry, Metabolic diseases).

Information on support for adults with Mitochondrial Cytopathies can be obtained from the Muscular Dystrophy Group (see entry, Muscular Dystrophy and neuromuscular disorders).

MOEBIUS SYNDROME

Background

Moebius syndrome was first described by von Graefe (1880) and Moebius (1888). It is a rare congenital disorder associated with abnormal development of the nerve supply to the head and neck which is divided into twelve cranial nerves. The main nerves affected are the sixth and seventh cranial nerves leading to congenital facial palsy (paralysis).

What are the symptoms?

Affected people have poor facial expression and eye movement. Localised mouth, face and limb malformations may be associated with the disorder. Involvement of other cranial nerves is common. Occasionally, the fifth, tenth, eleventh and twelfth cranial nerves are involved, resulting in difficulty of chewing, swallowing, and coughing, which often leads to respiratory complications. Learning disability (see entry) and Autistic Spectrum disorder (see entry) have been reported in some cases.

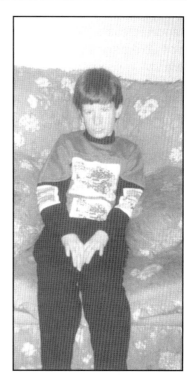

There is also a well documented association between Moebius and Poland syndrome (see entry), a disorder characterised by absence of pectoralis major (chest muscle) and congenital limb defects.

What are the causes?

It is thought that Moebius syndrome is due to a more general defect of brainstem development and studies of electrophysiologic (electrical aspects of body processes) abnormalities in a number of people with Moebius syndrome suggest defects can occur at various levels of the brain in different patients. It is, therefore, thought that Moebius syndrome is a complex regional developmental disorder of the brainstem. However, other theories, such as disruption of the subclavian (collar bone) artery supply have been considered as possible causes of Moebius syndrome.

How is it diagnosed?

Diagnosis of Moebius syndrome is by the identification of the known features of the disorder.

How is it treated?

Treatment of Moebius syndrome is symptomatic and supportive.

Inheritance patterns and prenatal diagnosis

Inheritance patterns

The majority of Moebius syndrome cases are sporadic, however there are reported cases of two or more affected members in one family suggesting a possible genetic basis to this syndrome. There are also reports of patients with Moebius syndrome and an associated chromosome defect; from this several chromosomal regions are been implicated of harbouring a gene responsible for this condition.

Prenatal diagnosis

Associated features such as limb defects may be diagnosed in obstetric scans, but there is no reliable prenatal diagnosis.

Medical text written May 2006 by Dr W Lam, Consultant Clinical Geneticist, Western General Hospital, Edinburgh and Senior Lecturer, Edinburgh University, Edinburgh, UK.

Further online resources

Medical texts in *The Contact a Family Directory* are designed to give a short, clear description of specific conditions and rare disorders. More extensive information on this condition can be found on a range of reliable, validated websites. Further information on these resources can be found in our **Medical Information on the Internet** article on page 21.

Support

Moebius Syndrome Support Group

R7, The Linskill Centre, Linskill Terrace, North Shields NE30 2AY   Tel: 0191 296 4050
The Support Group is a National Registered Charity No. 1073282, established in 1987. The group offers support and information to families and individuals, linking families with each other where possible. It has a quarterly newsletter and holds bi-ennial conferences. The group is in touch with approximately 150 families.
Group details last updated August 2007.

MOTOR NEURONE DISEASE

Background

The description of motor neurone disease (MND) is given to a group of closely related conditions where degeneration of the motor neurones (nerve cells which control muscles) in the brain and spinal cords causes progressive muscular wasting and weakness.

Precise figures of the incidence and prevalence of MND are not certain:

- incidence is thought to be 2 in 100,000 per year;
- prevalence thought to be 7 in 100,000;
- estimated number of people with MND in the UK is approximately five thousand.

What are the symptoms?

People affected by MND generally experience muscle wasting and weakness in the arms and/or legs causing difficulties with walking and personal care. Others may develop weakness and wasting in the face and throat muscles leading to difficulties speaking, chewing and swallowing.

There are four main types of motor neurone disease, namely Amyotrophic Lateral Sclerosis (ALS), Progressive Bulbar Palsy (PBP), Progressive Muscular Atrophy (PMA), and Primary Lateral Sclerosis (PLS).

Amyotrophic Lateral Sclerosis (ALS)

- Most common form of MND (approximately sixty-six per cent);
- Involving both upper and lower motor neurones (upper motor neurones descend from the brain to the brain stem and the spinal cord; lower motor neurones extend from the brain stem and the spinal cord to the muscles);
- Characterised by muscle weakness, spasticity, hyperactive reflexes (hyperreflexia – overactive or over responsive reflexes) and inappropriate emotional responses;
- Age of onset usually over fifty-five years (males are more affected than females in the ratio of 3 to 2);
- Average survival two to five years.

Progressive Bulbar Palsy (PBP)

- Affects approximately twenty-five per cent;
- Both upper and lower motor neurones may be involved;
- Characterised by dysarthria (difficulty in articulating words) and dysphagia (difficulty in swallowing). Lower motor neurone damage causing nasal speech, regurgitation of fluid via the nose, tongue atrophy (wasting away) and fasciculation (muscle twitching) and pharyngeal (tube between mouth and stomach) weakness. Upper motor neurone

damage characterised by a spastic tongue, explosive dysarthria and inappropriate emotional responses. Muscles in the upper limbs and shoulder girdle may also become progressively weaker;

- PBP mostly occurs in older people, slightly more common in women;
- Survival from onset of symptoms is usually between six months and three years.

Primary Lateral Sclerosis (PLS)
- A rare form which affects the upper motor neurones only;
- Characterised by spastic quadriparesis (spasms in all limbs), inappropriate emotions and spastic dysarthria;
- Age of onset fifty years;
- Average survival rate of twenty years.

Progressive Muscular Atrophy (PMA)
- Affects approximately seven point five per cent of people with MND;
- Predominantly lower motor neurone degeneration;
- Causes muscle wasting and weakness (often starting in the fine motor muscles of the hand) with loss of weight and fasciculation (muscle twitching);
- Age of onset is usually under fifty years (male are more affected than females in the ratio of 5 to 1);
- Majority of people surviving beyond five years.

There is considerable overlap between these forms of MND. In particular, in time, people with PMA develop upper motor neurone involvement, and in both PMA and ALS most people eventually experience speech and swallowing difficulties in varying degrees.

What are the causes?
All causes of Motor Neurone disease are not yet known but it is thought to be multi-factorial. Considerable research is being undertaken worldwide and encouraging advances are being made in understanding both the disease process and the way in which motor neurones function.

How is it treated?
Clinical trials have focused on treatments that might have a positive impact on the course of the disease by increasing life expectancy and/or slowing down the rate of progression of symptoms.

At present there is no cure for MND but much can be offered in the management of symptoms. Clinical trials have focussed on treatments that might have a positive impact on the course of the disease by increasing life expectancy and/or slow down the rate of progression of symptoms.

Inheritance patterns and prenatal diagnosis

Inheritance patterns

Ninety to ninety-five per cent of MND cases are sporadic with no family history of the disease. Familial MND (FMND) affects five per cent of MND cases. Clinically, sporadic and familial forms of MND are indistinguishable.

Approximately twenty per cent of FMND patients have an autosomal dominant mutation in the copper zinc superoxide dismutase 1 (SOD1) gene on chromosome 21. Over one hundred different SOD1 mutations have been reported to date; the presence of which may have significant differences in age of onset and disease prognosis.

Following the discovery of the SOD1 gene mutation in 1993, other genes that cause FMND have been discovered. As these mutations occur in a very small percentage of people with the familial form of MND, these discoveries are more significant for research than for clinical diagnosis.

The care and support required by someone with FMND is no different to a person who has the sporadic form of the disease and the MND Association has a range of services available to help. However, for the person affected and the extended family, increased emotional support and an understanding of the genetics involved may be required. Referral to a neurologist who understands the particular needs of people with FMND may be helpful, the GP or current neurologist can arrange this.

Prenatal diagnosis

None.

Medical text written August 2005 by Dr Brian Dickie PhD, Director of Research Development, MND Association, Northampton, UK.

Further online resources

Medical texts in *The Contact a Family Directory* are designed to give a short, clear description of specific conditions and rare disorders. More extensive information on this condition can be found on a range of reliable, validated websites. Further information on these resources can be found in our **Medical Information on the Internet** article on page 21.

Support

Motor Neurone Disease Association
PO Box 246, Northampton NN1 2PR   Tel: 01604 250505
MND Connect Tel: 08457 626 262 low cost call Helpline   Fax: 01604 624726
e-mail: enquiries@mndassociation.org   Web: http://www.mndassociation.org
The Association is a National Registered Charity No. 294354, established in 1979. It covers England, Wales, Northern Ireland and the Channel Islands. It offers support for people living with MND, their carers and health and social care professionals. It produces regularly updated information sheets on research and current clinical trials, details on request. The Association has over 6,000 members.
Group details last updated September 2007.

Scottish Motor Neurone Disease Association

76 Firhill Road, Glasgow G20 7BA   Tel: 0141 945 1077   Fax: 0141 945 2578
e-mail: info@scotmnd.co.uk   Web: http://www.scotmnd.org.uk
*The Association is a Scottish Charity Registration No. SCO 02662, established in 1981.
It is a member of the International Alliance of ALS/MND Associations representing 50
organisations in 40 countries working to achieve a Baseline of Services for ALS/MND. It
offers care and support to anyone diagnosed with MND living in Scotland. It has specialist
care advisers linked to neurology departments at hospitals in Glasgow, Edinburgh,
Dundee and Aberdeen. It publishes a quarterly Newsletter 'Aware' and has an equipment
loan service, library and information service for people with MND, family, friends and
professionals. The Association offers an education service for families, health and social
care professionals, a counselling service and has a holiday caravan facility. It runs
befriending services in Fife and Tayside. The Association responds to the needs of the
estimated 280 people living in Scotland with MND.*
Group details last updated February 2008.

"I find your internet site an excellent
source of information for parents and
often refer them to it. I think it is a vital
way of helping parents with accessible
and reliable information." Librarian.

MOWAT-WILSON SYNDROME

Mowat-Wilson syndrome: Hirschsprung's disease-Microcephaly-Mental Retardation syndrome

Background

Mowat-Wilson syndrome is a rare disorder which was first described in detail by Dr D R Mowat and Dr M J Wilson in 1998. Although individuals with the main characteristics of Hirschsprung's disease (see entry), learning disability (see entry) and typical facial features, had been described by a number of doctors in the preceding twenty years, it was suggested in 2002 that the syndrome be called Mowat-Wilson syndrome. The syndrome affects both males and females and by 2004, forty-seven cases of the syndrome had been reported in medical literature.

What are the symptoms?

The major features of Mowat-Wilson syndrome are:

- Hirschsprung's disease;
- Mild to moderate learning disability;
- Typical facial features that include:
    - Microcephaly (see entry);
    - Deep set, widely spaced eyes;
    - Characteristic ear shape with a turned-up ear lobe;
    - Broad nasal tip and short philtrum (the vertical central groove from the nose to the upper lip);
    - Small open mouth with a highly arched palate;
    - Prominent chin.
- Growth, and motor development delay – speech can be delayed or absent;
- Seizures in the majority of individuals (see entry, Epilepsy);
- Failure to thrive in early life.

Other features that have been observed in individuals with Mowat-Wilson syndrome include:

- Congenital heart disease (see entry, Heart defects);
- Cleft lip and/or palate (see entry);
- Genitourinary anomalies;
- Eye anomalies;
- White patches on the skin.

What are the causes?

The majority of patients with Mowat-Wilson syndrome have a mutation or a deletion of the ZFHX1B gene (also known as the SMADIP1 gene) on chromosome 2q22. There are, however, some affected individuals who do not have any detectable abnormality within this gene and this group of patients may either have an abnormality of ZFHX1B which is not detectable by current techniques or a different genetic basis for their condition.

How is it diagnosed?

Diagnosis of the syndrome is made by recognition of the clinical features and identification of a ZFHX1B gene change. Diagnosis of the syndrome has been made on clinical grounds alone in a number of individuals without the gene mutation.

How is it treated?

Mowat-Wilson syndrome cannot be cured. Treatment is symptomatic aimed at maintaining or improving quality of life.

Inheritance patterns and prenatal diagnosis

Inheritance patterns

Mowat-Wilson syndrome is usually a sporadic disorder (isolated with no other affected family members). Genetic advice or counselling is available for families.

Prenatal diagnosis

This may be possible in families with an affected child where a genetic change of ZFHX1B has previously been identified.

Medical text written November 2004 by Contact a Family. Approved November 2004 by Dr J Clayton-Smith, Consultant Clinical Geneticist, St Mary's Hospital, Manchester, UK.

Further online resources

Medical texts in *The Contact a Family Directory* are designed to give a short, clear description of specific conditions and rare disorders. More extensive information on this condition can be found on a range of reliable, validated websites. Further information on these resources can be found in our **Medical Information on the Internet** article on page 21.

Support

Mowat-Wilson Syndrome Support Group
13 Barry Avenue, Ingol, Preston PR2 3XL   Tel: 01772 760119
e-mail: support@mowatwilsonsyndrome.co.uk
Web: http://www.mowatwilsonsyndrome.co.uk
The Group is an informal network of families in the UK and overseas, set up in 2005. It provides information and mutual support.
Group details last updated April 2007.

MOYA MOYA DISEASE

Moya Moya disease: MMD; Moya Moya syndrome; Moyamoya disease

Background

This condition was first described by Takeuchi and Shimizu in 1957. Moya Moya is Japanese for a puff or cloud of smoke and refers to the characteristic appearance of the diagnostic angiogram for the condition.

What are the symptoms?

Moya Moya syndrome is a condition characterised by the narrowing of the major arteries to the brain. Half of all Moya Moya cases are found in patients under ten years of age, with females more affected than males. This extremely rare condition is more common in the Japanese population.

What are the causes?

Although the direct cause of Moya Moya is often uncertain it can be seen in a number of diseases that can affect arteries: Trisomy 21 (Down syndrome, see entry), Sickle Cell disorders (see entry), chronic Meningitis (see entry, Meningitis) and Neurofibromatosis (see entry).

The internal carotid artery is one of the major arteries to the brain. This artery branches into many smaller vessels in order to reach all areas of the brain. In patients with Moya Moya, there is narrowing of the internal carotid arteries and their major branches which reduces the blood supply to the brain. The brain responds by increasing the size of many smaller vessels to improve blood flow to deprived areas of the brain. In children, the first symptom is often stroke, which may cause paralysis of one side of the body or sometimes seizures. In some children development slows down or skills may be lost. Adults are more prone to acute bleeding in the head.

How is it diagnosed?

Following MRI, cerebral angiography, in which a dye is injected into the arteries of the brain, is the conventional method of diagnosis. In Moya Moya patients a characteristic pattern of narrowed arteries and the anastomotic (extra) arteries is seen.

How is it treated?

Surgical revascularisation of various types has been developed to attempt to restore blood supply to the brain. The main drugs used in childhood are antiplatelet agents such as aspirin.

Inheritance patterns and prenatal diagnosis

Inheritance patterns

Except where the underlying cause is genetic, MMD is usually sporadic (with no other affected family members). Occasionally, autosomal dominant inheritance has been found.

Prenatal diagnosis

None.

Medical text written October 2006 by Contact a Family. Approved October 2006 by Professor Brian Neville, Professor of Childhood Epilepsy, Institute of Child Health/ Great Ormond Street Hospital, London, UK.

Support

There is no support group for Moya Moya syndrome. Cross referrals to other entries in the Contact a Family Directory are intended to provide relevant support for those particular features of the disorder. Organisations identified in those entries do not provide support specifically for Moya Moya syndrome. Families can use Contact a Family's Freephone Helpline for advice, information and, where possible, links to other families. Contact a Family's web-based linking service Making Contact.org can be accessed at http://www.makingcontact.org

In 2004 Contact a Family and the Family Fund completed research into debt amongst families with disabled children. The research found 8.1% of families described themselves as in very serious financial difficulty whilst 17.5% described themselves as struggling financially with debts which were beginning to worry them. *Debt and Disability: The impact of debt on families with disabled children. Contact a Family and the Family Fund. 2004*

MUCOPOLYSACCHARIDE DISEASES and associated diseases

Background

These rare lysosomal diseases are each caused by a different enzyme deficiency. This results in Mucopolysaccharides being stored in cells of the body causing progressive damage.

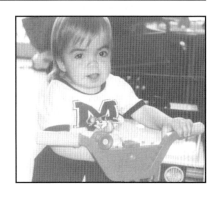

The Mucopolysaccharide diseases are classified as MPS I-IX. They are named after the doctor who first described them:

Hurler (MPS IH)	α-L-iduronidase deficiency
Hurler Scheie (MPS IHS)	α-L-iduronidase deficiency (formerly MPS V)
Scheie (MPS IS)	α-L-iduronidase deficiency
Hunter (MPS II)	α-L-iduronidase-2-sulphate-sulphatase deficiency
Sanfilippo (MPS III)	4 distinct enzyme abnormalities, same clinical patterns
Morquio (MPS IV) A	Galactosamine-6-sulphate sulphatase
Morquio (MPS IV) B	β-Galactosidase
Maroteaux Lamy (MPS VI)	N-acetyl galactosamine-4-sulphatase deficiency
Sly (MPS VII)	β-gluconidase deficiency
MPS IX	Hyaluronidase deficiency

The mucolipidoses and other storage diseases are as follows:

ML I	Neuramidase deficiency
ML II	I Cell disease (also known as Leroy syndrome)
ML III	Pseudo Hurler Polydystrophy
ML IV	
Sialidosis	
Fucosidosis	
Mannosidosis	
Sialic Acid Storage disease	
Multiple Sulphatase deficiency	
Aspartylglycosaminuria	
Winchester syndrome	
Fabry disease	

What are the symptoms?

In most children growth is restricted and some diseases cause progressive mental as well as physical disability. Many of the diseases are associated with death in childhood.

How is it treated?

At present there is no cure for these conditions. Bone marrow transplantation is an option for a small number of these conditions. Enzyme replacement therapy for Fabry disease and MPS I has been developed. Phase three human clinical trials for MPS II and MPS VI are currently taking place.

Inheritance patterns and prenatal diagnosis

Inheritance patterns

All these conditions are autosomal recessive except Hunter disease (MPS II) and Fabry disease which are X-linked.

Prenatal diagnosis

This is available for most types of Mucopolysaccharidoses and related conditions. Usually the procedure can take place at ten to twelve weeks using chorionic villus sampling (CVS). Alternatively amniocentesis may be performed at twelve to sixteen weeks.

Medical text written November 1991 by Contact a Family. Approved November 1991 by Professor M Patton, Professor of Medical Genetics, St Georges Hospital Medical School, London, UK and Dr J E Wraith. **Last updated February 2003 by Dr J E Wraith, Consultant Paediatrician, Willink Biochemical Genetics Unit, Royal Manchester Children's Hospital, Manchester, UK.**

Further online resources

Medical texts in *The Contact a Family Directory* are designed to give a short, clear description of specific conditions and rare disorders. More extensive information on this condition can be found on a range of reliable, validated websites. Further information on these resources can be found in our **Medical Information on the Internet** article on page 21.

Support

The Society for Mucopolysaccharide diseases

MPS House, Repton Place, White Lion Road, Amersham HP7 9LP   Tel: 0845 389 9901 Fax: 0845 389 9902 e-mail: mps@mpssociety.co.uk Web: http://www.mpssociety.co.uk *The Society is National Registered Charity No. 287034, established in 1982. It offers a needs-led service in areas of special educational needs, home adaptations, welfare benefits, palliative care and short breaks. The Society publishes a quarterly newsletter and a large range of printed material for affected families and professionals. The Society facilitates twelve regional MPS clinics throughout the UK. It holds the European Registry of Mucopolysaccharide and Related diseases and is able to demonstrate incidence and epidemiology for these diseases as well as specific anonymised data to researchers and the biotech industry. The Society represents approximately 1,200 individuals affected by MPS and Related diseases and their families. It is estimated that at any particular time there will be about 800 living sufferers, including those with Fabry disease, in the UK.* Group details last confirmed March 2007.

MULTIPLE ENDOCRINE NEOPLASIA TYPE I

Multiple Endocrine Neoplasia type I: Wermer syndrome; MEN I

Background

Multiple Endocrine Neoplasia type I is a rare genetic condition associated with tumours in the endocrine glands. The age of onset of MEN I is usually in the teenage years, although symptoms may not appear for several years. In most individuals, therefore, a diagnosis of MEN I is made by the fourth decade. MEN I affects men and women equally.

What are the symptoms?

Many of the health problems associated with MEN I occur frequently in the general population such as stomach ulcers, kidney stones, tiredness, headaches, low blood sugar, and high calcium levels. MEN I may, therefore, go undetected in families. Individuals may have tumours which are asymptomatic. The majority of tumours are slow growing and 'benign'. However, some are cancerous and so accurate diagnosis and treatment are essential. With early detection and treatment the potential problems caused by MEN I can be greatly reduced.

The range and severity of features associated with MEN I depends upon the glands in which tumours are located in any one individual. The location of the tumours varies among individuals, even within the same families. In most individuals, tumours in the parathyroids glands are the first sign of MEN I. The parathyroid glands control calcium in the blood, bones and urine. Over-activity of the parathyroid gland (hyperparathyroidism) is associated with high levels of calcium in the blood (hyercalcemia). The medical problems associated with hyperparathyroidism include tiredness, weakness, muscle or bone pain, indigestion, kidney stones or thinning of the bones, poor memory, irritability, ulcers and bone fractures.

The pancreas releases digestive juices into the intestines. Tumours in the pancreatic islet cells are associated with the release of excessive amounts of hormones such as gastrin, glucagons or vasoactive intestine polypeptide. Normally, gastrin causes the stomach to secrete enough acid needed for digestion. Over-secretion of gastrin in MEN I is associated with the formation of severe ulcers in the stomach and small intestine which may cause severe vomiting with blood and/or diarrhoea. About one third of individuals with MEN I have gastrin-releasing tumours (otherwise known as gastrinomas). If left untreated, these may cause rupture of the stomach or intestine. In some cases, they are fatal.

The pituitary gland plays a critical role in regulating growth and development, metabolism and reproduction. It releases prolactin and other key hormones. Symptoms associated with tumours in the pituitary gland include a loss or irregularity of the menstrual cycle, headaches and eye problems.

What are the causes?

MEN I occurs where two or more of the following endocrine glands develop tumours (hyperplasia or adenoma); the pancreas which is located behind the stomach; the parathyroid gland which is located in the neck; and the pituitary gland which is located in the head. Normally, hormones are secreted by endocrine glands in a carefully balanced way to regulate specific body functions and meet the body's needs. The presence of tumours in MEN I results in the over-production of hormones and this is associated with a range of medical problems. Over-activity of more than one endocrine gland may occur at the same time or later on in a person's life.

Inheritance patterns and prenatal diagnosis

Inheritance patterns

MEN I is inherited as an autosomal dominant trait. Changes in a gene on chromosome 11 (known as MEN I) are associated with the clinical features.

Prenatal diagnosis

This may be possible. Genetic counselling is advised for all individuals and families prior to genetic testing together with further specialist information and support.

Medical text written September 2003 by Contact a Family. Approved September 2003 by Professor R V Thakker. **Last updated January 2006 by Professor R V Thakkar, Head of the Molecular Endocrinology Group, John Radcliffe Hospital, Oxford, UK.**

Further online resources

Medical texts in *The Contact a Family Directory* are designed to give a short, clear description of specific conditions and rare disorders. More extensive information on this condition can be found on a range of reliable, validated websites. Further information on these resources can be found in our **Medical Information on the Internet** article on page 21.

Support

Information and support for Multiple Endocrine Neoplasia type I is available from AMEND (see separate entry, Multiple Endocrine Neoplasia type II).

MULTIPLE ENDOCRINE NEOPLASIA TYPE II

Multiple Endocrine Neoplasia type II: MEN II

Background

Multiple Endocrine Neoplasia type II is a rare genetic disorder characterised by tumours (growths) in particular endocrine glands including the thyroid, parathyroid and adrenal glands. The tumours secrete excessive amounts of hormones which are associated with a range of medical features. Some tumours are cancerous (see entry, Cancer). MEN II affects men and women equally and may occur at any age.

What are the symptoms?

There are three types of MEN II including Multiple Endocrine Neoplasia type IIA (MEN IIA); Multiple Endocrine Neoplasia type IIB (MEN II B) and Medullary Thyroid Cancer (MTC). Diagnosis of respective subtypes is based on the pattern of glands affected. Although each person's health is affected differently by MEN, the symptoms tend to follow the same pattern in a family (for example, families will either have MEN IIA or MEN IIB or MTC only).

Multiple Endocrine Neoplasia type IIA

MEN IIA, also known as Sipple syndrome, is the most common type of MEN II. It is characterised by thyroid cancer (medullary thyroid cancer), recurring tumours in the adrenal glands (pheochromocytoma) and hyperplasia (overgrowth) of the parathyroid gland. MTC is commonly the first sign of MEN IIA and appears as a lump in the neck or as neck pain between the ages of fifteen to twenty-five years. It is very aggressive and potentially fatal. Accurate diagnosis and treatment of MEN IIA, therefore, is essential as this may lead to cure. The development of MTC in MEN IIA is associated with excessive secretion of hormones in other glands. Pheochromocytoma is a tumour of the adrenal gland that secretes excessive amounts of hormones which regulate heart rate and blood pressure (epinephrine and norepinephrine). The symptoms of pheochromocytoma are high blood pressure, excessive sweating, rapid heartbeat and stroke. In most cases the tumours are benign. The tumours may occur at any age but are most common in young adult to mid-adult life. The development of MTC is also associated with hyperplasia of the parathyroid glands.

Multiple Endocrine Neoplasia type IIB

MEN IIB, also known as Mucosal Neuroma syndrome, is characterised by the early development of an aggressive form of MTC in all individuals. Tumours of the adrenal glands (pheochromocytoma) occur in approximately fifty per cent of individuals with MEN IIB. Tumours in the parathyroid glands are rare. Individuals with MEN IIB may be identified in infancy or early childhood by the presence of tumours in the mouth (mucosal neuromas). Individuals may also develop abdominal distension, constipation or diarrhoea and may be taller than average.

Medullary Thyroid Carcinoma

This form of medullary carcinoma is the least aggressive and is not associated with tumours in other glands.

Inheritance patterns and prenatal diagnosis

Inheritance patterns

All MEN II subtypes are inherited as an autosomal dominant trait. Changes in a gene on chromosome 10 (known as *RET*) are associated with the clinical features. Genetic testing is available in individuals who are unaffected with MEN II. Genetic counselling is advised for all individuals and families prior to genetic testing.

Prenatal diagnosis

This may be possible. Genetic counselling is advised for all individuals and families prior to genetic testing together with further specialist information and support.

Medical text written September 2003 by Contact a Family. Approved September 2003 by Professor R V Thakker. **Last updated January 2006 by Professor R V Thakkar, Head of the Molecular Endocrinology Group, John Radcliffe Hospital, Oxford, UK.**

Further online resources

Medical texts in *The Contact a Family Directory* are designed to give a short, clear description of specific conditions and rare disorders. More extensive information on this condition can be found on a range of reliable, validated websites. Further information on these resources can be found in our **Medical Information on the Internet** article on page 21.

Support

AMEND

PO Box 89, Tunbridge Wells TN2 9G
Tel: 01423 780594 MEN I enquiries   Tel: 01892 525308 MEN II enquiries
e-mail: info@amend.org.uk   Web: http://www.amend.org.uk
AMEND is a National Registered Charity No. 1099796. It is a patient support group run by volunteers for the benefit of everyone affected by the multiple endocrine neoplasia disorders and their associated familial and sporadic growths. In addition to providing worldwide e-mail and telephone support, AMEND runs a UK research database and produces patient information. With strong medical advisory team backup, AMEND has gone from strength to strength since it's inception as a registered UK charity in 2002, and in 2007 has recently formed a patient/professional partnership working group to look at ways of improving the care and management of MEN patients throughout the UK.
Group details last updated February 2008.

MULTIPLE EPIPHYSEAL DYSPLASIA

Background

Multiple Epiphyseal Dysplasia (MED) is a rare, inherited, skeletal dysplasia resulting from malformation of the growing ends of the long bones.

What are the symptoms?

The condition is characterised by mild to moderate short stature and painful joints. MED affects both males and females equally and onset is usually during childhood or early adolescence with most cases becoming apparent between the ages of two and ten. The incidence of MED is thought to be about 10 to 15 in 1,000,000.

The main features of MED may include:

- A waddling gait;
- Pain in the joints and fatigue after exercise;
- Normal intelligence;
- Progressive worsening of pain and joint stiffness and deformity;
- Reduced height in adults (in the lower normal range or mildly shortened) with limbs relatively short in comparison with the trunk.

Adults with MED are likely to have early-onset osteoarthritis which may lead to early joint replacement.

There is a rare form of Recessive MED that is characterised by joint pain, malformations of the hands, feet, and knees, and scoliosis. Stature is usually within the normal range prior to puberty; in adulthood, stature is only slightly diminished and is in the range of 150-180 cm. Functional disability is mild or absent.

What are the causes?

Mutations of a number of genes are known to cause MED. About thirty-five per cent of affected individuals have a mutation of the COMP gene on chromosome 19 while about fifteen per cent have mutations in other genes. However, in about fifty per cent, a mutation cannot be identified and there may be other, as yet unidentified, genes involved.

How is it diagnosed?

A diagnosis of MED will be made on the clinical presentation in the individual and radiographic (x-ray) evidence.

How is it treated?

Congenital disorders such as MED cannot be cured. The control of pain and the limitation of joint destruction that can lead to the development of osteoarthritis is important. A combination of analgesics and physiotherapy including hydrotherapy is helpful in many cases together with a referral to a pain specialist and a rheumatologist. Weight control and avoidance of exercise that causes repetitive strain on affected joints are beneficial. Consultation with an orthopaedic surgeon can determine if realignment osteotomy (an operation in which a bone is divided or a piece of bone is taken out to correct a deformity) and/or acetabular (hip socket) osteotomy may be helpful in slowing the progression of symptoms. In some cases, total joint arthroplasty (replacement) may be required.

Psychosocial support addressing issues of short stature, disability, employment, and risk to other family members is appropriate.

Inheritance patterns and prenatal diagnosis
Inheritance patterns
Autosomal Dominant or, rarely, an autosomal recessive form.
Prenatal diagnosis
This is possible in the case of families known to be affected by MED where the mutation responsible for the condition is known. Testing is by amniocentesis at sixteen to eighteen weeks or by Chorionic Villus Sampling at ten to twelve weeks.

Medical text written October 2005 by Contact a Family. Approved October 2005 by Dr M Wright, Consultant Clinical Geneticist, Institute of Medical Genetics, International Centre for Life, Newcastle upon Tyne, UK.

Further online resources
Medical texts in *The Contact a Family Directory* are designed to give a short, clear description of specific conditions and rare disorders. More extensive information on this condition can be found on a range of reliable, validated websites. Further information on these resources can be found in our **Medical Information on the Internet** article on page 21.

Support
Support for Multiple Epiphyseal Dysplasia is available from the Perthes Association (see entry, Perthes disease).

MULTIPLE SCLEROSIS

Background

Multiple sclerosis is the most common potentially disabling disease of the central nervous system affecting young adults. The lifetime risk is about 1 in 500 in the UK and there is a slight excess risk in females (it affects three times more females than males).

Multiple sclerosis is usually perceived as a disorder of adulthood but children and adolescents can be affected. Although childhood and adolescent onset is not common, it is thought that 2.7 to 4.4 per cent of people with Multiple sclerosis have onset before the age of sixteen. Of this figure, 0.2 to 1.6 per cent are affected before the age of ten years. The relapsing remitting form of Multiple sclerosis is more common in those having childhood onset. Common features in childhood onset Multiple sclerosis are sensory problems, movement difficulties such as poor co-ordination and tremor, and visual problems.

What are the symptoms?

In most patients the pattern is initially episodic but the disorder moves through characteristic phases of attacks which recover, episodes leaving persistent deficits and then slow progression; occasionally, multiple sclerosis is progressive from onset. This natural history usually evolves over many years and life expectancy is not significantly reduced. Disability relates to onset and duration of the progressive phase. Focal inflammation causes acute injury of the myelin sheath that coats many nerve fibres in the brain and spinal cord disrupting the normal rapid passage of electrical impulses (saltatory conduction). The symptoms and signs of multiple sclerosis reflect the functional anatomy of impaired saltatory conduction at the sites affected - the cerebrum, optic nerves, brain stem and cerebellum, and spinal cord - producing alterations in vision, balance and co-ordination, sensation, movement and control of the bowel and bladder. Although these effects are initially reversible, due to resolution of inflammation and (perhaps) remyelination, with time there is persistent demyelination, axonal (nerve fibre) loss and astrocytes (small star shaped cells) scarring causing the sclerosed (hardened) plaques from which the disease gets its name.

What are the causes?

The cause of the disease is unknown but epidemiological studies indicate an interplay between genetic susceptibility factors and environmental triggers.

Inheritance patterns and prenatal diagnosis

Inheritance patterns

Multiple sclerosis is a typical complex trait and susceptibility is genetically determined. Recurrence risk amongst the relatives of probands - the affected individual through whom a family with a genetic disorder is ascertained - identify a familial recurrence rate of approximately fifteen per cent. The age-adjusted risk is highest for siblings (three per cent), then parents (two per cent) and children (two per cent) with lower rates in second and third degree relatives. Recurrence in monozygotic twins is around thirty-five per cent. The frequency of multiple sclerosis in the social relatives of adoptees is no higher than the population risk and significantly lower than expected in biological relatives of index cases. The age-adjusted risk for half-siblings is also less than for full siblings. Recurrence is higher in the children of conjugal pairs with multiple sclerosis (six per cent; age-adjusted twenty per cent) than the offspring of single affecteds (two per cent).

Prenatal diagnosis

None.

Medical text written November 2002 by Professor A Compston. Last updated June 2005 by Contact a Family and approved by Professor A Compston, Professor of Neurology, University of Cambridge, Cambridge, UK.

Further online resources

Medical texts in *The Contact a Family Directory* are designed to give a short, clear description of specific conditions and rare disorders. More extensive information on this condition can be found on a range of reliable, validated websites. Further information on these resources can be found in our **Medical Information on the Internet** article on page 21.

Support

Multiple Sclerosis Resource Centre (MSRC)

7 Peartree Business Centre, Peartree Road, Stanway, Colchester CO3 0JN
Tel: 0800 783 0518 (24 hour MS telephone counselling service)   Tel: 01206 505444
Fax: 01206 505449   e-mail: info@msrc.co.uk   Web: http://www.msrc.co.uk
The Centre is a National Registered Charity No. 1033731, established in 1993. It is dedicated to supporting all those affected by MS, including friends, family, work colleagues and professionals. The MSRC publishes a bi-monthly magazine New Pathways which is also available on CD. It has a wide range of information and publications, details on request. The website has extensive information about all aspects of MS and includes a message board and chat room. The MSRC works closely with the many MS Therapy Centres throughout the country. The centre has over 6,000 magazine subscribers and gives advice and information to thousands of people from all over the world.
Group details last updated August 2007.

Contact a Family Helpline 0808 808 3555

Multiple Sclerosis Society
MS National Centre, 372 Edgware Road, London NW2 6ND
Tel: 0808 800 8000 Helpline (9am - 9pm, Mon-Fri)   Tel: 020 8438 0700
Fax: 020 8438 0701   e-mail: info@mssociety.org.uk   Web: http://www.mssociety.org.uk
The Society is a National Registered Charity No. 207495, established in 1953. It offers support and advice to people affected by MS, health and social care professionals. It promotes research to find the cause and a cure for MS. It offers short breaks and grants for individuals in need. It also has partnership funding for MS Nurse posts. It publishes 'MS Matters' a bi-monthly magazine for members of the Society and has a wide range of information available, details on request. Across the UK information and support is available to anyone affected by MS from a network of over 340 local branches.
Group details last confirmed February 2008.

Direct services for children and adults with Multiple Sclerosis are also provided by the National Institute of Conductive Education (see Foundation for Conductive Education, under separate entry, Cerebral Palsy).

"May I take this opportunity to say thank you to everyone at Contact a Family for being there for all the support groups. Your support and guidance is invaluable to us all. Group leaders may have the dedication, but without an organisation like yours we could waste valuable time pursuing aims and objectives that would be destined to fail without your advice." A parent support group leader.

MULTIPLE SYSTEMS ATROPHY

Background

Multiple System Atrophy is a neurological disorder caused by degeneration of cells in certain areas of the brain. These control a number of different body systems; hence the name of the disorder. Damage to them affects functions of the autonomic nervous system (that normally occur automatically, such as control of blood pressure, sweating, bladder function, temperature regulation) and the motor system (such as muscle activation, movement and balance). MSA affects both men and women.

What are the symptoms?

Symptoms usually start between forty to sixty years of age.

MSA can manifest in a variety of ways and progresses in an unpredictable sequence and time scale in each patient. It is important to understand that having a diagnosis of MSA does not mean that you will experience all the symptoms from the range below. Furthermore, one or more of these symptoms may not necessarily mean a diagnosis of MSA as there are other conditions which overlap.

There are three forms - the parkinsonian, the cerebellar and the mixed forms (the last with both parkinsonian and cerebellar signs). In each form, autonomic dysfunction, examples of which are provided below, is an integral component, and may occur before the parkinsonian and cerebellar features. Motor symptoms may resemble Parkinson's disease (see entry) with slowness of movement, stiffness of limbs and, occasionally, tremor. Balance difficulties occur when the cerebellum is involved. Those erroneously diagnosed with Parkinson's disease may have been given anti-parkinsonian drug treatment with mixed results. A poor response to these drugs and the following symptoms are suggestive of MSA:

- dizziness and/or fainting, especially when rising from a lying or sitting position. This can be worse in the morning, in hot weather, after a meal, or after even mild exercise;
- cold extremities;
- urinary problems, with difficulty initiating passing urine, increased frequency especially at night, or incontinence;
- in the male, disturbance of sexual function;
- constipation;
- inability to sweat;
- speech disturbance, hoarseness, weak voice;
- swallowing disturbance, difficulty chewing, choking episodes;
- increased snoring at night, noisy breathing during the day;

- restless sleep with difficulty turning in bed;
- increased emotional response to happy or sad events.

As emphasised above, there are many disorders with symptoms which overlap with those of MSA; therefore diagnosis is made by a hospital consultant such as a neurologist, ideally with expertise in such disorders, at the request of a GP. Information about the history of an individual's symptoms and an examination will be performed. There are also hospital tests needed to exclude other conditions and to confirm the diagnosis. Importantly, many autonomic tests help understand the basis of symptoms and the reasons for them, which aids effective treatment.

Many of the symptoms described can be treated with drugs with management supervised by the specialist, with the most effective results obtained in combination with appropriate therapists and specialist nurses. Hospitals or GPs can involve physiotherapists to help with mobility; occupational therapists to help with advice or equipment for home, work or leisure; speech therapists for speech or swallowing problems; dieticians for nutritional help especially for those with swallowing problems; and social workers for benefit and carer advice.

What are the causes?

The cause of MSA is not known, and importantly is neither inherited nor contagious.

How is it treated?

Currently there is no cure for MSA. However, advances in treatment reduce the disabling effect of the symptoms so that as full a life as possible can be led.

Medical text written November 2000 by Professor C J Mathias. **Last updated August 2005 by Professor C J Mathias, Professor of Neurovascular Medicine, Imperial College London, St Mary's Hospital, London, UK and National Hospital for Neurology and Neurosurgery, Queen Square, Institute of Neurology, University College London, London, UK.**

Further online resources

Medical texts in *The Contact a Family Directory* are designed to give a short, clear description of specific conditions and rare disorders. More extensive information on this condition can be found on a range of reliable, validated websites. Further information on these resources can be found in our **Medical Information on the Internet** article on page 21.

Support

Sarah Matheson Trust

Pickering Unit , St Mary's Hospital, Praed Street, London W2 1NY

Tel: 020 7886 1520 Adviceline (Mon-Fri, 9.30am–4.30pm & Answerphone)

Fax: 020 7886 1540   e-mail: office@msaweb.co.uk   Web: http://www.msaweb.co.uk

The Trust is a National Registered Charity Number 1062308, established in 1997 to support all people in the UK living with Multiple System Atrophy and their carers. The Trust employs specialist nurses to offer support to patients and their families, and also to provide an educational resource to professionals. The Trust also provides information on other autonomic disorders such as pure autonomic failure. Their services include an advice line, support meetings, a newsletter, SMarT News, written information and education sessions. The Trust also sponsors and promotes research into MSA. The Trust is funded entirely by donations.

Group details last confirmed September 2007.

The Welsh Assembly Government commissioned Contact a Family Wales to conduct a major consultation on the Children's National Service Framework in Wales. The reports are available on Contact a Family's website.

MUSCULAR DYSTROPHY and neuromuscular disorders

Background

The muscular dystrophies are a group of disorders, caused by a genetic abnormality, that cause progressive weakness. Although genetic in origin, there are various reasons why an affected individual might have no family history of a similar condition. Some are severe and limit life expectancy, others relatively mild.

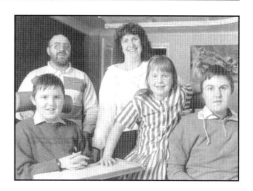

They belong to a broader group of conditions called neuromuscular disorders. These are defined as conditions affecting the nerves which pass from the brain and spinal cord to the muscles, for example spinal muscular atrophy and the peripheral neuropathies (see entries), the muscles themselves, and the complex junction between each nerve and muscle (myasthenic conditions). Most neuromuscular disorders cause weakness and it can be very difficult for even a specialist to identify the precise cause of the problem. Many, but not all, neuromuscular disorders are inherited. Accurate diagnosis is essential in order to offer the appropriate management and genetic advice.

Muscular dystrophies and neuromuscular disorders

Specific muscular dystrophies and neuromuscular disorders include:

- **Becker Muscular Dystrophy** (see entry). A muscular dystrophy associated with mutations in the dystrophin gene;
- **Charcot-Marie-Tooth disease** (see entry). An inherited nerve disorder causing muscle weakness around the ankles and of the hands;
- **Congenital Muscular Dystrophy** (see entry). A muscle weakness disorder showing at birth or within the first six months;
- **Congenital Myotonic Dystrophy** (see entry, Myotonic Dystrophy/ Congenital Myotonic Dystrophy). A form of Myotonic Dystrophy with early childhood onset;
- **Dermatomyositis and Polymyositis** (see entry). Rare auto-immune inflammatory muscle diseases (with skin involvement in dermatomyositis);
- **Duchenne Muscular Dystrophy** (see entry). A severe progressive life-limiting neuromuscular disorder;
- **Facioscapulohumeral Muscular Dystrophy** (see entry). A genetic

muscle wasting condition, the name describes the muscles involved;

- **Glycogen Storage diseases** (see entry). A group of metabolic diseases some of which affect the muscles;
- **Guillain-Barré syndrome** (see entry). An inflammatory syndrome of the peripheral nerves leading to muscle weakness;
- **Mitochondrial Myopathies** (see entry, Mitochondrial Cytopathies and related disorders). A group of disorders presenting at any age resulting from abnormal function of the mitochondria (power houses of the cell);
- **Myasthenia Gravis** (see entry, Myasthenia Gravis and other Myasthenic syndromes). An auto-immune disorder in which the body's own antibodies attack the muscles, causing fatigable weakness;
- **Myotonic Dystrophy** (see entry, Myotonic Dystrophy/Congenital Myotonic Dystrophy). A progressive muscle weakness disorder;
- **Myotubular Myopathy** (see entry). A muscle wasting and weakness disorder usually present at birth;
- **Spinal Muscular Atrophies** (see entry, Spinal Muscular Atrophy). A group of inherited disorders in which cells of the spinal cord degenerate causing progressive weakness around the hips and shoulders.

Inheritance and prenatal diagnosis

Inheritance patterns
As noted, not all neuromuscular disorders are inherited.

Prenatal diagnosis
This is available for some inherited disorders. Expert genetic counselling is essential. Tests used are chorionic villus sampling (ten to twelve weeks) and amniocentesis (sixteen weeks).

Medical text written September 2001 by Dr D Hilton-Jones. **Last updated December 2005 by Contact a Family. Approved December 2005 by Dr D Hilton-Jones, Clinical Director, Department of Clinical Neurology, University of Oxford, Oxford, UK.**

Further online resources

Medical texts in *The Contact a Family Directory* are designed to give a short, clear description of specific conditions and rare disorders. More extensive information on this condition can be found on a range of reliable, validated websites. Further information on these resources can be found in our **Medical Information on the Internet** article on page 21.

Support

Muscular Dystrophy Campaign
61 Southwark Street, London SE1 0HL   Tel: 0800 652 6352 information and support
e-mail: info@muscular-dystrophy.org   Web: http://www.muscular-dystrophy.org
The Campaign is a National Registered Charity No. 205395, established in 1959. It offers advice and support through MDC Care Advisers based in neuromuscular centres and hospitals throughout the UK. It has an Information and Advice Service and a network of local groups and representatives. It publishes a quarterly magazine 'Target MD' and has a wide range of information available, details on request. Membership is free.
Group details last updated August 2007.

MYASTHENIA GRAVIS and other myasthenic syndromes

Background

Myasthenia Gravis (MG) is an autoimmune disease usually caused by antibodies which attack the acetylcholine receptors on voluntary muscle, leading to receptor loss and a breakdown in communication between the nerve and the muscle.

What are the symptoms?

The condition is characterised by fluctuating weakness that becomes worse with increasing effort. Sometimes it affects only the eye muscles (ocular myasthenia) causing double vision and drooping of the eyelids. More commonly, the condition is generalised with weakness variously affecting not only the eye muscles but also the face, throat, neck, trunk, limbs, and breathing muscles. Some improvement in strength is achieved by rest. Generalised fatigue is not a feature of the condition.

Where muscles associated with swallowing and/or breathing are affected, patients may require assisted ventilation.

The **Lambert-Eaton Myasthenic syndrome** (LEMS) is also an autoimmune disease, caused by antibodies to calcium channels at the nerve terminal on which acetylcholine release depends. This results in a decrease in the amount of acetylcholine released by the nerve impulse. Patients typically have weakness of the legs and arms and there may also be disturbance of the autonomic nervous system: for example, causing a dry mouth and constipation.

In **Congenital Myasthenia** (CM) the immunological system is not implicated at all. It is a genetic condition in which a mutation that can occur at many different sites in the genes for the acetylcholine receptor interferes with their function. This causes muscle weakness which may be present at birth or evident soon afterwards.

Inheritance patterns and prenatal diagnosis

Inheritance patterns

There is a very weak familial susceptibility to MG and to other autoimmune diseases in the families of patients with MG of the LEMS. CM can be autosomal dominant, autosomal recessive or sporadic.

Prenatal diagnosis

This is not applicable to MG and the LEMS. It is now possible in some CM families, but only when the exact fault is known.

Medical text written November 1991 by Contact a Family. Approved November 1991 by Professor M Patton, Professor of Medical Genetics, St Georges Hospital Medical School, London, UK and Dr J E Wraith, Consultant Paediatrician, Royal Manchester Children's Hospital, Manchester, UK. **Last updated December 2003 by Professor J Newsom-Davis, Department of Clinical Neurology, University of Oxford, Oxford, UK.**

Further online resources

Medical texts in *The Contact a Family Directory* are designed to give a short, clear description of specific conditions and rare disorders. More extensive information on this condition can be found on a range of reliable, validated websites. Further information on these resources can be found in our **Medical Information on the Internet** article on page 21.

Support

Myasthenia Gravis Association
First Floor, Southgate Business Centre, Normanton Road, Derby DE23 6UQ
Tel: 0800 919922 Helpline   Tel: 01322 290219 Office   Fax: 01322 293641
e-mail: mg@mga-charity.org   Web: http://www.mga-charity.org
The Association is a National Registered Charity No. 1046443 established as the British Association of Myasthenics in 1976. Other conditions covered by the Association are Lambert-Eaton Myasthenia syndrome (LEMS) and Congenital Myasthenia. It offers mutual support through local groups. It publishes a quarterly newsletter and has information available, details on request. The Association has over 4,000 members (mainly adults). Group details last confirmed October 2007.

MYOTONIC DYSTROPHY/CONGENITAL MYOTONIC DYSTROPHY

Myotonic Dystrophy

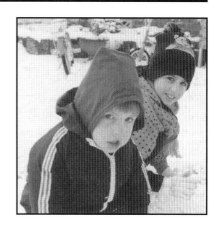

People with myotonic dystrophy, like those with other muscular dystrophies, experience muscle weakness and wasting which is usually progressive. There are many differences, though, in the type of problem that myotonic dystrophy patients may have. These may include the following:

- The types of muscles involved are usually in the face, jaw and neck area – the large, weight-bearing muscles of the legs and thighs are much less affected;
- The rate of deterioration is commonly slow, with little change over a long period – some patients never have significant muscle disability;
- Muscle stiffness or 'myotonia' is characteristic, especially affecting the hands;
- Involvement of other body systems is frequent; associated problems may include cataracts, disturbance of heart rhythm, hormonal problems and, in children, learning difficulties;
- Age at onset is very variable;
- Symptoms may appear at any time from birth to old age.

Operations and anaesthetics can be risky, even for mildly affected people. It is most important that any surgeon or anaesthetist should know a patient has myotonic dystrophy before surgery is planned.

An 'alert card' should be carried and is available from the UK Myotonic Dystrophy Support Group who also produce a valuable 'care sheet'.

Inheritance patterns

This condition follows a 'dominant' inheritance pattern which means that on average half of the children of an affected person are themselves affected. Both men and women are equally likely to be affected and to pass on the disorder, but affected women are more likely to have a severely affected child. In general (though not always) the disorder tends to be more severe in successive generations. This is because the mutation responsible for the condition (an expanded CTG repeat sequence) is unstable and tends to increase generation by generation. Healthy family members are not likely to pass on the condition, but should be thoroughly checked by an expert since minor features can easily escape detection.

Very few cases of myotonic dystrophy occur 'out of the blue.' Almost always, one parent proves to be affected, often very mildly. Careful study of the whole family often shows more members to be affected than would appear likely at first.

Prenatal diagnosis

In families known to have members with Myotonic Dystrophy, genetic testing is available which should be accompanied by full genetic counselling and clinical assessment. This permits accurate carrier detection and, if wished, prenatal diagnosis. Pre-implantation genetic diagnosis is becoming possible in a very few centres world-wide. A very small number of patients with similar features may show a different mutation - type 2 myotonic dystrophy or PROMM (Proximal Myotonic Myopathy).

Congenital Myotonic Dystrophy

Congenital myotonic dystrophy is the early childhood form of myotonic dystrophy (also known as Steinert's disease). Usually in myotonic dystrophy the symptoms begin to show in childhood or later in life, but symptoms of congenital myotonic dystrophy are evident from birth. It occurs only when the mother already has myotonic dystrophy (although she may not be aware of this) and she passes it on to the child in a more severe form. Congenital means 'from birth' because the condition is usually identified at birth or soon after; myotonic means 'involving muscle stiffness'; and dystrophy is 'muscle wasting and weakness'.

Congenital myotonic dystrophy can vary considerably in severity from child to child. If a child is diagnosed with the condition soon after birth, symptoms are likely to be severe.

Operations and anaesthetics can be risky. It is very important that any surgeon and anaesthetist should know a child has congenital myotonic dystrophy before surgery is planned.

Inheritance patterns

The condition follows a 'dominant' inheritance pattern which means that, on average, half of the children of a woman with myotonic dystrophy will be affected themselves. It affects both sexes, but the mother is usually the affected parent. Congenital Myotonic Dystrophy does not occur in the rare type 2 muscular dystrophy or PROMM (Proximal Myotonic Myopathy) families.

Prenatal diagnosis

Prenatal testing may be available at an early stage of pregnancy.

Psychological and behavioural characteristics

The psychological characteristics of individuals with classical myotonic dystrophy may depend to some extent on their age at onset of symptoms. As noted above, age at onset is very variable and may itself represent variation in the size of the genetic anomaly. Also, the effects may be more severe if the condition is inherited from the mother rather than the father. In any case, the psychological effects of myotonic dystrophy are usually thought to be developmental rather than progressive.

Even in adult-onset cases there may be psychological problems in some patients. Visuospatial skills may be more affected than verbal abilities. Some individuals also experience memory problems.

Individuals with myotonic dystrophy can seem apathetic or lacking in motivation even if the muscular weakness is relatively mild. They are also at risk of developing emotional problems such as depression and anxiety, and of social withdrawal.

Given the comments above regarding the significance of age at onset, it is unsurprising that the outcome for individuals with the congenital form of myotonic dystrophy is less favourable than that for the later onset form.

Most infants with congenital myotonic dystrophy show signs of early developmental delay. Babies may have difficulties in breathing, sucking and swallowing, and therefore in feeding. Muscle weakness may reduce facial expression and affect speech pronunciation. Acquisition of other self-care skills, such as toileting, can also be delayed.

In the longer term, most individuals display a learning disability, usually in the mild to moderate range.

Medical text written May 2001 by Professor Peter S Harper. **Last updated May 2004 by Professor Peter S Harper, Professor of Medical Genetics, University of Wales College of Medicine, Cardiff, UK. Psychological and behavioural characteristics information written March 2004 by Dr A Kuczynski, Child Clinical Psychologist, South London & Maudsley NHS Trust, London, UK and Dr O Udwin, Consultant Clinical Child Psychologist, West London Mental Health NHS Trust, London, UK.**

Further online resources

Medical texts in *The Contact a Family Directory* are designed to give a short, clear description of specific conditions and rare disorders. More extensive information on this condition can be found on a range of reliable, validated websites. Further information on these resources can be found in our **Medical Information on the Internet** article on page 21.

Support

Myotonic Dystrophy Support Group

35a Carlton Hill, Carlton, Nottingham NG4 1BG   Tel/Fax: 0115 987 0080 (for Fax call first)
e-mail: mdsg@tesco.net   Web: http://www.mdsguk.org

The Group is a National Registered Charity No. 1073211, established in 1989. It offers support by telephone and letter and contact with other families where possible. It has a network of Regional Co-ordinators and provides an 'ALERT' card to be carried by affected persons for use in emergency situations giving vital details about abnormal heart rhythm, anaesthetics, speech difficulties, extreme tiredness and muscle stiffness and weakness in people with myotonic dystrophy. Also available is a 'CARE' card; a personal record for health checks useful for individuals and professionals caring for them. It publishes a quarterly newsletter and has a wide range of information available, details on request. The Group has around 1,500 families in membership.

Group details last updated April 2007.

Contact a Family has a Dads' Zone on its website, which includes material on fathers' rights, employment rights, benefits and money matters, relationships and family life.

MYOTUBULAR MYOPATHY

Myotubular Myopathy: Centronuclear Myopathy

Background

Myotubular Myopathy is a congenital myopathy, one of a group of conditions causing weakness and wasting of the muscles with symptoms usually present at birth. The name 'myopathy' means muscle disorder and comes from the Greek words 'myo' meaning muscle and 'pathy' meaning disease.

Myotubular Myopathy is so called because the affected muscle fibres look like myotubes (muscle cells found only during fetal development when the fetus is between twelve to twenty weeks old). The condition is also known as 'centronuclear myopathy' because the nuclei of affected muscle cells are found in the centre of each cell instead of the periphery or edge of the cells (as occurs in healthy muscle cells).

What are the symptoms?

There are at least three different types of this condition. The types are defined by the way in which it has been inherited. The most severe form, which typically affects boys, presents at birth or even before birth, in contrast to the other two and milder forms which present later in childhood. The most severe type is called 'X-linked recessive' type and the milder types are called 'autosomal recessive' and 'autosomal dominant'. In all types, but particularly the severe type, the mother may notice a reduction in fetal movements during the pregnancy, or the doctors might have said that there was too much fluid (water) around the baby. The baby may also have a low birth-weight.

At birth, the symptoms are Hypotonia (see entry), breathing and swallowing difficulties. In the very severely affected cases, the baby may not survive for more than a few days or weeks. In others, there appears to be slowly progressive muscle weakness that affects the face, limbs and muscles involved in breathing. The affected muscles are weak and cannot function as well as normal (unaffected) muscles. As a result, children may have a variety of symptoms, including drooping of the eyelids, reduced movements of their eyes, drooling, swallowing difficulties and weakness of limbs and trunk. Some children are constipated and this may be as a direct result of the muscles in the gut being affected or caused by poor mobility. Hearing, vision and intelligence are usually unaffected.

The condition may be non-progressive, progress slowly or progress moderately quickly. In general the earlier the onset of the disease the more severe and progressive the disorder appears to be. In the form that presents at birth, there may be life-threatening breathing difficulties and severe hypotonia (floppiness). However, in most cases the disease is only slowly progressive and most patients become weaker in late adolescence or early adult life and may eventually lose the ability to walk. They may also develop droopy eyelids and the muscles that move the eyeballs may also be affected. Occasionally muscle weakness may progress quite rapidly and these patients experience serious breathing problems.

How is it diagnosed?

Diagnosis of Myotubular Myopathy can only really be made by doing a muscle biopsy – which means taking a piece of muscle, usually from the outer part of the thigh or sometimes from the upper arm and looking at this under a microscope (called histological diagnosis). In addition there is a genetic test that may be undertaken on blood that may diagnose the most severe type of myotubular myopthay – the X-linked type – the one that generally only affects boys. This genetic test looks for an abnormality in the MTM1 gene that is located on the X chromosome (MTM1 stands for 'myotubularin' which is the protein that is very important for making normal muscles).

How is it treated?

There is currently no cure for Myotubular Myopathy. However, there are other helpful measures which can certainly improve a person's quality of life and how they can live with this disorder. These include physiotherapy, the use of antibiotics to treat chest infections and nasogastric or feeding gastrostomy tubes if normal feeding is difficult. There is also treatment to help those children and teenagers who have problems with their breathing, particularly at night; this is called 'non-invasive ventilation' and may be very beneficial and make people feel better during the day. Regular but non-strenuous exercise such as swimming and cycling may help. It is also very important not to become overweight.

Inheritance patterns and prenatal patterns

Inheritance patterns

Myotubular Myopathy can be inherited in X-linked recessive, autosomal recessive and autosomal dominant types while some cases are sporadic. The X-linked recessive type that affects boys only typically presents at birth. The autosomal and autosomal dominant types affect boys and girls equally.

Prenatal diagnosis

This is only possible in those families where a previous child has been found to have the most severe type, 'X-linked recessive' myotubular myopathy and where the gene mutation has been found in this previously affected child.

Medical text written September 2002 by Contact a Family from information supplied by Dr R Appleton. Approved September 2002 by Dr R Appleton. **Last Updated September 2007 by Dr R Appleton, Consultant Paediatric Neurologist, Alder Hey Children's Hospital, Liverpool, UK**

Contact a Family Helpline 0808 808 3555

Further online resources

Medical texts in *The Contact a Family Directory* are designed to give a short, clear description of specific conditions and rare disorders. More extensive information on this condition can be found on a range of reliable, validated websites. Further information on these resources can be found in our **Medical Information on the Internet** article on page 21.

Support

There is an online support group for this condition, The Information Point for Centronuclear and Myotubular Myopathy, Web: http://www.centronuclear.org.uk e-mail: centronuclear.org@btinternet.com (information about the use of online groups is available in our 'Medical Information on the Internet: Seeking Quality' article). This group is moderated and refers affected adults, children and their families to relevant and trusted sources of information. It also puts families in touch with one another. They produce a newsletter three times a year for the Centronuclear and Myotubular Myopathy community which is also distributed to medical professionals, charities and other organisations. If you do not have internet access, please telephone our freephone helpline on 0808 808 3555. Group details last updated February 2007.

NAGER SYNDROME

Nager syndrome: Acrofacial Dysostosis

Background

Nager syndrome is probably not a single disorder but rather a group of disorders which all affect the development of the jaws, external ears and limbs.

What are the symptoms?

The milder type affects the face and ears in a similar way to Treacher Collins syndrome (see entry) with an under developed lower jaw and small external ears.

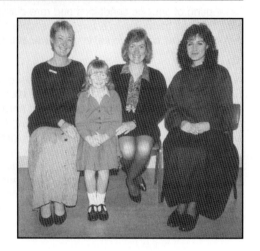

In some children this can lead to feeding and breathing difficulties. Cleft palate (see entry, Cleft Lip and/or Palate) may occur and hearing problems are frequent (see Deafness). The limb abnormalities are usually confined to the hands and forearms; the thumbs may be absent or under developed (see entry, Upper Limb Abnormalities). Intelligence is usually normal.

The severe types are likely to be due to different gene abnormalities. Most babies do not survive. The facial abnormalities are very severe and there is a shortening of all four limbs with digits missing.

Inheritance patterns and prenatal diagnosis

Inheritance patterns

- **Milder type**. Most cases are sporadic but there are well documented cases of parent to child transmission indicating autosomal dominant inheritance. There may be autosomal recessive types as well.
- **Severe types**. Most of these are likely to be autosomal recessive since affected siblings and cousin parents have been described.

Prenatal diagnosis

This is possible for these severe types by detailed ultrasound scanning from sixteen weeks of pregnancy. Genetic counselling is recommended to identify the type of Nager syndrome and the recurrence risks in individual families.

Medical text written September 1993 by Dr Dian Donnai. **Last reviewed September 2006 by Professor Dian Donnai, Consultant Clinical Geneticist, St Mary's Hospital, Manchester, UK.**

Support

The support group covering Nager syndrome is no longer in existence. Families can use Contact a Family's Freephone Helpline for advice, information and, where possible, links to other families. Contact a Family's web-based linking service Making Contact.org can be accessed at http://www.makingcontact.org

---

In December 2005 the means test was abolished in England for parents with disabled children applying for the Disabled Facilities Grant for help with the costs of adapting their homes.

NAIL-PATELLA SYNDROME

Nail-Patella syndrome (NPS): Hereditary-Osteo-Onycho-Dysplasia (HOOD); Fong's disease; Turner-Kieser syndrome

Background

This is a rare genetic condition, and those affected may have small or absent patellae (kneecaps), underdeveloped nails and an inability to fully straighten the elbows.

What are the symptoms?

NPS is extremely variable in its features and severity, even within members of the same family. X-rays may show small or absent patellae, dislocated elbows and

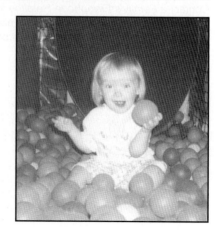

there may be small extra bony prominences on the rear of the pelvic bones called iliac horns. These do not cause any problems themselves, and can usually only be detected on X-ray. Other features can include talipes (club foot) or an inability to fully straighten the knees. Back pain may be a problem in adults and the small of the back may have an increased curve inwards. Surgery to correct joint problems may sometimes help but should be performed by an experienced surgeon, after scans have been done to investigate the anatomy of the joint which can be very abnormal.

Kidney problems (see entry, Kidney disease) can occur in people with NPS at any age, with leakage of protein in the urine. A person may not be aware of this but if protein leakage becomes more severe there may be associated swelling (see entry, Nephrotic syndrome). Occasionally, kidney failure can occur and it is important for anyone with NPS to have their urine checked every year.

In the eyes, people with NPS are more likely to develop Glaucoma (see entry), and at an earlier age than in the general population and so it is recommended that this should also be checked for on a regular basis. Other problems seen more frequently in NPS include Irritable Bowel syndrome (see entry), constipation and poor circulation in the hands and feet with occasional numbness and tingling. NPS does not affect intelligence but there may be a link with Attention Deficit Hyperactivity Disorder (ADHD).

Inheritance patterns and prenatal diagnosis

Inheritance patterns

Autosomal dominant. Most people will have inherited the condition from one of their parents but for some people the condition will have started for the first time in them and their parents will be unaffected. When inherited, the severity of the child's condition cannot be predicted. The gene which causes NPS is called LMX1B and it is located on Chromosome 9. The diagnosis is made based on clinical findings but genetic testing is possible if required.

Prenatal diagnosis

Genetic testing of a pregnancy for NPS is difficult as the severity to which the child would be affected cannot be predicted. Ultrasound in pregnancy is not a reliable test for NPS but may detect club foot, if present. Pre-eclampsia (see entry) is more common in pregnant women with NPS.

Medical text written July 2006 by Dr Elizabeth Sweeney, Consultant Clinical Geneticist, Royal Liverpool Children's Hospital, Alder Hey, Liverpool, UK.

Further online resources

Medical texts in *The Contact a Family Directory* are designed to give a short, clear description of specific conditions and rare disorders. More extensive information on this condition can be found on a range of reliable, validated websites. Further information on these resources can be found in our **Medical Information on the Internet** article on page 21.

Support

Nail-Patella Syndrome UK

PO Box 26415, East Kilbride, Glasgow G74 1YW   Tel: 0800 121 8298 freephone helpline
e-mail: dobbinsek@btinternet.com   Web: http://www.npsuk.org
Nail-Patella Syndrome UK is a National Registered Charity No. 1095621, established in 2003. It offers support and linking of affected families where possible. The group raises awareness about the condition, fundraises for research and holds a biennial conference. It publishes a newsletter and has information available, details on request. The group is in touch with approximately 150 families.
Group details last confirmed August 2007.

NARCOLEPSY

Background

Narcolepsy is a neurological disorder of the sleep/waking regulating mechanism.

What are the symptoms?

The primary symptoms are excessive day-time sleepiness and cataplexy. **Cataplexy** is characterised by short-lived (seconds to minutes) weakness or paralysis of the face, neck, jaw, trunk and limb muscles. Cataplexy is not always present at the outset of narcolepsy, but usually develops in time.

Other additional symptoms may include sleep paralysis, hypnapagogic (waking) hallucinations; automatic behaviour and disturbed night sleep.

What are the causes?

Evidence now suggests that narcolepsy is due to a deficiency of a brain chemical known as hypocretin.

Inheritance patterns and prenatal diagnosis

Inheritance patterns

No specific inheritance pattern has been established although there is a familial predisposition. There is also an association with the genetic marker HLA DR2 in the majority of cases.

Prenatal diagnosis

None

Medical text written November 1991 by Contact a Family. Approved November 1991 by Professor M Patton, Professor of Medical Genetics, St Georges Hospital Medical School, London, UK and Dr J E Wraith, Consultant Paediatrician, Royal Manchester Children's Hospital, Manchester, UK. **Last updated April 2004 by Professor A Zeman, Professor of Cognitive and Behavioural Neurology, Peninsula Medical School, Exeter, UK.**

Further online resources

Medical texts in *The Contact a Family Directory* are designed to give a short, clear description of specific conditions and rare disorders. More extensive information on this condition can be found on a range of reliable, validated websites. Further information on these resources can be found in our **Medical Information on the Internet** article on page 21.

Support

Narcolepsy Association UK (UKAN)
PO Box 13842, Penicuik EH26 8WX   Tel: 0845 4500 394   e-mail: info@narcolepsy.org.uk
Web: http://www.narcolepsy.org.uk
UKAN is a National Registered Charity No. 326361, established in 1981. It offers contact with others where possible. It publishes a quarterly newsletter and has information available, details on request. Please send SAE. The Association has over 800 members including the families of some children and young people.
Group details last updated May 2005.

NECROTISING FASCIITIS

Background

Necrotising Fasciitis is a rare, but serious soft tissue infection involving the skin, subcutaneous tissue and muscle.

There are several recognised risk factors. Patients who have compromised immunity such as patients with diabetes mellitus, cancer, peripheral vascular disease, intravenous drug users, those who have recently undergone surgery, receiving steroids or other immunosuppressive treatments are all predisposed. Healthy children whose skin is breached by minor trauma or skin infection are also at increased risk. In particular, children with recent Varicella Zoster virus infection (chicken pox) are prone and some investigators have suggested that the use of nonsteroidal anti-inflammatory drugs in these children increase the risk of necrotising fasciitis. Since the mid 1980's the number of cases have been increasing in healthy individuals with little or no compromise to their immunity or skin integrity.

What are the symptoms?

Necrotising Fasciitis commonly occurs on the extremities, abdomen and peripheral region but may occur anywhere on the body. It begins with local swelling, redness and tenderness and fever is often present. The pain is usually out of proportion with the clinical picture. The infection spreads beneath the skin so skin changes are delayed. Fluid filled blisters develop initially and later become blood filled. Loss of sensation and tissue gangrene then occur before the skin sloughs. Severe systemic toxicity can result in shock and multiple organ failure. Death can occur in up to twenty to fifty per cent of patients. Fortunately this is less common and carries a lower fatality in children.

What are the causes?

The commonest and most serious infections are caused by bacteria called Streptococcus pyogenes (Group A beta haemolytic Streptococcus). Occasionally it can be caused by Staphylococcus aureas, Clostridium perfringens, Clostridium septicum, Pseudomonas aeruginosa, Vibrio species and some fungi. Rarely it may be as a result of a non-group A streptococci, Streptococcus pneumonia or Haemophilus influenzae type b infection. Sometimes bacteria that are anaerobic (able to live without oxygen) and aerobic (needing oxygen) or facultative (having the ability to grow without oxygen) act together to cause tissue necrosis (death of a limited portion of tissue).

How is it diagnosed?

The definitive diagnosis is made by surgical exploration. MRI (Magnetic Resonance imaging) or CT (computerized tomography) helps to define the extent of the infection and microbiological investigations may identify the causative organism.

How is it treated?

A high index of suspicion, early supportive care, aggressive surgical debridement and broad-spectrum intravenous antibiotics are mandatory. The use of intravenous immunoglobulins have been associated with improved survival when associated with toxic shock. Long term surgical follow up may be required to treat disfiguring scars.

Inheritance patterns and prenatal diagnosis

Inheritance patterns

None.

Prenatal diagnosis

Not applicable.

Medical text written August 2002 by Dr P Salt, Registrar, Paediatric Intensive Care Unit, St Mary's Hospital, London, UK.

Support

Lee Spark NF Foundation

Moor Heys Farm, Knowle Green, Preston PR3 2XE   Tel: 01254 878 701 (Tel/Fax)
e-mail: info@nfsuk.org.uk   Web: http://www.nfsuk.org.uk

The Lee Spark NF Foundation is a National Registered Charity No. 1088094, established in 2000. The Foundation covers Necrotising Fasciitis and other Streptococcal infections. It offers support to affected families, carers and professionals; a range of information, an annual get-together, quarterly newsletter and a medical advisory panel.
Group details last updated August 2007.

NEPHROTIC SYNDROME

Background

Nephrotic syndrome is a serious kidney disorder where protein leaks into urine. Kidneys contain a large number of nephrons, the filtering elements that remove waste materials and fluid from the body. Nephrotic syndrome occurs when the filtering elements malfunction and allow large amounts of protein to leak into the urine. Normally, little or no protein appears in the urine. If there is excessive protein leaking into the urine, the protein in the blood is depleted and the liver has difficulty in replacing it quickly. The function of protein in blood is to retain its thickness and to draw water from the tissues. This process is needed to prevent the build up of fluid in the tissue spaces which can lead to infection.

The syndrome is slightly more likely to affect males than females.

Congenital Nephrotic syndrome is very rare and symptoms will manifest in the first few weeks or months of life.

What are the symptoms?

The main feature of the syndrome is oedema (swelling) of the tissues of the body. For example, fluid can build up in the abdomen and chest, can show around the eyes and can lead to weight gain. Fluid retention around the lungs can lead to breathlessness. The loss of protein can even cause malnutrition.

What are the causes?

In children the most common cause of Nephrotic syndrome is Minimal Change disease so called because the nephrons seem to be undamaged other than when an electron microscope is used. Nephrotic syndrome in children usually appears in early childhood.

In adults the most common cause is Membranous Nephropathy, a kidney disorder resulting in disruption of kidney function because of inflammation of the glomerulus - part of the filtering structures of the kidney.

How is it treated?

Early dialysis and transplantation are now used to treat patients with Congenital Nephrotic syndrome and are important features which can lead to a good outcome.

There are a number of complications of Nephrotic syndrome which necessitate careful monitoring. These include the risk of infection, formation of blood clots and the development of high cholesterol (a type of fat in the blood) and hypertension (high blood pressure) in those who have a persistent nephrotic condition.

Diuretic drugs are used to increase the urinary output of water and reduce the oedema. In children, treatment with high doses of steroids will stop the protein leak from the kidney in ninety per cent of cases. The effect is less good in adults. Drugs are also used to treat high cholesterol levels and hypertension. In the case of blood clots arising a blood thinner may be required. It is helpful to reduce the intake of salt and follow a healthy eating diet.

How is it diagnosed?

As the most common cause of water retention in adults is cardiac disease, this needs to be eliminated before considering Nephrotic syndrome as a diagnosis. The specific tests to diagnose Nephrotic syndrome include the measurement of the loss of protein in the urine and the levels of protein (albumin) in the blood. A biopsy (examination of a sample) of kidney tissue is likely to be necessary.

Inheritance and prenatal diagnosis

Inheritance patterns

Congenital Nephrotic syndrome is autosomal recessive. Other forms of Nephrotic syndrome are not genetic.

Prenatal diagnosis

Congenital Nephrotic syndrome may be diagnosed prenatally by elevated levels of alpha-fetoprotein in amniotic fluid.

Medical text written July 2004 by Contact a Family. Approved July 2004 by Dr A R Watson, Consultant Paediatric Nephrologist, Nottingham City Hospital, Nottingham, UK.

Further online resources

Medical texts in *The Contact a Family Directory* are designed to give a short, clear description of specific conditions and rare disorders. More extensive information on this condition can be found on a range of reliable, validated websites. Further information on these resources can be found in our **Medical Information on the Internet** article on page 21.

Support

Nephrotic Syndrome in Children Support Group
94 Bulford, Wellington, Somerset TA21 8DH Tel: 01823 652 886
e-mail: support@nephrotic.co.uk web: http://www.nephrotic.co.uk
The Group is a network, established in 1996. It offers support to families by telephone and e-mail, nationally and internationally. Enquiries from professionals are also very welcome. The group supports research. It is in touch with over 1,000 individuals and familes.
Group details last updated November 2007.

There is a small family support group for families of children with Nephrotic syndrome. Details can be obtained from Contact a Family's Freephone Helpline.

Information, support and advice are available for adults with the syndrome from a number of other organisations (see entry, Kidney Disease).

NETHERTON SYNDROME

Background

Netherton syndrome is a rare hereditary disorder in which the skin is red and scaly most, if not all, of the time. The characteristic features of Netherton syndrome include inflamed, red, scaly skin; a fragile hair condition, known as 'bamboo hair', and atopy (allergy problems). Individuals with Netherton syndrome may show some or all of these features and may be affected differently by the severity of their symptoms.

What are the symptoms?

At birth most infants with Netherton syndrome look 'scalded'. The skin is 'leaky' causing infants to loose heat, water and proteins - all of which are necessary for normal growth and development. Babies are slow to gain weight, especially in the first year of life. The defective skin makes the babies more at risk of infection. In some babies, infection may be life-threatening. Most suffer from a severe failure to thrive in the first year. For the most severely affected infants, the prognosis of Netherton syndrome is poor.

Later in childhood some develop a distinctive circular scaling on the skin known as ichthyosis linearis circumflexa (see entry, Ichthyosis). The skin condition tends to go through bouts of flaring and may be itchy, sensitive or raw and often thickened at the joints. Individuals may become distressed if the skin, especially the face, is constantly red and peeling. Between episodes, the skin may appear normal. In most children, Netherton syndrome improves gradually over time, although the basic problem persists. There is no specific treatment as yet available. The main issue is the skin barrier that can be improved by the regular daily application of an ointment based moisturiser.

In Netherton syndrome, the hair is fragile and spiky, so-called 'bamboo' hair, which affects the scalp, eyelashes, eyebrows and body hair. A diagnosis may be confirmed by the microscopic examination of the characteristic 'bamboo' swellings of hair. A diagnosis after birth may be delayed, as the hair may be sparse and not obviously characteristic of the condition. A recent development has been the successful use of an antibody test on a skin biopsy demonstrating the absence of LEKTI.

Individuals with Netherton syndrome have a higher risk of allergies (see entry) and anaphylaxis (see entry). Some individuals are allergic to foods such as fish and nuts, or are prone to hay fever, asthma and eczematous-like rashes. Children with Netherton syndrome have high levels of IgE (allergy antibody) in their blood and suffer attacks of angioedema (allergic skin disease).

Individuals with Netherton syndrome are usually shorter than average and may have difficulty gaining weight. Gastrointestinal problems also occur often as diarrhoea, especially in early infancy.

What are the causes?

The cause of the skin and hair abnormalities is associated with the lack of a specific protein called LEKTI (lympho-epithelial kazal type related inhibitor), which is a serine protease inhibitor. The absence of this protein leads to a profound defect in the outermost part of the skin, 'the skin barrier'.

Inheritance patterns and prenatal diagnosis

Inheritance patterns

Netherton syndrome is inherited as an autosomal recessive trait. The gene for this condition (SPINK5) is on chromosome 5.

Prenatal diagnosis

This is now available using molecular genetic analysis.

Medical text written October 2004 by Contact a Family. Approved October 2004 by Professor J Harper, Consultant in Paediatric Dermatology, Great Ormond Street Hospital, London, UK.

Further online resources

Medical texts in *The Contact a Family Directory* are designed to give a short, clear description of specific conditions and rare disorders. More extensive information on this condition can be found on a range of reliable, validated websites. Further information on these resources can be found in our **Medical Information on the Internet** article on page 21.

Support

As Netherton syndrome is an Ichthyosis, information, support and advice is available from the Ichthyosis Support Group (see entry, Ichthyosis).

NEUROACANTHOCYTOSIS DISORDERS

Background

The term Neuroacanthocytosis refers to a group of rare inherited disorders displaying abnormalities of the nervous system, often chorea (involuntary movements), and acanthocytosis (the presence of abnormal red blood cells that on examination can be seen to have a spur-like projection).

The disorders in the Neuroacanthocytosis group are:
- Chorea-acanthocytosis: Levine-Critchley syndrome (this is often just referred to as Neuroacanthocytosis);
- Abetalipoproteinemia: Bassen-Kornzweig syndrome;
- Hypobetalipoproteinemia (presents without chorea);
- McLeod Neuroacanthocytosis syndrome: McLeod syndrome.

Choreoacanthocytosis

Choreoacanthocytosis: Chorea-acanthocytosis; Levine-Critchley syndrome; ChAc

In 1967 Critchley et all described a rare inherited condition of neurological abnormalities in an adult and in 1970 Levine et al described a similar condition in a family of nineteen persons over four generations, the majority of whom had Acanthocytosis - the typical abnormal red blood cell with spur like projections found in Neuroacanthocytosis. The condition affects both males and females, with a slight predominance in males, and all ethnic backgrounds. Reports of about 200 to 250 individuals have appeared in medical literature.

There is a wide variation in how the disorder affects individuals but the features of Chorea-acanthocytosis can include:
- Acanthocytosis;
- Behaviour changes;
- Involuntary movements (chorea, faster, dancing movements; dystonia, more sustained movements and posturing) of the limbs, trunk, neck, face, or parkinsonism (slowed movements and stiffness of limbs);
- Impaired swallowing that can lead to weight loss;
- Lip and tongue biting;
- Difficulty with speech and communication, mostly due to Central Nervous System disease, leading in some persons becoming mute;
- Seizures in about fifty per cent of affected persons;
- Peripheral neuropathy;
- Enlargement of liver and spleen.

Mutations in the VPS13A gene on chromosome 9q21 are thought to cause

Chorea-acanthocytosis.

A diagnosis of Chorea-acanthocytosis can be made when the typical neurological features are seen, especially the movements of the face with lip and tongue biting. If there are other affected siblings this also suggests the diagnosis. Not all persons show the presence of Acanthocytosis. However, the majority of persons with Chorea-acanthocytosis will show an increased presence of muscle creatine phosphokinase. The VPS13A gene is the only gene known to be associated with the condition. As molecular genetic testing for the gene is only available on a research basis, availability of the test needs to be kept under review.

Chorea-acanthocytosis cannot be cured. Treatment is symptomatic for the features affecting the individual, and assessment for the best way of helping people with Chorea-acanthocytosis. This will include speech therapy and mechanical aids such as computer speech assistance and aids to ameliorate the effects of teeth grinding, head banging and constant falls. Seizure control with anti-epileptic drugs, alleviation of depression with antidepressants and drugs to slow cognitive loss such as those used in Alzheimer's disease are all used.

Inheritance patterns
Autosomal recessive. Reports from Japan, where it appears to be somewhat more common, also indicate autosomal dominant inheritance.
Prenatal diagnosis
This may be possible in families already known to be affected.

Abetalipoproteinemia

Abetalipoproteinemia; Bassen-Kornzweig syndrome; Acanthocytosis; Apolipoprotein B Deficiency

Abetalipoproteinemia was first described by Dr F A Bassen and Dr A L Kornzweig in 1950. It is characterised by inability to absorb dietary fats through the intestine, neuropathy (abnormality of the nerves) and ataxia (inability to co-ordinate voluntary muscular movements). Abetalipoproteinemia affects both sexes but predominantly males (seventy per cent).

Abetalipoproteinemia is caused by mutations in the APOB (Apolipoprotein B) gene and the MTP (microsomal triglyceride transfer protein) gene.

Features of Abetalipoproteinemia include:
- Pale, frothy, foul-smelling stools;
- Protruding abdomen;
- Developmental delay;
- Failure to thrive;
- Muscle weakness and later poor muscle co-ordination;
- Scoliosis;

- Slurred speech;
- Retinal degeneration;
- Balance problems.

Diagnosis of Abetalipoproteinemia is made on a number of tests:
- Blood tests showing Acanthocytosis (the typical abnormal red blood cell with spur like projections);
- Stool examination showing elevated fat levels, low levels of fat-soluble vitamins (A, B, E or K) and low levels of low-density lipoproteins (LDL), and very-low-density lipoproteins (VLDL);
- Identification of retinal degeneration;
- Electromyelogram (EMG) tests may show demyelination (destruction of the fatty nerve sheath) of the peripheral nerves;
- Gene mutation tests for the APOB or MTP genes;
- Absent or low apolipoprotein B blood levels.

Treatment of Abetalipoproteinemia should be under an expert dietician and is designed to boost vitamin intake of fat-soluble vitamins such as A, B, E or K and avoiding over consumption of foods containing triglycerides (fat compounds contained in lipoproteins). A daily diet should contain no more than 140g (5oz) of poultry, fish or lean meat. Skimmed milk should be used. As fats are needed for normal growth and development, the dietician or doctor will supervise their use in the diet.

Inheritance patterns

Autosomal recessive. Hypobetalipoproteinemia, in which the levels of low-density lipoproteins (LDL), and very-low-density lipoproteins (VLDL) are very low rather than essentially absent, is autosomal dominant.

Prenatal diagnosis

This may be possible in families already known to be affected.

McLeod Neuroacanthocytosis syndrome

McLeod Neuroacanthocytosis syndrome: McLeod syndrome

McLeod Neuroacanthocytosis syndrome is a rare inherited disorder affecting males. Rarely women carrying the gene may have symptoms. The syndrome is named after Hugh McLeod the blood donor involved in the 1961 report by Allen et al first documenting the syndrome. It is a disorder of neuromuscular, haematological, liver, spleen, heart and central nervous system features. About one hundred and fifty cases have been reported worldwide.

It is thought to be caused by mutations of the XK gene on the X-chromosome.

The features of McLeod Neuroacanthocytosis syndrome can develop singly or in variable combinations and include:
- Acanthocytosis;

- Presence of the Mcleod blood group phenotype (characteristics determined by the interaction between an individuals genes and the environment);
- Involuntary movements of the limbs, trunk, neck, face (but lip and tongue biting are not typical);
- Cardiac problems;
- Enlarged liver and spleen, and abnormal liver function tests;
- Development of psychiatric problems in about twenty per cent of affected individuals;
- Development of seizures in about forty per cent of affected individuals.

A diagnosis of McLeod Neuroacanthocytosis syndrome is made by establishing the following features:

- Presence of the Mcleod blood group phenotype;
- Family history consistent with X-linked inheritance;

and any combination of:

- Central Nervous System involvement;
  - Progressive chorea (involuntary movements) or parkinsonism (slowed movements and stiffness of limbs) and seizures;
- Neuromuscular involvement;
  - Myopathy (muscle abnormalities);
  - Sensorimotor axonopathy (disease of the nerves relating to the senses and motion);
- Heart manifestations;
  - Dilated cardiomyopathy (dilation and impaired pumping function of the main chambers of the heart);
  - Arrhythmia (alteration in rhythm of the heartbeat either in time or force);
- Enlarged liver and spleen.

McLeod Neuroacanthocytosis syndrome cannot be cured and treatment is symptomatic for the features affecting the individual. Drug therapy will be prescribed for the movement, cardiac problems and seizures. Multidisciplinary psychosocial support for both the affected individuals and their families should be provided. Care must be taken if blood transfusion is required, as transfusion reactions can occur following repeated transfusion of blood with Kell antigens (as most people have). The patient then makes antibodies to Kell and has a transfusion reaction if blood with Kell is transfused again similar to the rhesus reaction in newborns. Banking of autologous (patient's own) blood is recommended.

Inheritance patterns
X-linked dominant.

Prenatal diagnosis
This may be possible in families already known to be affected.

Pantothenate Kinase-associated Neurodegeneration (PKAN)

This further disorder was formerly known as Hallervordern-Spatz syndrome but this name is no longer used as Drs Hallervordern and Spatz were implicated in euthenasing children with learning disabilities before and during World War II. PKAN involves acanthocytosis in about eight per cent of affected individuals and can be included in the Neuroacanthocytosis grouping.

About fifty per cent of individuals thought to have PKAN as a result of clinical features are found to have mutations of the PANK 2 gene on chromosome 20p13-p12.3.

The signs, symptoms and progression of PKAN vary according to the PKAN type.

Features of Classic PKAN include:
- Onset as early as three years of age;
- Periods of rapid deterioration interspersed with periods of stability;
- Choreoathetosis (involuntary purposeless and uncontrollable movements), dystonia;
- spasticity (sudden, involuntary muscle spasms);
- ataxia (inability to coordinate movements);
- Intellectual impairment may or may not be present;
- Variable life span.

Features of Atypical PKAN include:
- Average age of onset is 13½ years;
- Slower rate of progression than in Classic PKAN;
- Speech defects including dysarthria, palilalia (repetition of words and phrases) and tachylalia/tachylogia (rapid speech of words and/or phrases);
- Parkinsonian type freezing while walking;
- Psychiatric problems of personality change, depression and violent outbursts.

A diagnosis of PKAN can be made on the basis of the presenting features, characteristic signs identified in magnetic resonance imaging (MRI) and the mutation of the PANK gene.

PKAN cannot be cured and treatment is symptomatic for the features affecting the individual. Treatment is designed to alleviate the effects of the involuntary movements and maintaining independence as much as possible. Regular assessment to identify adaptive aids as they become necessary should take place as well as identification of services for helping the affected individual, their carers and families.

Inheritance patterns
Autosomal recessive.

Prenatal diagnosis
This may be possible in families already known to be affected.

Medical text written February 2005 by Contact a Family. Approved February 2005 by Dr Ruth H Walker, MB, ChB, PhD, Assistant Professor, Department of Neurology, Department of Veterans Affairs, Bronx, New York and Mount Sinai School of Medicine, New York, USA.

Further online resources

Medical texts in *The Contact a Family Directory* are designed to give a short, clear description of specific conditions and rare disorders. More extensive information on this condition can be found on a range of reliable, validated websites. Further information on these resources can be found in our **Medical Information on the Internet** article on page 21.

Support

Advocacy for Neuroacanthocytosis Patients
32 Launceston Place, London W8 5RN   Tel: 020 7937 2938
e-mail: ginger@naadvocacy.org Web: http://www.naadvocacy.org
This is a patient group offering support and linking, where possible. The group is involved in research and in holding international symposia.
Group details last updated August 2007.

Support is also available from a group of families of children with Hallervordern-Spatz syndrome (Pantothenate Kinase-associated Neurodegeneration) under the umbrella of Climb (see entry, Metabolic diseases).

NEUROBLASTOMA

Background

Neuroblastoma is a highly malignant childhood cancer and leukaemia (see entries: Cancer, and Leukaemia and other allied blood disorders) of the sympathetic nervous system.

Most tumours arise from the centre (medulla) of the adrenal gland which lies above the kidney. Other sites of the disease include the chest, the spine and the pelvis. It can occur at any age during childhood, but mainly occurs in young children less than five years old. The tumour is potentially fatal due to widespread secondary deposits which are normally present at diagnosis.

Inheritance patterns and prenatal diagnosis

Inheritance patterns

None

Prenatal diagnosis

None.

Medical text last reviewed January 2004 by Dr B L Pizer, Consultant Paediatric Oncologist, Alder Hey Children's Hospital, Liverpool, UK.

Further online resources

Medical texts in The Contact a Family Directory are designed to give a short, clear description of specific conditions and rare disorders. More extensive information on this condition can be found on a range of reliable, validated websites. Further information on these resources can be found in our **Medical Information on the Internet** article on page 21.

Support

Neuroblastoma Society
2 Caesar Court, Moss Street, York YO23 1DD
Tel: 01344 442 302
e-mail: info@nsoc.co.uk (general e-mail, see website for specific e-mail addresses)
Web: http://www.nsoc.co.uk
The Society is a National Registered Charity No. 326385, established in 1982. It offers support and contact between parents where possible together with advice about the condition and its treatment. It fundraises for research into Neuroblastoma. It publishes a quarterly newsletter and has information available, details on request. The Society has 300-400 members.
Group details last updated August 2007.

NEUROFIBROMATOSIS

Background

Neurofibromatosis (NF) is an inherited genetic disorder causing tumours on nerve tissue anywhere in the body and often other effects.

There are two main types of neurofibromatosis: NF1 caused by a defect on Chromosome 17 (ninety per cent of cases) and NF2 caused by a defect on Chromosome 22.

What are the symptoms?

Major features of NF1 include Café au lait (CAL) spots on the skin, Dermal neurofibromas which show as lumps under skin, Lisch nodules (brown spots on iris) and axillary or inguinal freckling (in the armpits or groin area). Minor, occasional features of NF1 include short stature and mild macrocephaly (large head size). Complications of NF1 are mainly cosmetic, but in about a third of cases complications of varying severity may occur, including plexiform neurofibromas (deeper nerve growths), scoliosis (curvature of the spine) see entry, pseudarthrosis (stiffening) of the long bones, optic glioma (eye growths, often without symptoms), spinal neurofibroma, hypertension due to renal artery stenosis and phaeochromocytoma (a usually benign adrenal gland tumour). Various tumours may occur in a small proportion of patients. Learning difficulties may occur, for example short term memory problems, impulsive fidgety behaviour and difficulty concentrating.

Major features of NF2 include bilateral acoustic neuromas (Vestibular schwannomas) which usually begin to cause problems in the late teens or early twenties although rarely some are later onset. Minor features of NF2 include juvenile lenticular cataracts and possibly CAL spots (but fewer than in NF1). Complications of NF2 include brain tumours which are normally benign - the most common type being meningiomas, spinal tumours and skin tumours - Schwannomas which may be similar to neurofibromas in NF1.

Psychological and behavioural characteristics

The majority of children with NF1 have an intelligence that usually falls within the normal range. However, a substantial proportion (estimates vary between forty and sixty per cent) do have learning difficulties which can be specific, such as dyslexia, or generalised, such as intellectual disability.

A specific learning difficulty can be indicated when a child's academic achievement in particular skills falls significantly below their general intellectual ability. For children with NF1, their performance and perceptual abilities may fail to reflect their general intelligence. This can cause difficulties in areas such as reading, writing, listening and mathematics.

Once in school, it may be apparent that compared with their peers, children with NF1 can have difficulty with concentration, co-ordination affecting both fine and gross motor skills, memory, visuo-motor and visuo-spatial skills, organisation and processing. Social and language problems have also been documented.

Within the framework of the education system, additional help drawn from the resources of the Special Education Needs range of support can be effective in helping children with the diagnosis of NF1 to achieve their potential.

Children with NF1 can make a substantial degree of progress in response to appropriately targeted help.

Additional therapeutic services including physiotherapy, occupational therapy and speech therapy should be considered. Occasionally the services of a clinical psychologist or psychiatrist may prove to be necessary and useful.

Some children with NF1 can show characteristic patterns of behaviour such as impulsiveness, over-activity and socially imperceptive traits. Under-confidence can be an enduring legacy and adolescence, a particularly testing time as it is, is the stage that the neurofibromas may start to appear.

NF1 is a variable and unpredictable condition which imposes a psychological burden that is difficult for both parents, affected individuals and those professionals engaged in their care. Appropriate referral at an early age can be helpful.

In NF2 the psychological difficulties are in the main related to the consequence of the condition itself coupled with the effects of chronic illness. Sensory impairment, communication difficulties attendant on hearing loss, together with mobility problems can lead to social isolation and depression.

Inheritance patterns and prenatal diagnosis
Inheritance patterns
Autosomal dominant. Fifty per cent of cases result from spontaneous new mutations in families with no previous history of the disorder.

A third form of neurofibromatosis which is similar to NF2 called 'schwannomatosis' has recently been confirmed also due to a gene on chromosome 22. Vestibular schwannomas are rare in this condition as are meningiomas.

Prenatal diagnosis
Possible in both NF1 and NF2. Severity of effect cannot be predicted in NF1 but can sometimes be predicted in NF2. Brain scans or genetic studies may allow early diagnosis or presymptomatic diagnosis in NF2.

Medical text written December 1996 by Contact a Family. Approved December 1996 by Professor M Patton, Professor of Medical Genetics, St George's Hospital Medical School, London, UK. **Last updated September 2007 by Professor G Evans, Professor of Medical Genetics, Regional Genetics Service, St Mary's Hospital, Manchester, UK.** Information on the Psychological and Behavioural Characteristics provided by Professor J Turk. **Last updated December 2005 by Professor J Turk, Professor of Developmental Psychiatry and Consultant Child & Adolescent Psychiatrist, Department of Clinical Developmental Sciences, St. George's Hospital Medical School, London, UK.**

Further online resources

Medical texts in *The Contact a Family Directory* are designed to give a short, clear description of specific conditions and rare disorders. More extensive information on this condition can be found on a range of reliable, validated websites. Further information on these resources can be found in our **Medical Information on the Internet** article on page 21.

Support

The Neurofibromatosis Association
Quayside House, 38 High Street, Kingston upon Thames KT1 1HL
Tel: 0845 602 4173 Helpline (Mon, Tues and Weds, 9am-4pm)
Tel: 020 8439 1234   Fax: 020 8439 1200   e-mail: info@nfauk.org
Web: http://www.nfauk.org

The Association is a National Registered Charity No. 1078790, established in 1981. It offers support and information to affected individuals and families. It attempts to link those with NF with medical professionals and with other families where possible. It publishes a newsletter three times a year and has a wide range of information available, details on request. The Association has around 2,000 member families.
Group details last updated July 2007.

NEUTROPENIA (SEVERE CHRONIC)

Background

There are four main groups of Severe Chronic Neutropenia (SCN). Neutrophils are the most numerous white cells in the blood. In SCN, individuals have below normal numbers of neutrophils, the white blood cell which combat bacterial infections. The lack of neutrophils results in the individual having an impaired ability to fight infection. SCN affects people of both sexes and all ethnic groups with a possible predominance in Caucasian people. SCN is rare with an incidence thought to be about 1 to 2 in 1,000,000.

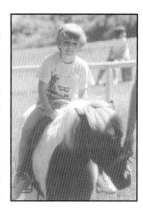

SCN types are:

- **Congenital Neutropenia** in which diagnosis is usually made soon after birth. Congenital Neutropenia can be inherited or sporadic (with no other affected family members but still of genetic cause);
- **Cyclical Neutropenia** is a form of SCN, with neutropenia occurring over a period of about three to seven days in a cycle of twenty-one days. Cyclical Neutropenia is often caused by mutations of the ELA2 gene on chromosome 19;
- **Idiopathic Neutropenia** is the name given to children and adults described as neutropenic in which no clear cause can be found. Affected people may have had a normal blood cell count in the past. Idiopathic Neutropenia is usually a relatively mild condition;
- **Autoimmune Neutropenia** is most common in infants and young children. The body identifies the neutrophils as enemies and makes antibodies to destroy them. Children usually grow out of it within two years of diagnosis.

What are the symptoms?

In SCN frequent infections can develop very rapidly due to the impaired ability of children to combat them. Infections include:

- Mouth ulcers and gingivitis (inflammation of the gums);
- Sore throat;
- Chest infections;
- Diarrhoea;
- Burning sensation when urinating;
- Unusual redness, pain, or swelling around a wound;
- High fevers and chills;
- Exhaustion and lethargy.

What are the causes?

The cause of SCN differs according to the specific type and can be hereditary, autoimmune (in which the body destroys its own neutrophils), related to bone marrow production or idiopathic (of unknown cause).

How is it diagnosed?

Diagnosis of the different types of SCN is made by blood tests and bone marrow aspiration and biopsy (examination).

How is it treated?

Granulocyte Colony Stimulating Factor (G-CSF) is used in the management of SCN and can significantly improve the quality of life by stimulating the bone marrow to produce neutrophils to fight infections. G-CSFs are given by an injection just under the skin using a very small needle. To make this less painful, a local anaesthetic cream can be applied to the site half an hour before the injection is due. Prophylactic antibiotics may be given in addition, or are often effective alone for less severely affected individuals.

Inheritance patterns and prenatal diagnosis

Inheritance patterns

Congenital Neutropenia is typically sporadic but autosomal dominant and recessive cases are also described. Cyclical Neutropenia is typically autosomal dominant but can be sporadic (with no other affected family members).

Prenatal diagnosis

This is theoretically possible if a causative mutation is identified. It is usual to find a mutation in around sixty to seventy per cent of cases of severe congenital neutropenia and cyclical neutropenia.

Medical text written October 2005 by Contact a Family. Approved October 2005 by Dr P Ancliffe, Consultant Haematologist, Great Ormond Street Hospital, London, UK.

Further online resources

Medical texts in *The Contact a Family Directory* are designed to give a short, clear description of specific conditions and rare disorders. More extensive information on this condition can be found on a range of reliable, validated websites. Further information on these resources can be found in our **Medical Information on the Internet** article on page 21.

Support

As Congenital Neutropenia is a primary immunodeficiency, information, support and advice is available from the Primary Immunodeficiency Association (see entry, Primary Immunodeficiencies).

NIEMANN-PICK DISEASE

Background

There are a number of types of Niemann-Pick disease all of which are characterised by an accumulation of fats in the liver, spleen and bone marrow. Most types of Niemann-Pick disease involve progressive neurological deterioration. Both sexes are equally affected.

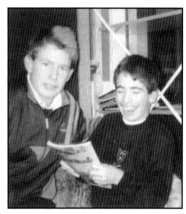

Niemann-Pick is a group of rare, inherited, metabolic conditions that normally affect children, but can sometimes occur in young adults. These conditions are caused by specific genetic mutations. There are three commonly recognised forms: Types A, B and C. Current medical opinion suggests that Types A and B may be opposite ends of a spectrum of the same disease. Type C is very different at both a genetic and a biochemical level and has also, in the past, been known by other names including: Nevilles Disease, Sphyngomyelin Lipidosis, DAF Syndrome and Juvenile Dystonic Lipidosis.

Nieman-Pick Types

Niemann-Pick Type A. NP-A is an acute form and normally reveals itself within the first few months of a baby's life. Caused by an enzyme deficiency, it is a severe neurological disease. Symptoms may include early feeding difficulties, failure to thrive and an abnormally large abdomen. It is a degenerative disease and there is a progressive loss of motor skills. Life expectancy rarely exceeds five years of age.

Niemann-Pick Type B. In NP-B there is generally little if any neurological involvement. Growth rate may be slow and puberty is often delayed, but patients generally survive into their teens and adulthood. Symptoms include an enlarged spleen, which can usually be detected in early childhood, and an enlarged liver, which normally happens a little later. Some patients develop repeated respiratory infections.

Niemann-Pick Type C. The presentation of NP-C is very variable and the onset of symptoms may occur at any time from early infancy to adulthood, though it most usually affects children of school age. Life expectancy varies considerably and there are a variety of symptoms. These may include an enlarged spleen and liver and, in newborn babies, there may be prolonged jaundice (see entry liver disease). The disease is neurologically degenerative leading to progressive loss of motor skills and difficulty with walking. Speech can become slurred and swallowing problems may develop. Patients may experience sudden loss of muscle tone, which can lead to falls, also epileptic seizures that are generally difficult to control. A symptom that is particularly suggestive of NP-C is difficulty with upward and downward eye movement. In those young adults, where onset is later, psychological problems and dementia can be major symptoms.

Niemann-Pick Type D is a form of Niemann-Pick Type C found in a population of Nova Scotia ancestry.

Biochemical Lesion NP-A and **NP-B** are primary deficiencies of sphingomyelinase. **NP-C/NP-D** is a totally different disorder with an, as yet, unidentified lesion in intracellular cholesterol transport.

Inheritance patterns and prenatal diagnosis
Inheritance patterns
Autosomal recessive.
Prenatal diagnosis
For Types A, B and most forms of Type C, this is possible by chorionic villus sampling at 10 to 12 weeks or amniocentesis at 16 weeks.

Medical text last updated July 2007 by Jackie Imrie SRN RSCN MSc, Clinical Nurse Specialist- Niemann-Pick Disease, Royal Manchester Children's Hospital, Manchester, UK. Approved by Dr J E Wraith, Consultant Paediatrician, Royal Manchester Children's Hospital, Manchester, UK.

Further online resources
Medical texts in *The Contact a Family Directory* are designed to give a short, clear description of specific conditions and rare disorders. More extensive information on this condition can be found on a range of reliable, validated websites. Further information on these resources can be found in our **Medical Information on the Internet** article on page 21.

Support
Niemann-Pick Disease Group (UK)
11 Greenwood Close, Washington NE38 8LR   Tel: 0191 415 0693
e-mail: niemann-pick@zetnet.co.uk   Web: http://www.niemannpick.org.uk
The Group is a National Registered Charity No. 1061881, established in 1991. The Group supports families of children with all forms of Niemann-Pick disease, which has also previously been known as Neville's disease, Sphingomyelin Lipidosis, DAF syndrome and Juvenile Dystonic Lipidosis. It offers contact with others in similar circumstances. It publishes a newsletter and has information available, details on request. The Group has 150 member families.
Group details last confirmed February 2008.

As Niemann-Pick disease is a metabolic disease, support and advice are also available from Climb (see entry, Metabolic diseases). Support for dementia in Niemann-Pick disease can be obtained from the Alzheimer's Society (see entry, Alzheimer's disease).

NOONAN SYNDROME

Background

Noonan syndrome is a genetic condition which is very variable in degree and so mildly affected individuals may remain undiagnosed.

There is an overlap between Noonan syndrome and LEOPARD syndrome. Some cases of LEOPARD syndrome may be caused by the same gene as Noonan syndrome. The term LEOPARD stands for Lentignes (freckles), ECG (minor abnormalities in the electrical activity of the heart), Ocular hypertelorisrn (widely spaced eyes), Pulmonary stenosis, Abnormalities of the male genitalia, Retardation of growth, Deafness.

What are the symptoms?

Additionally the characteristics, especially facial, appear to change as the individual ages.

Characteristics include:

- heart defects (see entry), the commonest being pulmonary valve stenosis – atrial septal defects and hypertrophic cardiomyopathy;
- facial features: ptosis (drooping eyelids); large downward slanting eyes; hypertelorism (widely spaced eyes), flat nasal bridge; short neck with or anterior rotations;
- short stature in correct proportion.

Additional features may include:

- excess oedema at birth and slow weight gain;
- feeding difficulties with poor sucking and weaning and frequent and/ or forceful vomiting in babies which may be assessed as failure to thrive;
- mild hearing loss;
- dental delay;
- elevated or depressed sternum;
- hypotonia (see entry);
- undescended testes;
- mild developmental delay in a minority of children;
- speech and behaviour problems.

Inheritance patterns and prenatal diagnosis

Inheritance patterns

Autosomal dominant. A gene PTPN11 on chromosome 12 has been found to account for half of all cases of Noonan syndrome.

Prenatal diagnosis

It is occasionally possible to diagnose the syndrome with ultrasound scanning.

Medical text written November 1991 by Contact a Family. Approved November 1991 by Professor M Patton and Dr J E Wraith, Consultant Paediatrician, Royal Manchester Children's Hospital, Manchester, UK. **Last updated October 2004 by Professor Michael Patton, Professor of Medical Genetics, St George's Hospital Medical School, London, UK.**

Support

The Noonan Syndrome Society is no longer functioning. The Family Services Officer of the Birth Defects Foundation (see Helpful Organisations) can provide information to families.

"We were at our wits end trying to cope when we called you and now, for the first time, we have hope and a possible future as a family." Parents.

NORMAL PRESSURE HYDROCEPHALUS

Background

Normal Pressure Hydrocephalus is increasingly being thought of as a misnomer, it may even have episodes of quite raised pressure. It is nothing to do with the Hydrocephalus that is seen following infections or intracranial haemorrhages nor the congenital types of Hydrocephalus predominantly in babies and children. Normal Pressure Hydrocephalus is a disease that affects generally the elderly population and is perhaps slightly more frequent in men than in women. Normal Pressure Hydrocephalus is a condition that can often be confused with other causes of Dementia (see entry) including alcoholism, Parkinson's disease (see entry) and Alzheimer's disease (see entry) for example. Therefore such diseases need to be excluded prior to a diagnosis of Normal Pressure Hydrocephalus being made. Clearly the treatments for these conditions are potentially quite different.

What are the symptoms?

Normal Pressure Hydrocephalus has a classic presentation pattern with dementia, gait disturbance and urinary incontinence. This is also know as Hakim's triad. The gait disturbance in Normal Pressure Hydrocephalus most commonly appears first, prior to any dementia or incontinence. Characteristically the gait can be wide based with short and shuffling steps and in particular unsteadiness when making turns. The dementia is primarily of a memory impairment pattern and there is slowness of thought and movement as well. Urinary incontinence is usually the last to appear in Normal Pressure Hydrocephalus but it must be remembered that any demented patient can have urinary incontinence.

What are the causes?

Hydrocephalus in this age group can be caused by many things and it is important to exclude other causes such as previous haemorrhages, trauma, infections, tumours etc in order to arrive at the diagnosis of Normal Pressure Hydrocephalus. Therefore there are no specific tests for Normal Pressure Hydrocephalus and the CT scans and MRI scans tend to show enlarged fluid cavities (ventricles) but often don't suggest that the pressure within the head is raised.

How is it diagnosed?

Tests for Normal Pressure Hydrocephalus include having a lumbar puncture to see if this improves the walking and memory faculties. Often patients will have a timed walking test whereby they walk a set distance, have some CSF (cerebral spinal fluid) taken off, and then have a further walking test. If the second test shows an improvement following the lumbar puncture this is an indication that they may benefit from having a shunt (a procedure to drain the fluid from the ventricles into the abdominal cavity). Other authorities suggest continuous CSF pressure monitoring which involves infusions and measuring whether there are any pressure changes within the cerebro-spinal fluid demonstrating the resistance within the system. If patients are found to have high resistance then they are thought to respond better to shunts than those without them. The scans must show Hydrocephalus (enlarged ventricles) but without any evidence of any other cause.

How is it treated?

Once the diagnosis has been established and no other treatments are appropriate then some sort of shunt procedure is indicated that will drain the fluid from the ventricles into the abdominal cavity. The most common procedure is a Ventriculoperitoneal (VP) shunt. Although lumbar peritoneal shunts have been used these tend to over-drain and therefore they are less frequently used than ventricular peritoneal shunts.

It is most likely that incontinence will improve, then gait, then lastly dementia and a response like this is more likely when the symptoms have been present for only a short period of time (a few months rather than a few years).

Inheritance patterns and prenatal diagnosis

Inheritance patterns

None.

Prenatal diagnosis

None as this is an acquired condition in the elderly.

Medical text written September 2004 by Mr Neil Buxton, Consultant Paediatric Neurosurgeon, Alder Hey Children's Hospital, Liverpool, UK.

Further online resources

Medical texts in *The Contact a Family Directory* are designed to give a short, clear description of specific conditions and rare disorders. More extensive information on this condition can be found on a range of reliable, validated websites. Further information on these resources can be found in our **Medical Information on the Internet** article on page 21.

Support

As Normal Pressure Hydrocephalus is a form of Hydrocephalus, information, support and advice is available from the Association for Spina Bifida and Hydrocephalus - ASBAH (see entry, Hydrocephalus)

NORRIE DISEASE

Background
Norrie disease is a rare inherited disorder which affects the eyes and can also lead to learning disability and deafness.

What are the symptoms?
The features of Norrie disease are:
- Visual problems (see entry, Vision Disorders in Childhood) affecting the development of the retina which is the light sensitive film at the back of the eye. Boys who have Norrie disease are usually born with severe visual problems and, on examination, an ophthalmologist will see an abnormal looking retina at the back of the eye and can make the diagnosis on this examination. Boys with Norrie disease may have retinal detachment and may also develop cataracts;
- Developmental delay (see entry, Learning Disability) which affects around one third of patients to some degree. In a small group of patients there is severe developmental delay which can be associated with behavioural problems;
- Hearing difficulty (see entry, Deafness) which affects around one third of patients. It is often progressive, starting in early childhood.

What are the causes?
Norrie disease is caused by a gene fault in the NDP gene on the X chromosome so it only affects boys. The mothers of affected boys may be carriers of the gene fault. If the mother carries the gene fault then there is a risk of other female relatives also carrying the gene fault and being at risk of having affected sons.

How is it diagnosed?
The diagnosis is made clinically by an ophthalmologist and can be confirmed now by gene testing of the NDP gene. If a gene fault is identified in the affected boy then it is possible to test his mother for carrier status and to offer testing to other female family members.

How is it treated?
There is currently no cure for Norrie disease but making the diagnosis is important, as understanding how a child interacts with the world may help to develop ways of working with the child to make sense of the world.

Inheritance patterns and prenatal diagnosis
Inheritance patterns
X-linked.
Prenatal diagnosis
It is possible to offer prenatal diagnosis to known carrier females.

Medical text written October 2005 by Contact a Family. Approved October 2005 by Professor D Trump, Professor of Human Molecular Genetics and Hon. Consultant in Clinical Genetics, University of Manchester, Manchester, UK.

Further online resources

Medical texts in *The Contact a Family Directory* are designed to give a short, clear description of specific conditions and rare disorders. More extensive information on this condition can be found on a range of reliable, validated websites. Further information on these resources can be found in our **Medical Information on the Internet** article on page 21.

Support

There is no support group for Norrie disease. Cross referrals to other entries in the Contact a Family Directory are intended to provide relevant support for these particular features of the disorder. Organisations identified in those entries do not provide support specifically for Norrie disease. Families can use Contact a Family's Freephone Helpline for advice, information and, where possible, links to other families. Contact a Family's web based linking service Making Contact.org can be accessed at http://www.makingcontact.org

NYSTAGMUS

Background

Nystagmus is a term used for spontaneous oscillations of the eyes. The most common form of nystagmus in young children is **Congenital nystagmus** (also called **Infantile nystagmus**) occurs at birth or in the first few months of life.

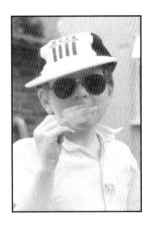

The incidence of nystagmus is unclear, but probably occurs in approximately 1 in 1,000 births. Some of these children will, however, have multiple disabilities.

Congenital nystagmus occurs at birth or in the first few months of life. It is usually associated with an underlying visual disorder, such as albinism in which there is poor pigmentation of the eyes, skin and hair. Congenital nystagmus may occur, however, in association with a wide range of infantile visual disorders.

Rarely in young children nystagmus may be secondary to a neurological disorder.

How is it diagnosed?

Accurate diagnosis for nystagmus is necessary to ensure the child has adequate help to deal with the disorder. Occasionally no visual disorder can be detected and the nystagmus is called **congenital idiopathic nystagmus** or **congenital motor nystagmus**.

Inheritance patterns and prenatal diagnosis

Inheritance patterns

These depend upon the underlying visual disorder. Congenital idiopathic nystagmus may also be inherited. Genetic counselling may be sought in cases of nystagmus.

Prenatal diagnosis

None

Medical text written November 1991 by Contact a Family. Approved November 1991 by Professor M Patton, Professor of Medical Genetics, St Georges Hospital Medical School, London, UK and Dr J E Wraith, Consultant Paediatrician, Royal Manchester Children's Hospital, Manchester, UK. **Last updated December 2007 by Professor C Harris, Professor of Neurosciences, Institute of Neurosciences, Plymouth University, Plymouth, UK.**

Support

Nystagmus Network

13 Tinsley Close, Claypole, Newark NG23 5BS   Tel: 0845 634 2630 Helpline
Tel: 01636 627004 Office   e-mail: info@nystagmusnet.org
Web: http://www.nystagmusnet.org

The Network is a National Registered Charity No. 803440, established in 1985. It offers self help support and information for people with Nystagmus, their families and professionals. It publishes a quarterly newsletter 'FOCUS' and has a wide range of information available, details on request. The Network encourages research into Nystagmus and has around 1,000 members.

Group details last updated February 2008

Contact a Family has a support pack for health professionals working with families affected by a disability or health condition from pregnancy to pre-school.

OBSESSIVE COMPULSIVE DISORDER

Background

Obsessive Compulsive Disorder (OCD) is the name given to a condition in which people experience repetitive and upsetting thoughts and/or behaviours. OCD has two main features: obsessions and compulsions.

Obsessions refer to involuntary thoughts, often unpleasant, about things such as contamination and harm to others; sometimes these thoughts are sexual, aggressive or religious.

Compulsions are repetitive, stereotyped, unnecessary behaviours such as constant checking and repeating actions, e.g. washing. Compulsions can also be mental rituals such as repeating words or phrases, counting or saying a prayer. These thoughts and actions are behaviours that people feel they have to do, even when they do not want to. Often people try to stop themselves from doing these things, but feel frustrated or worried unless they can finish.

The cause of OCD is unknown. Anxiety is a central symptom. The latest research suggests that the brain chemical serotonin may be involved.

OCD in children

Studies have shown that OCD may affect one per cent of young people. Problems with obsessions or compulsions can begin to affect young people in their families, at school and with their friends. Many children have obsessions or compulsions at some time, but when it becomes a problem for the young person and their family, it is diagnosed as OCD.

Usually the first treatment to try for OCD in children and young people is cognitive-behaviour therapy (CBT). This is usually undertaken with a specially trained cognitive behavioural therapist, but can be self-help, guided by a book or computer. CBT helps the person with OCD understand anxiety, and gradually learn to confront their feared situation/trigger without carrying out a ritual/compulsion. The aim of the treatment is to teach people to get in control of their OCD. Beginning with understanding the role of anxiety within OCD, CBT equips young people with tools to tackle their difficulties in manageable steps. CBT usually takes place over a number of sessions.

Most young people should obtain significant benefit from either psychological or medication treatment, or a combination of the two. Medication can help some people with OCD. These medications act on the brain chemical serotonin; the ones most often used in children are Sertraline and Fluvoxamine. Occasionally, a second medication may be added. Medication for OCD should be initiated by a specialist and carefully monitored.

OCD in adults

It is thought that between one to two per cent of the UK population has OCD. In very severe cases OCD may reach such proportions, that individuals' entire lives, and those of their families, are centred upon them. Behavioural programmes including exposure therapy (CBT) are again useful, particular when combined with 'response prevention' strategies, which encourage people with OCD to tolerate situations which are increasingly stressful to them while remaining calm and resisting the urges. In extreme instances modern antidepressants which have strong anti-obsessional properties are prescribed.

OCD is generally a treatable disorder and some people with OCD get better on their own, but most need help by working with a psychiatrist or a psychologist/cognitive behaviour therapist . Self-help groups, books, leaflets can be very helpful. As in children and young people, Selective Serotonin Reuptake Inhibitors (SSRI's) medications are also used.

Inheritance patterns and prenatal diagnosis

Inheritance patterns

OCD can run in families, and seems to be genetically related to tic disorders and Tourette syndrome.

Prenatal diagnosis

None.

Medical text written July 2005 by Contact a Family. Approved July 2005 by Dr I Heyman, Consultant Child and Adolescent Psychiatrist, Institute of Psychiatry, London, UK.

Support

OCD Action

Aberdeen Centre, 22 - 24 Highbury Grove, London N5 2EA
Tel: 0845 390 6232 Help and Information Line (local rate)
Tel: 0870 360 6232 Office (national rate)   Fax: 020 7288 0828
e-mail: info@ocdaction.org.uk   Web: http://www.ocdaction.org.uk
Web: http://www.ocdyouth.info
OCD Action is a National Registered Charity No: 1035213, established in 1991. It provides information, advice and support for people with OCD and their families, friends and carers, as well as interested professionals and the media. OCD Action also promotes awareness and understanding of OCD and related disorders.
Group details last updated August 2007.

OHDO SYNDROME

Ohdo syndrome: Ohdo Blepharophimosis syndrome

Background

Ohdo and his colleagues from Japan first described two sisters and a cousin with learning disabilities associated with congenital heart disease, blepharophimosis (small eye openings), blepharoptosis (drooping eyelid) and small teeth. Following this report, doctors from various countries have described children with similar problems. All the reports, apart from those in the original report, have concerned single affected children without any family history.

There are clinical similarities to BPES syndrome (Blepharophimosis-Ptosis-Epicanthus Inversus syndrome), now known to be due to a gene change or deletion but Ohdo patients do not have these changes. The condition called Young-Simpson syndrome is so similar that many doctors consider them to be the same.

What are the symptoms?

Affected children are often very floppy at birth and have major feeding problems requiring tube feeding. They have generally decreased movements, particularly facial movements. Some, but not all, children have heart problems and some have an absent part of the brain called the corpus callosum. When the teeth erupt they are often very small. Many older children have had joint problems ranging from mild bending of a finger to more severe hip disorders.

Progress in the first year of life is slow, and head control, sitting and walking occur late. However, ultimate progress is often better than was anticipated at first although all children have mild to moderate learning difficulties. Some children do not survive, due to the severity of their heart defects or to major respiratory problems.

Inheritance patterns and prenatal diagnosis

Inheritance patterns

Apart from the original report, all cases have been single cases, other than one possible case of a parent to child transmission. It is possible that Ohdo syndrome represents a microdeletion syndrome of chromosome material.

Prenatal diagnosis

Recurrence risk seems to be very low. The risk for the offspring of affected individuals may be higher, approaching fifty per cent. Detailed ultrasound scanning in subsequent pregnancies, looking particularly for heart and brain defects and for hydramnios due to impaired swallowing, may be offered.

Medical text last updated January 2003 by Professor Dian Donnai, Consultant Clinical Geneticist, St Mary's Hospital, Manchester, UK.

Support

Ohdo Syndrome Family Network

36 Borrowdale Avenue, Gatley, Cheadle SK8 4QF   Tel: 0161 428 8583

e-mail: patseville@btinternet.com   Web: http://www.seville44.fsnet.co.uk

The Network was, established in 1997. It offers support by telephone and letter and linking families where possible. It has information available, details on request. Please send SAE. The Network is in touch with over 25 families. The network offers an e-mail group at http://uk.groups.yahoo.com/group/ohdosyndrome (information about the use of online groups is available in our 'Medical Information on the Internet: Seeking Quality' article). Group details last updated July 2005.

The Children's National Service Framework (NSF) for England sets standards for children's health and social services, and the interface of those services with education. Order a leaflet from our helpline on how to use it to improve local services.

OHTAHARA SYNDROME

Ohtahara syndrome: Early Infantile Epileptic Encephalopathy

Background

Ohtahara syndrome is a rare childhood epilepsy first described by Ohtahara et al in 1976. Ohtahara syndrome is one of several severe epilepsy syndromes including West syndrome and Lennox-Gastaut syndrome that have been defined by the age of onset. Seizures often begin in the first ten days of life and usually before the age of three months. It is thought that Ohtahara syndrome affects about 0.2 per cent of children with epilepsy. Boys are thought to be slightly more affected than girls.

What are the symptoms?

The signs of Ohtahara syndrome are:

- Tonic seizures (stiffening of the extremities);
- Psychomotor development delay (delay in development of skills involving mental and motor development);
- There may be later development of other neurological difficulties such as diplegia (spasticity and weakness in the legs), hemiplegia (spasticity and weakness of one side of the body), tetraplegia (spasticity and weakness of both sides of the body), ataxia (unsteady gait), or dystonia (abnormal movements with increased tone).

What are the causes?

Ohtahara syndrome can be caused by a cerebral (brain) malformation and occasionally as a result of glycine encephalopathy (metabolic disorder). It is not, therefore, a single disease.

How is it diagnosed?

Ohtahara syndrome is diagnosed by age of onset of seizures and confirmation of suppression burst patterns on an electroencephalogram (EEG) showing the brain wave pattern of an individual. Suppression burst patterns alternate between showing electrical activity and suppression of activity.

The condition may progress to West syndrome over the first six months of life. Some authorities are uncertain about the separate distinct nature of Ohtahara syndrome regarding it as an early presentation variant of the much commoner West syndrome (infantile spasms).

How is it treated?

There is no cure for Ohtahara syndrome; treatment is symptomatic. Control of the seizures is difficult and the balance of the advantages (extending the times between seizures) and disadvantages (sleepiness) of using such drugs as phenobarbitone has to be considered. Use of anticonvulsants will not halt the psychomotor development deterioration.

Inheritance patterns and prenatal diagnosis

Inheritance patterns

Research has shown that some children found to have Ohtahara syndrome have been diagnosed with a range of disorders including cerebral malformations and metabolic disorders which may be genetic and incur a risk of recurrence.

Prenatal diagnosis

None.

Medical text written August 2004 by Contact a Family. Approved August 2004 by Professor B Neville. **Last updated April 2006 by Professor B Neville, Professor of Childhood Epilepsy, Institute of Child Health, London, UK.**

Further online resources

Medical texts in *The Contact a Family Directory* are designed to give a short, clear description of specific conditions and rare disorders. More extensive information on this condition can be found on a range of reliable, validated websites. Further information on these resources can be found in our **Medical Information on the Internet** article on page 21.

Support

There is no support group for Ohtahara syndrome but general support can be obtained from support organisations for Epilepsy (see entry). Families can use Contact a Family's Freephone Helpline for advice and information, and where possible, links to other families of children with Ohtahara syndrome.

OLLIER DISEASE

Ollier disease: Enchondromatosis

Background

An Enchondroma is an island of unossified hyaline cartilage situated within bone (cartilage is the precursor of bone). They are usually multiple, affecting one or several bones. Characteristically, it is an asymmetric disorder, confined to one side of the body. The bones most commonly affected are the long bones, pelvis and bones of the hand. The islands of cartilage appear early in childhood and can develop, but it is very unusual for additional lesions to appear after puberty.

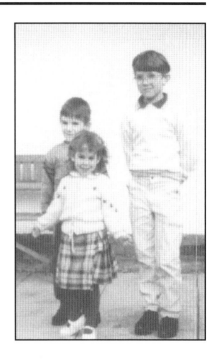

What are the symptoms?

Ollier disease is a very rare disorder which affects both sexes. It presents either as a lump or swelling or deformity of the long bone in early childhood. As the bones are weakened, they may fracture but healing is normal. The severity varies but otherwise the child develops normally. The main complications are the nature of the lump or swelling, the deformity of the affected bone and the shortening of the affected bone.

How is it treated?

The deformity can be corrected by osteotomy and the shortening can be addressed by leg lengthening in the knowledge that the bones will heal normally. Differential diagnoses of fibrous dysplasia and diaphyseal aclasis need to be considered. It is recognised that malignancy can occur but it is extremely rare. Maffucci syndrome in which there are cutaneous haemangionates associated with the enchondromas does carry a definite risk of malignancy. However, this is a separate and even rarer condition.

Inheritance patterns and prenatal diagnosis

Inheritance patterns

None

Prenatal diagnosis

None

Medical text written September 2000 by Mr M Smith. **Last updated April 2005 by Mr M Smith, Consultant Orthopaedic Surgeon, Guy's Hospital, London, UK.**

O

Support

A support group for Ollier disease is currently being formed. Families can use Contact a Family's Freephone Helpline for advice, information and, where possible, links to other families. Contact a Family's web-based linking service Making Contact.org can be accessed at http://www.makingcontact.org

---

Each year, our staff and volunteers give talks at over 470 meetings attended by over 9,750 parents and professionals.

OPITZ G/BBB SYNDROME

Opitz G/BBB syndrome; G syndrome; Hypertelorism-Hypospadias syndrome; Opitz-Frias syndrome

Background

Professor John Opitz, an eminent North American geneticist, and colleagues first drew attention to these conditions in 1969 and subsequently. Professor Opitz did not wish to follow the practice of naming syndromes after the medical authors who report the condition, so he suggested conditions are represented by the initials of the names of families who first present. However, with an increasing number of newly reported syndromes, this system fell out of favour.

What are the symptoms?

In Opitz G/BBB syndrome the clinical features mainly affect midline structures of the body. Increased spacing between the eyes (hypertelorism) is often apparent but this is less important than difficulties in swallowing or breathing due to malformation of the larynx (voicebox), trachea (the main airway) or oesophagus (the gullet) or bottom (imperforate anus). Kidney abnormalities (see entry, Kidney disease) and hypospadias (displacement of the orifice at the tip of the penis) (see entry) are common. Other complications are present less frequently.

What are the causes?

It is now generally agreed that Opitz G/BBB syndromes are clinically indistinguishable, but it is likely that in different families the condition may arise from different genetic changes. This phenomenon is termed genetic heterogeneity and it is important for families because it complicates genetic risk prediction and makes gene testing more difficult.

Probably, there is an Opitz G/BBB gene fault or mutation located on chromosome 22. In a few cases only, a larger chromosome 22q11 deletion has been diagnosed by a special (FISH) chromosome test.

In yet other families, the Opitz G/BBB syndrome gene is located at the tip of the X chromosome in a gene called midline (MID1).

Note that the Opitz G/BBB syndrome is different from another X chromosome condition called Opitz-Kaveggia/FG syndrome, sometimes caused by a change in the MED12 gene.

Inheritance patterns and prenatal diagnosis

Inheritance patterns

This may be very difficult to assess, especially if only one person in a family is affected. Specialist genetic counselling is advisable. Without evidence from the family tree, it might be difficult to estimate the risk of recurrence of the syndrome in a family. Parents and other close relatives may need to be examined for minor features of the syndrome. Rarely, the family tree indicates clear-cut autosomal dominant or X-chromosome linked inheritance that carries high risk of recurrence.

Prenatal diagnosis

Gene tests are not routinely available but in some families a causative gene change is identified that does permit prenatal testing after chorion villus sampling or amniocentesis. In other families, prenatal diagnosis by ultrasound examination may demonstrate a rare complication associated with the presence of the syndrome in the fetus.

Medical text written October 2001 by Dr J Tolmie. **Last updated September 2007 by Dr J Tolmie, Consultant Clinical Geneticist, Ferguson-Smith Centre for Clinical Genetics, Glasgow, UK.**

Further online resources

Medical texts in *The Contact a Family Directory* are designed to give a short, clear description of specific conditions and rare disorders. More extensive information on this condition can be found on a range of reliable, validated websites. Further information on these resources can be found in our **Medical Information on the Internet** article on page 21.

Support

A support group for specific Opitz syndromes has not yet been established. However, a one-to-one linking system between parents who have children with Opitz G syndrome and Opitz-Frias syndrome is offered within Contact a Family. This service has been formulated and adapted to provide a confidential and sensitive service aimed to meet individual needs.

Only the form of Opitz G/BBB resulting from a chromosome 22q11 deletion is supported by the Max Appeal (see entry, 22q11 Deletion syndromes).

Further information and support for specific features of the syndromes are covered by cross referrals in the above text.

OPITZ-KAVEGGIA / FG SYNDROME

FG syndrome: Opitz-Kaveggia syndrome; Opitz FG syndrome; Keller syndrome

Background

FG syndrome was first described by Professor Opitz and Dr Kaveggia in 1974. It became known as FG syndrome according to the system used at that time by Dr Opitz, who preferred to name conditions with the initials of the names of the first presenting families, rather than eponymously, after the name of the doctors who wrote the first medical reports. Nevertheless, the Opitz-Kaveggia name is now preferred by some doctors and the name Keller syndrome is a name that is seldom used. Note Opitz-Kaveggia/FG syndrome has subtle clinical and important genetic differences from the Opitz G/BBB syndrome (see entry).

What are the symptoms?

The main signs and symptoms Opitz-Kaveggia/FG affect male infants and include hypotonia (reduced muscle tone) with global developmental delay and subsequent learning disability; imperforate or narrowed anus (skin covered or blocked bottom) or severe constipation; high prominent forehead with larger than average head circumference and somewhat widened and flattened appearing thumbs and great toes. Brain scan may show a lesion called agenesis of the corpus callosum that is not in itself harmful. As the imperforate anus is not present in each case and constipation is a non-specific sign, Opitz-Kaveggia/FG can be hard to diagnose and it may therefore have gone unrecognised in the past

As mentioned above, the clinical features of FG syndrome can vary in different affected individuals and can include:

- learning disability (see entry) in males;
- imperforate anus or severe constipation;
- reduced or lax muscle tone in childhood; increased tone in adulthood;
- minor changes in appearance such as high broad forehead with upsweep of the hairline (cow's lick), wide-apart eyes, smallish external ears, broad thumbs and great toes;
- congenital heart defect (see entry, Heart defects);
- short stature (see entry, Restricted Growth);
- seizures (see entry, Epilepsy);
- hearing loss (see entry, Deafness);
- hyperactivity and tantrums (see entry, Attention Deficit Hyperactivity Disorder);
- friendly or out-going personality.

What are the causes?

Opitz-Kaveggia/ FG syndrome is sometimes due to a mutation in a gene called MED12 that is located on the X chromosome. Female carriers are generally unaffected but a few carriers may have some symptoms or signs. Because MED12 gene mutations have been identified recently, DNA-based postnatal and prenatal diagnosis may be possible in the future in some but not all families.

How is it diagnosed?

Diagnosis of Opitz-Kaveggia/FG syndrome is usually made by observation of affected individuals with clinical features of the disorder, and its inheritance in an X-chromosome linked fashion within the family lends further support. Families should be offered genetic counselling.

How is it treated?

Multidisciplinary treatments and support are required for the child who has complex or severe learning disabilities and surgical treatment is required to correct an imperforate or narrowed anus.

Inheritance patterns and prenatal diagnosis

Inheritance patterns

X-chromosome linked but it is likely that there is more than one FG syndrome gene on the X-chromosome.

Prenatal diagnosis

This will be possible by DNA testing if the Opitz-Kaveggia/FG syndrome gene mutation has already been identified in an affected relative. Otherwise, an affected fetus might be identified in mid-pregnancy through identification by a detailed ultrasound examination of a particular pattern of abnormalities including a corpus callosum (structure in the brain) abnormality.

Medical text written August 2005 by Contact a Family. Approved August 2005 by Dr J Tolmie. **Last updated August 2007 by Contact a Family and by Dr J Tolmie, Consultant Clinical Geneticist, Ferguson-Smith Centre for Clinical Genetics, Glasgow, UK.**

Further online resources

Medical texts in The Contact a Family Directory are designed to give a short, clear description of specific conditions and rare disorders. More extensive information on this condition can be found on a range of reliable, validated websites. Further information on these resources can be found in our **Medical Information on the Internet** article on page 21.

Support

There is no support group for FG syndrome in the UK. Cross referrals to other entries in the Contact a Family Directory are intended to provide relevant support for those particular features of the disorder. Organisations identified in those entries do not provide support specifically for FG syndrome. Families can use Contact a Family's Freephone Helpline for advice, information and, where possible, links to other families. Contact a Family's web-based linking service Making Contact.org can be accessed at http://www.makingcontact.org

There is a US based support group, FG Syndrome Family Alliance, Inc Web: http://www.fg-syndrome.org
Group details last confirmed February 2008.

"It means so much to me having information on my daughter's rare condition and to know that people like yourselves care." Parent.

OPTIC NERVE HYPOPLASIA

Optic Nerve Hypoplasia: Optic Nerve Head Hypoplasia

Background

Optic Nerve Hypoplasia (ONH) is a congenital condition (present at birth) in which there is underdevelopment of the optic nerve. ONH can be unilateral (affecting one eye) or bilateral (affecting both eyes) in both males and females. ONH is thought to be one of the three most common causes of visual impairment in children.

What are the symptoms?

The optic nerve carries visual information from the eye to the brain which interprets it and allows people to 'see' objects and the surrounding world. This process can be interrupted to a greater or lesser degree depending on the amount of underdevelopment of the optic nerve. If the nerve in only one eye is affected in a minor way vision can be almost normal but if both eyes are affected in a more major way, the individual may only be able to see large objects and bright lights.

Other features of ONH may include:
- Nystagmus (see entry) (jerky movements of the eyes);
- Mild photophobia (light sensitivity);
- Problems of peripheral vision (inability to see objects to the side);
- Poor depth perception.

ONH may also be associated with other conditions such as Septo-optic dysplasia (see entry) due to incorrect development of the pituitary gland (see entry, Pituitary disorders).

What are the causes?

The cause of ONH is not known but in a few cases there may be an association with maternal diabetes. It is believed that at some stage of the growth of the fetus there is a loss of nerve fibre resulting in underdevelopment of the optic nerve.

How is it diagnosed?

ONH is diagnosed on examination of the optic nerve and observation of its size and that of the nerve head.

How is it treated?

There is no cure for ONH and treatment is symptomatic for the specific difficulties it causes. Families and teachers can help children by providing appropriately sized books and toys. Children with ONH often have to learn aspects of vision, depth and perception to allow them to play and carry out many of the ordinary activities of childhood. In this, families can provide important assistance by teaching activities such as using slides, climbing stairs and water play.

Ongoing assessment of a child's needs and educational path should take place.

Inheritance patterns and prenatal diagnosis
Inheritance patterns
Most cases of ONH occur sporadically without any other affected family members.

Prenatal diagnosis
ONH is very rarely inherited. Prenatal diagnosis is not available. However, it is possible to image the septum pellucidum, a structure in the brain, antenatally by ultrasound. Absence of this structure may be an indicator of ONH. Obstetricians should be made aware if a previous child has ONH so that this can be checked carefully but absence of the structure does not have to be associated with ONH.

Medical text written October 2005 by Miss Isabelle Russell-Eggitt FRCS FRCOphth, Consultant Ophthalmic Surgeon, Great Ormond Street Hospital, London, UK.

Support
Support for Optic Nerve Hypoplasia is available from the SOD/ONH Network (see entry, Septo-optic dysplasia).

ORGANIC ACIDAEMIAS

Background

The organic acidaemias (also known as organic acidurias) are a group of inherited disorders that affect the way the body is able to metabolise protein. In each disorder there is a genetic deficiency of a particular enzyme involved in the breakdown of one or more aminoacids and this leads to a build up of harmful acidic chemicals in the body. Individual disorders are usually named after the type of chemical that accumulates in the blood or urine or, alternatively, according to the enzyme that is deficient. For example in propionic acidaemia there is an accumulation of propionic acid in blood but the condition is also called propionyl - CoA carboxylase deficiency since it is the enzyme propionyl - CoA carboxylase that is deficient.

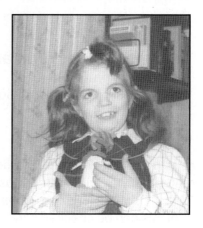

What are the symptoms?

Before birth a baby with an organic acidaemia is usually protected from harm as the placenta is able to remove any harmful acids. Soon after delivery these acids begin to accumulate and may cause a severe illness. Characteristic symptoms include general malaise, reluctance to feed, breathing problems, vomiting, hypotonia (see entry) and/or spasticity (stiffness).

How is it diagnosed?

The diagnosis is most often made by organic analysis of urine using gas chromatography/mass spectrometry (GCMS) or by analysis of acylcarnitines in blood using tandem mass spectrometry (TMS).

How is it treated?

Because the defect in the manufacture of the particular enzyme is permanent, and no effective enzyme replacement is yet possible, there is no cure for any of the organic acidaemias. However treatment may be effective, particularly in those with less severe disease. Treatment is mainly directed at trying to prevent the accumulation of the harmful acidic chemicals by reducing the intake of protein in the diet, to increase the removal of acidic chemicals using various medicines and to ensure that the diet of other essential nutrients is as complete as possible.

Inheritance patterns and prenatal diagnosis

Inheritance patterns

Autosomal recessive.

Prenatal diagnosis

Chorionic villus sampling at ten to twelve weeks is now the usual method of testing although on occasions amniocentesis at sixteen to eighteen weeks is also used.

Medical text last updated November 2004 by Dr J Walter, Consultant Paediatrician in Metabolic Disorders, Willink Biochemical Genetics Unit, Royal Manchester Children's Hospital, Manchester, UK.

Support

Due to the increasing number of conditions identified as coming under the umbrella of Organic Acidaemias, it is not possible to include them all in this entry. Individual conditions can be found listed individually in the index and are updated regularly. Where there is an alternative parent support network for individual conditions this is indicated.

As these conditions are also metabolic diseases support, advice and information are also available from Climb (see entry, Metabolic diseases).

OSTEOPETROSIS

Background

Osteopetrosis is a rare genetic disease which affects osteoclasts. These are cells which dissolve bone, so that it can be reshaped during growth or repaired after injury. This defect causes bones throughout the body to become excessively dense and to fracture easily. Nerves which sit in bony channels (such as those which pass through the skull to the eye or ear) can be damaged since these channels do not enlarge as the nerves grow.

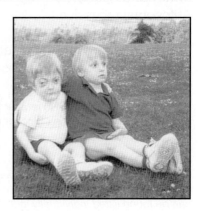

What are the symptoms?

Infantile ('malignant') Osteopetrosis is the most severe form of the disease. Affected children tend to be short but with relatively large heads. They often sustain birth fractures and may be jittery or have convulsions during the first month of life due to a low blood calcium. Subsequently they develop persistent snuffles (narrow nasal passages) and are prone to infections. Bone marrow cavities are reduced: blood is then, established in the liver and spleen, causing swelling of these organs and a low blood count may result. Many children become blind (see entry, Vision Disorder in Childhood) by six months of age, deafness and hydrocephalus (see entries) may develop later. A variety of different forms of the disease have been described, although the genetic cause is only known in approximately fifty per cent of affected children.

Adult ('benign') Osteopetrosis tends to be diagnosed in late adolescence or early adulthood when bones are X-rayed due to a fracture. Some people may go on to develop bone pain, dental problems and deafness or facial nerve paralysis. There is no specific treatment.

How is it treated?

Without treatment many affected children die before adolescence. However, in those for whom suitable donors can be found, bone marrow transplantation may be curative. Alternatively, injections of gamma interferon may alleviate some symptoms of the disease.

Inheritance patterns and prenatal diagnosis

Inheritance patterns

There has been rapid increase in the understanding of the genetics of osteopetrosis since 2000. Now it is known that mutation in any one of four genes (CAII, ATP6i, ClCN7, GL) is responsible for over three quarters of cases, with no causative gene having so far been identified in the remaining quarter. Autosomal recessive disease may result from mutation of any of these genes. Autosomal dominant disease results from mutations of ClCN7 in most cases.

Prenatal diagnosis

Accurate antenatal diagnosis is possible in families with known gene mutations by either chorionic villus sampling or amniocentesis from ten weeks of pregnancy onwards. For other families prenatal diagnosis is less reliable and depends on detection of changes in the fetus by X-ray or ultrasound in the last third of pregnancy.

Medical text written November 2000 by Dr C G Steward. **Last updated October 2005 by Dr C G Steward, Reader in Stem Cell, Bristol Children's Hospital, Bristol, UK.**

Further online resources

Medical texts in *The Contact a Family Directory* are designed to give a short, clear description of specific conditions and rare disorders. More extensive information on this condition can be found on a range of reliable, validated websites. Further information on these resources can be found in our **Medical Information on the Internet** article on page 21.

Support

Osteopetrosis Support Trust – OST

26 Doniford Road, Williton, Taunton TA4 4SE   Tel: 01984 639416

e-mail: alison@osteopetrosis.co.uk   Web: http://www.osteopetrosis.co.uk

The Trust is a National Registered Charity No. 1013052, established in 1991. OST is a parent-run support group offering support after diagnosis and bereavement and linking families where possible. It is supported by medical and scientific advisers and has information available for families and professionals, details on request (please send SAE). As this is such a rare disease the trust is run by the parents and families of Osteopetrosis sufferers and anyone is welcome to join and support at anytime.

Group details last updated October 2007.

OSTEOPOROSIS (ADULT)

Background

Osteoporosis literally means 'porous bones.' The bones in the skeleton are made of a thick outer shell and a strong inner mesh filled with collagen (protein), calcium salts and other minerals. The inside looks like honeycomb, with blood vessels and bone marrow in the spaces between bone. Osteoporosis occurs when the holes between bone become bigger, making it fragile and liable to break easily. Osteoporosis usually affects the whole skeleton but it most commonly causes breaks (fractures) to bones in the wrist, spine and hip.

What are the cause?

Osteoporosis affects 1 in 2 women and 1 in 5 men during their lifetime. Bone loss occurs as individuals get older with increased incidence seen as life expectation in the population increases. There are also many other factors which can increase the risk of osteoporosis:

For women:
a lack of oestrogen, caused by
- early menopause (before the age of forty-five);
- early hysterectomy (before the age of forty-five), particularly when both ovaries are removed (oophorectomy);
- missing periods for six months or more (excluding pregnancy) as a result of over-exercising or over-dieting.

For men:
- low levels of the male hormone, testosterone (hypogonadism).

For men and women:
- long-term use of high dose corticosteroid tablets (for conditions such as arthritis and asthma);
- close family history of osteoporosis (mother or father), particularly if an individual's mother has suffered a hip fracture;
- other medical conditions such as Cushing's syndrome, intestinal diseases and liver and thyroid problems;
- malabsorption problems (Coeliac disease, Crohn's disease, gastric surgery);
- long-term immobility;
- heavy drinking;
- smoking.

The presence of one or more of these factors puts an individual at increased risk of developing osteoporosis. Such individuals should discuss prevention and treatment with their doctor.

How is it treated?

There is much that can be done to try to build and maintain strong, healthy bones that will help to prevent osteoporosis. An individual's genes determine the potential height and strength of the skeleton but lifestyle factors have an influence.

It is vitally important to try to maximise peak bone mass during childhood, adolescence and early adulthood, when the skeleton is increasing in bone density. Such maximisation of peak bone mass increases ability to withstand the natural bone loss that occurs later in life. Individuals in their mid-thirties or older should aim to maintain bone strength.

Healthy bones need a well-balanced diet, incorporating minerals and vitamins from four different food groups, including bread and cereals; fruit and vegetables; milk and dairy products; meat, fish, eggs, pulses, nuts and seeds. It is especially important to ensure that the diet is rich in calcium. Calcium is the most abundant mineral found in bones and helps to give them strength and rigidity and is found a variety of products including cheese, yogurt, green leafy vegetables and baked beans.

Bones, like muscles and other parts of the body, suffer if they are not used. They need regular weight-bearing exercise that exerts a loading impact and stretches and contracts the muscles, stimulating bone to strengthen. Good bone building exercise includes running, skipping, aerobics, tennis and weight-training.

Smoking has a toxic effect on bone in men and women. It can cause women to have an earlier menopause and may increase the risk of hip fracture in later life. Stopping smoking will benefit bones and general health and fitness.

Drinking too much alcohol is damaging to bone turnover. Alcohol intake should be limited to a maximum of twenty-eight units per week for men and twenty-one units for women. One unit of alcohol is equivalent to a glass of wine; a measure of spirits; or half a pint of normal strength beer or cider. The moderate intake of one or two glasses of wine a day may have beneficial effects on the skeleton as well as the heart.

Osteoporosis causes more than two hundred thousand fractures each year in the UK, and there are over three million people with the disease. There are 70,000 hip fractures each year: up to twenty per cent of hip fracture patients may die prematurely and fifty per cent are unable to live independently. Research has shown that treating osteoporotic fractures annually costs the NHS and Government over £940 million.

Inheritance patterns and prenatal diagnosis
Inheritance patterns
None.
Prenatal diagnosis
None.

Medical text written November 2000 by the National Osteoporosis Society. Approved November 2000 by Professor Anthony Woolf, Consultant Rheumatologist, Royal Cornwall Hospital, Truro UK. **Last updated May 2005 by Professor D M Reid, Professor of Rheumatology, University of Aberdeen Medical School, Aberdeen, UK.**

Further online resources
Medical texts in *The Contact a Family Directory* are designed to give a short, clear description of specific conditions and rare disorders. More extensive information on this condition can be found on a range of reliable, validated websites. Further information on these resources can be found in our **Medical Information on the Internet** article on page 21.

Support
The National Osteoporosis Society
Camerton, Bath BA2 0PJ   Tel: 0845 450 0230 Helpline   Tel: 01761 471771
Fax: 01761 471104   e-mail: info@nos.org.uk   Web: http://www.nos.org.uk
The Society is a National Registered Charity No. 292660, established in 1986. Its aim is to ensure that all people with osteoporosis receive appropriate treatment and that all preventable osteoporosis is prevented. The Society has a member of staff who responds to parents of children with juvenile osteoporosis (see entry). It has a wide range of information available, details on request. The Society has around 27,000 members.
Group details last confirmed July 2004.

OSTEOPOROSIS (JUVENILE)

Background

In Osteoporosis there is a reduction in both the quantity and quality of bone in the skeleton leading to an increased risk of fracture. Osteoporosis causes more than 200,000 fractures each year which result in pain, deformity and sometimes premature death. It affects 1 in 3 women and 1 in 12 men in the UK and although uncommon it can present in childhood and early adolescence. Bone is lost due to the natural ageing process but in addition this is also influenced by the effect of hormones (particularly oestrogen in women), dietary factors especially calcium intake, physical inactivity and excess tobacco and alcohol consumption. The chance of developing osteoporosis is also increased by specific drugs, notably corticosteroids and other diseases, for example an untreated over active thyroid gland.

When osteoporosis develops in childhood it may be as a result of one of these factors but it is also possible that no underlying cause is found and the term idiopathic juvenile osteoporosis is used to describe this condition.

How is it treated?

Although there are several drugs used for the treatment of osteoporosis in adults there is little known about the effects of these drugs in children and it is therefore important that a child with osteoporosis is under the care of a specialist. The long term outlook for children with osteoporosis remains uncertain but spontaneous improvement appears to occur in a proportion of cases.

Inheritance patterns and prenatal diagnosis

Inheritance patterns

Familial incidence has been recognised but genetic causes have not yet been fully established.

Prenatal diagnosis

Not applicable.

Medical text written November 1996 by Dr R M Francis. Last updated August 2001 by Dr R M Francis, Consultant Physician, Freeman Hospital, Newcastle upon Tyne, UK. **Last reviewed May 2005 by Professor D M Reid, Professor of Rheumatology, University of Aberdeen Medical School, Aberdeen, UK.**

Support

Support and advice about Juvenile Osteoporosis are available from the National Osteoporosis Society – see entry, Osteoporosis (Adult).

PEHO SYNDROME

PEHO syndrome is a rare neurodegenerative condition which usually begins within the first few weeks of life. The condition takes its name from the following features: **P**rogressive encephalopathy with (O)**E**dema, **H**ypsarrhythmia and **O**ptic atrophy (PEHO).

Progressive encephalopathy is the term used to describe degenerative changes which take place in brain tissue; in PEHO syndrome, these changes characteristically occur in the cerebellum. The cerebellum is important for maintaining posture, co-ordinating head and eye movements and fine-tuning of muscles. Infants with PEHO syndrome may become increasingly floppy (see entry, hypotonia) and lose control of their muscles. The muscles supporting the head become floppy and weak and rolling over, sitting, standing and walking are rarely accomplished. Oedema or swelling of the hands, feet and face is also a feature of PEHO syndrome which may be transient or permanent.

Another feature of PEHO syndrome is infantile spasms. These are characterised by brief, but often repetitive, muscle contractions usually involving the head, trunk, and extremities. They occur in association with a particular pattern on EEG examination known as hypsarrhythmia. Seizures are also typical in PEHO syndrome and may begin from birth to twelve months. Infants with PEHO syndrome gradually lose their ability to see (optic atrophy). Visual fixation is either absent at birth or lost during the first months of life, leaving infants with wandering and upward turning eyes. Learning difficulties have also been associated with PEHO syndrome. These become apparent at an early stage and usually affect language skills.

At birth, neonates are severely floppy, have feeding difficulties and are very drowsy. Their appearance is characterised by an expressionless, pear shaped face with narrow forehead, broad, puffy cheeks and receding chin. The nose is small and upturned and the mouth is constantly open with a curved upper lip. Earlobes are outward turning. Although the head size is normal at birth, it usually becomes smaller (microcephaly) during the first year and the face becomes narrower with time.

The major diagnostic criteria for PEHO syndrome are changes in the brain originating in the cerebellum (cerebellar atrophy) and progressing to the brain stem. These may be identified by magnetic resonance imaging (MRI scan) or at post-mortem. A diagnosis of PEHO-like syndrome may be given to those infants who look similar to infants with PEHO syndrome but who may have milder clinical features. Brain scan investigations of infants with PEHO-like syndrome do not show the progressive cerebellar atrophy diagnostic of PEHO syndrome.

A number of conditions share similar features with PEHO syndrome including Joubert syndrome, autosomal recessive hypoplasia (Norman syndrome), olivo-pontine cerebellar atrophies and carbohydrate-deficient glycoprotein (CDG).

Inheritance patterns and prenatal diagnosis

Inheritance patterns

PEHO syndrome is thought to be inherited as an autosomal recessive trait.

Prenatal diagnosis

None available.

Medical text last updated September 2002. Written by Contact a Family and approved by Dr S Robb, Consultant Paediatric Neurologist, Hammersmith Hospital, London, UK.

Further online resources

Medical texts in *The Contact a Family Directory* are designed to give a short, clear description of specific conditions and rare disorders. More extensive information on this condition can be found on a range of reliable, validated websites. Further information on these resources can be found in our **Medical Information on the Internet** article on page 21.

Support

There is no support group for PEHO syndrome. Families can use Contact a Family's Freephone Helpline for advice, information and, where possible, links to other families. Contact a Family's web-based linking service Making Contact.org can be accessed at http://www.makingcontact.org

PAGET DISEASE

Paget disease; Paget's disease

Background

Paget's Disease of Bone was first described by Sir James Paget in 1877. This is a late onset disorder, mainly presenting in individuals over forty years of age. Paget Disease is more commonly found in males, with about three times more men affected than women.

What are the symptoms?

Most people with Paget disease are not aware that they have it. For others, the most common symptom of Paget's disease is bone pain. The specific areas of pain depend on the bones affected. Features may include headaches, back pain, pain in the shin bone and hip pain. Individuals may show some or all of these features and in addition may be differently affected by the severity of their symptoms. Thus individuals may be so mildly affected that they are unaware of their symptoms and the diagnosis only comes to light by chance on an X-ray or blood test. In some people the affected bone can cause nerve compression - the most common instance of this is deafness due to Paget disease of the skull.

In the advanced stages of Paget disease, bowed limbs and increased head size may be evident. If there is damage to joint cartilage, arthritis can develop. Some symptoms may initially seem to indicate other conditions such as arthritis.

What are the causes?

Normally, bone tissue is renewed continuously by a process of being broken-down and generated over the course of an individual's life. This process is maintained by a complex series of metabolic processes. In Paget disease, the metabolic equilibrium is upset. As a result, newly formed bone is thicker and yet softer than normal, causing weight bearing bones to bend.

How is it diagnosed?

Paget disease may be diagnosed by X-ray or a bone scan. Furthermore a blood test for a metabolic screen may indicate an elevated level of an enzyme produced in bone - alkaline phosphatase.

How is it treated?

Treatment is mainly in the form of drug therapy. Surgery may be necessary if the bone fractures or arthritis develops. The goal of medication is to relieve pain and halt the progress of the disorder. However, gentle exercise will maintain health and joint mobility.

Inheritance patterns and prenatal diagnosis

Inheritance patterns

The precise cause of Paget disease remains unknown. However, genetic factors are thought to be involved. There is a large genetic component in cases of familial Paget disease but this is very uncommon. When familial Paget disease does occur it tends to occur in younger (less than forty years) age groups.

Prenatal diagnosis

Not available.

Medical text written March 2004 by Contact a Family. Approved March 2004 by Dr P Helliwell, Senior Lecturer in Rheumatology, Rheumatism and Rehabilitation Unit, Leeds University, Leeds, UK.

Further online resources

Medical texts in *The Contact a Family Directory* are designed to give a short, clear description of specific conditions and rare disorders. More extensive information on this condition can be found on a range of reliable, validated websites. Further information on these resources can be found in our **Medical Information on the Internet** article on page 21.

Support

National Association for the Relief of Paget's Disease

323 Manchester Road, Walkden, Worsley, Manchester M28 3HH   Tel: 0161 799 4646   Fax: 0161 799 6511   e-mail: director@paget.org.uk   Web: http://www.paget.org.uk
The National Association for the Relief of Paget's Disease (NARPD) is a National Registered Charity No. 266071, established in 1973. NARPD provides support and information to individuals with Paget's disease, funds research and publishes a quarterly newsletter. It holds awareness weeks and patient days and has a range of information available, details on request with SAE. NARPD has over 2,800 members.
Group details last confirmed October 2007.

PALLISTER-HALL SYNDROME

Pallister-Hall syndrome: Ano-Cerebro-Digital syndrome; CAVE Lethality Multiplex syndrome; Cerebro-Acro-Visceral Early Lethality Multiplex syndrome; Hypothalamic Hamartoblastoma syndrome

Background

Pallister-Hall syndrome (PHS) is a developmental disorder that was first recognised in 1980. It is rare, with about one hundred cases recognised worldwide. It usually affects only one person in a family but may be inherited in some families.

What are the symptoms?

The condition is very variable - individuals with mild PHS may only have one extra digit; more severe PHS is manifest by severe birth defects that can be lethal. The main features of PHS include:

- **Hypothalamic hamartoma** (see entry), previously called hamartoblastoma. This is a benign brain tumour that arises from the hypothalamus (a region of the brain). Its presence can sometimes cause hormonal disturbance (see below). It is usually picked up on an MRI scan (neither cranial CT nor ultrasound scanning is adequate in looking for this tumour). No treatment is usually necessary and the hamartoma should not in most circumstances be removed or biopsied because of the risk of surgical complications.

- **Pituitary gland abnormalities**. The pituitary gland sits below the hypothalamus (see above). It is sometimes called "the master gland" in that it produces a number of hormones that control different metabolic and growth functions in the body. In PHS there may be a spectrum of abnormalities: at the mildest end the pituitary gland is located in the wrong place but works normally; at the more severe end of the spectrum the pituitary gland does not produce any hormones. Any baby with PHS needs urgent assessment by a paediatric endocrinologist (a doctor who specialises in looking after children with hormone problems) as they may need hormone replacement. Long-term endocrinology follow-up is necessary to monitor for hormone deficiency and to look for signs of precocious puberty.

- **Polydactyly** (extra fingers and/or toes). In PHS the extra digits typically arise between the second to fifth digits or at the outside edge of the fifth digit (called central and post-axial polydactyly respectively). Occasionally there may be some webbing between the digits (called syndactyly). A referral to an appropriate surgical team may be necessary.

- **Dysplastic nails** (small or unusual growing nails).
- **Bifid Epiglottis**. The epiglottis is a leaflet of tissue at the back of the throat that helps prevent food going down the windpipe. In PHS there is a cleft (split or opening) in the epiglottis but in general it does not cause problems. If the affected person's history suggests aspiration of food or breathing problems then an ENT opinion should be sought. It is an important feature in making a diagnosis of PHS, as it appears to be rare in other conditions.
- **Imperforate Anus**. This means the back passage has not opened during development and results in a newborn baby being unable to pass stool. It requires surgery soon after birth.

Other features may include congenital heart defects, renal and genitourinary abnormalities and seizures. A small number of children will have learning difficulties. The long-term outcome for affected individuals depends on the presence or absence of life-threatening malformations (such as the presence of hormone deficiencies) but, if mildly affected, is good.

Inheritance patterns and prenatal diagnosis
Inheritance patterns
Pallister-Hall syndrome is caused by an alteration or fault in the GLI3 gene that is on chromosome 7. Usually this fault has arisen at conception in the child but occasionally it is inherited from one parent (who may have mild features of the condition). It is important that families are referred to a clinical geneticist who can accurately assess and counsel the family on the diagnosis, inheritance pattern, recurrence risk and the possibility of prenatal diagnosis in future pregnancies.
Prenatal diagnosis
This may be possible and the advise of a clinical geneticist should be sought.

Medical text written January 2006 by Dr E McCann, Specialist Registrar in Genetics, Royal Liverpool Children's Hospital, Liverpool, UK.

Further online resources
Medical texts in *The Contact a Family Directory* are designed to give a short, clear description of specific conditions and rare disorders. More extensive information on this condition can be found on a range of reliable, validated websites. Further information on these resources can be found in our **Medical Information on the Internet** article on page 21.

Support
A support group for Pallister-Hall syndrome has not yet been, established in the UK. However, a one-to-one linking system between parents who have children with Pallister-Hall syndrome is offered within Contact a Family. This service has been formulated and adapted to provide a confidential and sensitive service aimed to meet individual needs.

A number of organisations provide information and support services about conditions which may be associated with Pallister-Hall syndrome. There are links to these organisations in the medical text.

PALLISTER-KILLIAN SYNDROME

Background

Pallister-Killian syndrome (PKS) is a very rare chromosomal condition. A chromosome is a thread-like structure (divided into a short arm and a long arm) which is present in the nucleus of all body cells. The chromosomes carry the genes which are the instructions about how to make a new baby from a sperm and an egg. Usually individuals have twenty-three pairs of chromosomes (forty-six chromosomes in each cell). Individuals with PKS have an extra chromosome made up of material from the twelfth pair of chromosomes in some cells. This means there are forty-seven chromosomes in these cells rather than forty-six. The extra chromosome comprises two short arms of chromosome 12 (often referred to as isochromosome 12p). Because the affected person has extra genes, this causes the distinct features associated with PKS. The extra isochromosome 12 is not present in all body cells but only in part of them, with the other cells having a normal chromosome number. The condition is therefore described as a mosaic. It makes the diagnosis of PKS frequently difficult as the extra isochromosome is usually not present in blood cells. The extent to which an individual is affected by PKS depends in part upon the proportion of cells containing the isochromosome 12p throughout the body.

PKS affects both males and females equally. The condition is present at birth and the oldest known individuals with PKS are in their forties.

What are the symptoms?

The major symptoms of PKS include a characteristic facial appearance, learning difficulties (see entry), seizures (see entry, epilepsy), loss of muscle tone (see entry, hypotonia) and streaks of skin in which there is no colour (hypopigmentation) or darker skin colour than normal (hyperpigmentation) anywhere on the body. Individuals may show some or all of these features and, in addition, may be differently affected in the severity of their symptoms.

Typically individuals with PKS have a high forehead, sparse hair on the temple region of the scalp and eyebrows, an abnormally wide space between the eyes, a fold of skin over the inner corner of the eyes and a flat nose.

At birth infants with PKS are profoundly hypotonic (floppy) and this may persist into later life. Between the ages of five to ten years, children may have stiffness of joints (contractures). Children are almost always developmentally delayed with learning difficulties and minimal speech. Seizures may occur during infancy. Difficulties with vision (see entry, Vision Disorders in Childhood) and hearing (see entry, deafness) may also occur. Affected individuals usually have to go to special schools and may not be able to live independently as adults.

A number of other features may be associated with PKS including congenital heart defects (see entry), gastro-oesophageal reflux (see entry, Gut Motility Disorders), cataracts (see entry) and extra nipples. Diaphragmatic problems may occur in newborn babies with PKS, and in these cases babies may die shortly after birth, although some cases can be treated with operations. PKS is rare, and therefore it is not easily diagnosed.

Inheritance patterns and prenatal diagnosis

Inheritance patterns

PKS occurs sporadically. In other words, no other family member, brother and sister, is usually affected.

Prenatal diagnosis

PKS is sometimes suggested by ultrasound examination if major malformations are present or by examination of chorionic villus sampling (CVS) or amniotic fluid.

Medical text written September 2002 by Contact a Family. Approved July 2002 by Professor R Hennekam. **Last updated July 2007 by, Professor R Hennekam , Professor in Clinical Genetics and Dysmorphology, Institute of Child Health, London, UK.**

Further online resources

Medical texts in *The Contact a Family Directory* are designed to give a short, clear description of specific conditions and rare disorders. More extensive information on this condition can be found on a range of reliable, validated websites. Further information on these resources can be found in our **Medical Information on the Internet** article on page 21.

Support

Support and advice for Pallister-Killian syndrome is available from Unique, the Rare Chromosome Support Group (see entry, Chromosome Disorders).

PANCREATITIS

Background

The pancreas is a gland situated deep in the abdomen, lying behind the stomach, that secretes digestive juices into the duodenum (the first part of the intestine) and this helps with the break down of food into the small molecules that can be absorbed by the body's digestive system. It also secretes insulin into the bloodstream to keep the concentration of glucose in the blood at the right level (endocrine function).

When the pancreas becomes inflamed, its own enzymes are released into the blood, as well as within the organ itself. Although the highly active enzymes are usually contained in protected ductal areas, in the inflamed pancreas they start to 'digest' the pancreas itself causing further inflammation.

What are the symptoms?

Almost all people with acute pancreatitis suffer very severe mid and upper abdominal pain, frequently radiating straight through to the back. Vomiting is common, and often early signs of shock are seen. Large amounts of fluid may pour into the abdominal cavity which, when combined with the vomiting and an inability to drink fluids as normal, leave the circulation with inadequate volumes to maintain a normal blood pressure. Ultimately, shock and death may occur. The intensely tender abdomen may mimic that seen in many other conditions, and requires careful differentiation from surgically treatable diseases; surgery in the presence of pancreatitis is very dangerous.

Recurrent attacks of acute pancreatitis are referred to as chronic pancreatitis.

What are the causes?

There are a number of possible causes of pancreatitis including alcohol abuse, biliary stone disease and the effects of a range of medications and infections.

How is it treated?

Treatment is aimed at replacing large amounts of body fluid by vein. The pancreas and digestive system in general should be 'shut down' to minimize enzyme production through the use of a stomach tube and/or regular antacids to neutralize acid production. Large doses of injected narcotic pain relievers may be necessary.

In a minority of patients, infection may set in from bacteria in the intestinal tract, requiring massive antibiotic treatment, which is not always successful. Still others develop severe bleeding from the raw and inflamed pancreas, or develop a highly aggressive pus-forming pancreatic involvement. With these complications, up to ninety per cent of patients may die.

Inheritance patterns and prenatal diagnosis

Inheritance patterns

This is poorly understood. There are several types of pancreatitis that run in families (familial or hereditary pancreatitis) but these are not common. Some types begin in early childhood and can be very difficult to diagnose. Much work is being done at present on discovering patterns of inheritance. In the UK, this work is co-ordinated by EUROPAC at Alder Hey Children's Hospital, Liverpool.

Prenatal diagnosis

Not applicable.

Medical text last updated April 2002 by Professor M Larvin, Professor of Surgery, University of Nottingham, Derby, UK.

Further online resources

Medical texts in *The Contact a Family Directory* are designed to give a short, clear description of specific conditions and rare disorders. More extensive information on this condition can be found on a range of reliable, validated websites. Further information on these resources can be found in our **Medical Information on the Internet** article on page 21.

Support

Pancreatitis Supporters Network

PO Box 8938, Birmingham B13 9FW

Tel/Fax: 0121 449 0667 (Minicom available by prior arrangement)

e-mail: psn@pancreatitis.org.uk   Web: http://www.pancreatitis.org.uk

The Network is a National Registered Charity No. 1027443, established in 1997. It offers support to affected people and their families. It publishes a bi-annual newsletter, has a wide range of information and offers free loans of ENM devices, details on request. It also has access to a list of all the pancreatitis specialists in the UK. The Network has over 350 members and responds to over 1,000 enquiries a year.

Group details last confirmed February 2008.

PARKINSON'S DISEASE

Background

Parkinson's disease is a progressive, neurological disorder, which is treated mainly with drug therapy although physiotherapy, occupational therapy and speech therapy have important contributions. It can affect all activities of a person's life, including talking, walking, swallowing, and writing.

Approximately one hundred and twenty thousand people in the UK have Parkinson's, 1 in 500 of the general population. This increases to 1 in 100 over the age of sixty-five and 1 in 50 over the age of eighty. Ten thousand people are diagnosed each year. Most people are diagnosed over the age of sixty, but it is estimated that 1 in 20 are under forty when diagnosed.

What are the symptoms?

Each person with Parkinson's is different, and the ability to perform movements may differ from one day to the next. Early symptoms could be mild but as the condition advances, more and more symptoms are experienced. Parkinson's has a dramatic effect on a person's quality of life. It can affect everything they do, from getting out of bed in the morning to hugging and kissing a partner, or even being able to smile at them.

What are the causes?

It occurs because Parkinson's affects a part of the brain known as the substantia nigra which plays a vital role in the control of movements. The substantia nigra has nerve cells (neurones) which produce a chemical called dopamine. In Parkinson's, these cells undergo progressive degeneration leading to progressive reduction of available dopamine. Dopamine is a chemical messenger that plays an important role in enabling people to initiate and perform smooth co-ordinated movements.

It is not known why the cells that produce dopamine die. Once eighty per cent of these cells have been destroyed the symptoms of Parkinson's will occur. Symptoms include shaking, muscle stiffness, and slowness of initiating and movement. There is no known cure.

How is it treated?

Drug treatment is aimed at restoring the imbalance in neurotransmission (the way messages are passed between different parts of the brain) caused by the lack of Dopamine. Dopamine interacts with various other neurotransmitters and manipulating these chemicals can limit the symptoms. Various approaches are used. Drugs which reduce the amount of another neurotransmitter called acetyl choline can produce mild relief of symptoms. The most effective treatment is directed at increasing the amount of dopamine available by various means. These include: using drugs such as Co-caryldopa

(Sinemet®), Co-benyldopa (Madopar®) which increase the dopamine in the brain; using drugs such as Entacapone, Tolcapone, Selegeline and Rasagiline which interfere with the disposal of dopamine and thereby increase the levels of dopamine; and using drugs such as Ropinirole, Cabergoline and Pramipexole which mimic dopamine and "fool" the brain into thinking they are Dopamine (called dopamine agonists).

These drugs have varying degrees of efficacy and they all have side effects. If they are prescribed wisely under the supervision of a specialist, they can significantly ameliorate the symptoms of Parkinson's and give many years of satisfactory life.

Parkinson's people will need drugs for life and it is very important that this should be managed properly as long term use of drugs could lead to problems such as increasing side effects, erratic control and unpredictable variations in efficacy. These need to be anticipated and carefully managed.

Much more work is needed to help improve the treatment offered to people with Parkinson's.

Young Onset Parkinson's disease

Although the majority of people diagnosed with Parkinson's will be aged over 60; it is estimated that 1 in 7 people diagnosed will be aged under fifty at diagnosis. One in twenty people will be aged under forty at diagnosis. Medically a person is usually said to have young onset Parkinson's disease when the symptoms develop after the age of twenty-one and before the age of forty. Theories about the nature of young onset Parkinson's vary. The general medical opinion suggests that young onset Parkinson's disease is idiopathic Parkinson's disease occurring at a younger age, although some doctors have suggested it may be a different but related condition.

Clinically most people with young onset Parkinson's disease present with classic symptoms of the condition, such as rigidity, slowness of movement and the characteristic resting tremor. No two people with young-onset Parkinson's will be exactly the same and the presentation and rate of progression of the condition will vary considerably from person to person.

As Parkinson's is often wrongly identified as being a condition affecting only older people, younger people with Parkinson's have often found it difficult to get an accurate diagnosis because of their age.

Generally younger people respond well to the drugs, such as levodopa, used to treat Parkinson's. However, a large proportion of people with young onset Parkinson's disease may develop side-effects much earlier on in the course of the treatment.

People with young onset Parkinson's will have to live with the condition for thirty to forty years. Decisions about treatment options need to take into account the person's current level of ability and quality of life, as well as personal circumstances and needs. It is important that young people with Parkinson's are under the care of a neurologist or other specialist doctor with a special interest in Parkinson's.

Psychological and behavioural characteristics
Psychological, emotional and social aspects

Where diagnoses of Parkinson's will probably have the most impact on a younger person with Parkinson's and their family is with regard to the psychological, emotional and social effects they experience.

As the condition occurs at an earlier age, the effect on a younger person's life and that of their family can be profound. Diagnosis often comes at a time when many young people are still leading a very active life, perhaps developing a chosen career and raising a family.

The period after diagnosis can often be a particularly difficult time. There can be many different and conflicting emotions. Many people feel devastated. Some feel relief that a name has been given to the problems they have, particularly if they have had trouble getting a diagnosis. Others try to cope by trying to deny what is happening. Others hide it or have trouble telling their families or friends. Many people feel angry or ask 'Why me?' Many people also feel anxious and depressed.

Communication difficulties, loss of self-esteem and confidence can have a marked affect on the person's relationships and social life. There can be a tendency to withdraw from social activities and relationships with family and friends may be affected. Some people experience problems with the emotional and sexual relationship with their partner. Many young people are also raising children and are concerned about the effect that the Parkinson's will have on their children.

Practical matters such as employment and finance are often also of greater concern to younger people. These include staying in work, paying mortgages, insurance and benefits.

Medical text written October 2000 by the Parkinson's Disease Society. Approved October 2000 by the Parkinson's Disease Society Medical Advisory Board: Chair, Professor A Williams, Professor of Neurology, Queen Elizabeth Hospital, Birmingham, UK. **Last updated June 2005 by the Parkinson's Disease Society. Approved June 2005 by the Parkinson's Disease Society Medical Advisory Board: Chair, Dr. Mahendra Gonsalkorale, Consultant Physician and Clinical Director, Hope Hospital, Salford, UK.**

Further online resources

Medical texts in *The Contact a Family Directory* are designed to give a short, clear description of specific conditions and rare disorders. More extensive information on this condition can be found on a range of reliable, validated websites. Further information on these resources can be found in our **Medical Information on the Internet** article on page 21.

Support

Parkinson's Disease Society of the UK

215 Vauxhall Bridge Road, London SW1V 1EJ
Tel: 0808 800 0303 Helpline (Mon-Fri, 9.30am-9pm, Sat 9.30am-5.30pm)
Tel: 020 7963 9380 Text phone
Tel: 020 7931 8080   Fax: 020 7233 9908   e-mail: enquiries@parkinsons.org.uk
Web: http://www.parkinsons.org.uk
The Society is a National Registered Charity No. 258197, established in 1969. It aims to achieve the conquest of Parkinson's disease, and the alleviation of the suffering and distress it causes, through effective research, education, welfare and communication. It offers support and advice for people with Parkinson's, their carers and families. It gives advice to health and social care professionals on models of good practice, including residential care and short breaks. It has a network of local Parkinson's Disease Society branches. It publishes a quarterly magazine and has a wide range of information available, details on request. The Society has around 28,000 members.
Group details last updated September 2007.

YPN – Younger Parkinsons Network

c/o Parkinson's Disease Society, contact details as above
YPN is a branch of the Parkinson's Disease Society UK. It aims to support and represent the needs of younger people with Parkinson's disease who are likely to have different needs from older people. Support groups exist in many areas of the UK and there are around 510 members.
Group details last updated July 2006.

Direct services for adults with Parkinson's disease are also provided by the National Institute of Conductive Education (see Foundation for Conductive Education, under separate entry, Cerebral Palsy)

PAROXYSMAL EXTREME PAIN DISORDER

Paroxysmal extreme pain disorder: Familial rectal pain

Background

Paroxysmal extreme pain disorder is a rare disorder of abnormal pain sensation which presents in the first year of life with episodes of severe rectal pain following bowel movements which is often accompanied by Reflex Anoxic Seizures (see entry). Eventually there is a colour change down one half of the body; this may also be horizontally from the waist down. Older patients are also affected by painful eye and jaw crises.

What are the symptoms?

The condition is hallmarked by the four different types of episode/crises which are outlined below and patients may have any or all of them.

Birth episode

Affected babies are born red and stiff. This abates within minutes and is presumably secondary to 'the pain of birth'. No apnoeas (cessation of breathing) or bradycardias (heart beat slowness) are noted at the time of birth.

Rectal episode

The episode which defines the phenotype is the rectal or lower body episode. Defecation is almost always the sole trigger in infants and children. From birth until about eight years of age these children have paroxysms (episodes) of pain following defecation. They often become restless for a few hours prior to opening their bowels. After opening their bowels they experience a severe burning pain which starts in the anus, ascends up the rectum and spreads all over their bodies but is especially severe in the abdominal area. This pain is often accompanied by apnoea and bradycardia resembling Reflex Anoxic Seizures which lasts up to several minutes. EEG recordings during an episode show no seizure activity. Following the Reflex Anoxic Seizures there is the classical flushing as described above.

Although children eventually outgrow defecation induced rectal episodes, affected adults fear defecating in case an episode is triggered. Adults experience similar attacks albeit rarely. Triggers include unexpected falls, fights, sexual activity and vivid dreams but not defecation.

Ocular crisis

These are the most frequent of the crises and occur in adults and children. They are mostly paroxysmal in nature (sudden attacks); however, if provoked, a change in temperature and a cold wind are the commonest triggers. Some individuals have up to twenty a day. They describe the pain as if someone is poking red hot needles into the back of one eye. This lasts for up to thirty seconds and resolves spontaneously. After this the eye waters, the pupil dilates and there is flushing on that side of the face.

Mandibular/facial crisis

Typically these occur in older children and adults and are often triggered by the first mouthful of food at a meal. Yawning is also a common trigger. Patients may experience a burning pain over the jaw area on one side of the face. It may spread round the back of the neck, and up to the ipsilateral eye (on the same side). In these instances there is an overlap with the ocular crisis. Once the pain abates the skin over the jaw area flushes and the nostril on the same side runs.

How is it diagnosed?

Diagnosis is based on a careful history, a normal examination and normal EEG (electroencephalogram), ECG (electrocardiogram)and nerve conduction studies.

How is it treated?

In children, it has been important to manage the inevitable constipation that ensues from stool withholding secondary to fear of defecation. The episodes themselves respond to medication useful in the management of chronic neuropathic pain disorders - namely anticonvulsants. Carbamazepine is the most effective of these.

Inheritance patterns and prenatal diagnosis

Inheritance patterns

Autosomal dominant. Mutations in the sodium channel gene SCN9A cause paroxysmal extreme pain disorder in several families.

Prenatal diagnosis

In a particular family where the mutation is known it is possible to offer prenatal diagnosis.

Medical text written November 2002 by Dr C Fertleman. **Last updated February 2007 by Dr C Fertleman, Honorary Senior Lecturer, Royal Free and University College London Medical School, London, UK.**

Further online resources

Medical texts in *The Contact a Family Directory* are designed to give a short, clear description of specific conditions and rare disorders. More extensive information on this condition can be found on a range of reliable, validated websites. Further information on these resources can be found in our **Medical Information on the Internet** article on page 21.

Support

There is no support group for Paroxysmal extreme pain disorder. Cross referrals to other entries in The Contact a Family Directory are intended to provide relevant support for these particular features of the disorder. Organisations identified in these entries do not provide support specifically for Paroxysmal extreme pain disorder. Families can use Contact a Family's Freephone Helpline for advice, information and, where possible, links to other families. Contact a Family's web-based linking service Making Contact.org can be accessed at http://www.makingcontact.org

---

"Young disabled people had similar aspirations to their non-disabled peers. Most wanted to leave the parental home and most did not regard their first house as a home for life." A study, produced by the Joseph Rowntree Foundation and published in 2003, exploring the housing aspirations and experiences of thirty young disabled people in Scotland who had a physical or sensory impairment or a learning difficulty.

PATAU SYNDROME

Trisomy 13: 13+ syndrome; Patau syndrome

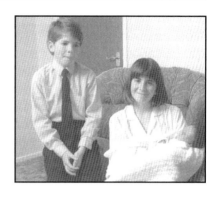

Background

Patau syndrome is a severe chromosomal abnormality in which the child has an extra chromosome 13. This is usually present in every cell.

Chromosome are rod-like structures present in the nucleus of all body cells, with the exception of the red blood cells. They are made up of several thousand genes which store genetic information. Normally humans have 23 pairs of chromosomes, the unfertilised ova and each sperm carrying a set of 23 chromosomes. On fertilisation the chromosomes combine to give a total of 46 (23 pairs). A normal female has an XX pair and a normal male an XY pair.

What are the symptoms?

Patau syndrome is characterised by low birth weight, heart defects, structural eye defects, cleft lip and/or palate, meningomyelocele (a spinal defect), omphalocele (abdominal defect), abnormal genitalia, low set ears, abnormal palmar crease patterns, scalp defects, extra digits and overlapping of fingers over thumb. Between 80 per cent and 90 per cent of babies do not survive infancy and in those that do survive learning disability (see entry) is present.

What are the causes?

When children have the mosaic form some cells carry the extra 13 chromosome while others have the normal chromosome pair. The extent and severity of the condition depends upon the ratio of normal to abnormal cells and is very difficult to predict if this finding is made before birth by a test such as chorionic villus sampling or amniocentesis. Generally, children with mosaic Patau syndrome are less severely affected than those with the full syndrome, which is caused by the presence of an additional chromosome 13 in every cell.

Other chromosome 13 defects are partial trisomy 13 where an unbalanced translocation or ring formation occurs. In an unbalanced translocation a chromosome or part of a chromosome is absent from its pair and exchanges position with a chromosome from another pair. The results of such translocations are extremely variable depending upon the other chromosome involved. Even where the chromosome involved is the same, individual cases may present with very different problems.

Inheritance patterns and prenatal diagnosis

Inheritance patterns

Most cases represent isolated events within a family. However a balanced translocation in a parent can give rise to an unbalanced translocation in a child. When parents have had one child with full trisomy 13, the risk that a future child will be affected is approximately 1 in 200. If Patau syndrome has been caused by an unbalanced translocation or any other unusual rearrangement, then it is very important that parents seek professional guidance from a clinical geneticist to determine if there is a significant risk of recurrence in a future pregnancy.

Prenatal diagnosis

Chorionic villus sampling at ten to twelve weeks or amniocentesis at sixteen weeks. Parents who have had a baby with trisomy 13 are usually offered a test such as chorionic villus sampling or amniocentesis in all future pregnancies even though the risk of recurrence is relatively low (1 in 200). Alternatively, non-invasive screening based on nuchal translucency and a maternal blood test may be offered.

Medical text written November 1991 by Contact a Family. Approved November 1991 by Professor M Patton, Professor of Medical Genetics, St Georges Hospital Medical School, London, UK and Dr J E Wraith, Consultant Paediatrician, Royal Manchester Children's Hospital, Manchester, UK. **Last updated December 2005 by Professor I Young, Department of Clinical Genetics, Leicester Royal Infirmary, Leicester, UK.**

Support

SOFT UK, St. Jude, Dixton Road, Monmouth NP25 3PP
Tel: 0121 351 3122 (24 Hour Helpline)   e-mail: enquiries@soft.org.uk
Web: http://www.soft.org.uk
The Group is a National Registered Charity No. 1002918, established in 1990. It offers support and information to enable informed choices. It also offers support and contact with other families where possible together with bereavement support and prenatal befrienders. It encourages research into causes, cures, new medical procedures and breakthroughs in care and support. It publishes a biannual newsletter and has information available, details on request. The Group has over 500 families in membership.
Group details last confirmed February 2007.

PATHOLOGICAL DEMAND AVOIDANCE SYNDROME

Pathological Demand Avoidance syndrome: PDA

Background

PDA is a pervasive developmental disorder related to, but significantly different from, autism and Asperger syndrome (see entry, Autism Spectrum disorders including Asperger syndrome). First identified as a separate syndrome at the University of Nottingham, research has continued at the Early Years Diagnostic Centre, which now holds a database of more than one

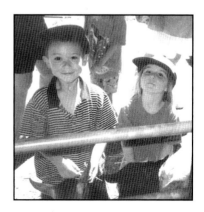

hundred and fifty children and adults. These children would previously have been diagnosed as having 'non-typical autism/asperger' or 'pervasive developmental disorder not otherwise specified'; but it is important to diagnose them separately since they do not respond well to the educational and treatment methods that are helpful with autistic and Asperger children, and since appropriate guidelines for education and handling are now available from the Early Years Diagnostic Centre.

- Passive early history in first year: ignores toys, often delayed milestones, 'just watches.' This passivity becomes active resistance to the ordinary demands on small children; a few actively resist from the start;

- Continues to resist and avoid normal demands to a pathological extent; seems to feel under intolerable pressure from these, does everything on own terms. This is not a 'difficult phase' but continues into adulthood (so far as follow-up research has yet shown). As language develops, strategies of avoidance are essentially socially manipulative: this is an important diagnostic feature. If frustrated in avoidance, major outbursts occur, often violent, apparently panic attacks;

- Surface sociability, but apparent lack of social identity, pride or shame. Seems sociable, but doesn't identify with other children, and shocks them by complete lack of normal boundaries. No sense of responsibility, seems very naughty, but parents and others recognise as confused. Praise and punishment ineffective;

- Lability of mood, impulsive, led by need to control situations. Many seem constantly on the edge of violence or loud excitability. May apologise but re-offend at once, or totally deny the obvious. Rules and routine do not help; better with variety and novelty;

- Comfortable in role-play and pretending: some appear to lose touch with reality. May take over roles as coping strategy; parents often confused as to 'who s/he really is.' May behave as teacher to control other children, or as baby or disabled person to avoid demands; often more animated when pretending than in real life. Interest in fantasy persists in adulthood;
- Early language delay, perhaps result of passivity: good degree of catch-up, often sudden. Eye contact often over-strong, and facial expression over vivacious. Speech content usually odd or bizarre;
- Obsessive behaviour. Much of child's behaviour carried out in obsessive way, especially demand avoidance and role play. This results in underachievement. Some target other people obsessionally, either harassing or showing overpowering liking;
- Neurological involvement. Soft neurological signs: clumsiness, awkwardness; many never crawled. Some absences, fits or episodic dyscontrol. Most show barely controlled excitability and impulsivity. Research currently in progress on PDA combined with epilepsy.

Fifty per cent of children with PDA are girls; this compares with about twenty per cent girls in autism and less than ten per cent girls in Asperger syndrome, both clearly significantly different from PDA figures.

What are the causes?

As in all pervasive developmental disorders, the underlying cause of PDA is believed to be organic brain dysfunction with genetic factors.

How is it diagnosed?

A provisional diagnosis is possible before the age of four, but diagnosis is more difficult than in autism because the child usually shows more social interest, more normal language development and better imaginative play by four or five than autistic children do.

Inheritance patterns and prenatal diagnosis

Inheritance patterns

It seems likely that genetic factors are similar to those in autism, but refer to inheritance of a pervasive developmental disorder rather than PDA specifically: thus perhaps six per cent of children with PDA are known to have a sibling with either PDA or Autism/Asperger. Preliminary research is currently underway.

Prenatal diagnosis

None at present.

Medical text last update October 2001 by Professor Elizabeth Newson, Consultant in Developmental Psychology, Early Years Diagnostic Centre, Nottingham, UK.

Contact a Family Helpline 0808 808 3555

Support

PDA Contact Group
c/o Contact a Family, 209-211 City Road, London EC1V 1JN
Tel: 0808 808 355 Freephone Helpline Textphone: 0808 808 3556
Tel: 020 7608 8700 Admin Tel: 0114 2589670 (evenings only, after 8.30pm)
e-mail: margaret.duncan@pdacontact.org.uk Web: http://www.pdacontact.org.uk
The PDA Group is a small parent support group, established in 1997. It offers listening ear support and a web based international eGroup for families and professionals. The group is in touch with over 60 families and a similar number of professionals.
Group details last updated November 2007.

Contact a Family was established in the London Borough of Wandsworth in early 1974 and became a registered charity in 1979.

PELIZAEUS-MERZBACHER DISEASE

Background

Pelizaeus-Merzbacher is a neurological disorder involving myelin where there is a loss of the white matter in the brain which affects the central nervous system

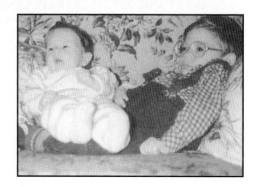

What are the symptoms?

Features of the disorder are flickering of the eyes (nystagmus), laboured breathing (stridor), spasticity and cognitive delay. The age of onset and progression of the disorder is very variable.

What are the causes?

The disorder is usually caused by mutations in an important and abundant gene in myelin, proteolipid protein. In most cases the affected boys have an extra copy of the proteolipid protein (PLP) gene although the sequence of both copies is normal. In a minority of cases there is a mutation in the coding sequence of the PLP gene.

It is rare for a female with a mutation in the PLP gene to be affected and affected females with apparently similar clinical symptoms may have mutations in other, as yet unknown, genes.

Inheritance patterns and prenatal diagnosis

Inheritance patterns

It is often inherited in an X-linked fashion, i.e. boys are affected and their female relatives, who are not themselves affected, may be carriers. The gene duplication can be detected by cytogenetic and molecular analysis in Regional Genetics Centres where counselling is also available.

Prenatal diagnosis

Prenatal diagnosis is available and has been carried out in a number of cases.

Medical text written April 2002 by Professor S Malcolm, Head of the Department of Molecular Genetics, Institute of Child Health, London, UK.

Further online resources

Medical texts in *The Contact a Family Directory* are designed to give a short, clear description of specific conditions and rare disorders. More extensive information on this condition can be found on a range of reliable, validated websites. Further information on these resources can be found in our **Medical Information on the Internet** article on page 21.

Contact a Family Helpline 0808 808 3555

Support

Pelizaeus-Merzbacher Support Group
c/o Contact a Family, 209-211 City Road, London EC1V 1JN
Tel: 0808 808 3555 Freephone Helpline   Tel: 020 7608 8700 Office   Fax: 020 7608 8701
e-mail: pmdsupport@dsl.pipex.com
This is a small family support group offering support to families, newsletters and occasional events with a network of 50 families in touch.
Group details last updated August 2007.

As Pelizaeus-Merzbacher is a metabolic disease, support and advice are also available from Climb (see entry, Metabolic diseases).

"She was our baby. She was our first. To us, whether there was something wrong or not, she was still a baby. She still needed us, and so we just got on with it." Parent.

PEMPHIGUS VULGARIS

Background

Pemphigus vulgaris (PV) is a condition which causes blistering of the outer layer of the skin (epidermis) and mucosal membranes. It is a very rare condition and occurs almost exclusively in middle-aged or older people of all races and ethnic groups.

What are the symptoms?

PV causes the skin to separate easily and peel easily. For many individuals, PV usually begins with blistering in the mouth and throat (a sensation likened to that of a candle burning in the throat). This is followed by blistering or erosions of the skin, including the groin, underarm, face, scalp and chest areas. PV lesions may cover extensive portions of the body. In some affected people the lesions are relatively asymptomatic. However, in the healing stage following treatment, the lesions often crust over but they no longer itch or burn and leak fluid. In some people the skin lesions may itch and burn continuously and rupture which may leave red erosions of the skin surrounded by a crust and scaling. Affected areas usually heal without scarring, unless the lesions become infected. Blisters in the mouth may make it difficult to eat and drink, leading to problems with weight loss and dehydration.

What are the causes?

PV is one of a group of chronic, relapsing conditions in which the immune system produces antibodies against specific proteins in the skin and mucous membrane, leading to the inability of the skin cells to bind together. It is thought that PV may be triggered by a range of factors. Thus, a few cases of PV have occurred following reactions to medications, including penicillamine and captopril. Individuals are probably genetically predisposed to PV. Specific information about a gene change(s) will not, however, indicate the certainty with which an individual will become affected with PV in the future.

How is it diagnosed?

PV is very rare and this may lead to misdiagnosis of the condition. It is one of the three main types of pemphigus, the others are:

Pemphigus Foliaceus (PF) In pemphigus foliaceus, blisters and sores do not occur in the mouth. Crusted sores or fragile blisters usually first appear on the face and scalp and later involve the chest and back. The blisters are superficial and often itchy, but are not usually as painful as PV. In PF, disfiguring skin lesions can occur, but the mortality rate from the disease is much lower than in PV.

Paraneoplastic Pemphigus (PNP) PNP is the most serious form of pemphigus. It occurs most often in someone who has already been diagnosed with cancer (see entry). Fortunately, it is also the least common. Painful sores of the mouth, lips and oesophagus are almost always present; and skin lesions of different types occur. PNP can affect the lungs. In some cases, the diagnosis of the disease will prompt doctors to search for a hidden tumour. In some cases the tumour will be benign and the disease will improve if the tumour is surgically removed. It is important to know that this condition is rare and looks different than the other forms of pemphigus. The antibodies in the blood are also different and the difference can be determined by laboratory tests.

Diagnosis of these diseases is made by skin biopsy and immunopathology.

How is it treated?

There is no cure available for PV but in most cases available treatments are successful in reducing symptoms and preventing complications. PV is controlled with high dose steroids and immunosuppressive drugs. Response to medication varies from individual to individual. For some individuals, lesions may not heal for extended periods of time. The main risk from PV is life-threatening infection and complications, resulting from medication aimed at suppressing the immune system.

Inheritance patterns and prenatal diagnosis

Inheritance patterns

None detectable but familial cases occur very rarely.

Prenatal diagnosis

None available and not appropriate.

Medical text written September 2002 written by Contact a Family. Approved September 2002 by Professor M M Black, Consultant Dermatologist, St John's Institute of Dermatology, Guy's, King's and St. Thomas' School of Medicine, London, UK.

Support

Pemphigus Vulgaris Network

Flat C, 26 St Germans Road, London SE23 1RJ   Tel: 020 8690-6462 (8.30am - 10am; owing to lack of funding they are unable to return phone calls)
Web: http://www.pemphigus.org.uk
The Pemphigus Vulgaris Network is a small voluntary network offering support to affected individuals, a forum for affected persons and professionals, contact with others, where possible, and information on the disorder (please send SAE).
Group details last updated July 2007.

As Pemphigus conditions can give rise to pain in affected individuals, details of sources of information can be found in the Pain Management section on the Helpful Organisations pages.

PENDRED SYNDROME

Pendred syndrome: goiter-deafness syndrome: deafness with goiter

Background

Pendred syndrome (PS) was clinically recognized in 1896 by Vaughan Pendred. A century later, the gene for this condition was discovered by Coyle, Sheffield and colleagues.

PS is characterized by sensorineural (sense perception mediated by nerves) hearing loss, developmental abnormalities of the cochlear (part of the inner ear concerned with hearing and balance), and goiter (enlargement of the thyroid in the front of the neck). Individuals and families are affected differently by the severity of their symptoms; goiter is a particularly variable feature.

What are the symptoms?

The deafness associated with PS is caused by an improper development of the inner ear (otherwise known as labyrinth). Typically hearing loss is severe to profound, bilateral (both ears are involved) and congenital (present at birth) or at least before the child starts to talk. Rarely does hearing loss progress after speech has been acquired.

Not all individuals with PS develop goiter. Goiter is rarely present at birth and if it appears in the newborn period, then this may result in upper airway obstruction and respiratory distress. Goiter commonly develops in late puberty or adulthood but may develop in late childhood or early puberty. Goiter arises due to a defect in the making of thyroid hormone.

The abnormality of the inner ear associated with PS is evident on a CT (computer tomography) scan of the temporal bone in the skull. PS is associated with a distinctive malformation of the cochlear. This leads to balance problems in individuals.

Individuals with PS may have is an increased risk of thyroid cancer and learning difficulties may occur due to congenital thyroid defect.

Inheritance patterns and prenatal diagnosis

Inheritance patterns

PS is inherited as an autosomal recessive trait. The condition results from changes (or mutations) in the PDS gene on chromosome 7. The normal PDS gene makes a protein, called pendrin, which is found at significant levels in the thyroid gland only. The symptoms of PS are associated with changes in the PDS gene.

Most affected individuals have no family history of PS. However, when the altered gene for PS is detected in an individual, carrier testing for at-risk family members and prenatal testing for at-risk pregnancies is possible.

Prenatal diagnosis

Prenatal testing may be available for individuals with PS where the altered gene has been identified.

Medical text written May 2004 by Contact a Family. Approved May 2004 by Dr V Das, Consultant in Audiological Medicine, Manchester Royal Infirmary, Manchester, UK.

Further online resources

Medical texts in *The Contact a Family Directory* are designed to give a short, clear description of specific conditions and rare disorders. More extensive information on this condition can be found on a range of reliable, validated websites. Further information on these resources can be found in our **Medical Information on the Internet** article on page 21.

Support

A support group for Pendred syndrome is being formed. Details can be obtained from Contact a Family's Freephone Helpline. As Pendred syndrome causes deafness, information, support and advice are also available from a range of deafness organisations (see entry, Deafness).

PERIPHERAL NEUROPATHY

Background

Peripheral Neuropathy is not a specific disease but rather a manifestation of many conditions that cause damage to the peripheral nerves.

Peripheral Neuropathy is a generic phrase denoting functional disturbances and/or pathological changes in the peripheral nervous system. If the involvement is in one nerve it is commonly referred to as **mononeuropathy**, in several nerves, **mononeuritis multiplex** and if diffuse and bilateral, **polyneuropathy**.

What are the symptoms?

The symptoms of peripheral neuropathy tend to vary depending upon the location and types of nerves affected. In most people the problems seem to commence with numbness, pain and/or weakness. Common characteristics, depending on the type of neuropathy may include muscle weakness, neuropathic pain (including - numbness, sensory disturbance, pins & needles, burning sensations etc.), and paralysis.

How is it treated?

The treatment of Peripheral Neuropathy is dependent on diagnosing the underlying cause; therefore early recognition and intervention is paramount. If the neuropathy is diagnosed quickly then there is likely to be less damage to the nerves and obviously an increased chance that the neuropathy can be slowed down, halted or reversed.

Diabetic neuropathy. One of the most common known causes of Peripheral Neuropathy is diabetes mellitus. It is estimated that approximately ten per cent of diabetics develop neuropathic symptoms. In diabetes the development of neuropathy may be slowed down by close control of the underlying disorder.

Vitamin deficiency derived neuropathies. These may be corrected by supplementing the deficient vitamins, either orally or by injection.

Autoimmune and inflammatory neuropathies. These are normally treated by immunomodulating or immuno-suppressive medicines (e.g. corticosteroids). However, this is a very complex area of medicine and the treatment varies widely according to the underlying condition.

Toxic & drug induced neuropathies. These are treated by eliminating the poison or agent.

Inheritance patterns and prenatal diagnosis
Inheritance patterns

The underlying causes for some peripheral neuropathies are sometimes successfully determined; however in many cases the underlying cause remains undiagnosed and this is what is called cryptogenic or idiopathic.

Recent studies suggest that between a third and a half of all undiagnosed neuropathies eventually turn out to be hereditary type neuropathies not recognised because of the lack of information about relatives or because symptoms have not yet started in any family members. This clearly demonstrates the importance of early recognition, referral to an appropriate specialist, improved communication, greater awareness and further education amongst all parties.

Prenatal diagnosis

Not applicable

Medical text written February 2001 by Dr S Ellis, Consultant Neurologist, North Staffordshire Hospital, Stoke on Trent, UK. **Last reviewed June 2006 by Professor R A C Hughes, Professor of Neurology, King's College London School of Medicine, London, UK.**

Further online resources

Medical texts in *The Contact a Family Directory* are designed to give a short, clear description of specific conditions and rare disorders. More extensive information on this condition can be found on a range of reliable, validated websites. Further information on these resources can be found in our **Medical Information on the Internet** article on page 21.

Support
The Neuropathy Trust

PO Box 26, Nantwich CW5 5FP   Tel/Fax: 01270 611828
e-mail: admin@neurocentre.com   Web: http://www.neurocentre.com
The Trust is a National Registered Charity No. 1071228, established in 1998. It offers support and information to affected people, their carers and professional workers. It has a regional Local Contact Network and participates in national and international awareness, education, research and information exchanges. It publishes a journal 'RELAY' three times per year and has a wide range of information available, details on request. The Trust responds to the needs of the estimated two million people who are affected by Peripheral Neuropathies and Neuropathic Pain in the UK. The Trust also receives many overseas enquiries.
Group details last updated August 2007.

PERTHES DISEASE

Perthes disease: Calvé-Perthes disease; Legg-Calvé-Perthes disease; Coxa Plana; Osteochondritis of the upper femoral epiphysis

Background

This condition is a disease of the epiphysis (growing head) of the femur (thigh bone) at the hip joint. The cause of the condition is unknown. It occurs due to an interruption of the blood supply to the head of the femur, part, or all of which, softens and is deformed by weight bearing. A number of factors, both local and general, act together to result in the above which can result in deformation of the shape of the femur at maturity.

The age of onset of the condition is between two to 14 years of age and occurs mainly in boys rather than girls. Affected children are often a little shorter than average and their bone maturity a little delayed. There is no specific evidence of hormonal deficiencies.

What are the causes?

Environmental factors may play a role and there is some circumstantial evidence that parental smoking may be a contributory factor.

How is it treated?

The main principle of treatment is to attempt to preserve movement of the affected hip. This is usually achieved with a combination of conservative measures which can include rest, physiotherapy or anti-inflammatory medications. Another principle of treatment is to "contain" the head of the femur within the socket. Conservatively this can be achieved by the use of splints or braces. This can also be achieved surgically, altering the angle of the bones at the hip. Sometimes this is done to the upper femur and sometimes to the bone around the socket of the hip. Newer treatments are being tried and these can include distraction of the hip with an external frame.

The outcome in this condition is variable. Sometimes the shape of the hip remains excellent and at other times the hip can become flattened and movement reduced. The most important factor appears to be how much of the hip is affected by the loss of the blood supply. The more of the hip that is involved the worse the prognosis. Another major factor is how old the patient is at the onset of Perthes disease. The younger the patient the better, as the body has time to adapt and remodel with further growth. In those patients younger than five years there is often, but not always, a reasonable prognosis.

If the final shape of the femoral head is disturbed, movement of the hip may be reduced and the possibility of early degenerative changes (osteoarthritis) increase.

The other hip may be involved at a different time in childhood in up to 10% of patients.

Inheritance patterns and prenatal diagnosis

Inheritance patterns

In families with an affected child the risk of other children of other children developing the condition is slightly increased.

Prenatal diagnosis

Not applicable.

Medical text last updated September 2002 by Mr A Moulton, Consultant Orthopaedic Surgeon, Kingsmill Centre for Health Care Services NHS Trust, Sutton in Ashfield, UK and Professor R G Burwell, Emeritus Professor and former Hon. Consultant in Orthopaedics.

Support

Perthes Association

PO Box 773, Guildford GU1 1XN   Tel: 01483 306637   e-mail: info@perthes.org.uk
Web: http://www.perthes.org.uk

The Association is a National Registered Charity No. 326161, established in 1976. The Association also supports families of children with Multiple Epiphyseal Dysplasia (MED), Osgood Schlatter disease, Severs disease, Kohlers disease and Scheurmanns disease. It offers contact with local families of same age/sex/treatment where possible together with information and advice about management of the condition. A limited number of wheelchairs/buggies and hand propelled trikes are available for loan to members. It has information available, details on request. The Association has around 1,000 members and has helped over 8,000 families since it was founded.

Group details last updated September 2007.

PETERS ANOMALY/PETERS PLUS SYNDROME

Peters anomaly

Peters anomaly: Anterior Chamber Cleavage syndrome

Peters anomaly was first described in 1906 by a German Ophthalmologist, Dr Alfred Peters. The anomaly affects the eyes of people of both genders and from all ethnic groups. Peters anomaly is a developmental error of early pregnancy (10-16 weeks).

Normally, the cornea, which is the transparent 'window' of the eye, focuses light through the lens onto the retina (a light sensitive film at the back of the eye). Signals are then sent by the optic nerve to the brain for interpretation. The cornea, lens, retina and optic nerve need to work perfectly in harmony for clear vision.

In Peters anomaly the central part of the cornea is hazy and white. This may affect one or both eyes. The corneal opacity is the obvious feature that Dr Peters described but this is now known to be part of a spectrum of abnormal development of the front of the eye. The eye may be abnormal in other ways including the drainage angle of the eye which may be underdeveloped so there is a risk of glaucoma (see entry) and the lens of the eye may be cloudy (see entry, cataracts). The fellow eye may have a milder developmental anomaly or be more severely affected where only a rudimentary small eye has developed.

What are the symptoms?

A number of features will lead to the actual way the child is affected:

- If the centre area of the cornea is white or cloudy, the cornea will not allow the eye to obtain a clear picture of the world. Light enters the eye but, if both eyes are affected, the child will not be able to clearly see what an object is. They will just be aware that something is there and aware of colours.
- Peters anomaly can be associated with other eye problems that contribute further to reduced vision including glaucoma, nystagmus (see entry), microphthalmia, cataracts and retinal detachment.
- As the cloudy area usually affects the centre of the cornea, then even if the cornea is later grafted with a clear donor cornea the eye will be amblyopic (lazy eye). The area of the developing infant brain that responds to signals from the eyes needs to be given information of good quality about the world very early in life for normal eyesight to develop.

In one study, sixty per cent individuals with Peters anomaly of the eye had abnormalities of other organs, in particular the heart or central nervous system. Twenty per cent of cases had developmental delay. Some of the anomalies associated with Peters anomaly occur in a particular pattern and form a recognisable syndrome such as Peters Plus syndrome.

What are the causes?

Most cases occur sporadically with no other members of the family having an associated ocular abnormality, but it can be inherited. Peters anomaly is not a single disorder and can be the result of an error in one or more genes or possibly due to environmental influences on the developing eye. Errors (mutations) in several different genes including PAX6, PITX2, CYP1B1, and FOXC1 (Rieger syndrome gene) have been found in individuals with Peters anomaly.

How is it diagnosed?

A diagnosis of Peters anomaly will be made by examination by an ophthalmologist. Usually, the eye abnormality is detected soon after birth but there may be a delay before the correct diagnosis is made. The clouding of the front of the eye may spontaneously improve over the first few months but it is most important that the child is examined as soon as possible by an ophthalmologist. It is very rare for an ophthalmologist to require a baby to have a general anaesthetic to make a diagnosis but occasionally this may be necessary to make a thorough examination. It is difficult for both parents and specialists to predict how well the child will see. This will become more apparent as the child develops and interacts with their environment.

How is it treated?

In cases where Peters anomaly is bilateral (affecting both eyes), surgical intervention may be possible by way of a cornea transplant. However, the process is complicated and very difficult for a child to handle with constant hospital visits and daily eye drops. Great improvement in vision cannot be guaranteed. Other surgery such as an optical iridectomy (making a small window in the iris of the eye under a clear area of cornea) may be helpful in selected cases. Spectacles, with dark lens to help with sun glare, or contact lens can improve use and comfort of eyesight.

Inheritance patterns and prenatal diagnosis

Inheritance patterns

Peters anomaly can be inherited in autosomal dominant or autosomal recessive mode as well as occurring sporadically (with no other associated family members).

Prenatal diagnosis

In most cases there will be no prenatal diagnosis possible. However, in the minority where a gene defect can be identified, there may be a possibility.

Peters Plus syndrome

Peters Plus syndrome: Krause-Kivlin syndrome

Peters Plus syndrome is a rare disorder in which Peters anomaly is usually associated with short limb dwarfism and learning disability.

The cause of the syndrome is not known.

Features of Peters Plus syndrome associated with Peters anomaly may include:

- learning disability in over eighty per cent of cases;
- cleft lip and/or palate (see entry) in over forty per cent of cases;
- a short or broad head, thin upper lip with smooth philtrum;
- hydrocephalus (see entry);
- short hands with tapering or webbing of the fingers;
- heart anomalies (see entry, heart defects);
- cataracts;
- genitourinary abnormalities;
- hearing abnormality;
- hypotonia and lax joints.

Inheritance patterns
Autosomal recessive.

Prenatal diagnosis
As no gene defect has been identified in Peters Plus syndrome, molecular prenatal diagnosis is not yet possible. However, in some cases, dysmorphic features of the fetus can be detected by ultrasound by twenty weeks gestation.

Medical text written January 2006 by Contact a Family. Approved January 2006 by Miss Isabelle Russell-Eggitt FRCS FRCOphth, Consultant Ophthalmic Surgeon, Great Ormond Street Hospital, London, UK.

Further online resources

Medical texts in *The Contact a Family Directory* are designed to give a short, clear description of specific conditions and rare disorders. More extensive information on this condition can be found on a range of reliable, validated websites. Further information on these resources can be found in our **Medical Information on the Internet** article on page 21.

Support

There is no support group for Peters anomaly or Peters Plus syndrome. Cross referrals to other entries in The Contact a Family Directory are intended to provide relevant support for these particular features of the disorder. Organisations identified in these entries do not provide support specifically for Peters anomaly or Peters Plus syndrome. Families can use Contact a Family's Freephone Helpline for advice, information and, where possible, links to other families. Contact a Family's web-based linking service Making Contact.org can be accessed at http://www.makingcontact.org

PHENYLKETONURIA

Background

Phenylketonuria (PKU) is an inherited metabolic condition where there is a defect in phenylalanine hydroxylase. This enzyme normally converts the phenylalanine in the body into tyrosine. Where there is an enzyme block the phenylalanine accumulates in the body tissues and affects the normal development of the brain causing learning difficulties.

Phenylalanine is an essential amino acid in dietary protein. In phenylketonuria the body is unable to make phenylalanine into other amino acids. A small quantity is required to ensure normal growth. The diet of an affected child is carefully controlled so that only the small amounts of phenylalanine necessary for growth is given. With a phenylalanine-restricted diet PKU children develop normally. It is imperative that women with PKU should be on a low phenylalanine diet before or from early pregnancy to reduce the risk of fetal abnormality.

How is it diagnosed?

The heel prick test (Guthrie test) is now done on all newborn babies at six to ten days of age and can identify PKU at an early age.

Inheritance patterns and prenatal diagnosis

Inheritance patterns

Autosomal recessive. Genetic advice is available for families with the condition.

Prenatal diagnosis

May be made by genetic studies on chorionic villus samples in families already studied.

Medical text last updated January 2004 by Dr D C Davidson, Consultant Paediatrician, Alder Hey Children's Hospital, Liverpool, UK.

Further online resources

Medical texts in *The Contact a Family Directory* are designed to give a short, clear description of specific conditions and rare disorders. More extensive information on this condition can be found on a range of reliable, validated websites. Further information on these resources can be found in our **Medical Information on the Internet** article on page 21.

Support

National Society for Phenylketonuria (UK) Ltd
PO Box 26642, London N14 4ZF   Tel: 020 8364 3010 Helpline   Fax: 0845 004 8341
e-mail: info@nspku.org   Web: http://www.nspku.org
*The Society is a National Registered Charity No. 273670, established in 1973. It offers
support to families and individuals and linking where possible. It has several local support
groups. It publishes a quarterly newsletter and has a wide range of information available,
details on request. The Society has around 1,200 members (this represents 1,000 families
and 200 medical members).*
Group details last updated March 2007.

*As Phenylketonuria is a metabolic disease, support and advice are also available from
Climb (see entry, Metabolic diseases).*

"Having such a valuable resource as
the team at Contact a Family to draw
on means that charities such as ours
are able to develop quickly to meet the
challenging needs of our members.
They've been fantastic." Group leader.

PIERRE ROBIN SYNDROME

Pierre Robin syndrome: Robin Anomalad; Pierre Robin sequence

Background

The condition is rare. Estimates range from 1 in 8,000 to 30,000.

The only features of Pierre Robin are:

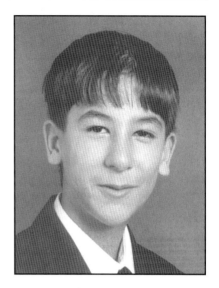

Micrognathia - a small lower jaw

Glossoptosis - a tendency for the base of the tongue to ball up and fall backwards into the throat causing obstruction and, therefore, breathing difficulties.

Cleft Palate - a cleft palate (see entry, Cleft Lip and/or Palate), or a high arched palate without a cleft may be present. The jaw bone continues to grow during childhood and will usually fully correct by adult life.

What are the symptoms?

All babies with Pierre Robin have some difficulties. Some have no problems with breathing and minor feeding difficulties. Others have moderate difficulties, which require them to be in hospital until breathing and feeding patterns can be established. A smaller group of babies has great difficulties in both areas, which can persist for several months. These babies require assistance with breathing which might include the use of a nasal prong or a tracheotomy.

If a cleft palate is present, repair can take place anytime between six to nineteen months of age, depending both on the severity of breathing difficulty and on the preference of the plastic surgeon. The operation normally takes about two hours, and a stay in hospital of several days is usually required.

What are the causes?

It is generally thought that this is a sequence of events arising from the jaw being compressed which then leads to the tongue being projected upwards and this in turn interferes with the closure of the palate. However, it is not fully known why the condition occurs. Maternal virus in the early stages of pregnancy and folic acid deficiency are other areas that have been researched, but nothing conclusive has been determined. Pierre Robin Sequence usually occurs in isolation, but it can also feature in other syndromes/conditions that have genetic links, such as Stickler syndrome (see entry). Careful investigation is therefore required by experienced doctors to ensure that a correct diagnosis and appropriate care is given to babies born with the Pierre Robin Sequence.

Inheritance patterns and prenatal diagnosis

Inheritance patterns

Most are sporadic events; some cases may be due to Stickler syndrome which is caused by a type II collagen defect and has autosomal dominant inheritance.

Prenatal diagnosis

Where a cleft palate is present it may be able to identify this using ultrasound scanning.

Medical text written June 2000 by Professor Michael Patton. **Last updated August 2005 by Professor Michael Patton, Professor of Medical Genetics, St George's Hospital Medical School, London, UK.**

Support

There is currently no effective support group covering Pierre Robin syndrome. This medical description is retained for information purposes. However, the Cleft, Lip and Palate Association (CLAPA) may be able to link families (see entry, Cleft Lip and/or Palate). Families can also use Contact a Family's Freephone Helpline for advice, information and, where possible, links to other families.

PITUITARY DISORDERS

Background

Pituitary disorders fall into the category of endocrine disease. The pituitary gland is situated beneath a part of the brain known as the hypothalamus. Together, the pituitary and hypothalamus regulate certain target organs and tissues, including the thyroid, adrenals and gonads, maintaining the body's delicate hormonal balance.

Although over forty thousand people in the UK are thought to suffer from pituitary disorders, many of the illnesses are little known outside specialist clinics.

What are the causes?

Disorders of the hypothalamic/pituitary axis are generally due to benign pituitary tumours (adenomas) which cause either over- or under- secretion of pituitary hormones, leading to specific illnesses. Some adenomas, described as 'non-functioning', do not produce hormones but can cause local pressure effects resulting in headache or compression of adjacent anatomical structures such as the optic chiasm, causing a visual field disturbance.

How is it diagnosed?

Diagnostic laboratory tests are available through a GP or an Endocrinologist. The type of test performed is usually indicated by the presenting signs and symptoms. Radiological imaging (MRI and CT scans) is also commonly used to detect the presence of pituitary adenomas.

Inheritance patterns and prenatal diagnosis

Inheritance patterns

Pituitary Disorders can affect any age group and with the exception of certain familial syndromes, are not generally thought to be hereditary in origin.

Prenatal diagnosis

None

Medical text last reviewed March 2004 by Dr J Webster, Consultant Physician and Endocrinologist, Northern General Hospital, Sheffield, UK.

Further online resources

Medical texts in *The Contact a Family Directory* are designed to give a short, clear description of specific conditions and rare disorders. More extensive information on this condition can be found on a range of reliable, validated websites. Further information on these resources can be found in our **Medical Information on the Internet** article on page 21.

Support

The Pituitary Foundation

PO Box 1944, Bristol BS99 2UB   Tel: 0845 450 0375 Helpline (Mon-Fri, 9am-5pm)
Fax: 0117 933 0910   e-mail: helpline@pituitary.org.uk   Web: http://www.pituitary.org.uk
*The Foundation is a National Registered Charity No. 1058968, established in 1994. It
offers the services of an endocrine nurse counsellor, a network of regional support groups,
covering England, Scotland, Wales, Northern Ireland and the Republic of Ireland, offering
support to members at a local level, and a network of telephone buddies. It publishes a
quarterly newsletter and has a wide range of information available, details on request.
Please send SAE.*
Group details last updated July 2007.

A donation of £10 a month with Gift Aid
would enable a disabled child to attend
one of our summer playschemes each
year. A donation form is on page 1088

POLAND SYNDROME

Background

This syndrome was described in 1841 by Sir Alfred Poland. It is a rare developmental disorder (1 in 20,000 live births) which is present at birth (congenital). It consists of underdevelopment of some or all of the chest, shoulder girdle and upper limb on one side of the body. It affects males more frequently than females.

What are the symptoms?

The severity and extent of abnormalities varies between individuals, and it is rare to have all the features of Poland syndrome. There is hypoplasia (underdevelopment) of the ribs and chest wall. The most common abnormality of the shoulder girdle and chest wall is absence of part of the chest muscle (pectoralis major) which makes the anterior (front) fold of the armpit. In girls, this may be associated with undergrowth or complete absence of a breast, and a small or absent nipple and areola (the areola is the pink or brown circle around the nipple). There may also be absence (agenesis) or hypoplasia of other chest muscles (including pectoralis minor).

The affected arm may be underdeveloped. Abnormalities of the hand vary from a mild change in skin crease patterns to complete absence of some fingers. In some cases the skin, and sometimes bone, has not separated during development and is still joined together (Syndactyly). Short fingers can also occur (Brachydactyly).

What are the causes?

The cause of Poland syndrome is thought to be due to a temporary alteration in blood flow in the developing shoulder girdle and upper limb during pregnancy, at approximately seven weeks. Individuals affected by Poland syndrome have a normal life expectancy and intelligence is within the normal range.

Inheritance patterns and prenatal diagnosis

Inheritance patterns

In most individuals, Poland syndrome occurs sporadically as a result of an error in development in the womb. There is no increased risk of recurrence for the affected family when neither parent has Poland syndrome. There may be a genetic component in a minority of families, and genetic counselling is suggested in such cases. Poland syndrome may occur as part of the Möbius syndrome.

Prenatal diagnosis

When the limb and chest abnormalities are severe, ultrasound scanning may identify the syndrome before birth.

Medical text written July 2003 by Contact a Family. Approved July 2003 by Mr R Dunn, Specialist Registrar in Plastic Surgery, St James's University Hospital, Leeds, UK.

Support

Poland Syndrome Support Group (UK)

c/o Contact a Family, 209-211 City Road, London EC1V 1JN   Tel: 01283 551113

e-mail: polandsyndrome@hotmail.com

The Group is a National Registered Charity No. 1100794, established in 2002. It offers support by letter, telephone and e-mail to individuals and families of affected children. It has information available, publishes a newsletter and has access to a medical adviser. The Group has a membership of over 100.

Group details last confirmed June 2007.

"My child has a behaviour problem and can find it hard to make friends because he can seem aggressive to others. But the first time I left him at the Contact a Family playscheme, they rang me twice during the day to tell me all was well. Now I know that they will help him mix in and keep him safe. It is very reassuring and provides a welcome break for me." Parent.

POLIOMYELITIS

Poliomyelitis: Polio: Infantile Paralysis

Background

Poliomyelitis is caused by an infection with the Poliomyelitis virus, which is an enterovirus. Polio can appear at any age, but used to be more common in young children hence the name Infantile Paralysis. It occurred in widespread epidemics particularly after the Second World War, but these have largely disappeared with the advent on effective immunization in 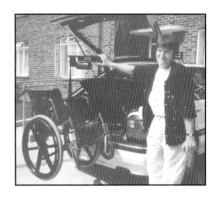 thelate 1950's. Occasional new cases do, however appear even in developed countries.

What are the symptoms?

The majority of infections are characterized by a mild fever often with vomiting or diarrhoea. Weakness or complete paralysis of any of the skeletal muscles appears in a minority of subjects, but this may develop rapidly. After a few days or weeks the weakness begins to improve and may continue to do so for one to two years.

Post-Polio syndrome

It has recently been recognized that after an interval of at least thirty-five years after the acute infection a condition known as the Post-Polio syndrome may develop. This is due to dying back of the peripheral nerve fibres which were damaged, but regenerated after the acute illness. This causes weakness, pain and fatigue in muscles which were previously affected. The Post-Polio syndrome occurs in around fifty per cent of those who have had polio, but in eighty per cent of these it is either static or only slowly progressive. Specialist advice about how to adapt the lifestyle to minimize the risk of the progression of this syndrome is often effective. Respiratory support usually with a non-invasive ventilator system used at night may be needed if the respiratory (breathing) muscles are affected. The Post-Polio syndrome should be distinguished from similar symptoms which may be due to degenerative changes in the joints or soft tissues, peripheral nerve entrapment, or aging.

How is it treated?

In the most severely affected patients all the limb and trunk muscles as well as the breathing and swallowing muscles may be affected and treatment with mechanical respiratory support is required to maintain life. The most common long term effect is weakness of one or more limbs.

Inheritance patterns and prenatal diagnosis
Inheritance patterns
Not applicable
Prenatal diagnosis
Not applicable

Medical text last reviewed January 2004 by Dr J M Shneerson, Consultant Physician, Director of the Respiratory Support and Sleep Centre, Papworth Hospital, Cambridge, UK.

Further online resources
Medical texts in *The Contact a Family Directory* are designed to give a short, clear description of specific conditions and rare disorders. More extensive information on this condition can be found on a range of reliable, validated websites. Further information on these resources can be found in our **Medical Information on the Internet** article on page 21.

Support
British Polio Fellowship
Eagle Office Centre, The Runway, Ruislip HA4 6SE   Tel: 0800 0180586 Freephone
Fax: 020 8842 0555   e-mail: info@britishpolio.org.uk   Web: http://www.britishpolio.org.uk
The Fellowship is a National Registered Charity No. 1108335, established in 1939. It was the first organisation to be started by disabled people for disabled people. It offers support, including financial assistance, for affected persons, together with accessible holiday accommodation and advocacy on welfare benefits and post-polio syndrome. It has a national network of groups and branches. It publishes a newsletter 6 times a year. The Fellowship has approximately 8,000 members including a small number of affected children.
Group details last updated November 2007.

POLYCYSTIC KIDNEY DISEASE

Background

The kidneys (see entry, Kidney disease) are the body's blood filter system. They act as specialised organs that filter and purify the blood, ridding the body of excess water, salts and waste products. The filtered fluid is processed as it passes down through thin long tubes called the tubules, leaving only the excess water and waste to be eliminated from the body via the bladder, as urine.

Autosomal Dominant Polycystic Kidney disease (ADPKD)

At least 1 in 1,000 people have inherited Polycystic Kidney disease (PKD). The underlying fault in PKD is not confined to the kidneys, but they are the organs that show the most obvious changes. The kidney tubules in part expand into many balloon-like cysts containing filtered fluid. These cysts gradually increase in size and number, pressing on the surrounding kidney tissue, damaging it.

Cysts may also develop in the liver and pancreas. However, they usually cause relatively little trouble in these organs. The damage to the kidneys is progressive and affects their ability to maintain water and chemical balance, excrete waste products and control the blood pressure. The conditions almost always affect both kidneys equally.

Other than some loin discomfort and occasional pain most individuals with PKD have relatively few problems in the first twenty to thirty years of life. Symptoms of PKD include:

- High blood pressure which is an early and common complication of PKD;
- Passing blood in the urine (haematuria);
- Kidney stones;
- Infections in the kidney and/or urine;
- Difficulties in conserving water, salt and other chemicals in the body.

Complete kidney failure develops in forty to fifty per cent of affected individuals by the age of sixty years.

A rare complication of PKD is the development of weaknesses in the walls of the arteries that lie just under the brain and supply it with blood. This occurs in about ten per cent of PKD patients. These areas of weakness can form fragile, balloon-like pouches (aneurysms) that may press on surrounding nerves or actually rupture, causing a stroke. It is thought that this complication may run in families.

Inheritance patterns

Autosomal dominant.

Prenatal diagnosis

For adult polycystic kidney disease, two genes have been identified. These are PKD1 (eighty-five per cent of cases), and PKD2 (fifteen per cent of cases). Mutation analysis is not widely available, and testing is technically difficult. Prenatal diagnosis is possible using a technique known as 'linkage analysis', usually in specialised genetic centres. However, the clinical variability of ADPKD, even within families means that demand for prenatal diagnosis is low.

Autosomal Recessive Polycystic Kidney disease (ARPKD)

Autosomal Recessive Polycystic Kidney Disease (ARPKD) is an inherited kidney condition where children have enlarged kidneys with or without cysts, often with liver enlargement and high blood pressure. There is often progressive scaring of the bile ducts, which is called Congenital Hepatic Fibrosis (CHF). Almost all children with ARPKD are diagnosed during infancy or childhood, but the first signs of the disease are variable.

About half of infants with ARPKD die at birth or shortly thereafter, primarily as the result of underdeveloped lungs because the kidneys often reach quite a large size which prevents the lungs from growing normally. Survival is possible and the prognosis is much better for babies that survive the new born period. If supported, which often involves mechanical ventilation until babies are able to breath on their own, the five year survival rate may be as high as eighty to ninety-five per cent.

High blood pressure is a very common complication and is one factor thought to be important in the progression of the kidney disease, and subsequent kidney failure, which many of these children develop within a few months or years of life.

A small proportion of children with ARPKD do appear to be perfectly normal until later childhood or adolescence. This particular group primarily have liver involvement with enlarged livers and relatively small kidneys.

Inheritance patterns

Autosomal recessive. In ADPKD, the features of the condition when inherited by children only manifest themselves in adulthood.

Prenatal diagnosis

For ARPKD there is one gene, but mutation analysis is not widely available. Linkage analysis can be used for prenatal testing, usually in specialised centres.

Medical text written November 2003 by Dr A K Saggar, Consultant in Clinical Genetics and General Medicine, St George's Hospital Medical School, London, UK.

Further online resources

Medical texts in *The Contact a Family Directory* are designed to give a short, clear description of specific conditions and rare disorders. More extensive information on this condition can be found on a range of reliable, validated websites. Further information on these resources can be found in our **Medical Information on the Internet** article on page 21.

Support

The Polycystic Kidney Disease Charity
PO Box 141, Bishop Auckland DL14 6ZD   Tel: 01388 665004 (Mon-Fri, 7-9pm)
e-mail: support@pkdcharity.org.uk   Web: http://www.pkdcharity.org.uk
The PKD Charity is a national registered charity number 1085662. It offers information, a newsletter and linking where possible. It has over 300 members.
Group details last confirmed October 2007.

POLYCYSTIC OVARY SYNDROME

Polycystic Ovary syndrome: Polycystic Ovarian disease: PCOS: Stein-Leventhal syndrome

Background

Polycystic Ovary syndrome is a condition in which women with polycystic ovaries also have one or more additional symptoms. It was first 'discovered' in 1935 by Doctors Stein and Leventhal and for many years was known as the Stein-Leventhal syndrome. Polycystic ovaries are common affecting twenty to thirty per cent of women and PCOS affects about ten to fifteen per cent.

The ovaries are a pair of female reproductive organs that produce eggs and female sex hormones. In individuals affected by PCOS hormonal inbalances in the production of oestrogens, progesterones and androgens lead to the presence of many small cysts in the ovaries. The cysts, usually no bigger than 8 millimetres each, are egg-containing follicles that have not developed properly and are arranged just below the surface of the ovaries.

What are the symptoms?

The symptoms of PCOS can include:

- irregular periods, or a lack of periods altogether;
- irregular ovulation, or no ovulation at all;
- reduced fertility: difficulty in becoming pregnant, recurrent miscarriage;
- unwanted facial or body hair (hirsutism);
- oily skin, acne;
- thinning hair or hair loss from the scalp (alopecia);
- weight problems: being overweight, rapid weight gain, difficulty in losing weight;
- depression and mood changes.

What are the causes?

The effects of PCOS can vary with some women having mild symptoms and others having a wider range of the more severe symptoms. It is not yet fully understood what causes the hormonal imbalances in PCOS and it is possible that there are several causes which could explain why different women have such different symptoms.

How is it diagnosed?

PCOS is usually diagnosed using a combination of an ultrasound scan to check for polycystic ovaries and blood tests to detect hormone imbalances. Blood pressure levels are checked and in overweight individuals the blood sugar level is checked. On diagnosis, an individual is likely to be referred to a gynaecologist or an endocrinologist.

How is it treated?

As PCOS cannot currently be cured, treatment aims to manage the symptoms which can be successfully achieved without medical intervention through good nutrition, exercise, and adopting a generally healthy lifestyle. There are a number of methods to help women affected by PCOS who are having fertility problems. These should only be provided by a specialist centre that can monitor all of the above treatments in order to prevent the risks of multiple pregnancy and a condition called Ovarian Hyperstimulation syndrome. This is a particular risk for women with PCOS who may be very sensitive to the drugs used.

Inheritance patterns and prenatal diagnosis

Inheritance patterns

It is thought that there is a hereditary link, whereby some women inherit a greater chance of having PCOS, but whether or not these women actually develop the syndrome depends on a number of additional factors which may include diet and lifestyle.

Prenatal diagnosis

Not available.

Medical text written March 2004 by Contact a Family. Approved March 2004 by Mr Adam Balen, Consultant Obstetrician and Gynaecologist and Subspecialist in Reproductive Medicine and Surgery, Leeds General Infirmary, Leeds, UK.

Further online resources

Medical texts in *The Contact a Family Directory* are designed to give a short, clear description of specific conditions and rare disorders. More extensive information on this condition can be found on a range of reliable, validated websites. Further information on these resources can be found in our **Medical Information on the Internet** article on page 21.

Support

Verity

Unit AS20.01, The Aberdeen Centre, 22-24 Highbury Grove, London N5 2EA
Web: http://www.verity-pcos.org.uk
Verity is a National Registered Charity No. 1097599, established in 1997 to provide support for women with Polycystic Ovary Syndrome. It holds conferences with speakers on medicine, research, complementary health, nutrition and lifestyle information. Verity publishes a bi-annual newsletter, "In Touch", and a range of factsheets dealing with specific symptoms and ways of managing the syndrome. Please send a SAE for details or sign up as a member via the website. The website now includes discussion boards for additional support. Verity is managed entirely by part-time volunteers so please allow 4-6 weeks for receipt of information packs.
Group details last confirmed October 2007.

POMPE DISEASE

Pompe disease; Glycogen storage disease type II; α 1,4-glucosidase deficiency; Acid Maltase deficiency

Background

Pompe disease is a rare inherited metabolic disorder caused by the deficiency of an enzyme that removes excess glycogen from cells within the body. In this condition glycogen accumulates and causes damage, particularly to muscle.

What are the symptoms?

Within the first few months of life children with the most common form of this disorder become floppy, have an enlarged tongue and develop a weak heart muscle. The condition is usually fatal within the first eighteen months of life.

Milder forms of this disorder exist in which the heart is not affected and where symptoms develop later in childhood or in adult life.

How is it treated?

Enzyme replacement treatment is now available and early results of treatment look positive. Some individuals with the milder forms of the disorder have been helped by a diet high in protein.

Inheritance patterns and prenatal diagnosis

Inheritance patterns

Autosomal recessive.

Prenatal diagnosis

This is available.

Medical text written May 2000 by Dr J Walter, Consultant Paediatrician, Willink Biochemical Genetics Unit, Royal Manchester Children's Hospital, Manchester, UK. **Last updated May 2006 by Dr J E Wraith, Consultant Paediatrician, Willink Biochemical Genetics Unit, Royal Manchester Children's Hospital, Manchester, UK.**

Further online resources

Medical texts in *The Contact a Family Directory* are designed to give a short, clear description of specific conditions and rare disorders. More extensive information on this condition can be found on a range of reliable, validated websites. Further information on these resources can be found in our **Medical Information on the Internet** article on page 21.

Support

As Pompe disease is a Glycogen Storage disease, information and support is available from the Association for Glycogen Storage Diseases (UK) (see entry, Glycogen Storage diseases).

PORENCEPHALY

Porencephaly: Porencephalic Cyst

Background

This is a condition whereby there are isolated cavities within the cerebral hemisphere. They may or may not be single and there may be communication with ventricles and other subarachnoid space.

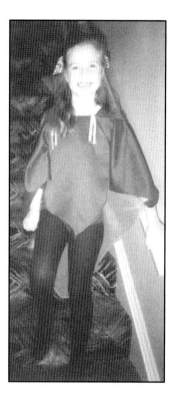

What are the causes?

The aetiology is thought to be that there is a localised destruction of brain tissue due to a number of causes but potentially including toxaemia, maternal injuries, infection, hypoxic injury or even intra-uterine intra-cerebral haemorrhage. Its overall incidence is unknown, aetiology must be multi-factorial and some series suggest that there is a risk that a patient with porencephaly has at two to four per cent chance of having a child with a neural tube defect.

How is it treated?

There is no specific treatment other than symptomatic for conditions that may have caused it . There may be seizures but most of the time these present as incidental findings.

Inheritance patterns and prenatal diagnosis

Inheritance patterns

None.

Prenatal diagnosis

None is available at present. Cysts can sometimes be detected by ultrasound scanning.

Medical text written February 2003 by Mr N Buxton, Consultant Paediatric Neurosurgeon, Alder Hey Children's Hospital, Liverpool, UK.

Further online resources

Medical texts in *The Contact a Family Directory* are designed to give a short, clear description of specific conditions and rare disorders. More extensive information on this condition can be found on a range of reliable, validated websites. Further information on these resources can be found in our **Medical Information on the Internet** article on page 21.

Support

There is no support group for Porencephaly. Families can use Contact a Family's Freephone Helpline for advice, information and, where possible, links to other families. Contact a Family's web-based linking service Making Contact.org can be accessed at http://www.makingcontact.org

Disabled children in England and Wales are missing out on leading ordinary lives because public services are failing to meet their real needs, according to a report launched in 2003 by the Audit Commission. If you feel your child is missing out, and would like information about support available call the Contact a Family Helpline.

PORPHYRIA

Background

The porphyrias are a group of diseases that have a strong hereditary basis that result from a partial failure of the formation of the pigment haem (a component of haemoglobin in the blood and of many proteins and tissue enzymes.) The porphyrias are principally 'over-production diseases' where the build-up of intermediate compounds that cannot be completely converted to haem leads to clinical manifestations. Many of the intermediate compounds or their derivatives, the porphyrins, interact with light and their accumulation leads to various types of light sensitivity of the skin. This is shown by pain, scarring, occasional blistering, altered pigmentation and fragility in the exposed skin. Over-production of some of the other intermediates including the early chemical compounds that form haem lead to the so-called neurovisceral manifestations of the porphyrias. These may or may not be accompanied by excess porphyrin formation and so light sensitivity may or may not occur as well.

What are the symptoms?

The neurovisceral manifestations constitute the 'acute' porphyric attack. Characteristically these attacks consist of clinical episodes of abdominal pain, limb pain, vomiting, constipation, seizures or rarely diarrhoea and the intermittent appearance of dark urine which may on occasion go brown, pink, port-wine or burgundy-coloured or occasionally the colour of blackcurrant juice - particularly on standing in the light. The urinary changes are by no means inevitable. Very severe attacks may be accompanied by paralysis of the muscles of breathing and swallowing as well as limb paralysis and severe neuralgic (nerve) pain.

Occasionally psychological manifestations and seizures occur during the course of acute attacks of porphyria which are accompanied by changes in the blood salt composition (low sodium - hyponatraemia) and high blood pressure (hypertension) that can be severe. Life-threatening acute porphyric attacks may occur.

Acute attacks are usually precipitated by starvation, injury (including surgery with or without anaesthetics), intercurrent illnesses and fevers and hormonal changes (particularly sex hormone changes in women). Alcohol and many hundreds of drugs prescribed for good medical reasons often trigger porphyric attacks and all doctors who prescribe for patients with porphyria need to refer carefully to recommended lists of drugs before prescribing safely. Such lists of drugs are present in standard medical reference books and an abbreviated version is available in the British National Formulary.

The consumption of alcohol as well as herbal remedies and simple pain-relieving drugs available across the counter may also precipitate acute porphyric attacks.

Individual Disorders

Cutaneous porphyrias

1.   **Porphyria cutanea tarda (PCT)**.
2.   **Congenital porphyria** (a severe disorder that usually presents in infancy and associated with extreme light-induced skin and tissue damage).
3.   **Erythropoietic protoporphyria** (very rarely complicated by liver disease and obstructed bile flow).
4.   **Variegate porphyria** (also accompanied by acute attacks).
5.   **Hereditary coproporphyria** (acute attacks also).

Skin (cutaneous porphyrias): sun screens and light avoidance; ß-carotene may benefit erythropoietic protoporphyria. Bone marrow transplantation may be indicated for severe congenital porphyria.

Acute Porphyrias

1.   **ALA dehydratase deficiency**.
2.   **Acute intermittent porphyria**.
3.   **Variegate porphyria** (skin reactions occur).
4.   **Hereditary coproporphyria** (skin reactions occur).

How is it treated?

Acute Porphyrias: Avoiding precipitating factors; maintaining regular meals and a balanced diet is important and wide dissemination of prohibited agents is recommended. Avoid alcohol, starvation and unwarranted physical or surgical strain. Acute attacks can also be managed by the use of increased calorie intake either by mouth or parenterally, scrupulous attention to fluid balance is required for the management of hyponatraemia (due to syndrome of inappropriate anti-diuretic hormone release); safe control of intercurrent hypertension. In severe attacks parenteral administration of haem arginate is recommended which suppresses the haem formation pathway and reduces the biochemical abnormalities that underpin the acute attack. Seizure control requires special consideration since many conventional anti-convulsants are porphyrinogenic.

Acute attacks should be rapidly evaluated and hospital admission considered for assessment. In the patient with progressive acute disease, ventilation and intensive care therapy followed by active rehabilitation may be needed for paralysis.

An updated list of safe drugs is available from the Welsh Medicines Information

Centre, University Hospital of Wales, Tel: 029 2074 3877

e-mail: welshmedicines.information@cardiffandvale.wales.nhs.uk

The Information Centre's list is available to patients and their health care professionals. Advice can be sought on the safe use of medicines for Porphyria.

See also MedicAlert, Web: http://www.medicalert.org.uk the Emergency Identification System for people with hidden medical conditions.

Inheritance patterns and prenatal diagnosis

Inheritance patterns

Most of the porphyrias are inherited as dominant complaints with variable features and expressivity. One cutaneous porphyria (PCT) has a relationship to iron overload and the HFE gene that determines iron storage in haemochromatosis (see entry, Haemochromatosis) is frequently observed in patients with this disorder. Viral infections, such as hepatitis C, B and HIV may incidentally also provoke expression of PCT in predisposed individuals. Erythropoietic protoporphyria, which is principally a cutaneous porphyria, shows di-allelic inheritance. ALA dehydratase deficiency, a very rare acute porphyria exacerbated by exposure to light, is inherited as a recessive condition. Congenital porphyria is inherited as a recessive disorder.

Prenatal diagnosis

In severe cases of porphyria, prenatal diagnosis may be undertaken in selected families at risk.

Medical text written February 2001 by Professor T Cox. **Last updated December 2005 by Professor T Cox, Professor of Medicine, University of Cambridge School of Clinical Medicine, Cambridge, UK.**

Further online resources

Medical texts in *The Contact a Family Directory* are designed to give a short, clear description of specific conditions and rare disorders. More extensive information on this condition can be found on a range of reliable, validated websites. Further information on these resources can be found in our **Medical Information on the Internet** article on page 21.

Support

British Porphyria Association

136 Devonshire Road, Durham DH1 2BL   Tel: 0191 3862146

e-mail: helpline@porphyria.org.uk   Web: http://www.porphyria.org.uk

The Association is a National Registered Charity No 1089609, established in 1999. It offers support to families and individuals affected by Porphyria. It publishes a newsletter twice a year and has information available, details on request. Please send SAE. The Association has over 250 individuals, family groups and interested medical professionals in membership.

Group details last confirmed February 2008.

POTTER SYNDROME

Background

Potter syndrome was first described by Dr Edith Potter in 1946. It is an extremely rare condition involving a total absence (agenesis) or severe malformation (dysgenesis or dysplasia) of both infant kidneys. The normal function of the kidneys is to filter waste products from the blood, eliminating them as urine. Absence of one kidney (unilateral) is compatible with life whereas absence of both kidneys (bilateral) is incompatible with life.

What are the symptoms?

The first signs of Potter syndrome are evident in the womb before one month of development. At this stage, the ureteral bud, which forms the kidneys, fails to develop and as a result little womb amniotic fluid is produced. The production of amniotic fluid during pregnancy is vital to the development of the baby's lungs. In Potter syndrome, the lungs of the baby do not develop fully because of a lack of amniotic fluid (also known as oligohydramnios). During pregnancy, babies may appear to have normal weight and size for their age because the placenta performs the filtering work of the kidneys. However, babies die either during birth or very shortly thereafter mainly because of underdevelopment of the lungs (pulmonary hypoplasia).

Another function of amniotic fluid is to 'cushion' the developing baby as it grows in the womb. If there is oligiohydramnios (reduced amounts of amniotic fluid), the baby may be compressed against the uterine wall. In addition, compression may cause growth retardation, a 'squashed' facial appearance and/or torso. Other features of Potter syndrome may include clubbing of the hands and feet and contractures (shortening of the muscle or of fibrous tissue).

How is it treated?

Potter syndrome occurs twice as frequently in males. There is no known treatment for Potters syndrome and it is always fatal.

Inheritance patterns and prenatal diagnosis

Inheritance patterns

In most cases, Potter syndrome occurs sporadically in which case it is not likely to happen again in the same family. In some cases, Potters syndrome may be inherited as an autosomal dominant trait. Potter syndrome is more common in infants born of a parent who has a kidney malformation, particularly unilateral renal agenesis (absence of one kidney). Genetic counselling is recommended after the birth of a baby with Potter syndrome.

Prenatal diagnosis

Potter syndrome may be identified on ultrasound examination in subsequent pregnancies. As Potter syndrome is frequently associated with clinically silent anomalies of the kidneys, ultrasound examination of the kidneys and urinary tract would be recommended for the parents in the first instance.

Medical text written August 2003 by Contact a Family. Approved August 2003 by the medical advisor in paediatric nephrology to the National Kidney Research Fund UK.

Further online resources

Medical texts in *The Contact a Family Directory* are designed to give a short, clear description of specific conditions and rare disorders. More extensive information on this condition can be found on a range of reliable, validated websites. Further information on these resources can be found in our **Medical Information on the Internet** article on page 21.

Support

Potter Syndrome Support Group
c/o Contact a Family, 209-211 City Road, London EC1V 1JN
Tel: 0808 808 3555 Freephone Helpline   Tel: 020 7608 8700 Admin   Fax: 020 7608 8701
e-mail: helpline@cafamily.org.uk
This is a small informal support group offering information about the condition and a listening ear.
Group details last confirmed September 2007.

PRADER-WILLI SYNDROME

Prader-Willi: cryptorchidism- shortness of stature- obesity- subnormal mentality; Prader-Willi Labhart

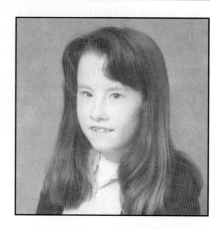

Background

Prader-Willi syndrome is characterised by two phases. At birth and in infancy, hypotonia (see entry), sleepiness and feeding difficulties are usually present. Thereafter, hypotonia becomes less, feeding difficulties stop and hyperphagia (over eating) begins, usually between the ages of two to four.

What are the symptoms?

Other features of Prader-Willi syndrome include:

- Hypogonadism (undescended testicles in males, reduced or lacking menstruation in females);
- mild to moderate intellectual disabilities;
- obesity (in the absence of food restrictions this appears to be universal).

The syndrome often includes:

- short stature;
- developmental delay in walking and speech;
- obsessive behaviour;
- strabismus (squint);
- almond-shaped eyes;
- very small hands and feet;
- skin picking;
- scoliosis;
- diabetes;
- behavioural problems.

Psychological and behavioural characteristics

Prader-Willi syndrome is characterised by a number of distinctive psychological and behavioural features. Motor and language development are significantly delayed, and there are difficulties with gross motor skills, co-ordination and balance, voice problems (primarily hypernasality) and multiple articulation errors resulting in reduced intelligibility. These speech production problems are likely to be due at least partly to the early hypotonia and also the facial abnormalities associated with the syndrome. Spoken language is often considerably poorer than comprehension of language. Overall, cognitive abilities range from moderate learning difficulties through borderline abilities to average abilities or better, but usually with multiple learning disabilities. Severe learning difficulties are not commonly found.

The children tend to have an unusual cognitive profile, with particular strengths in visual organisation and perception, and in academic achievement tasks such as reading and vocabulary. Unusual skill with jigsaw puzzles is often noted. In contrast, auditory information processing and sequential processing are relatively weak, and most individuals have specific difficulties with arithmetic, writing, visual and auditory short-term memory and auditory attention.

Behaviourally, children with Prader-Willi syndrome tend to be floppy, sleepy and passive in the first year. Their muscle tone begins to improve towards the end of the first year and they become more active and alert. They are often described as easy-going, friendly and affectionate; but behavioural difficulties become increasingly apparent and severe with age. These are often related to the insatiable desire to obtain food, which develops between one and four years of age and is accompanied by excessive or rapid weight gain, and is physically, emotionally and socially debilitating. Excessive intake of food may cause life-threatening obesity and often involves foraging for food, stealing and hoarding food. Research shows that people with Prader-Willi syndrome think a lot more about food than other people, and may continue to eat at a steady rate as long as food is available.

Dietary management is the corner stone of managing the obesity. Typically, carers have to limit access to food and take over total control of food intake. Behaviour modification methods which rely on reinforcement and self-monitoring as part of weight control and exercise programmes, are also required. Long-term maintenance of weight loss is difficult to achieve, and problems with weight control can become worse in adult life when, with increased independence, food is more readily available.

Outbursts of rage and aggression, stubbornness and belligerence, are common in affected individuals, beginning around age three to five, becoming more marked later in childhood and persisting into adulthood. Tantrums and aggression may be related to wanting access to food, but typically extend also to situations unrelated to food (for example in response to changes in routine), and may occur with little provocation. Between the episodes of difficult behaviour, individuals with Prader-Willi syndrome are usually described as being good natured, placid and co-operative. They may be over friendly, with impulsive chatter, but most are also reported to be immature and socially isolated. Compulsive/obsessive behaviours and anxiety-based difficulties, excessive worry, and self-injury by deliberately picking or scratching the skin, are further common difficulties. The above behaviours are believed to result from the combination of the physical aspects of the syndrome, the relentless hunger, and the psychosocial pressures of being obese, sexually immature and cognitively limited. Physical inactivity and passivity are commonly reported, as are various sleep disorders, for example frequent waking in the night due to breathing difficulties (sleep apnoea) and excessive daytime sleepiness. In addition, psychiatric symptoms such as hallucinations, paranoia, agitation, anxiety and depression have been described in some adolescents and adults with the syndrome.

Inheritance patterns and prenatal diagnosis
Inheritance patterns
Prader-Willi syndrome is due to the loss of expression of maternally imprinted (paternally expressed) genes on the chromosome 15 of paternal origin. In approximately seventy per cent of cases this is due to a deletion, 15q11-q13, and in most other cases both copies of chromosome 15 are maternal in origin (maternal disomy) with no paternal copy. Rarely, it will arise as a result of a chromosomal translocation or a mutation in the imprinting centre, which may be transmitted through unaffected carriers. Genetic testing is undertaken using DNA and parental blood samples may be requested to confirm maternal disomy.

Prenatal diagnosis
Usually none at present. There may be reduced fetal movement. In the very rare known carrier families, amniocentesis may be recommended.

Medical text written November 1991 by Contact a Family. Approved November 1991 by Professor M Patton, Professor of Medical Genetics, St Georges Hospital Medical School, London, UK and Dr J E Wraith, Consultant Paediatrician, Royal Manchester Children's Hospital, Manchester, UK. Psychological and behavioural characteristics written November 1998 by Dr O Udwin, Consultant Clinical Child Psychologist, Society for the Study of Behavioural Phenotypes. **Medical text last updated November 2004 and Psychological and behavioural characteristics last reviewed November 2004 by Dr J Whittington, Senior Research Associate, Section of Developmental Psychiatry, Department of Psychiatry, University of Cambridge, Cambridge, UK.**

Further online resources
Medical texts in The Contact a Family Directory are designed to give a short, clear description of specific conditions and rare disorders. More extensive information on this condition can be found on a range of reliable, validated websites. Further information on these resources can be found in our **Medical Information on the Internet** article on page 21.

Contact a Family Helpline 0808 808 3555

Support

Prader-Willi Syndrome Association (UK)
125a London Road, Derby DE1 2QQ   Tel: 01332 365676   Fax: 01332 360401
e-mail: admin@pwsa-uk.demon.co.uk   Web: http://www.pwsa.co.uk
The Association is a National Registered Charity No. 284583, established in 1981. It offers support, advice and contact with others. It organises multi-disciplinary training days for professional workers from health, education, social services and residential and community care. Local and regional group meetings are sometimes organised. It publishes a quarterly newsletter and has a wide range of information available, details on request. The Association has over 800 family members, over 200 adult members with Prader-Willi syndrome and over 800 professional members.
Group details last updated May 2007.

'Behavioural phenotype' is a medical term which describes behaviour associated with specific disorders. Contact a Family has produced a guide on understanding your child's behaviour – free from the helpline.

PRE-ECLAMPSIA

Pre-eclampsia: Pre-eclamptic Toxaemia (PET); EPH Gestosis

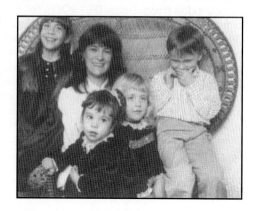

Background

Pre-eclampsia is a complication of the second half of pregnancy, labour or the first few days after delivery. New hypertension (raised blood pressure) and proteinuria (abnormal amounts of protein in the urine) are its main features. Oedema (swelling) is an inconsistent part of the condition. As its name suggests pre-eclampsia may precede eclampsia, when epileptic-like convulsions occur.

Pre-eclampsia affects about five per cent of first pregnancies. Eclampsia is much rarer. In very rare circumstances mothers can die. The babies can also suffer by growing poorly, needing early delivery or by dying before birth of asphyxia. About five per cent of women, having the condition in a first pregnancy, go on to have a recurrence in the next pregnancy.

What are the causes?

Susceptibility to pre-eclampsia is increased:

- in a first pregnancy;
- in a woman who has been pregnant before with a history of pre-eclampsia in any of those previous pregnancies;
- in twin or multiple pregnancies;
- in very overweight women;
- in women who suffer long term hypertension, kidney disease, diabetes or some other medical conditions.

Increasing age is also a factor.

There is no known single cause for pre-eclampsia. It is detected and managed by careful and thorough ante-natal care and induced delivery if needed. There is no certain way to prevent or predict the condition.

Inheritance patterns and prenatal diagnosis

Inheritance patterns

This is, in part, a familial condition with the daughters of eclamptic women being six to eight times more likely to have pre-eclampsia. However the majority of women who get pre-eclampsia cannot identify another member of their families who has similarly suffered.

Prenatal diagnosis

None. The condition is detected by repeated antenatal checks after twenty weeks of pregnancy.

Medical text written August 2001 by Professor C Redman. **Last updated December 2005 by Professor C Redman, Professor in Obstetric Medicine, Oxford University, Oxford, UK.**

Further online resources

Medical texts in *The Contact a Family Directory* are designed to give a short, clear description of specific conditions and rare disorders. More extensive information on this condition can be found on a range of reliable, validated websites. Further information on these resources can be found in our **Medical Information on the Internet** article on page 21.

Support

Pre-Eclampsia Society (PETS)

Rhianfa, Carmel, Caernarfon LL54 7RL   Tel/Fax: 01702 205088
e-mail: dawnjames@clara.co.uk e-mail: dawnrose@clara.co.uk
Web: http://www.pre-eclampsia-society.org.uk
The Society is a National Registered Charity No. 326206 established in 1981. It is a self help and support group also offering information about the latest research. It publishes a quarterly newsletter and has information available, details on request. Please send SAE. The Society has 1,000 members worldwide and an autonomous group in Germany with 300 members.
Group details last confirmed February 2008.

APEC (Action On Pre-Eclampsia)

84-88 Pinner Road, Harrow HA1 4HZ   Tel: 020 8863 3271
Tel: 020 8427 4217 Helpline (Mon - Fri, 10am - 1pm)   Fax: 020 8424 0653
e-mail: info@apec.org.uk   Web: http://www.apec.org.uk
APEC is a National Registered Charity No. 1013557, established in 1992. It offers support and advice for families and a befriending system. It publishes a twice yearly newsletter and has information available, details on request.
Group details last confirmed October 2007.

PREMATURE SEXUAL MATURATION

Background

Premature sexual maturation occurs when any signs of sexual development occur under the age of eight in a girl and nine in a boy. There are three common causes. Precocious puberty almost always requires careful medical investigation and treatment.

What are the symptoms?

Isolated premature thelarche is a condition of young girls which involves only breast development and usually resolves after a year or two and does not require treatment.

Premature adrenarche is a common condition between the ages of six and nine years of age with early activation of the adrenal glands involving pubic hair development, and increased rate of growth which only requires reassurance.

What are the causes?

There are many other very rare causes of premature sexual maturation and these require the involvement of a specialist. Many of these conditions involving the early secretion of sex hormones are associated with psychological and educational difficulties which may require extra support.

Inheritance patterns and prenatal diagnosis

Inheritance patterns

This is dependent on the underlying diagnosis

Prenatal diagnosis

None

Medical text written November 1995 by Dr R Stanhope. **Last reviewed July 2006 by Dr R Stanhope, Consultant Paediatric Endocrinologist, Great Ormond Street Hospital, London, UK.**

Support

The PSM Support Group works under the umbrella of the Child Growth Foundation, from which support and advice is available (see entry, Restricted Growth).

PREMATURITY and sick newborn

Background

Pre-term infants are those which are born before thirty-seven weeks gestation.

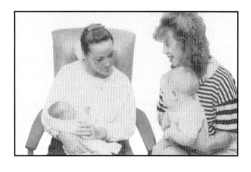

With modern perinatal and neonatal intensive care it is now possible for many babies born prematurely to survive. The majority of these babies do so without significant long term problems; a few babies are now surviving from as little as twenty-three weeks gestation although at these extreme gestations there is more concern about long term problems and their developmental outcomes.

Sick full term babies and babies requiring surgery are also treated in neonatal units. Some pre-term or sick newborns may remain in the baby unit for many weeks or even months. The birth of a premature or sick newborn baby can therefore be a traumatic event for a family. The prolonged stay in hospital which may be necessary can place tremendous strains on a family, disrupting the normal pattern of family life over an extended period. Many neonatal units will have family support strategies in place to help the families concerned.

Inheritance patterns and prenatal diagnosis

Inheritance patterns

Inapplicable in most cases. Some inherited disorders contribute to the premature birth of a baby.

Prenatal diagnosis

The likelihood of a premature birth may occasionally be predicted earlier in the pregnancy but generally, the cause of premature birth is often unclear. Pre-eclampsia (see entry) is an established reason for a baby needing to be delivered early; other factors contributing to premature births are smoking, acute or prolonged stress, poor diet, drug abuse and certain infections.

Medical text written November 1991 by Contact a Family. Approved November 1991 by Professor M Patton, Professor of Medical Genetics, St Georges Hospital Medical School, London, UK and Dr J E Wraith, Consultant Paediatrician, Royal Manchester Children's Hospital, Manchester, UK. **Last updated November 2004 by Dr R Rivers, Consultant Paediatrician, Special Care Baby Unit, St Mary's Hospital, London, UK.**

Support

BLISS – The Premature Baby Society

2nd & 3rd Floors, 9 Holyrood Street, London SE1 2EL   Tel: 0500 618140 Helpline (Mon-Fri, 10am-5pm)

Tel: 020 7378 1122   Fax: 020 7403 0673   e-mail: information@bliss.org.uk

Web: http://www.bliss.org.uk

BLISS is a National Registered charity No.1002973, established in 1979. BLISS exists to give everybody the best possible start to life. For information, advice and support, or to arrange to speak to another parent with a similar experience, call the BLISS Family Support Team Helpline.

Group details last updated September 2007.

"I wanted to thank you for listening to me when I telephoned. I was feeling quite low and isolated. I am now in contact with the local group of mothers you told me about and it has been wonderful." Parent.

PRIMARY CILIARY DYSKINESIA

Primary Ciliary Dyskinesia: PCD

Background

Primary ciliary dyskinesia is a relatively rare genetic condition. Several genes for the condition have been found, and more are being sought. The prevalence is almost certainly underestimated. Late diagnosis is common, as are mild cases picked up by screening siblings of an index case. Even given a prevalence of 1 in 15,000,

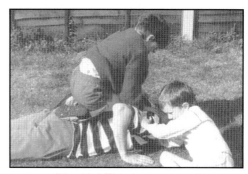

'No, No! This is supposed to be chest physiotherapy!'

there will be around seventy new cases born per year, and three thousand cases in the UK in total. The diagnosis has implications for many aspects of upper and lower respiratory tract disease, in particular the avoidance of inappropriate ear nose and throat (ENT) procedures and the assessment and treatment of deafness.

A diagnosis of PCD should be considered under a number of circumstances; no one feature is an absolute indication, and a combination of signs and symptoms may be more suggestive than one single indication on its own.

What are the symptoms?

At least half the PCD patients have symptoms when first born. These include unexplained tachypnoea (unusually rapid breathing) or neonatal pneumonia, rhinorrhea (runny nose), dextrocardia (heart positioned too far to the right) or complete mirror image arrangement with structurally normal heart; other heterotaxy (body structures arranged unusually); complex congenital heart disease, oesophageal atresia or other severe defects of oesophageal function (see entry, Tracheo-Oesophageal Fistula), biliary atresia (see Liver disease), hydrocephalus (see entry) and positive family history.

In the infant and older child, symptoms include 'asthma' that is atypical or not responsive to treatment, chronic particularly wet cough, sputum production in the older child who is able to expectorate, very severe gastro-oesophageal reflux; bronchiectasis; rhinosinusitis (inflammation of the nose and sinus) and chronic and severe secretory otitis media (ear infection).

In the adult, presentation is as in the older child, but also impaired female fertility including ectopic pregnancy and male infertility.

How is it diagnosed?

Diagnosis is first suspected by history and physical examination. Attention must be paid to the timing of onset of symptoms (particularly the onset at birth, which is highly suggestive of the diagnosis). Diagnostic tests are performed in three centrally funded units, at Leicester Royal Infirmary; Royal Brompton Hospital, London; and Southampton General Hospital. Testing includes measurement of the out put of a gas called nitric oxide from the nose (very low in people with PCD), and examination of structure and function of cilia from a nasal brushing.

How is it treated?

There is no cure for the condition. The aim is to prevent lung damage and bronchiectasis by chest physiotherapy, exercise and the aggressive use of antibiotic. Hearing problems usually improve by the teenage years, and tympoanostomy tubes should be avoided if possible.

Inheritance patterns and prenatal diagnosis

Inheritance patterns

PCD is mainly inherited as an autosomal recessive, but with other inheritance patterns possible.

Prenatal diagnosis

In a few patients, the responsible genes have been identified, opening up the possibility of antenatal testing in selected couples.

Medical text written February 2002 by Professor Andrew Bush. **Last Updated September 2007 by Professor Andrew Bush, Professor of Paediatric Respirology, Royal Brompton Hospital, London, UK.**

Further online resources

Medical texts in *The Contact a Family Directory* are designed to give a short, clear description of specific conditions and rare disorders. More extensive information on this condition can be found on a range of reliable, validated websites. Further information on these resources can be found in our **Medical Information on the Internet** article on page 21.

Support

PCD Family Support Group

15 Shuttleworth Grove, Wavendon Gate, Milton Keynes MK7 7RX   Tel: 01908 281635
e-mail: webcontact@pcdsupport.org.uk   Web: http://www.pcdsupport.org.uk
The Group is a National Registered Charity No. 1049931, established in 1990. It provides support to people with PCD and parents/families of affected children, and ensures that the condition is bought to the attention of the medical profession and public. The Group provides up-to-date information in the form of newsletters and via the web. The Group has over 200 members (affected children and adults).
Group details last confirmed September 2004.

PRIMARY IMMUNODEFICIENCIES

Background

Primary Immunodeficiencies are the result of defects in the immune system. Many distinct disorders have been discovered, most have a genetic base.

The most common primary immunodeficiency is Hypogammaglobulinaemia in which antibody production is deficient. This has several causes but prominent are **X- linked Agammaglobulinaemia (XLA)**, also known as Bruton's disease, and **Common Variable Immunodeficiency (CVID)**.

What are the symptoms?

Boys with XLA become unwell after their mother's antibody protection wears off at around six months old. CVID can occur at any age when an individual suddenly stops producing antibodies. The result of antibody deficiency is severe, recurrent and unusual infections with poor response to antibiotic treatment. These infections can cause permanent damage and may become life threatening without correct treatment.

How is it treated?

Hypogammaglobulinaemia cannot presently be cured but replacement antibody treatment is available and must be continued for life. The management of this treatment is specialised and should be in the hands of a clinical immunologist.

Certain primary immunodeficiencies such as **Severe Combined Immune Deficiency (SCID)** are so severe that careful protection of the patient from infection until they can be treated with early bone marrow or stem cell transplantation is essential. Gene replacement therapy is also considered for certain diseases but is in its infancy. Effective treatments are available for the various different primary immunodeficiencies and early referral to a clinical immunologist is essential in all cases.

Inheritance patterns and prenatal diagnosis

Inheritance patterns

X-linked inheritance is the commonest but some PID's are autosomal recessive.

Prenatal diagnosis

This is possible for some PID's. Expert genetic guidance should be sought.

Medical text written August 1996 by Dr T B Wallington. Last updated October 1999, Dr T B Wallington Consultant Immunologist, Southmead Hospital, Bristol UK. **Last reviewed February 2004 by Dr A Cant, Consultant Paediatric Immunologist, Newcastle General Hospital, UK and Dr M Helbert, Consultant Immunologist, St Mary's Hospital, Manchester, UK.**

Support

The Primary Immunodeficiency Association

Alliance House, 12 Caxton Street, London SW1H 0QS   Tel: 020 7976 7640
Tel: 0845 603 9158 Family After Hours Line (Mon - Thurs, 7pm - 10pm)
Fax: 020 7976 7641   e-mail: info@pia.org.uk   Web: http://www.pia.org.uk
*PiA is a national registered charity, number 1107233, and is the only patient support
charity in the UK representing the interests of those people suffering from serious inherited
disorders of the immune system. Genetically based, primary immunodeficiencies are
treatable, but as yet, not curable. The World Health Organisation recognises over 100 of
these conditions, ranging in severity from life limiting to life threatening. Some of the more
common conditions are listed in the index but please contact the PiA for further information
on conditions not mentioned. The Charity has over 3,500 patient and family members plus
a substantial number of medical, professional, pharmaceutical and corporate supporters.
PiA provides funding for important medical research into PID and actively campaigns
for greater awareness, improved diagnosis and treatment for PID patients. They provide
patient support and advice, including; an online discussion forum; After Hours Helpline;
patient days; young member activity holidays; and information and advice on social
and welfare benefits. PiA publishes a regular newsletter, Insight, and a wide range of
supporting literature, which is available on request.*
Group details last updated October 2007.

PRIMARY PULMONARY HYPERTENSION

Background

Hypertension is the medical term for an abnormally high blood pressure. Primary Pulmonary Hypertension (PPH) is a rare progressive disorder in which blood pressure in the lungs rises far above normal levels. PPH may affect individuals at any age, including new born babies and infants of either gender, and all races and ethnic origins. Most commonly, however, PPH affects women in their thirties and forties.

The UK National Specialist Commissioning Group includes a pulmonary hypertension service. Services are based at: the Papworth Hostpital, Cambridge; the Western Infirmary, Glasgow; the Hammersmith Hospital, London; the Freeman Hospital, Newcastle-upon-Tyne; and the Royal Hallamshire Hospital, Sheffield.

What are the symptoms?

The most common presenting symptom of PPH is breathlessness (dyspnea) and this is often associated with tiredness and lethargy. Dizziness and fainting spells (syncope) are also typical early symptoms. Individuals may experience chest pain, palpitation (a feeling of rapid heart beats in the chest) and a dry cough. The range and severity of symptoms varies between individuals and can occur at rest, whilst walking or during periods of mild exercise. In the more advanced stages, an individual is able to perform only minimal activity and has symptoms even when resting. In general, the more severe the symptoms, the more advanced the disease.

The symptoms of PPH are non-specific, in other words, they may be due to a number of other conditions. PPH is, therefore, difficult to diagnose at both early and later stages. In the later stages, PHH can be confused with other conditions affecting the heart and lungs. Because of this, individuals with PPH may experience a lengthy delay between the time they first experience symptoms to the time they receive a diagnosis.

What are the causes?

Primary pulmonary hypertension occurs when no cause is found. Pulmonary hypertension may be associated with other conditions such as severe sleep apnoea, emphysema, pulmonary emboli, some congenital heart defects, left heart failure and autoimmune disorders.

PPH involves both the heart and the lungs and starts in the lungs. Normally, oxygen-poor blood is pumped from the right ventricle, one of the pumping chambers of the heart, to the lungs via a blood vessel known as the pulmonary artery. When blood reaches the lungs, it collects oxygen and flows to the left ventricle, another pumping chamber of the heart. Oxygenated blood is pumped to the rest of the body through a blood vessel known as the aorta.

In an individual with PPH, the blood pressure in the pulmonary artery (the blood vessel which carries oxygen-poor blood from the heart to the lungs) is far higher than normal. The high blood pressure is a consequence of the disease of the blood vessels in the lungs. This causes a high resistance to blood flow. In order to maintain adequate blood flow through the lungs, the heart works harder to try to force blood through the lungs. This places a strain on the right ventricle of individuals with PPH. The overworked right ventricle expands in size but gradually loses its ability to pump enough blood to the lungs.

Inheritance patterns and prenatal diagnosis

Inheritance patterns

Changes in a gene (known as BMPR2) have been associated with familial pulmonary hypertension and a small number of cases of sporadic PPH. However, many carriers of this gene change do not develop PPH and so it has been suggested that an environmental trigger may be necessary. It is not clear what these environmental triggers are. Another gene (known as ALK1) has also been associated with pulmonary hypertension. There is still a considerable amount of research required to understand the genetics of this condition.

Prenatal diagnosis

None at present.

Medical text written April 2003 by Contact a Family. Approved April 2003 by Dr S Gibbs, Consultant Cardiologist, Hammersmith Hospital, London, UK.

Further online resources

Medical texts in *The Contact a Family Directory* are designed to give a short, clear description of specific conditions and rare disorders. More extensive information on this condition can be found on a range of reliable, validated websites. Further information on these resources can be found in our **Medical Information on the Internet** article on page 21.

Support

PHA-UK (Pulmonary Hypertension Association UK)
PO Box 2760, Lewes, East Sussex, BN8 4WA
Tel: 0800 389 8156 Helpline Tel: 01709 761450 General Fax: 01709 760265
e-mail: enquiries@pha-uk.com Web: http://www.pha-uk.com
The Association is a National Registered Charity No. 1120756, established in 2000. It offers support and information to families, carers and professionals. It holds an annual conference, regional meetings for families and professionals and an annual family weekend for affected children. The PHA-UK has a range of leaflets and videos and publishes a quarterly newsletter. The website provides information, a chat room and bulletin board and receives over 3,500 visitors a month.
Group details last updated February 2008.

PROGRESSIVE SUPRANUCLEAR PALSY

Progressive Supranuclear Palsy: PSP; Steele Richardson Olszewski syndrome

Background

PSP, otherwise known as Steele Richardson Olszewski syndrome after the three Canadian Doctors, who first described it in 1962 as a distinct disorder, is a neurodegenerative disease, which involves the progressive death of neurons, mainly in the basal ganglia and brainstem. In pathological examination of brain tissue, characteristic neurofibrillary tangles of a protein called tau distinguishes this disorder from other neurodegenerative disorders, particularly from Parkinson's disease (see entry) where lewy body deposits are a characteristic hallmark. However, in the early stages PSP can mimic Parkinson's disease and be misdiagnosed as such. The two disorders have historically been linked.

Average life expectancy is some seven years from onset, the last two often wheelchair-bound, with twenty-four hour care becoming necessary. The onset of PSP is mainly in the fifty to seventy age bracket, but patients as young as late thirties have been diagnosed. Recent studies indicate a prevalence of 5 in 100,000, which is nearly four times as many as earlier studies had indicated. Leading neurologists now assess there could be as many as five to ten thousand cases in the UK alone, many misdiagnosed or undiagnosed.

What are the symptoms?

PSP is a very individual disease and can present in different ways making diagnosis very difficult, particularly early in the disease. In the early stages, symptoms can include loss of balance and unexpected falls, often backwards, and difficulties with vision, particularly in upgaze and downgaze. Bright lights can be painful and the patient often presents with a characteristic 'Mona Lisa' type stare. Difficulty in walking, with a resulting broad-based unsteady shuffling gait can be observed in many cases. As the disease progresses, slurring of speech with a growly, guttural tone, together with increasing problems in swallowing can be noticed. These problems can also lead to loss of communication ability and the need for a gastrostomy for tube feeding. Other symptoms, may include dry eyes, stiff neck and incontinence.

How is it treated?

At present, there is no effective treatment and no cure for PSP, but with care, therapy and support, patients can live well into old age.

Inheritance patterns and prenatal diagnosis

Inheritance patterns

Although the cause is not yet known, there may well be a genetic component to PSP. This is currently being intensively researched. However, the probability of inheriting this disease is extremely low. There are only a handful of families across the world where siblings of a PSP patient can be shown to have the disease. This is similar to the patterns seen in Parkinson's disease and Alzheimer's, where there appears to be a small familial element, but the majority of cases are seen to be generic.

Prenatal diagnosis

Not applicable

Medical text written October 2000 by Professor A J Lees. **Last reviewed January 2005 by Professor A J Lees, Consultant Neurologist, The National Hospital for Neurology, London, UK and Director of Research, Reta Lila Weston Institute of Neurological Studies, London, UK and Chairman of the PSP Association Medical Advisory Panel.**

Further online resources

Medical texts in *The Contact a Family Directory* are designed to give a short, clear description of specific conditions and rare disorders. More extensive information on this condition can be found on a range of reliable, validated websites. Further information on these resources can be found in our **Medical Information on the Internet** article on page 21.

Support

The Progressive Supranuclear Palsy [PSP Europe] Association
PSP House, 167 Watling Street West, Towcester, Northamptonshire NN12 6BX
Tel: 01327 322 410
Fax: 01327 322 412   e-mail: psp@pspeur.org   Web: http://www.pspeur.org
The PSP Association is a National Registered Charity No. 1037087, established in 1994. It offers support to patients, their carers and their families across Europe. It has a nationwide network of local support groups and aims to raise awareness of the disease amongst relevant medical professionals, mainly in the UK. It also promotes worldwide research into the cause, effective treatment and eventual cure of PSP. It publishes three newsletters 'Bulletins' each year and has information available, details on request.
Group details last updated June 2007.

PROTEUS SYNDROME

Background

Proteus syndrome is a rare disorder first identified in 1979 but with cases described in the literature since 1856.

The clinical features of Proteus syndrome are overgrowth/enlargement of soft tissue and bone which can affect any area of the body but often involving the hands and/or the feet, the skull and sometimes the whole of one side of the body (hemihypertrophy) and blood vessel (vascular) abnormalities. Superficial warty birthmarks (epidermal naevi), soft deeper (subcutaneous) lumps, thickening of the skin on the soles and bony problems, in particular, of the skull, hand/feet and curvature of the spine may also be present.

The abnormalities seen in Proteus syndrome are present at birth but may become more apparent and develop with age. The clinical features described may not all be present in any one affected individual and the severity can vary widely. The nature of the varied complications of the disorder depend on the site and severity of the problem.

How is it treated?

Medical care requires a multidisciplinary approach covering orthopaedic, dermatological, genetic, surgical, dental, ophthalmological, radiological and psychological management.

Inheritance patterns and prenatal diagnosis

Inheritance patterns

The cause of Proteus syndrome is unknown

Prenatal diagnosis

None

Medical text written November 1998 by Dr J Harper. **Last reviewed October 2004 by Professor J Harper, Consultant in Paediatric Dermatology, Great Ormond Street Hospital, London, UK.**

Further online resources

Medical texts in *The Contact a Family Directory* are designed to give a short, clear description of specific conditions and rare disorders. More extensive information on this condition can be found on a range of reliable, validated websites. Further information on these resources can be found in our **Medical Information on the Internet** article on page 21.

Support

Proteus Family Network (UK)

31 Baswich Lane, Weeping Cross, Stafford ST17 0BH   Tel: 01785 254953

e-mail: info@proteus-uk.org   Web: http://www.proteus-uk.org

The Network is a National Registered Charity No. 1098608, established in 1997. It offers support by telephone and letter and linking families where possible. The Network has a Medical Advisory Board and supports research in the UK into Proteus syndrome It publishes a newsletter three times a year and has information available, details on request. Please send SAE. The Network is in touch with over 40 families in the UK and overseas. It can also provide support and information for families of those with associated conditions including Klippel-Trenaunay syndrome.

Group details last confirmed October 2006.

Proteus Syndrome Foundation (UK)

2 Watermill Close, Bexhill-on-Sea TN39 5EJ   Tel/Fax: 01424 736640 (evenings/weekends)

e-mail: tracy.whitewood_neal@virgin.net   Web: http://www.proteus-syndrome.org.uk

The Foundation is a National Registered Charity No. 1077796, established in 1997. It offers support to families by telephone, letter and e-mail and links families where possible. It has medical advisory panel, publishes a newsletter twice a year and has a library of medical articles available. The PSF UK also provides grants to families principally to improve the quality of life for affected children and their families. The Foundation is in touch with over 80 families in the UK and overseas. It has strong links with the PSF in the USA and supports families to attend research programmes and Family Conferences.

Group details last updated October 2007.

PRUNE BELLY SYNDROME

Prune Belly syndrome: Eagle Barrett syndrome

Background

Prune Belly syndrome is an extremely rare condition which, in most cases, affects males. It is characterised by a triad of distinctive features including weak or missing abdominal muscles, an abnormal expanded bladder and problems in the upper urinary tract which may include the bladder, ureters and kidneys and, in most males, bilateral cryptorchidism (failure of both testes to descend in the scrotum).

What are the symptoms?

Prune Belly syndrome affects indviduals to varying degrees. The prognosis may be serious and often life-threatening including in utero death, stillbirth or death within the first few weeks of life. Alternatively, the prognosis may involve a combination of congenital anomalies in infancy. For others, the outcome may be a near-normal life expectancy, with varying degrees of urinary tract pathology.

As the name implies, Prune Belly syndrome is characterised by an abdomen with a wrinkly or 'prune-like' appearance with multiple folds of skin. The cause of this is a blockage in a part of the unborn's urinary tract, resulting in other parts of the tract developing abnormally. The obstruction may occur in the urethra (the tube that drains urine from the bladder to the outside of the body for elimination). The effect of this is that the urine 'reverse flows', causing an expanded bladder. Fluid subsequently develops in the abdomen which stretches larger and larger. The fluid is reabsorbed before birth and when the infant is born, it has a sagging or wrinkled abdomen (thus the 'prune belly' name). Infants may have a range of severity from a complete absence of musculature to an abdomen of normal appearance. Infants may have difficulties in sitting upright.

The range of urinary tract anomalies varies widely in Prune Belly syndrome ranging from an inability to completely empty the bladder to a more serious impairment associated with the bladder, ureter and kidney. The urinary tract organs may be easy to feel through the abdominal area. A child may experience frequent urinary tract infections if an obstruction is present. Characteristic features of urinary tract anomalies in Prune Belly syndrome include dilation (abnormal widening) of the tubes that bring urine to the ureters (bladder), hydroureter (accumulation of urine in the ureters) and hydronephrosis (in the kidneys) and/or vesicoureteral reflux (backflow of urine from the bladder into the ureters). Ultrasound and x-rays may identify the type of urinary tract abnormalities present after birth.

In some affected males, the testes are present and are commonly small and intra-abdominal in location. In others, the testes in the scrotum are absent. Sperm are thought to be absent, and rarely neoplasia (malignant change) has been reported in the testes.

Complications associated with Prune Belly syndrome may include pulmonary hypoplasia (underdevelopment of the lungs), heart anomalies, gastrointestinal anomalies and musculoskeletal abnormalities. Girls may have defects in their external genitalia.

Inheritance patterns and prenatal diagnosis

Inheritance patterns
The exact cause of Prune Belly syndrome remains unknown.

Prenatal diagnosis
Prune Belly syndrome may be diagnosed by ultrasound examination from abnormal development of the bladder and urinary tract. Mothers carrying an unborn baby with Prune Belly syndrome may develop varying degrees of oligohydramnios (insufficient amniotic fluid) increasingly the liklihood of lung problems after birth.

Medical text written July 2004 by Contact a Family. Approved July 2004 by Mr D Wilcox, Consultant Paediatric Urologist, Great Ormond Street Hospital, London, UK.

Further online resources
Medical texts in *The Contact a Family Directory* are designed to give a short, clear description of specific conditions and rare disorders. More extensive information on this condition can be found on a range of reliable, validated websites. Further information on these resources can be found in our **Medical Information on the Internet** article on page 21.

Support
A support group for Prune Belly syndrome is currently being formed. Details can be obtained from Contact a Family's Freephone Helpline.

PSEUDOXANTHOMA ELASTICUM

Background

Pseudoxanthoma Elasticum (PXE) is a rare inherited disorder of connective tissue mainly affecting the skin and the eye. It is thought that PXE affects about 1 in 25,000 to 100,000 people. PXE is known in all ethnic groups but in a female-to-male ratio of 2 to 1. Although onset can be infancy up to old age, the average age of onset is in adolescence.

Connective tissue forms the supporting and connecting structures of the body. It is formed of collagen and elastin. In PXE the elastic fibres in the skin, the retina and the blood vessels degenerate and calcify.

What are the symptoms?

The main features of PXE include:

- Papules (small yellow-white raised areas) and laxity of the skin in flexures (folds) such as the neck and the arm pits. Although not painful, the altered appearance of the skin can cause upset.
- Visual impairment in over fifty per cent of people with PXE, caused by angioid streaks (tiny breaks in the elastin-filled tissue), bleeding and scarring of the retina. This can lead to loss of central vision and significant loss of sight.

Other features of PXE include:

- Possible heart attacks or stroke resulting from blood vessels being affected;
- Leg pain as blood cannot easily reach the muscles;
- Gastro-intestinal bleeding in some people.

What are the causes?

PXE is caused by mutations of the ABCC6 gene on chromosome 16.

How is it diagnosed?

Diagnosis of PXE is considered when the typical skin and eye features are found in an individual. The severity of the condition is very variable, even between members of the same family. A skin biopsy (examination of tissue) may be necessary to confirm the diagnosis.

How is it treated?

PXE cannot be cured. For the skin effects, camouflage can be used (see Procedures and Management section) and some people will undergo plastic surgery. Dietary and life style choices may lead to better outcomes.

People with the condition can be helped by effective management which can include:

- Regular eye examinations;
- Cardiovascular and gastrointestinal checks;
- Weight and blood pressure control – smoking avoidance may help;
- Use or avoidance of certain medications under doctor's guidance.

Inheritance patterns and prenatal diagnosis
Inheritance patterns
Autosomal recessive or, more rarely, autosomal dominant. Genetic counselling should be sought in families with an already affected member.
Prenatal diagnosis
This may be available for families in whom a PXE gene mutation has already been identified in an affected family member.

Medical text written December 2005 by Contact a Family. Approved December 2005 by Dr C Moss, Consultant Paediatric Dermatologist, Head of Dermatology Department, Birmingham Children's Hospital, Birmingham, UK and Mr S Kheterpal, Consultant Ophthalmic Surgeon, Prince Charles Eye Unit, King Edward VII Hospital, Windsor, UK.

Further online resources
Medical texts in *The Contact a Family Directory* are designed to give a short, clear description of specific conditions and rare disorders. More extensive information on this condition can be found on a range of reliable, validated websites. Further information on these resources can be found in our **Medical Information on the Internet** article on page 21.

Support
The PseudoXanthoma Elasticum Support Group – PiXiE
15 Mead Close, Marlow SL7 1HR   Tel: 01628 476687   e-mail: pxeeurope@aol.com
Web: http://www.pxe.org.uk
PiXiE is a National Registered Charity No. 1055465, established in 1984. It offers help and encouragement to people with PXE and aims to raise awareness of PXE to the medical community and the general public. It has information about the condition, publishes a newsletter and hold meetings for members. PiXiE has over 500 members.
Group details last confirmed February 2008.

PSORIASIS

Background

Psoriasis is a non-infectious disease affecting up to one person in twenty. The causes of Psoriasis are unknown. The majority of cases have minimal disease activity with scaling on elbows or knees. However, Psoriasis can present with red silvery scaly patches at any body site.

In Psoriasis the surface skin cells migrate rapidly through the surface layers of the skin causing a build up of scaly skin. Psoriasis can be triggered at injury sites, possible five to six weeks after the injury. In children it can also be triggered by streptococcal throat infections and present with a widespread pattern of small scaly patches known as guttate Psoriasis.

When no triggering factor can be found for causing Psoriasis there is a tendency amongst the medical profession to blame physical or emotional stress, but for the majority of individuals this is not relevant. A small proportion of people with Psoriasis will notice that when they go through a stressful patch their Psoriasis will flare, but for the majority of individuals stress has no aggravating contribution.

How is it treated?

Psoriasis can start at any age although it frequently first presents during adolescence or early adult life. The condition can wax and wain. With treatment it is possible to clear Psoriasis but the natural tendency is that of relapse at sometime in the future. Once cleared one person in five will probably not experience any relapse for five years while others may experience recurrence.

There are many treatments available for Psoriasis including ultra violet light in the form of sunshine (UVB) combined with the sensitizing drug, Psoralens. This needs to be monitored carefully due to the potential for ultra violet to damage the skin. This form of treatment is not, therefore, a first line treatment of choice.

Traditionally Psoriasis on the body is treated with tar containing preparations which in addition to helping treat the Psoriasis also have an anti-inflammatory effect on the skin with an anti-itching effect.

When it affects the scalp Psoriasis can be quite stubborn. In addition to regular shampooing and the application of steroid scalp applications, agents that lift off the dead skin cells may have to be used. These are based on salicylic acid and coconut oil and can be quite messy to use. When Psoriasis effects the face or the flexures (bends such as the armpits, groin or umbilicus) then a topical steroid cream may be indicated. Often this requires the short term use of a potent steroid and then weaning back onto a mild steroid to keep the Psoriasis under control.

With treatment it should be possible to control most patients' Psoriasis but it does require a commitment from the patient to use treatment on a regular basis.

The statement that Psoriasis cannot be cured is often misleading. When Psoriasis has been cleared it can never be predicted whether it is going to break out again in the future.

Inheritance patterns and prenatal diagnosis

Inheritance patterns

One third of individuals can identify an immediate relative within the family with Psoriasis and therefore it is thought that it is a genetically inherited disease, but no clear inheritance patterns have been determined. There is no genetic link to suggest that any of the offspring of a individual with severe Psoriasis will also be severely affected.

Prenatal diagnosis

None.

Medical text written June 2002 by Dr I S Foulds, Clinical Director in Dermatology, Birmingham Skin Centre, City Hospital, Birmingham, UK.

Further online resources

Medical texts in *The Contact a Family Directory* are designed to give a short, clear description of specific conditions and rare disorders. More extensive information on this condition can be found on a range of reliable, validated websites. Further information on these resources can be found in our **Medical Information on the Internet** article on page 21.

Support

The Psoriasis Association
Dick Coles House, 2 Queensbridge, Northampton NN4 7BF
Tel: 0845 676 0076 Helpline (Mon-Thu, 9.15am-4.45pm; Fri, 9.15am-4.15pm)
Tel: 01604 711129   Fax: 01604 792894   e-mail: mail@psoriasis-association.org.uk
Web: http://www.psoriasis-association.org.uk
The Association is a National Registered Charity No. 257414, established in 1968. It offers information to affected individuals, their families and health professionals. It has a small number of local support groups. It publishes a journal 4 times per year. The Association receives over 7,000 enquiries a year.
Group details last updated November 2007.

PSORIATIC ARTHROPATHY

Background

Psoriatic Arthropathy is a form of arthritis which accompanies the skin disorder psoriasis (see entry) and which is distinct from rheumatoid arthritis and can at times closely resemble it. It may be found in people with a family history of psoriasis even if they do not currently have any skin problems themselves. There is an increased likelihood of developing the arthritis if other members of the family with psoriasis have it too. There is more than one variety:

- **Peripheral type** Psoriatic Arthropathy which affects mostly the small joints of the hands and feet and is commonly associated with psoriatic changes in the nails;
- **Psoriatic spondylitis** in which the spine and sacroiliac joints are affected and which closely resembles ankylosing spondylitis. As in that condition the patient more often than not is of the B27 tissue type;
- A **mixed pattern** of spondylitis and arthritis of large or small joints, a combination in one individual of the two forms described above;
- A severe and fortunately rare form of psoriatic arthritis sometimes called **arthritis mutilans** because of the damage done to the joints and which affects large and small joints severely and leads to disability of varying degree.

Because rheumatoid arthritis and psoriasis are both common diseases it will happen from time to time that a patient has both. By definition the arthritis of psoriasis in all its forms is negative for rheumatoid factor and so cases with positive tests are not included in the remit of psoriatic arthropathy. In the early stages it may be difficult to decide how to characterise the disease of such patients and the Alliance will offer support and advice in such cases.

Inheritance patterns and prenatal diagnosis

Inheritance patterns

There is often a hereditary predisposition which is tissue type related in part.

Prenatal diagnosis

None.

Medical text written March 1995 by Dr A G White. **Last updated January 2002 by Dr A G White, Consultant Rheumatologist, Royal Free Hospital, London, UK.**

Further online resources

Medical texts in *The Contact a Family Directory* are designed to give a short, clear description of specific conditions and rare disorders. More extensive information on this condition can be found on a range of reliable, validated websites. Further information on these resources can be found in our **Medical Information on the Internet** article on page 21.

Support

Psoriasis and Psoriatic Arthritis Alliance
PO Box 111, St Albans AL2 3JQ   Tel: 0870 7703212   Fax: 0870 7703213
e-mail: info@papaa.org Web: http://www.papaa.org
The Alliance is a National Registered Charity No. 1118192, established in 1993. It
publishes a twice-yearly news journal and has information available, details on request.
The Alliance responds to approximately 5,000 calls a year.
Group details last updated June 2007.

The Carers (Equal Opportunities)
Act was implemented in England and
Wales on 1st April 2005. The Act gives
carers more choice and opportunities
to lead a more fulfilling life, by ensuring
that carers receive information about
their rights and to ensure that their
assessments consider leisure, training
and work opportunities.

PULMONARY HYPERTENSION OF THE NEWBORN

Background

Persistent Pulmonary Hypertension of the newborn (PPHN) is a rare disorder of the lungs which occurs at birth or shortly thereafter. The symptoms include cyanosis (blue cast of the skin due to deficient oxygenation of the blood), respiratory distress, tachypnea (increased rate of respiration), and minimal retractions (movement of an organ) during the first day of life.

The circulation of the unborn baby differs from that of an infant outside the womb. The unborn baby does not use its lungs to oxygenate its blood supply, but instead receives oxygen and gets rid of carbon dioxide via the placenta. All the many thousands of blood vessels in the lung are thick walled and have a small lumen (cavity of the blood vessel) so that the resistance to flow through the lungs is high. Also, the structure of the heart in the unborn functions slightly differently from newborns and adults because the fetus does not use the lung to breathe and obtain oxygen from the air (oxygen comes from the placenta) and blood is diverted away from the lungs through two channels. One channel is a small hole between the two chambers in the upper part of the heart, called the foramen ovale. The other channel is a connection between the two main blood vessels leaving the heart (aorta and pulmonary artery) and this communication is called the ductus arteriosus. Both channels normally close soon after birth.

Birth acts as a signal for changes to take place so that blood can be pumped to and from the lungs and the baby can take its first breath. As the baby breathes in, the lungs inflate for the first time, the blood vessels in the lungs widen, and blood rushes into the lungs from the heart. The pressures between the right and left sides of the heart becomes unequal. The pressure in the left side is now greater than that in the right. This causes the patent foramen ovale to close like a trap door. The ductus arteriosus constricts and eventually closes up after a few days.

Although the pattern of blood flow in the newborn baby is now the same as that of the adult the structure of the blood vessels within the lung are still very different. It takes several weeks for the walls of the blood vessel to become thin and for the resistance to flow to decrease. Sometimes this fails to happen. The resistance to the flow of blood through the lungs remains high and the pulmonary arterial pressure remains high after birth. This is called Persistent Pulmonary Hypertension of the newborn.

What are the causes?

Pulmonary hypertension can persist after birth in the presence of a heart which is normal although this is unusual. More commonly, the high pressure is secondary to abnormalities or diseases of the heart or lungs. The child may have a congenital abnormality of the heart (see entry, Heart defects) in which too much blood goes to the lungs at a high pressure. Or the baby may have difficulties in breathing and be short of oxygen as a result of Lung disease (see entry). In any child with Persistent Pulmonary Hypertension of the newborn, it is essential that an accurate diagnosis be made as rapidly as possible and appropriate treatment given. The UK National Specialist Commissioning Advisory Group includes a pulmonary hypertension service; the paediatric service is based at Great Ormond Street Hospital, London.

Inheritance patterns and prenatal diagnosis

Inheritance patterns

None.

Prenatal diagnosis

None.

Medical text written September 2004 by Contact a Family. Approved September 2004 by Professor S Haworth, British Heart Foundation Professor of Developmental Cardiology & Lead Clinician for the UK Network for the care of children with Pulmonary Hypertension, Institute of Child Health, London, UK.

Support

Information, support and advice for Pulmonary Hypertension of the Newborn is available from the Pulmonary Hypertension Association UK (see entry, Primary Pulmonary Hypertension).

PURINE & PYRIMIDINE METABOLIC DISEASES

Background

Purines are the source of our energy, ATP (Adenosine Triphosphate), and with pyrimidines are the building blocks of our DNA. Their production, recycling and breakdown involves a number of steps, each initiated (catalysed) by a different chemical called an enzyme. These rare disorders result when one of these enzymes is deficient. To date, twenty-seven enzyme deficiencies have been described, but some appear relatively benign with no obvious clinical problems or symptoms.

What are the symptoms?

For those purine and pyrimidine disorders that do present with symptoms, almost any system can be affected. Particular problems include kidney stones and renal disease (see entry, Kidney disease), recurrent infections and severe immune deficiency, severe recurrent anaemia, muscle cramps and wasting, arthritis (see entry, Arthritis (Adult)), neurological problems such as developmental delay, autism (see entry) and seizures (see entry, Epilepsy). They may also be responsible for adverse reactions to chemotherapy in patients undergoing treatment for cancer (see entry). Although originally thought to be childhood problems, it is clear that they may present at any age.

Symptoms may be severe and life-threatening.

How is it treated?

Specific treatment is only available for a small number of these conditions at present.

Inheritance patterns and prenatal diagnosis

Inheritance patterns

The mode of inheritance of these disorders is autosomal recessive, except Lesch Nyhan Lesch Nyhan (HPRT deficiency) and Phosphoribosylpyrophosphatesynthetase superactivity (PRPS) which are X-linked conditions, and familial juvenile hyperuricaemic nephropathy which is dominant. The degree of severity may be highly variable, even within the same family.

Prenatal diagnosis

Prenatal diagnosis is available for some of the purine and pyrimidine disorders.

Medical text written October 2002 by Dr M Champion. **Last reviewed September 2007 Dr M Champion, Consultant in Paediatric Metabolic Medicine, Evelina Children's Hospital, London, UK.**

Support

PUMPA (Purine Metabolic Patients Association)

Purine Research Unit, 3rd Floor, Block 7, South Wing, St Thomas' Hospital,
London SE1 7EH   Tel: 020 7188 1276   Fax: 020 7188 1280
e-mail: bebax@sgul.ac.uk or lynette.fairbanks@kcl.ac.uk

The Association is a National Registered Charity No. 1019792, established in 1993. Due to the large number of Purine & Pyrimidine Metabolic diseases the description given here is of a general nature. Information on the specific conditions which are listed in the index can be obtained from the Association. It offers support to affected families and funds research. It has information available, details on request.

Group details last updated September 2007.

Contact a Family has information for families in many community languages. Visit our website or phone the helpline for more information.

RASMUSSEN'S ENCEPHALITIS

Rasmussen's Encephalitis: Rasmussen's syndrome

Background

Rasmussen's Encephalitis (RE) is a progressive inflammation of the part of the brain called the cerebral cortex, which is made up of a right and a left hemisphere. The disease starts at one site in one hemisphere and spreads to adjoining areas on the same side. Curiously, it does not spread to the other hemisphere. The inflammation leads to loss of nerve cells and scar formation and usually results in severe disability. Although RE is most often diagnosed in children under the age of ten years, it can also start in adolescence and adulthood. It is a rare disorder and probably affects 1 in 500,000 to 1,000,000.

What are the symptoms?

The clinical problems in RE are determined by which areas of the affected hemisphere are inflamed as each area has different functions. As the disease spreads, more areas are damaged and the greater the severity and range of the disabilities. Typically, the disease progresses relentlessly until most of one hemisphere is affected. The inflammation burns out by itself but only rarely before severe disability has occurred. However, the speed of the spread varies between patients. At one end of the spectrum, the disease advances rapidly over a few weeks or months but at the other end, progression occurs slowly over several years. This slower clinical variant seems to be more common in adolescents and adults than in children. It is possible that there are milder forms of RE that fail to be recognized.

The typical clinical features of RE are epilepsy and neurological deficits such as hemiparesis (paralysis affecting one side of the body), hemianaesthesia (loss of touch-sense down one side of the body), visual loss, speech problems and cognitive deficits such as memory problems, intellectual impairment, and other neuropsychological deficits.

What are the causes?

It is thought that in most patients RE is an autoimmune disorder. Many patients have antibodies in their blood that bind to nerve cells and are capable of damaging the brain. In most patients, it is not clear what triggers the abnormal immune response, although sometimes RE has followed an otherwise minor bacterial or viral infection, or head injury.

How is it treated?

Surgery is the traditional treatment for advanced RE, and is used mainly to improve seizure control in patients with established disability. The extent of the surgery is determined by the severity, duration, rate of progression, the age of the patient and site of the disease. In patients with severe disease, all of the affected hemisphere may be removed (hemispherectomy). As epilepsy in RE is usually difficult to control, it can take time to find the best combination of anti-epileptic drugs. These drugs have no effect on progression of the underlying encephalitis.

There are now many reports that various combinations of powerful drugs that suppress the immune system (such as prednisolone, azathioprine, methotrexate, and cyclophosphamide) and therapies that modulate the function of the immune system (plasma exchange and intravenous immunoglobulin) may help at least some patients with RE. When more is known about the best use of immune therapy in RE, it is likely that fewer patients will need surgery.

Anti-viral drugs are only useful when the patient has a viral encephalitis rather than autoimmune RE.

Inheritance patterns and prenatal diagnosis
Inheritance patterns
None.
Prenatal diagnosis
None.

Medical text written April 2002 by Dr Ian Hart, Senior Lecturer and Consultant Neurologist, University Department of Neurological Science, Walton Centre for Neurology and Neurosurgery, Liverpool, UK.

Further online resources
Medical texts in *The Contact a Family Directory* are designed to give a short, clear description of specific conditions and rare disorders. More extensive information on this condition can be found on a range of reliable, validated websites. Further information on these resources can be found in our **Medical Information on the Internet** article on page 21.

Support
Support and information for Rasmussen's Encephalitis is provided by the Encephalitis Support Group (see entry, Encephalitis).

RAYNAUD'S PHENOMENON

Background

Raynaud's Phenomenon may be primary - occurring on its own - or secondary - occurring in association with disorders such as systemic lupus erythematosus (SLE), rheumatoid arthritis (RA) and scleroderma (systemic sclerosis). It has been estimated that some ten per cent of women suffer from Raynaud's. Some ninety-five per cent of scleroderma patients suffer from Raynaud's, but it must be stressed that only a small number of people with Raynaud's go on to develop scleroderma.

What are the symptoms?

The key feature of Raynaud's is colour changes associated with exposure to cold or any change in temperature. These changes occur most commonly in the hands, but may also affect the feet and occasionally other extremities, such as the nose or the tips of the ears. Raynaud's hands turn white, then blue, then later red as the circulation improves. In severe Raynaud's there may be considerable pain, ulceration or gangrene.

Raynaud's can occur in children, although it is rare. The symptoms are the same as those of the adult disease.

Inheritance patterns and prenatal diagnosis

Inheritance patterns

Raynaud's can be hereditary

Prenatal diagnosis

None

Medical text written May 1992 by Dr Carol Black. **Last reviewed August 2002 by Professor Carol Black, Consultant Rheumatologist, Royal Free Hospital, London, UK.**

Further online resources

Medical texts in *The Contact a Family Directory* are designed to give a short, clear description of specific conditions and rare disorders. More extensive information on this condition can be found on a range of reliable, validated websites. Further information on these resources can be found in our **Medical Information on the Internet** article on page 21.

Support

The Raynaud's & Scleroderma Association
112 Crewe Road, Alsager, Stoke-on-Trent, Cheshire ST7 2JA   Tel: 0800 917 2494 Helpline
Tel: 01270 872776 (office hours) e-mail: info@raynauds.org.uk
Web: http://www.raynauds.org.uk
The Association is a National Registered Charity No. 326306, established in 1982 as the Raynaud's Association and renamed to include Scleroderma in 1990. The Association also covers associated conditions such as Vibration White Finger, Systemic Lupus Erythematosus, Erythromelalgia and Sjögren's syndrome. It offers support to families of affected children and adults. It publishes a quarterly newsletter and has a wide range of information available, details on request. The Association has around 6,000 members. Group details last updated August 2007.

"It is nice to know that there is some help available and I am not alone."
Parent.

REFLEX ANOXIC SEIZURES

Background

Reflex Anoxic Seizure is the term used to describe a particular type of fit which is neither epileptic nor due to breath-holding. It is a particular type of severe syncope or 'faint' which is the result of a temporary cutting off of the supply of oxygenated blood to the brain.

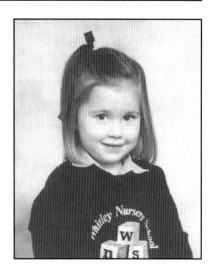

What are the symptoms?

Reflex Anoxic Seizures can occur in children as young as just a few days old. It is most common in toddlers, who usually grow out of it, but can reoccur in adolescents and adults. Any unexpected stimuli, such as pain, fear, fright or even a pleasant surprise, causes the heart to stop, the eyes to roll, marked pallor of the skin, and clenching of the jaw. The body also stiffens and there may be jerking movements of the arms and legs. After a few seconds to half a minute the heart starts and the body relaxes. The child may remain unconscious for anything from a few minutes to well over an hour as children often fall into a deep sleep afterwards. The frequency of attacks varies from child to child and Reflex Anoxic Seizure can be caused by even a mild pain if unexpected.

How is it diagnosed?

Reflex Anoxic Seizure is often misdiagnosed as breath holding, temper tantrums or as epilepsy. The associated marked pallor of the skin has led to these attacks being called Pallid Infantile Syncope or White breath-holding but some people now prefer the term Reflex Asystolic Syncope.

Medical text written October 1999 by Professor J B P Stephenson, Consultant in Paediatric Neurology, Royal Hospital for Sick Children, Glasgow, UK. **Last updated October 2005 by Dr W Whitehouse, Senior Lecturer in Paediatric Neurology and Consultant Paediatric Neurologist, University of Nottingham, Nottingham, UK.**

Further online resources

Medical texts in *The Contact a Family Directory* are designed to give a short, clear description of specific conditions and rare disorders. More extensive information on this condition can be found on a range of reliable, validated websites. Further information on these resources can be found in our **Medical Information on the Internet** article on page 21.

Support

Syncope Trust and Reflex Anoxic Seizures (STARS)
PO Box 175, Stratford upon Avon CV37 8YD   Tel: 0800 028 6362 Freephone Helpline
Tel: 01789 450564   Fax: 01789 450682   e-mail: trudie@stars.org.uk
Web: http://www.stars.org.uk
*STARS is a National Registered Charity No. 1084898, established in 1993. It offers
telephone, e-mail and letter support to affected families together with linking with similarly
affected families where possible. It also aims to raise awareness about the condition in
the public and among medical professionals. It publishes a half-yearly newsletter and has
information available, details on request. The group represents the interests of over 4,000
families and over 3,000 professional workers.*
Group details last confirmed September 2007.

Contact a Family produces a monthly
e-newsletter about our work and news
relevant to families with disabled
children.

REFLEX SYMPATHETIC DYSTROPHY

Reflex Sympathetic Dystrophy: Complex Regional Pain syndrome

Background

Reflex Sympathetic Dystrophy (RSD) is a chronic pain condition that is often localised to one area of the body. Somewhat confusingly it is also known as Complex Regional Pain Syndrome (CRPS) and, more generally, as Localised Pain Syndrome (LIPs).

Pain sensitivity varies substantially among humans. A significant part of the human population develops chronic pain conditions that are characterized by heightened pain sensitivity.

What are the symptoms?

It is not unusual for the pains to start in a localised area of the body (such as the ankle following sporting injury). The pains quickly intensify and there is a reluctance to move round. Often the painful area expands, spreading over time to involve larger areas of the body. In describing the pain, words such as 'stabbing, throbbing, burning or aching' are used. The discomfort increases and becomes constant. As the pains continue the young person tries not to use the area of body affected, this leads to muscular spasms, odd positioning or style of walking (gait) and greatly reduced fitness. This in turn further amplifies the pain. Unfortunately pain has a direct affect on other systems, leading to symptoms that can be as disabling as the pain itself (these include blurred vision, nausea, dizziness, headaches, extreme coldness, tummy pains and areas of numbness). Localised idiopathic pain syndrome simply describes pain that remains in a localised area (such as a limb). Within this descriptive diagnostic group are the complex regional pain syndromes (reflex sympathetic dystrophy).

What are the causes?

As with other chronic pain conditions CRPS is widely believed to be multifactoral in origin some of the factors which may contribute to the cause of the condition are:

Trauma

It is not unusual for an adolescent with a localised chronic pain to recall a sporting injury, operation or other trauma around the time that the chronic pain commenced. Whether or not this is causal is not clear. Excessive joint movement (hypermobility) has also been associated with falls and subsequent pain problems. There may often be a period of enforced immobilisation; this may be an additional factor in the development of a chronic pain syndrome.

Psychosocial Factors

Although often tempting to cite psychosocial distress as a trigger to chronic pain in adolescents, the data is lacking. Undoubtedly the pain associated disability and impact on lifestyle that follows has an enormous effect on psychosocial wellbeing.

Genetics

There is some evidence that CRPS may have a genetic predisposition in Caucasian women, but the underlying genomics are far from clear. Most young people with CRPS have no other relative with the same condition.

Environmental

It has been reported that girls have lower pain thresholds, poor sleep patterns and a tendency to hypermobility when compared with boys. This may, in part, explain the greater number of females with pain conditions. With CRPS there is a small, but significant, number of boys who present.

Pathophysiological

Once more there is very little data on how body functions are related to the condition (pathophysiology) of childhood chronic pain. It has been widely postulated that, in childhood CRPS, there is either overactivity of the sympathetic nervous system or under-responsiveness of the alpha adrenergic pathways. This is unproven.

How is it diagnosed?

The diagnosis of CRPS 1 remains based on observation of symptoms (clinical). There is often a precipitating trauma (not always). The pain is usually out of proportion to the inciting event. Autonomic changes are present; these include swelling, reduced skin perfusion and difficulty in distinguishing between hot and cold. There is also a marked reduction in range of movement and, in severe cases, ulceration. In adolescents the legs are more commonly affected. Occasionally more than one limb may be affected at presentation. It is not unusual for a hand or other leg to develop CRPS months after a leg has been affected. This may be due to the use of crutches and subsequent pain amplification but may also have no obvious trigger. Young people with CRPS may also develop low mood and overwhelming fatigue. This further complicates the clinical picture.

How is it treated?

One of the most important aspects of rehabilitation is that of inclusion. A dedicated team that works consistently with the adolescent and family will facilitate communication and enable goals to be reached earlier. It is essential that the young person is worked up medically to ensure no ongoing disease process or trauma is present. If the pain is coexisting with a known illness then it is important that this is as stable as possible before rehabilitation.

Medical therapies

The number of analgesics and interventions used is a sign that there are no well controlled therapeutic trials in the arena of childhood chronic pain. It is becoming widely accepted, however, that any analgesic intervention should be alongside multidisciplinary therapy. It is unusual for analgesia to work alone.

Complementary therapies are commonly utilised by patients with chronic pain. The evidence supporting many of these therapies in children and adolescents is poor but many young adults find certain therapies such as acupuncture, massage and aromatherapy helpful.

Multidisciplinary rehabilitation

The aim of treatment is to enable the young person to return to age appropriate activities and lifestyle. Ideally this would be pain free but, in many cases, this is initially with the pain.

Physiotherapists, occupational therapists and psychologists are key players in the team. They will be the primary professionals supporting the young person and the family. The physician is there to provide support if needed, occasional analgesic advice and very rarely, direct intervention. Intensive physiotherapy may be given for a set period of time. The aim of this is accelerated mobilisation. However many cases of pain will require a gentle, paced approach. In all cases the increase of activity should be consistent despite the pain. Where possible the young person should work to devise their own 'fitness plan'. Fun games can be included with an aim to return gradually to activities the young person previously enjoyed. Using a local gym rather than a hospital physiotherapy gym allows them to start to return to a more normal environment.

Working in this consistent, paced manner is extremely hard for the young person and their parents. The pain invariably continues at the beginning (if not throughout) and motivation is poor. Parental anxiety is understandably high and there is a fear that damage will be done. Psychological support during this time is key. The young person will need help setting goals, learning how to communicate pain to peers and family, keeping up motivation on 'bad days', managing low mood, dealing with anger and frustration and overcoming fears. Often they have not been at school for a long period of time and need help in preparing again for this difficult environment. In some cases there may be other mental health needs that can be identified and appropriately treated. Relaxation, advice on sleep and eating and advice on how to pace other areas of life can all be given by members of the team.

Most cases of complex regional pain syndromes in children have a favourable prognosis if early physiotherapy is initiated (with psychological support). A prolonged time to treatment and the presence of marked autonomic changes are not good prognostic indicators. Relapses of pain are relatively common but, in our experience, if the young person and their family recognise the onset of similar pains and put into practice physical and emotional strategies that have previously been taught then the impact of the pains can be significantly reduced.

Inheritance patterns and prenatal diagnosis

Inheritance patterns

As far as we can ascertain inherited predisposition to this syndrome is unclear.

Prenatal diagnosis

None.

Medical text written July 2007 by Dr Jacqui Clinch, Consultant paediatric rheumatology and adolescent chronic pain, Bristol Children's Hospital/ Royal National Hospital for Rheumatic Diseases, UK

Further online resources

Medical texts in *The Contact a Family Directory* are designed to give a short, clear description of specific conditions and rare disorders. More extensive information on this condition can be found on a range of reliable, validated websites. Further information on these resources can be found in our **Medical Information on the Internet** article on page 21.

Support

There is no *support group for Reflex Sympathetic Dystrophy*. Families can use Contact a Family's Freephone Helpline for advice, information and, where possible, links to other families. Contact a Family's web-based linking service Making Contact.org can be accessed at http://www.makingcontact.org

RELAPSING POLYCHONDRITIS

Background

Relapsing polychondritis (RP) is a rare episodic or progressive condition caused by inflammation of cartilage or other connective tissue, such as the ears, nose, throat, joints, kidney and heart. The damage caused by RP may lead to impaired use of these organs. RP occurs equally in middle-aged males and females and mainly occurs in white individuals.

What are the symptoms?

The initial symptoms of RP may begin suddenly. The most common first symptom is pain and swelling of the ear. Both ears may turn red or purple and are tender to the touch. Swelling may extend into the ear canal causing loss of hearing, ear infections, balance disturbances with vertigo and vomiting, and eventually a droopy ear. Throat pain may occur leading to hoarseness and difficulty talking. The nose may be affected and deterioration may lead to a flattened nose bridge (sometimes known as a 'saddle nose'). Inflammation of the eye occurs causing impaired vision. Fatigue and weight loss are common symptoms in RP and fever frequently accompanies acute flares.

During the later stages, the symptoms of RP may become more debilitating and life-threatening. RP may cause deterioration of the cartilage holding the windpipe open and this may lead to difficulties breathing. Deterioration of the rib cartilage can lead to the collapse of the chest, again hindering breathing. Joints everywhere are involved in episodes of arthritis (see entry, Arthritis (Juvenile Idiopathic)), with pain and swelling. As the disease progresses over a period of years, the mortality rate increases. Kidney failure (see entry, Kidney disease) may lead to death.

The disease may occur episodically with complete remission between episodes, or it may continue over time, causing progressive destruction (atrophy) of organs. Individuals may have persistent symptoms between acute flares or the pattern of disease may be more limited. The severity and the frequency of symptoms associated with RP varies between people and with time. Furthermore, the areas affected by RP may either remain constant or be completely unpredictable for each person.

What are the causes?

Cartilage is a tough, flexible tissue that changes into bone in many places in the body. Before birth, all bones start out as cartilage. Although children have more cartilage than adults, cartilage persists in adults in the linings of joints, the nose, the ears, the airway and the ribs near the breast bone. All these areas of the body may be affected by RP.

For many individuals, the cause of their condition remains unknown. However, RP is thought to be related to an underlying immune problem.

How is it diagnosed?

Individuals may have a wide array of symptoms that often pose major diagnostic dilemmas and RP may be misdiagnosed or under-diagnosed. RP is frequently diagnosed along with rheumatoid arthritis (see entry, Arthritis (Adult)), systemic lupus erythematosus (see entry, Lupus), and other connective tissue diseases.

How is it treated?

Although there is no cure for RP, in many patients the disease is well controlled with methotrexate, acute flares being controlled with steroids.

Inheritance patterns and prenatal diagnosis

Inheritance patterns

RP occurs sporadically.

Prenatal diagnosis

None available.

Medical text written October 2002 by Contact a Family. Approved October 2002 by Dr G Hughes. **Last updated March 2006 by Professor G Hughes, Consultant Rheumatologist, London Lupus Centre, London Bridge Hospital, London, UK.**

Support

Relapsing Polychondritis Support Group (UK)
21 Staneway, Leam Lane, Gateshead NE10 8LR   Tel: 0191 469 2342
e-mail: UK-Anne@polychondritis.com
The Relapsing Polychondritis Support Group (UK) offers support and information about this very rare disease. The group also aims to raise awareness of Relapsing Polychondritis among the public and medical profession and will link individuals where possible. The group is affiliated to the Polychondritis Education Society,
Web: http://www.polychondritis.com and has an increasing number of people in touch due to its Internet presence.
Group details last confirmed March 2007.

RESTRICTED GROWTH

Background

Restricted growth is exhibited as a common factor in over a hundred specific medical conditions. The resultant short stature in affected persons may be marked. Restricted growth falls into two main categories: **proportionate** and **disproportionate** short stature.

What are the symptoms?

In **proportionate** short stature, growth is limited throughout the body. Specific conditions exhibiting this form of growth pattern are hormone deficiencies where hormones produced by the thyroid and pituitary glands may be deficient, damaged, absent or else the body is unable to process the substance. Early recognition of hormone deficiency is vital to subsequent development. In chromosome defects such as Turner syndrome restricted growth may be the only symptom prior to puberty. Chronic heart, lung, kidney or liver disease may be associated with restricted growth.

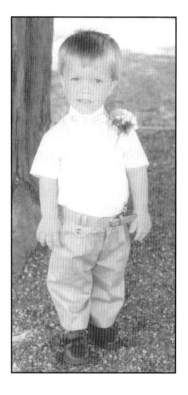

In **disproportionate** short stature (and sometimes proportionate short stature), the problem is often due to a disturbance in the growth of bones and cartilage. In some conditions this is evident at birth: in others evidence arises later. Specific disorders include: achondroplasia (see entry) with shortening of the limbs especially the upper arm and thigh; hypochondroplasia (see entry), a distinct condition with less severe growth restriction; diastrophic dysplasia (see entry) growth restriction affects the trunk and limbs, is apparent at birth and may be serious and progressive; in multiple epiphyseal dysplasia (MED) disorders of the epiphyses (growing ends of the long bones) occur; spondylo epiphyseal dysplasia (SED) the epiphyses of the long bones and the spine are affected (there are two main types: SED congenita; SED tarda); pseudoachondroplasia has several types, which have differing characteristics; Morquio disease is a mucopolysaccharide disease (see entry) which causes restricted growth.

Inheritance patterns and prenatal diagnosis
Inheritance patterns
Sporadic mutations, autosomal dominant, autosomal recessive and X-linked all occur. The specific type of inheritance will vary with the condition. For example achondroplasia has autosomal dominant inheritance, while in diastrophic dysplasia it is autosomal recessive. Genetic advice should be offered.

Prenatal diagnosis
Amniocentesis at fourteen to six teen weeks, chorionic villus sampling at ten to twelve weeks and ultrasound scanning at around twenty weeks are available depending upon the condition.

Medical text written November 1991 by Contact a Family. Approved November 1991 by Professor M Patton, Professor of Medical Genetics, St Georges Hospital Medical School, London, UK and Dr J E Wraith, Consultant Paediatrician, Royal Manchester Children's Hospital, Manchester, UK. **Last reviewed September 2005 by Dr R Stanhope, Consultant Paediatric Endocrinologist, Great Ormond Street Hospital, London, UK.**

Further online resources
Medical texts in *The Contact a Family Directory* are designed to give a short, clear description of specific conditions and rare disorders. More extensive information on this condition can be found on a range of reliable, validated websites. Further information on these resources can be found in our **Medical Information on the Internet** article on page 21.

Support
Restricted Growth Association
PO Box 4008, Yeovil BA20 9AW
Tel: 01935 841364 (Mon, Wed &Thur, 9am-5pm; Tues, 9am-9pm; Fri, 9am-12noon)
Fax: 01935 841364   e-mail: office@restrictedgrowth.co.uk
Web: http://www.restrictedgrowth.co.uk
The Association is a National Registered Charity No. 261647, established in 1970 as the Association for Research in Restricted Growth (ARRG). It offers support for affected families and individuals. It has welfare and counselling services together with a regional contact network. It gives information about clothing, employment, mobility and home aids. It publishes a quarterly newsletter and has information available, details on request. The Association has over 2,500 members.
Group details last confirmed April 2007.

Child Growth Foundation
2 Mayfield Avenue, Chiswick, London W4 1PW   Tel: 020 8994 7625   Tel: 020 8995 0257
Fax: 020 8995 9075   e-mail: jenny.cgf@btopenworld.com
Web: http://www.childgrowthfoundation.org
The Foundation is a National Registered Charity No. 274325, established in 1977. It acts as an umbrella organisation for Silver Russell syndrome, Sotos syndrome, Growth Hormone Insufficiency/MPHD, Bone dysplasia (Achondroplasia and other Bone dysplasia's), Premature Sexual Maturation and Turner syndrome. It offers support and advice to families of children with growth conditions and adults. It also offers contact with other families if required. It publishes a bi-annual newsletter and holds an annual convention for its members. Information booklets are available on request. Please send large SAE.
Group details last updated April 2007.

RETINITIS PIGMENTOSA

Background

Retinitis Pigmentosa (RP) is the name given to a group of hereditary diseases of the retina, the light sensitive tissue at the back of the eye in which the first stages of 'seeing' take place.

What are the symptoms?

In these conditions the retina slowly degenerates losing its ability to transmit images to the brain. In advanced stages of the conditions characteristic clumps of pigment appear in the retina. Often the first symptom is night blindness, followed by narrowing of side vision leading to 'tunnel' vision.

Inheritance patterns and prenatal diagnosis

Inheritance patterns

For retinitis pigmentosa inheritance may be autosomal dominant, autosomal recessive or X-linked.

In other related conditions inheritance patterns depend upon the specific condition. For example Best disease, butterfly-shaped dystrophy, and Bull's-eye dystrophy are autosomal dominant. Choroideremia is X-linked, and Usher and Refsum (see Metabolic diseases), Bardet-Biedl syndromes are autosomal recessive.

Many of the genes causing the various forms of Retinitis Pigmentosa and related disorders have now been identified and genetic testing for some of these conditions is now available.

Prenatal diagnosis

Prenatal diagnosis is now possible in some forms of Retinitis Pigmentosa and other inherited retinal disorders but only in those cases where the genetic change causing the condition has been identified.

Medical text written November 1991 by Contact a Family. Approved November 1991 by Professor M Patton, Professor of Medical Genetics, St Georges Hospital Medical School, London, UK and Dr J E Wraith, Consultant Paediatrician, Royal Manchester Children's Hospital, Manchester, UK. **Last updated August 2006 by Professor A T Moore, Duke-Elder Professor of Ophthalmology, Institute of Ophthalmology, London, UK.**

Further online resources

Medical texts in *The Contact a Family Directory* are designed to give a short, clear description of specific conditions and rare disorders. More extensive information on this condition can be found on a range of reliable, validated websites. Further information on these resources can be found in our **Medical Information on the Internet** article on page 21.

Support

British Retinitis Pigmentosa Society

PO Box 350, Buckingham MK18 1GZ   Tel: 0845 123 2354 Helpline   Tel: 01280 821334
Fax: 01280 815900   e-mail: info@brps.org.uk   Web: http://www.brps.org.uk
The Society is a National Registered Charity No. 271729, established in 1975. Other conditions covered by the Group are Macular dystrophy, Best disease, Butterfly-shaped dystrophy, Stargardt disease, Bull's-eye Dystrophy, Central Areolar Choroidal dystrophy, Inherited Disciform Macular Degeneration and Choroideremia. The eye problems presented by Usher syndrome; Refsum disease and Laurence-Moon-Bardet-Biedl syndrome are also covered by the Group. It offers support and contact through a network of branches. It publishes a quarterly newsletter and has a wide range of information available, details on request. The Society has around 3,000 members.
Group details last confirmed February 2008.

Working Tax Credit can be claimed by anyone who is responsible for a child and who works for at least 16 hours a week. Certain other workers who do not have children can also apply. The Child Tax Credit can be claimed by families with children regardless of whether you work or not. For more advice about tax credits, and a copy of the 'Tax credits guide', call the Contact a Family Helpline.

RETINOBLASTOMA

Background

Retinoblastoma is a malignant tumour which develops at the back of the eye. It originates in the cells of the retina, the light sensitive lining of the eye.

It affects babies and young children and is very rare after the age of five years. Retinoblastoma may be unilateral (affecting one eye) or bilateral (both eyes involved). The unilateral form is more common and accounts for approximately sixty per cent of all cases.

What are the symptoms?

When a unilateral tumour is diagnosed in very young children, particularly during the first year of life, a tumour may subsequently develop in the other eye so regular eye checks must be undertaken to detect any new tumours at an early stage.

If only one eye is affected, the child is likely to have normal vision in the other eye and will not need any special help at school. Where both eyes are affected, low vision aids are sometimes necessary to enable the child to attend a mainstream school.

What are the causes?

The cause of Retinoblastoma is a genetic defect, usually a mutation, affecting the Retinoblastoma gene on chromosome 13. In approximately 1 in 20 children with retinoblastoma, a small deletion of chromosome 13 can be detected by cytogenetic analysis looking at a chromosome preparation under the microscope. These children may have other features including a characteristic facial appearance with bushy eyebrows and they are sometimes delayed in reaching their milestones. This is known as the 13q deletion syndrome.

How is it treated?

More than ninety-five per cent of children with Retinoblastoma can be cured. Treatment of Retinoblastoma may include surgery to remove the eye, chemotherapy, laser therapy, freezing treatment, plaque or external beam radiotherapy. Often a combination of treatments is needed.

Inheritance patterns and prenatal diagnosis

Inheritance patterns

There are two types of Retinoblastoma, a genetic or hereditary form and a non-genetic or non-hereditary form. Parents of children with Retinoblastoma should have their own eyes examined to check for signs of a spontaneously regressed tumour which has gone undetected. If this is present, then the parent carries the defective Retinoblastoma gene and all of their subsequent children have approximately a 1 in 2 chance of being affected. If the parents are unaffected, there is no family history of Retinoblastoma and the child is the first affected member of the family, then the chances of another child being affected are less than 1 in 20. All patients with bilateral tumours and approximately fifteen per cent of patients with unilateral tumours carry the defective Retinoblastoma gene and can pass the gene on to their children.

Prenatal diagnosis

Where there is a family history of Retinoblastoma, it is possible to carry out genetic studies of individual family members, to see who is carrying the defective gene and who is not. It is also possible to do the test during the early part of pregnancy, usually at about eleven weeks, or on the cord blood once the baby has been born. In most bilaterally affected individuals, it is possible to identify the genetic mutation and to offer pre- or post- natal screening for their offspring and other members of the family. It is now also possible to offer this service to some unilaterally affected individuals, particularly when surgery has been undertaken and where tumour tissue is available for analysis.

Medical text written October 2001 by Dr J Kingston. **Last updated December 2005 by Dr J Kingston, Consultant Paediatric Oncologist, St Bartholomew's Hospital, London, UK.**

Support

Childhood Eye Cancer Trust (CHECT)
The Royal London Hospital, Whitechapel Road, London E1 1BB   Tel: 020 7377 5578
Fax: 020 7377 0740   e-mail: info@chect.org.uk   Web: http://www.chect.org.uk
The Trust is a National Registered Charity No. 327493, established in 1987. Through its network of families and individuals, the Trust offers support and information to those with the rare eye cancer, Retinoblastoma. It publishes a newsletter four times a year, raises funds for research and raises awareness amongst the public and with health professionals. It is in touch with over 1,000 families.
Group details last updated February 2008.

RETT SYNDROME

Background

Rett syndrome is the clinical expression of the Rett disorder, a complex, genetic, neurological condition which affects far more girls than boys. Although signs may not be initially obvious, it is present at birth. It usually becomes more evident during the second year. People with Rett syndrome are almost always profoundly and multiply disabled and totally dependent on others for all their needs throughout their lives but severity may vary considerably.

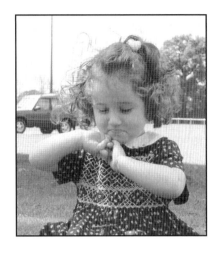

What are the symptoms?

The baby with classic (easily recognised) Rett syndrome is usually placid and rather inactive. Learning may be slow but progress may reach the nine or twelve month stage, occasionally beyond. Within a few weeks of birth the child's head size may fail to increase at the normal rate indicating failure of the brain to grow normally, although head size may remain within normal limits. Strange finger movements develop with the hands twisting and squeezing rather than reaching out to explore. Usually between one to three years the abnormal hand movements become more obvious and purposeful use is reduced or lost. During this time of regression the child may be agitated and distressed and breathing rhythm becomes irregular.

Brain scans may confirm poor growth of the brain and after some months the electroencephalogram may show abnormal electrical activity in the brain cells (an electroencephalogram is the tracing which shows the electrical activity due to the neurones on the surface of the brain). There is disturbance of several substances involved in brain development and mature function.

Later problems include poorly regulated muscle tension (reduced initially and increased later), with a tendency to develop joint contractures and curvature of the spine (scoliosis); involuntary movements including the hand stereotypies and abnormal movements of the limbs and face; feeding difficulties; periodic agitation and severe intellectual disability. Breathing rhythm is disturbed, an indication of poor brain control of heart and respiratory activity. This often leads to short non-epileptic vacant spells. There may also be epilepsy. Facial appearance is attractive with liking for human contact, good vision and hearing.

The disorder itself does not appear progressive. However there are serious health risks due to the tendency for muscle tone to increase, leading to worsening scoliosis and other joint contractures and increasing difficulty in feeding, leading to poor nutrition. The poor cardio-respiratory control probably contributes to some sudden deaths, although the estimated overall death rate is less than for many other profoundly disabling conditions (one point two per cent of UK recorded cases each year). In less severe cases, healthy survival into adult life with good retention of the early skills is well documented.

How is it diagnosed?

The diagnosis is confirmed by detecting a mutation (fault) on MECP2, a gene at the tip of the X chromosome. In just a few people with all or most of the clinical signs of Rett a mutation has not been found and it is possible that these people have a fault affecting control of MECP2 or of genes whose activity should be regulated by MECP2.

A young child with the Rett disorder may require many investigations because there are many disorders which may cause failure to develop and loss of skills in infancy. However, poor early progress in spite of a normal appearance should alert the physician to test for Rett mutations and a reduction in skills at one to two years is highly suggestive.

Inheritance patterns and prenatal diagnosis

Inheritance patterns

The Rett disorder affects more than 1 in 10,000 females and probably far fewer males. Most cases are solitary (sporadic). A case of Rett syndrome is believed to be due to the development of a fresh dominant mutation in a germ cell of one parent. The individual who inherits the affected gene is almost invariably affected and at high risk to transmit the disorder to any offspring. Families should seek advice from the regional clinical genetic centre but can usually be reassured that recurrence is very unlikely. The cause of Rett syndrome is mutations of a gene, MECP2, on the X-chromosome. Another gene, CDKL5, on the X-chromosome causes a rare form of the syndrome which a clinical geneticist will bear in mind when advising families.

Prenatal diagnosis

Prenatal diagnosis is possible where the mutation has been identified in an individual family. However, the risk of recurrence is very low, although not zero, except in the rare situation where the mother carries the mutation, or either of the parents is mosaic for the mutation (either parent carrying the mutation in a small proportion of their own cells). The possibility of prenatal diagnosis is best investigated in advance of a pregnancy. Advice may be obtained from a regional genetics centre.

Medical text written February 2002 by Dr Orlee Udwin, Consultant Clinical Psychologist, Society for the Study of Behavioural Phenotypes and Dr Alison Kerr. **Last updated August 2005 by Dr Alision Kerr, Consultant Paediatrician and Senior Lecturer, Department of Psychological Medicine, University of Glasgow and Gartnavel Royal Hospital, Glasgow, UK with material on prenatal diagnosis by Professor Angus Clarke, Professor in Medical Genetics, Institute of Medical Genetics University of Wales College of Medicine, Cardiff, UK.**

Further online resources

Medical texts in *The Contact a Family Directory* are designed to give a short, clear description of specific conditions and rare disorders. More extensive information on this condition can be found on a range of reliable, validated websites. Further information on these resources can be found in our **Medical Information on the Internet** article on page 21.

Support

Rett Syndrome Association UK

113 Friern Barnet Road, London N11 3EU

Tel: 0870 770 3266 (Mon-Fri 9am-5pm, 24hr answerphone) Fax: 0870 770 3265

e-mail: info@rettsyndrome.org.uk   Web: http://www.rettsyndrome.org.uk

The Association is a National Registered Charity No. 327309, established in 1985. It offers telephone support 7 days a week and has self-help support groups and a network of contact supporters. It publishes a quarterly magazine 'Rett News' and has a wide range of information available, details on request. The Association has over 1,000 members.
Group details last updated September 2007.

Rett Syndrome Association Scotland

Blackthorn, 12 Ailsa View, West Kilbride KA23 9GA   Tel: 01294 829100
 e-mail: rettsyndrome@btconnect.com

The Association is a Scottish Registered Charity No. SCO16645, formerly known as the National Rett Syndrome Association. It offers support through correspondence, telephone and one to one contact where possible. It has a bereavement counsellor and holds Therapy Days and regular Open Clinics. It publishes a quarterly newsletter 'RS News' and has information available, details on request. The Association has over 100 members.
Group details last confirmed March 2007.

REYE SYNDROME

Background

Reye syndrome is a rare sudden acute illness which affects children and, occasionally, adults when they appear to be recovering from a viral illness such as influenza, chicken pox or diarrhoea.

Some rare metabolic diseases such as Medium Chain Acyl Co - enzyme Dehydrogenase Deficiency (MCAD) (see entry, Metabolic diseases) may cause illnesses which are very similar to Reye syndrome.

What are the symptoms?

The child develops frequent or persistent vomiting and becomes drowsy. There may also be a personality change, clouding of consciousness or coma. Large amounts of fat develop in the liver. The detection of this helps to diagnose the condition. The brain becomes swollen and increased pressure in the skull can cut off the blood supply causing death, or irreversible brain damage in some survivors.

How is it treated?

There is substantial evidence that aspirin, given for the viral illness symptoms, initiates the onset of the syndrome. From June 1986 all aspirin containing medications in the UK were required to carry warning labelling cautioning against their use in children under twelve years except on medical advice. In April 2003 the Medicines and Healthcare Products Regulatory Agency issued new advice that would be applicable to all UK products containing aspirin from October 2003. This stated that the warning should now say: 'Do not give to children under sixteen years unless on the advice of a doctor.'

Inheritance patterns and prenatal diagnosis

Inheritance patterns

No evidence to suggest that 'true' Reye syndrome has any inheritance patterns. Some metabolic diseases which present Reye-like features may be either X-linked or autosomal recessive.

Prenatal diagnosis

None for Reye syndrome, but this is available for some metabolic diseases where the enzyme identification has been made through chorionic villus sampling or amniocentesis.

Medical text written November 1991 by Contact a Family. Approved November 1991 by Professor M Patton, Professor of Medical Genetics, St Georges Hospital Medical School, London, UK and Dr J E Wraith, Consultant Paediatrician, Royal Manchester Children's Hospital, Manchester, UK. **Last updated April 2003 by Dr S Hall, Sheffield Children's Hospital, Sheffield, UK.**

Further online resources

Medical texts in *The Contact a Family Directory* are designed to give a short, clear description of specific conditions and rare disorders. More extensive information on this condition can be found on a range of reliable, validated websites. Further information on these resources can be found in our **Medical Information on the Internet** article on page 21.

Support

National Reye's Syndrome Foundation of the UK

15 Nicholas Gardens, Pyrford, Woking GU22 8SD   Tel: 01932 346843
e-mail: Gordon.Denney@ukgateway.net   Web: http://www.reyessyndrome.co.uk
The Foundation is a National Registered Charity No. 288064, established in 1983. It offers advice to parents of affected children and those with a Reye-like illness. It funds research at several UK centres, publishes an occasional newsletter and has information available, details on request. The Foundation has around 150 families in membership.
Group details last confirmed October 2006.

Make 2008 a year to remember with an amazing trek to the Mount Everest Base Camp in aid of Contact a Family. To take part in this experience of a lifetime, call our fundraising team, Tel: 020 7608 8731.

RUBELLA

Rubella: German measles

Background

Rubella is no longer a common disease of childhood in the UK. This is a result of the Mumps, Measles and Rubella (MMR) vaccination programme (see Immunisation article) - although there are concerns that if MMR vaccination rates continue to drop then cases of rubella will reappear.

What are the symptoms?

Those born with congenital rubella infection may have congenital defects, generally involving the heart, eye and ear.

Common problems:

- Many children have sensorineural hearing loss (see entry, Deafness) in one or both ears. This is because the inner ear, which links the ear to the brain, has been damaged. Hearing loss is the most common manifestation of congenital rubella and often occurs in isolation and may not be obvious at birth. A child's hearing may also get worse over time. Before the MMR vaccination was introduced, fifteen to twenty per cent of cases of children born with sensorineural hearing loss were caused by rubella;
- Babies may be born with cataracts (cloudy lenses, see entry) in one or both eyes. Others may have rarer visual conditions or find that their sight gets worse as they get older. Children with congenital rubella cataract usually have associated defects of the heart and hearing, a syndrome referred to as 'congenital rubella syndrome'. This follows exposure to rubella infection early in pregnancy;
- Rubella can affect the heart in many different ways. Children may have heart problems (see entry, Heart defects) from birth and require hospital treatment;
- Rubella can also affect a child's brain and nervous system. Difficulties can vary from mild to severe (see entry, Learning disability) .

If a woman catches rubella in the later stages of pregnancy then this can cause hearing loss.

Worldwide rubella epidemics prior to the introduction of rubella vaccine, such as that in the 1960's, resulted in many babies being born with Congenital Rubella Defects. Those babies are now adults and even though rubella epidemics are now less common in the UK, the ongoing effects of congenital rubella remain. In fact, many individuals with Congenital Rubella may go on to develop additional problems to the ones they were born with - such as diabetes, declining vision and hearing, and disturbances in behaviour.

What are the causes?

Rubella is caused by a virus which is spread in the air as droplets - through close contact and by coughing and sneezing. Infection acquired after birth rarely causes any problems and is often without symptoms, but if caught by a woman in the early stages of pregnancy it poses a substantial risk to the unborn baby.

Inheritance patterns and prenatal diagnosis

Inheritance patterns

None.

Prenatal diagnosis

This depends on whether specific abnormalities can be identified by a scan.

Medical text written September 2004 by Sense. Approved October 2004 by Professor Catherine Peckham, Professor of Paediatric Epidemiology, Institute of Child Health, London, UK.

Further online resources

Medical texts in *The Contact a Family Directory* are designed to give a short, clear description of specific conditions and rare disorders. More extensive information on this condition can be found on a range of reliable, validated websites. Further information on these resources can be found in our **Medical Information on the Internet** article on page 21.

Support

Information, support and advice is available from Sense (see entry, Deafblindness).

RUBINSTEIN TAYBI SYNDROME

Rubinstein Taybi syndrome: Broad Thumb-Great Toe syndrome

Background

Children with Rubinstein-Taybi syndrome (RTS) usually have normal birthweights, but subsequent growth is poor, with most children being of short stature with a small head size.

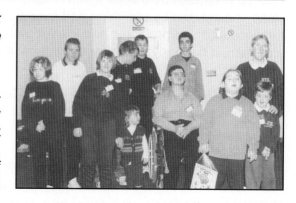

What are the symptoms?

Developmental delay is usual, but varies from mild to severe. The most striking physical feature is broad, sometimes angulated thumbs and first toes. The facial features vary with age and include a prominent beaked nose and downslanting eyes. Undescended testes occur in males. Other variable features include congenital heart disease and kidney abnormalities, eye and hearing problems, feeding difficulties in infancy and constipation. Seizures may occur. Most people with Rubinstein-Taybi syndrome have friendly and loving personalities.

Psychological and behavioural characteristics

The information below has been drawn up by Dr Orlee Udwin of the Society for the Study of Behavioural Phenotypes.

Children with Rubinstein-Taybi syndrome show similarities in their intellectual profiles and behaviour. Most have moderate to severe learning difficulties, though some have mild learning difficulties. Overall, visuo-spatial and motor abilities tend to be better than verbal abilities. Expressive language is particularly limited, and some affected children do not develop speech at all, although they can benefit from signing and a 'total communication' approach to language teaching. In general affected individuals are able to use their limited speech communicatively, and show overall good language competency. Poor concentration and distractibility are further common features.

The children are frequently described as happy, loving and easy to get on with. They are very sociable, even over-friendly, and love adult attention. They are reported to be particularly responsive to music and are very interested in manipulating objects such as electronic appliances and dials. Most become self-sufficient in eating, dressing and toileting. Severe sleep disturbance is reported in some cases and may be the result of frequent waking in the night due to breathing difficulties.

Over half of the children are said to engage in self-stimulatory behaviours such as rocking, hand flapping and spinning. Many also show resistance to environmental change, intolerance to loud noises and self-injurious behaviours. Older individuals may show sudden changes in mood and temper outbursts.

Inheritance patterns and prenatal diagnosis

Inheritance patterns

Rubinstein-Taybi syndrome, although a genetic disorder, usually affects only a single person in the family. Changes (mutations or deletions) in a gene called CREBBP located on chromosome 16 are found in a significant number of people with RTS. These changes are sometimes seen on chromosome analysis but often will require special laboratory techniques to be found. These are usually new genetic changes in just the affected person. If the parents of a child with RTS have normal chromosomes, the chance of a second affected child is small, around one per cent. If, however, an individual with RTS has children of their own, the chance for a similarly affected child may be as high as fifty per cent.

Prenatal diagnosis

If the genetic change is known in an affected child, pre-natal diagnosis may be possible to reassure parents.

Medical text written July 1998 by Dr Bronwyn Kerr. **Last updated October 2003 by Dr Bronwyn Kerr, Consultant Clinical Geneticist, Royal Manchester Children's Hospital, Manchester, UK. Psychological and behavioural characteristics written by Dr Orlee Udwin of the Society for the Study of Behavioural Phenotypes.**

Further online resources

Medical texts in *The Contact a Family Directory* are designed to give a short, clear description of specific conditions and rare disorders. More extensive information on this condition can be found on a range of reliable, validated websites. Further information on these resources can be found in our **Medical Information on the Internet** article on page 21.

Support

Rubinstein Taybi Syndrome Support Group

162 Buckfield Road, Leominster HR6 8UF   Tel: 01568 616149
e-mail: magsruck@blueyonder.co.uk   Web: http://www.rtsuk.org
The Group is a National Registered Charity No. 1037043, established in 1986. It offers support to families and linking with others where possible. It also has an area family network. It publishes a newsletter twice a year and has information available, details on request. The Group has over 200 UK and overseas families on its mailing list.
Group details last confirmed November 2007.

SACRAL AGENESIS

Background

The sacrum is a bone at the base of the spinal column that is formed following the fusion of five vertebrae. It lies in the region of the buttocks and just below it is another small series of bones called the coccyx. The presence of the sacrum gives rise to the normal 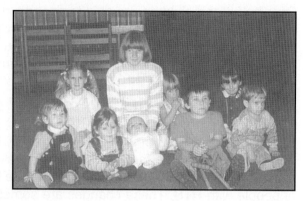 rounded contour of the buttocks and the shape of the pelvis. Nerves from the spinal cord pass through a bony canal within the sacrum and exit the sacrum in a number of places to provide nerve supply to the bowel and the anal sphincters, the bladder and the bladder sphincters and, also, to the muscles and sensory organs in the lower limbs. Sacral agenesis is a condition that exists when either part or all of the sacrum is absent. It is possible for two of the five sacral segments to be absent without causing problems with the nerve supply. However, if three or more of the sacral segments are absent, it is probable that there will be some abnormality of the nerves coming out of the sacrum.

What are the symptoms?

If there is an abnormality of the nerves coming out of the sacrum, this can have a number of different effects. It may affect the bowel and the bowel sphincters, which can give rise to constipation and/or faecal incontinence. It may affect the bladder and the urinary sphincters and this may give rise to urinary incontinence and urinary tract infections. It is possible that in patients with sacral agenesis the bladder will store urine at abnormally high pressure and thus may pose a risk of causing kidney damage. The final problem that may exist, if the nerves coming from the sacrum are abnormal, is varying degrees of paralysis affecting the lower limbs. This can vary from minor problems with gait to total paralysis requiring the permanent use of a wheelchair.

How is it diagnosed?

All patients with sacral agenesis will need to be assessed by a medical specialist with an interest in bowel and bladder problems, the neurology of the lower limbs and, probably, a specialist paediatric orthopaedic surgeon.

How is it treated?

There are a wide variety of treatments available to improve and control all of the disabilities arising from the complications of sacral agenesis, particularly with reference to the incontinence problems. With modern therapy it is now possible to achieve both faecal and urinary continence. It is also possible to safely protect the kidneys from damage due to the abnormal bladder.

Inheritance patterns and prenatal diagnosis

Inheritance patterns

There is an increased association between the development of sacral agenesis and maternal diabetes. However, most cases arise sporadically and no genetic linkage has been noted. Like all abnormalities of the development of the spine and spinal cord, however, if a parent has one child affected, there is an increased risk of further children being affected with the same condition. The parents would be advised to seek genetic counselling, which can be arranged through their local family doctor.

Prenatal diagnosis

Prenatal diagnosis is possible but is unusual. Most cases are only detected following delivery. Sometimes the presentation may be delayed until the child is older and presents with problems relating to incontinence, urinary tract infections or abnormalities with gait.

Medical text written May 2001 by Mr P Malone. **Last reviewed October 2005, by Mr P Malone, Consultant Paediatric Urologist, Southampton General Hospital, Southampton, UK.**

Support

Sacral Agenesis Contact Group
15 Elizabeth Gardens, Dibden Purlieu, Southampton SO4 5NF   Tel/Fax: 023 8084 2661
The Group is Contact Group, established in 1987. It offers mutual support by telephone and letter and through sharing of experiences. It has information available, details on request. The Group has around 20 members.
Group details last updated July 2004.

SARCOIDOSIS

Background

Sarcoidosis is a multisystem disorder of unknown cause which can affect any organ of the body taking the form of cells which cluster together in tiny nodules, or sarcoid granulomas. The word sarcoid comes from the Greek meaning 'flesh like'.

Sarcoidosis can develop in almost any organ. Most commonly it attacks the lungs, eyes, skin, more rarely the brain and nervous system. It can also spread to other organs such as the liver, heart and kidneys. The disease can range from a mild, self-limiting condition which needs no treatment, to a severe, chronically progressive illness.

What are the symptoms?

Initially, most affected persons have symptoms of fever, fatigue and weight loss. Other common symptoms include chronic cough, skin rash, shortness of breath, fatigue, joint pains and swelling and hypertension (high blood pressure). Indeed, sarcoidosis can cause almost any combination of symptoms and signs.

Although Sarcoidosis usually affects adults in the age range 20-40, children (rarely) and elderly persons can be affected. Research so far has identified a higher rate of occurrence in the following racial groups: the black population in the United States and the Caribbean regions, Scandinavians, Puerto Ricans, Irish and Japanese. It is more common in women than men.

Sarcoidosis may mimic many other diseases such as Lupus, Chronic Fatigue syndrome/Myalgic Encephalomyelitis, Tuberculosis and Arthritis (see entries).

What are the causes?

Diagnosis is usually by exclusion as the cause has not yet been identified.

Sarcoid granulomas result from chronic inflammation. The acute inflammatory response to an infection is usually beneficial, walling off the infection in order to contain and destroy it. If the infection persists despite the body's response, then the chronic build up of inflammatory cells may lead to granuloma formation. An example of this is Tuberculosis (see entry). It must be stressed that although sarcoid granulomas look like a response to chronic infection, no causative germ or virus has been found.

How is it treated?

The majority of patients recover without treatment and many do not have relapses. In the most severe cases the disease can be life threatening. Some affected people do need medication and for these individuals steroids can be effective usually given directly; for example, eye drops for eye symptoms.

Inheritance patterns and prenatal diagnosis

Inheritance patterns

There are clearly genetic factors which are important. How genes interact with other factors to produce Sarcoidosis is not known.

Prenatal diagnosis

None.

Medical text written March 2004 by Contact a Family. Approved March 2004 by Professor A Bush, Professor of Paediatric Respirology, Royal Brompton Hospital, London, UK.

Further online resources

Medical texts in *The Contact a Family Directory* are designed to give a short, clear description of specific conditions and rare disorders. More extensive information on this condition can be found on a range of reliable, validated websites. Further information on these resources can be found in our **Medical Information on the Internet** article on page 21.

Support

Sarcoidosis and Interstitial Lung Association (SILA)

c/o Chest Clinic Office, 2nd Floor Admin Block, Kings College Hospital, Denmark Hill, London SE5 9RS   Tel: 020 7237 5912   e-mail: info@sila.org.uk
Web: http://www.sila.org.uk
SILA is a National Registered Charity No. 1063986, established in 1993. It offers telephone, postal and e-mail support to individuals affected by Sarcoidosis, their families, carers and professionals. SILA holds monthly support meetings on the first Thursday in the month, except August, at King's College Hospital, London and pulishes a newsletter. It has information and a video available, details on request. SILA has over 100 members.
Group details last confirmed February 2008.

SCHIZOPHRENIA

Background

Schizophrenia is a serious mental illness which affects one person in a hundred. It usually develops in the late teens or early twenties, though it sometimes starts in middle age or even much later in life. The earlier it begins, the more potential it has to damage the personality and the ability to lead a normal life. About twenty-five per cent of people will make a good recovery within five years, two thirds will have multiple episodes with some degree of disability in between and ten to fifteen per cent will be severely incapacitated.

What are the symptoms?

When someone has schizophrenia their thoughts, feelings and actions are somewhat disconnected from each other so that what they do may be out of keeping with what they say or feel. The symptoms are divided into positive and negative symptoms.

Positive symptoms include: hallucinations, that is hearing, seeing, feeling or smelling something which is not actually there; and delusions which are false and normally unusual beliefs, for example, believing that you are someone famous.

Negative symptoms affect someones interest, energy and emotional life. As a result, the person with schizophrenia may not bother to get up or go out, they may not wash and they may find it hard to talk to other people.

New ways of producing pictures of the brain shows that some people with schizophrenia have larger spaces in the brain than people who do not suffer from the illness. This suggests that parts of the brain may not have developed quite normally. The two main theories to explain this are complications during birth and a virus infection during the early months of pregnancy.

Inheritance patterns and prenatal diagnosis

Inheritance patterns

No-one knows for sure as yet what causes schizophrenia but causation is likely to be genetic rather than up-bringing. In people with a parent who has Schizophrenia, there is a 1 in 10 risk of developing the condition. Whereas the risk factor in the general population is 1 in 100. It is believed that heredity provides about half the explanation of the illness but as yet the gene or combination of genes responsible has yet to be discovered.

Prenatal diagnosis

None

Medical text written July 1999 by Professor Julian Leff. **Last updated September 2007 by Professor Julian Leff, Institute of Psychiatry, London, UK.**

Contact a Family Helpline 0808 808 3555

Further online resources

Medical texts in *The Contact a Family Directory* are designed to give a short, clear description of specific conditions and rare disorders. More extensive information on this condition can be found on a range of reliable, validated websites. Further information on these resources can be found in our **Medical Information on the Internet** article on page 21.

Support

Rethink

28 Castle Street, Kingston upon Thames KT1 1SS   Tel: 0845 456 0455 New enquiries
Tel: 020 8974 6814 Advice Service (Mon, Wed & Fri, 10am - 3pm; Tue & Thur,
10am - 1pm)   Fax: 020 8547 3862   e-mail: advice@rethink.org
Web: http://www.rethink.org
Web: http://www.mentalhealthshop.org (publications website)
Rethink is a National Registered Charity No. 271028, established in 1972, formerly known as the National Schizophrenia Fellowship. It works to help everyone affected by severe mental illness recover a better quality of life by providing quality support, services and information and by influencing local, regional and national policies. Rethink is the largest mental health voluntary organisation in Europe. It offers advice and advocacy services, day care schemes, employment projects, registered nursing or residential care homes, supported accommodation projects and training courses. It also campaigns to influence the national and local decision makers about mental health issues. It publishes a quarterly magazine and has a wide range of information available, details on request. Rethink has around 7,000 members.
Group details last confirmed October 2006.

NSF (Scotland)

Claremont House, 130 East Claremont Street, Edinburgh EH7 4LB   Tel: 0131 557 8969
Fax: 0131 557 8968   e-mail: info@nsfscot.org.uk   Web: http://www.nsfscot.org.uk
NSF (Scotland) is a Scottish Registered Charity No. 13649, established in 1984. It offers support to people affected by mental illness including carers. It has a network of local support groups, provides a range of information (details on request), manages drop-in centres, employment support officers, Carers' Officers and an online Carers' Forum. NSF (Scotland) information services respond to over 3,000 calls a year and 3,000 people also use the project services annually.
Group details last confirmed October 2007.

SCLERODERMA

Background

Scleroderma (hard skin) is a little-known disease of the connective tissue, immune system and blood vessels which primarily affects women in the child-bearing years, though it can affect anyone of any age. It results in taut, hard, discoloured skin and may also affect the internal organs.

What are the symptoms?

Scleroderma is divided into localised forms (morphoea, linear scleroderma) and generalised scleroderma (systemic sclerosis, SSc). SSc has a severe form with patients having wide spread skin involvement and a mild form with patients having skin involvement only in the hands, lower arms, feet, lower legs and face. The severe form, diffuse cutaneous SSc, affects forty per cent of sufferers; the mild form, limited cutaneous SSc, sixty per cent. In the **severe** form, wide areas of the skin are affected and internal organ involvement occurs early. Scleroderma can be fatal, with lung disease as the chief cause of death. Survivors may have a reduced quality of life with breathlessness, kidney disease, heart disease, digestive problems and reduced function in joints, muscles and hands. In the **mild** form, there is limited skin involvement with the later development of gut disease (and thus difficulty in swallowing and eating) and lung problems, usually pulmonary hypertension. Additionally there may be calcinosis (deposits of calcium which mass under the skin and protrude), dry eyes and mouth, ulceration and a very poor circulation.

Juvenile scleroderma differs from the adult disease in that localised forms predominate. The juvenile disease attacks particularly the skin, muscles, joints, tendons and bones, with internal organ involvement a rarity. Childhood morphoea may last three to four years then resolve spontaneously, but the linear form may lead to growth defects. The UK Scleroderma Childhood Register is based at the ARC Epidemiology Unit, University of Manchester. The register is funded by the Raynaud's & Scleroderma Association which supports children with Scleroderma and Raynaud's Phenomenon.

Inheritance patterns and prenatal diagnosis

Inheritance patterns

None.

Prenatal diagnosis

None.

Medical text written March 1992 by Professor Carol Black. **Last updated August 2002 by Professor Carol Black, Consultant Rheumatologist, Royal Free Hospital, London, UK.**

Contact a Family Helpline 0808 808 3555

Further online resources

Medical texts in *The Contact a Family Directory* are designed to give a short, clear description of specific conditions and rare disorders. More extensive information on this condition can be found on a range of reliable, validated websites. Further information on these resources can be found in our **Medical Information on the Internet** article on page 21.

Support

The Scleroderma Society

PO Box 581, Chichester PO19 9EW   Tel: 0800 311 2756 Advice Line
 e-mail: info@sclerodermasociety.co.uk   Web: http://www.sclerodermasociety.co.uk
The Society is a National Registered Charity No. 286736, established in 1982. It offers support to all people with scleroderma, including families of children, by patient information leaflets, a telephone advice line, website with message board and e-mail. It has a number of area groups and contact persons. It publishes a quarterly newsletter and has information available, details on request. The Society responds to approximately 600 enquiries a year. Group details last updated May 2007.

Support is also available from the Raynaud's and Scleroderma Association (see entry, Raynaud's Phenomenon).

SCOLIOSIS

Background

Scoliosis is a lateral (sideways) curvature of the spine associated with rotation so that in the thoracic spine the ribs on the convex side are displaced backwards. It is very common with twenty-five per cent of the population having some degree of spinal asymmetry in childhood. Curves over 20° occur in 1 to 2 in 1,000 boys and 4 to 5 in 1,000 girls. Sixty-five per cent of all cases are idiopathic (cause not known). Most scoliosis occurs in girls at the start of adolescence.

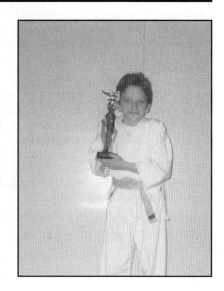

When idiopathic curvature occurs at or shortly after birth (infantile curves), the ratio is reversed and boys are often slightly more affected than girls. Interestingly, adolescent curve tends to be more convex to the right whereas infantile ones are to the left. In babies early diagnosis and treatment is particularly important.

What are the causes?

Scoliosis may also develop as a result of congenital malformations of the spine such as hemi-vertebra or fused vertebrae, or in association with spina bifida (see entry).

Scoliosis may develop as the result of neurological disease for example poliomyelitis or Friedreich's Ataxia (see entries). It may also occur in brittle bone disease, or in specific syndromes such as Marfan, Rett syndrome and Neurofibromatosis (see entries).

Inheritance patterns and prenatal diagnosis

Inheritance patterns

There is evidence that idiopathic scoliosis is familial. Where the cause of scoliosis is specific, the pattern of inheritance will depend upon the disorder concerned.

Prenatal diagnosis

None, except where specific conditions are concerned: for example, in spina bifida where amniocentesis at sixteen weeks is used. Ultrasound scanning can also identify spinal cord and vertebral defects.

Medical text written November 1991 by Mr M Edgar. **Last updated April 2002 by Mr M Edgar, Consultant Orthopaedic and Spinal Surgeon, Middlesex Hospital, London and Royal National Orthopaedic Hospital, Stanmore, UK.**

Further online resources

Medical texts in *The Contact a Family Directory* are designed to give a short, clear description of specific conditions and rare disorders. More extensive information on this condition can be found on a range of reliable, validated websites. Further information on these resources can be found in our **Medical Information on the Internet** article on page 21.

Support

Scoliosis Association (UK)
Unit 4, Ivebury Court, 325 Latimer Road, London W10 6RA
Tel: 020 8964 1166 Helpline (Mon-Thur, 10am-3pm)
Tel: 020 8964 5343 (Mon-Thur, 10am-3pm)   e-mail: sauk@sauk.org.uk
Web: http://www.sauk.org.uk
The Association is a National Registered Charity No. 285290, established in 1981 as the Scoliosis Self Help Group. It offers contact with other families and individuals and it has a nationwide network of voluntary branches. It publishes a newsletter twice a year and has information available, details on request. The Association has over 3,000 members.
Group details last updated October 2007.

SELECTIVE MUTISM

Background

A crucial diagnostic element of selective mutism (SM) is that the child has the ability to both comprehend spoken language and to speak, but yet fails to do so in select settings. Children with SM persistently lack the ability to speak in some settings (for example, school) but not in others (for example, home). In most children, SM is a passing phase and the ability to communicate in all settings is regained by adulthood. SM may, however, continue throughout adolescence or prevent the young person from acquiring age-appropriate social skills.

What are the symptoms?

SM may affect a child's ability to talk with specific members of the immediate family at home as well as teachers or peers at school or in other social situations. Children respond or make their needs known by nodding their heads, pointing or by remaining expressionless or motionless until someone correctly guesses what they want. SM may affect a child's educational performance but progress at school is not impeded in those situations where speaking is not required.

What are the causes?

SM is often not recognised because a child's behaviour is attributed to shyness or embarrassment. In the past, there was a tendency to perceive SM children as stubborn and oppositional. More recent research, however, indicates that in most cases SM is the result of crippling anxiety. Stressful early experiences, a clash of cultures between home and school, language difficulties, and/or unaccustomed expectations at school, may predispose a child to SM.

When under stress, children may become physically rigid and eye-contact increases their discomfort. Children may have the desire to speak but are over-come by 'stage-fright' and hence remain silent. In some cases, SM is known to be preceded by delayed milestones and speech and language difficulties. A psychological assessment may be useful to exclude the presence of learning problems. The usual onset of SM is around three years when the child enters a play-group. SM may commence later after a trauma or post-operatively and is then known as 'traumatic mutism.'

How is it treated?

Treatment is more likely to be successful if started early before the child assumes a 'non-speaking identity.' The most effective way of helping can be through a programme in which teachers and parents participate. Such a programme is based on a 'step-by-step' approach which aims at reducing the child's anxiety about speaking through a technique known as 'stimulus fading'. This involves moving the child by manageable small steps from a situation where there has been no speech to a situation where there is speech. The child's co-operation is essential and is gained by making the exercise enjoyable and rewarding. Another method which may be effective is play therapy and play with puppets.

Inheritance patterns and prenatal diagnosis
Inheritance patterns

Although SM may occur in any family, there may a familiar component in some families.

Prenatal diagnosis

Not applicable.

Medical text written July 2002 by Contact a Family. Approved July 2002 by Alice Sluckin, Hon. Visiting Fellow, Department of Psychology, University of Leicester, Leicester, UK.

Support
SMIRA (Selective Mutism Information and Research Association)
13 Humberstone Drive, Leicester LE5 0RE   Tel: 0116 212 7411 (Tue,Wed & Fri, 4-7pm)
e-mail: smiraleicester@hotmail.com
Web: http://www.selectivemutism.co.uk
SMIRA is a National Registered Charity No. 1022673, established in 1992. It supports families and offers advice to parents, teachers, speech therapists, psychologists and other interested professionals. SMIRA is based in Leicester, where it holds national parents meetings on an annual basis. It aims to put families in touch on a regional basis, hosts an e-mail discussion group and publishes a newsletter three times a year. It has information leaflets available and also a number of publications, including a video - details on request. The Association has over 200 members.
Group details last confirmed September 2007.

SEPTO-OPTIC DYSPLASIA

Background

Septo-optic dysplasia (SOD) is the commonest of the midline cerebral/cranial abnormalities involving the spectrum of holoprosencephaly (see entry), absence of the corpus callosum (see entry, Agenesis of the Corpus Callosum) and midline cleft palate and also involving the hypothalamopituitary region.

It comprises two out of the three features of optic nerve hypoplasia (ONH) (see entry) unilateral or bilateral, absence of the septum pellucidum and pituitary dysfunction. Because fifty per cent of patients with this condition have a septum pellucidum present, the older name of De Morsier's syndrome may be preferable.

What are the symptoms?

The loss of vision is extremely variable. Although the optic nerve and cerebral abnormalities are fixed, the pituitary dysfunction (see entry, Pituitary Disorders) is often variable and may well evolve with time. It also has the unusual characteristic of being commonly associated with diabetes insipidus, as well as anterior pituitary dysfunction. The anterior pituitary function commonly evolves with time and may well also be associated with retention of gonadotrophin secretion with either normal or precocious puberty (see entry, Premature Sexual Maturation)

All children with midline cerebral or cranial abnormalities should be seen by an endocrinologist. Epilepsy (see entry) in such children is often due to the endocrinopathy (abnormal plasma sodium concentration in diabetes insipidus and hypoglycaemia associated with growth hormone deficiency and/or cortisol deficiency) rather than due to the structural brain abnormality.

How is it diagnosed?

Since SOD can be highly variable in terms of its endocrine phenotype, with the possibility of evolution of other hormonal deficiencies over time, a child with the condition needs to be carefully evaluated with close monitoring and follow up. In particular, cortisol deficiency is not always easy to diagnose, and a careful evaluation of the hypothalamo-pituitary-adrenal axis is mandatory, as missing the diagnosis may lead to hypoglycaemia particularly at times of intercurrent illness. Other features of SOD include obesity, behavioural and learning difficulties, and sleep disorders.

Inheritance patterns and prenatal diagnosis

Inheritance patterns

Septo-optic dysplasia is largely thought to be a sporadic disorder. However, in the light of the recent identification of the HESXI gene, it is now clear that genetic mutations in this gene may account for some cases of SOD.

Additionally, there is increasing evidence to suggest that septo-optic dysplasia is a multigenic disorder, with other genes being involved, and possible interaction with environmental factors, ultimately leading to a phenotype.

Prenatal diagnosis

At present, this is only available for those rare families with an autosomal recessive form of SOD due to HEXSI mutations.

Medical text written October 2001 by Dr R Stanhope and Dr M Dattani. **Last updated September 2005 by Dr R Stanhope, Consultant Paediatric Endocrinologist, Great Ormond Street Hospital, London, UK and Dr M Dattani, Reader and Hon. Consultant in Paediatric Endocrinology, Institute of Child Health, London, UK.**

Further online resources

Medical texts in *The Contact a Family Directory* are designed to give a short, clear description of specific conditions and rare disorders. More extensive information on this condition can be found on a range of reliable, validated websites. Further information on these resources can be found in our **Medical Information on the Internet** article on page 21.

Support

SOD/ONH Support Network

Corpus Christi Barge, Meadow Lane, Oxford OX4 4BJ   Tel: 07930 627 144
e-mail: arvatec@tesco.net   Web: http://www.focusfamilies.org

The Network is a family support network, established in 2000. It offers support for families and linking where possible. It publishes a newsletter and has information available, details on request. The Network has over 50 UK families in membership. Over 300 families world wide link through Focus Families which has groups in Australia, Canada, the USA as well as in the UK.

Group details last updated February 2008.

SHWACHMAN-DIAMOND SYNDROME

Shwachman-Diamond syndrome: Shwachman syndrome

Background

Shwachman-Diamond syndrome is a rare, multi-system disorder in which affected individuals have a defective pancreas that fails to secrete digestive enzymes, poor growth and a predisposition to recurrent infection and blood disorders.

What are the symptoms?

The digestive defects results in diarrhoea and fatty stools with fat soluble vitamin and mineral deficiency. Poor growth is an integral part of the condition in about fifty per cent of individuals. Specific skeletal defects are present including metaphyseal dysostosis and a thoracic dystrophy. Dental problems are common and can be severe. Mild to moderate learning difficulties are present as well as behavioural and feeding problems in up to fifty per cent of affected children.

Expression of the disorder is variable and ranges from mild pancreatic insufficiency to a serious life-threatening disorder. Some spontaneous improvement in symptoms may occur, usually after the age of eight years.

Recurrent infection, which may be life threatening, is due to both minor immunodeficiency and neutrophil defects. In about sixty per cent of cases, neutropenia is present and this may be cyclical. In severe cases more serious haematological disorder may occur with aplastic anaemia (anemia - US) myelodysplasia and possibly acute myeloid leukaemia. Rarely, hepatic fibrosis and ichthyotic skin lesions may occur.

How is it diagnosed?

Diagnosis requires specialist gastroenterological and haematological investigation.

How is it treated?

Treatment is by pancreatic enzyme replacement and multi-vitamin supplements with prophylactic antibiotics to prevent infection and aggressive treatment of infections when they occur. Haematological and immunological defects may require appropriate specific treatment. Psychological intervention and feeding interventions may also be needed.

A register of patients is maintained in the Department of Gastroenterology, Great Ormond Street Hospital for Children, London WC1N 3JH.

Inheritance patterns and prenatal diagnosis
Inheritance patterns

Autosomal recessive but may occur sporadically. The gene affected is the SBDS gene found on chromosome 7. five per cent of all known cases have a common compound heterozygote mutation. Genetic testing following careful clinical evaluation is available at the North West Regional Genetics Reference Laboratory, St. Mary's Hospital, Hathersage Road, Manchester M13 0JH, Tel: 0161 276 6122 / 6605, contact Dr Martin Schwarz, Consultant Clinical Molecular Geneticist.

Prenatal diagnosis

Available for those with confirmed mutations in the SBDS gene.

Medical text written December 1993 by Professor P Milla. **Last updated October 2005 by Professor P Milla, Professor of Paediatric Gastroenterology and Dr N Shah, Consultant Paediatric Gastroenterologist, Great Ormond Street Hospital, London, UK.**

Further online resources

Medical texts in *The Contact a Family Directory* are designed to give a short, clear description of specific conditions and rare disorders. More extensive information on this condition can be found on a range of reliable, validated websites. Further information on these resources can be found in our **Medical Information on the Internet** article on page 21.

Support
Shwachman-Diamond Support

9 Tippett Close, Nuneaton, Warwickshire CV11 4SU   Tel: 02476 345199
e-mail: enquiries@shwachman-diamondsupport.org
Web: http://www.shwachman-diamondsupport.org
The Group is a National Registered Charity No. 1081122, established in 2000. It offers support for affected persons and their families and promotes research initiatives. It aims to raise awareness of Shwachman syndrome among the medical profession, support agencies and the public. It offers an information booklet and bi-annual family conferences. The group has a medical advisory board.
Group details last updated January 2008.

SICKLE CELL DISORDERS

Sickle Cell disorders: Sickle Cell disease

Background

Sickle Cell disorders are a group of inheritable genetic conditions in which there is an abnormality of the haemoglobin. Haemoglobin carries oxygen to the various organs of the body and is contained in the red blood cells. In the sickle cell disorders some of the red blood cells assume a sickle shape following the release of oxygen. This abnormal shape causes the cells to clump together making their passage through smaller blood vessels difficult, which may lead to blockage of these small blood vessels and an associated inflammatory reaction.

The most common Sickle Cell disorder is Sickle Cell anaemia, Hb SS, and in the UK the next most common are Hb SC disease (also called Sickle Hb C disease or Hb SC) and sickle beta thalassaemia (Hb S/beta thal).

What are the symptoms?

Symptoms are rarely apparent before the age of three months due to the continuing effect of fetal (baby) haemoglobin. The most common symptoms are episodic pain in the bones, joints, abdomen and other parts of the body and these are known as "painful crises." They may be precipitated by cold, dehydration, or infections. Other problems associated with the condition may affect the spleen or cause jaundice, strokes, blood in the urine, leg ulcers, problems with the hips and/or shoulders, eye problems, lung problems, priapism (an abnormal, sometimes persistent and often painful erection), enuresis (incontinence of urine) and delayed puberty.

If strokes occur, they usually do so during childhood and they may be recurrent. If a child has had a stroke, treatment with regular blood transfusions may reduce the chance of a further stroke. However, if any person has regular blood transfusions they will also need regular treatment to avoid iron overload from the blood transfusions. This is because iron overload can cause considerable harm if it is allowed to develop.

The painful crisis can be extremely variable. First, it may occur frequently, or it may occur only rarely. Second, the severity of the pain can vary a lot from one episode to another and from one person to another.

How is it diagnosed?

Sickle Cell disorders mainly occur in people whose ancestors are of African, African-Caribbean, Mediterranean, Middle East or Indian origins. Tests which can identify carriers or individuals with sickle cell disorder may be undertaken in high risk groups in pregnancy and before anaesthesia.

How is it treated?

Painful crises usually disappear spontaneously within a few days and most can be helped by simple measures at home such as rest, fluids and simple pain killers (such as paracetamol and ibuprofen). Unfortunately some painful crises are associated with severe pain requiring treatment with strong pain killers and these situations usually need admission to hospital. Although we know some of the situations that precipitate painful crises (see above) there is still a lot that is not known and they often occur in an unpredictable way. Damage to the hips or shoulders may cause severe chronic pain and disability and may need treatment with artificial joints. This chronic pain is different from a painful crisis and is often more difficult to treat.

Inheritance patterns and prenatal diagnosis

Inheritance patterns

Sickle cell disorders are autosomal recessive.

Prenatal diagnosis

Chorionic villus sampling (CVS) at any time after ten weeks of pregnancy or Fetal blood tests later in pregnancy (approximately nineteen to twenty weeks) can be used to diagnose sickle cell disorders prenatally. For CVS samples it is also important to have blood samples from both parents.

Medical text written August 2002 by Dr A Stephens. **Last updated August 2005 by Dr A Stephens, Consultant Haematologist, King's College Hospital, London, UK.**

Further online resources

Medical texts in *The Contact a Family Directory* are designed to give a short, clear description of specific conditions and rare disorders. More extensive information on this condition can be found on a range of reliable, validated websites. Further information on these resources can be found in our **Medical Information on the Internet** article on page 21.

Support

The Sickle Cell Society
54 Station Road, London NW10 4UA   Tel: 0800 0015660 (24 hour helpline)
Tel: 020 8961 7795   Fax: 020 8961 8346   e-mail: info@sicklecellsociety.org
Web: http://www.sicklecellsociety.org
The Society is a National Registered Charity No. 1046631, established in 1979. The Society offers a Regional Care Support Service supported by the Community Fund which provides care outside of statutory provisions and helps to create and strengthen support groups that will provide a forum for advice, discussion and community involvement. It also offers support through contact with others, where possible, together with welfare, educational grants and holiday schemes for affected children. It publishes a quarterly newsletter and has information available, details on request. Please send SAE. The Society has around 600-700 members.
Group details last updated November 2007.

Sickle Cell & Young Stroke Survivors

801 Old Kent Road, London SE15 1NX   Tel: 0800 528 2785 Helpline (Mon-Fri, 12-3pm)
Tel: 020 7635 9810   e-mail: info@scyss.org   Web: http://www.scyss.org

SCYSS is a parent support group, established in 2005 by the mother of a child with Sickle Cell disorder who had a stroke. Children with Sickle Cell disorder are a great risk of one or more strokes. SYCSS offers support to families and advice to professionals by telephone, e-mail and letter. It has information available, details on request.
Group details last updated January 2007.

Across the UK, a child is diagnosed with a severe disability every 25 minutes and over 98% of disabled children are cared for at home by a parent or other family member who didn't "apply for the job" but who has quickly had to become an expert.

SILVER-RUSSELL SYNDROME

Silver-Russell syndrome: Asymmetry Dwarfism; Russell-Silver syndrome; Silver's syndrome

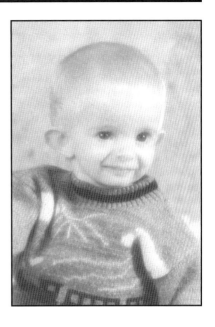

Background

This syndrome is a congenital condition characterised by significant asymmetry and short stature.

What are the symptoms?

Other characteristics may include a short incurved 5th finger, triangular facial features, turned down corners of the mouth, café au lait spots and syndactyly. In a small minority of cases mild neurological delay can occur. In the first year of life excessive sweating, particularly at night is common and may be a reflection of chronic hypoglycaemia (low blood sugar). This is extremely important to recognise and may well be the cause of the educational difficulties that have been identified in such children.

How is it treated?

Continuous overnight feeds using gastric tubes or gastrostomy may need to be considered and growth hormone treatment may also be helpful.

Intra-uterine growth retardation without dysmorphic features is also covered by the group.

Inheritance patterns and prenatal diagnosis

Inheritance patterns

This is not yet fully determined. It has been suggested that while many cases are sporadic, about ten per cent of cases are due to inheriting two copies of Chromosome 7 from their mother. Another fifty per cent have an abnormality on Chromosome 11.

However there is a congenital association between siblings which may result from placental insufficiency. Such placental problems may be hereditary.

Prenatal diagnosis

There is no biochemical diagnosis but serial ultrasound assessments starting from early pregnancy will confirm intra-uterine growth retardation

Medical text written November 1991 by Contact a Family. Approved November 1991 by Professor M Patton, Professor of Medical Genetics, St Georges Hospital Medical School, London, UK and Dr J E Wraith, Consultant Paediatrician, Royal Manchester Children's Hospital, Manchester, UK. **Last updated July 2006 by Dr R Stanhope, Consultant Paediatric Endocrinologist, Great Ormond Street Hospital, London, UK.**

Further online resources

Medical texts in *The Contact a Family Directory* are designed to give a short, clear description of specific conditions and rare disorders. More extensive information on this condition can be found on a range of reliable, validated websites. Further information on these resources can be found in our **Medical Information on the Internet** article on page 21.

Support

The Silver-Russell Support Group works under the umbrella of the Child Growth Foundation (see entry, Restricted Growth), from which support and advice is available.

Do you run a local or national support group? Thinking of setting one up? Find the information you need in the Contact a Family Group Action Pack, Tel: 020 7608 8700 for details.

SJÖGREN SYNDROME

Background

Sjögren syndrome (SS) is a condition in which the immune system attacks salivary and tear (lachrymal) glands leading to dryness of the eyes and the mouth.

What are the symptoms?

In common with other auto-immune diseases, it can have more general (systemic) effects including tiredness, fatigue and aching joints and muscles. Kidneys, brain or heart are rarely affected. SS is unlikely to lead to serious disability or reduced lifespan.

The disorder is extremely variable in its severity, presentation and disease associations. There are two main types of the syndrome:

Non-systemic Sjögren syndrome. The features of Sjögren syndrome are limited to dryness of the eyes and mouth without involvement of the other body systems.

Systemic Sjögren syndrome. There are associated problems of joints, blood vessels and/or skin. Only a minority of people will experience other associated problems, even after many years of the disease.

Almost everyone with SS has dryness of mouth and grittiness of the eyes, but other secretions can be affected such as dryness of the air passages including nose and trachea. This tends to make the airways hypersensitive to irritants so very few people with SS tend to smoke.

SS also affects the sweat glands. This causes the skin to become dry and sensitive to strong sunlight and sun block creams are usually recommended during summer. In addition, regular application of moisturising creams is appropriate. Dry hair is one of the less common manifestations of the disease and may be alleviated with specially formulated shampoos.

Some people with SS may experience irritable bowel syndrome (see entry). This can cause lower abdominal pain and alteration in bowel habit. In some ways, it is similar to the 'irritable airways' and may be associated with low volume intestinal mucous secretions. Lack of mucus production in the bowel may cause constipation in some people, however, a high fibre diet may be sufficient to control for these problems.

Women with SS may experience vaginal dryness. In menopausal women, hormone replacement therapy (HRT) alleviates this, as well as relieving hot flushes and improving a sense of overall well-being. Fertility is not affected by SS and complications in pregnancy, which may include problems in the baby's heart, affects only a minority (two per cent) of women. Cardiac anomalies may be detected on routine ultrasound scans from about twelve weeks. Expert treatment and the involvement of a paediatrician from an early stage of pregnancy is recommended if this abnormality is detected.

Tiredness, lethargy and malaise are features common to many people with SS and may lead to feelings of complete exhaustion. Because these features are rarely associated with other clinical symptoms, they may be the source of social frustration given that an individual otherwise 'looks well.' Sometimes the tiredness follows a cyclical course during the day and may also be worse premenstrually. In such instances, laboratory tests for other causes of tiredness e.g. thyroid disease and anaemia (anemia - US) should be ordered, though the results are frequently normal. Medical treatment, particularly hydroxycholoroquine, has a modest therapeutic effect on fatigue in some people. Most sufferers use a 'coping strategy' that works for them, such as a period of rest during the mid-afternoon. Recent research has shown that graded exercise regimes, with a view to increasing physical fitness, can have substantial benefit both in improving quality of sleep as well as treating tiredness.

Arthritis of the joints is common but usually follows a relatively mild course. Small joints in the hands and feet tend to be affected. Pain is often more troublesome than swelling, and inflammation of the joints leading to destruction and deformity is rare in primary Sjögren syndrome. True inflammation of the muscles (myositis) is very rare but is recognised as causing pain, tenderness and weakness of the muscles, particularly around the shoulders and pelvis. Increased sensitivity of blood vessels to the cold causing Raynaud's phenomenon (see entry) is common. Rarely the kidney (see entry) may be involved.

True inflammation of blood vessels may occur and is termed 'vasculitis'. This tends to cause rash or ulceration of the skin in the legs.

Migraine (see entry) does appear to be more common in people with SS and some affected people develop true inflammation of the lungs not due to infection. This can cause breathlessness on exertion and a nonproductive cough.

Inheritance patterns and prenatal diagnosis
Inheritance patterns
Sjögren syndrome is not a true genetic disease, though the risk is inherited. This means that if you have the disease, the chances that a close relative will also get the disease is about 1 in 20. Some of the genes that are associated with SS are known. Chief amongst these is DR3 (a gene which is involved in the immune system) which increases the chance of getting SS about four-fold. However there are many people who are DR3 positive who do not have the disease.

Prenatal diagnosis

None.

Medical text written February 2002 by Professor P Venables. **Last updated February 2008 by Professor P Venables, Professor of Viral Immunorheumatology, Kennedy Institute of Rheumatology Division, Imperial College School of Medicine, London, UK.**

Further online resources

Medical texts in *The Contact a Family Directory* are designed to give a short, clear description of specific conditions and rare disorders. More extensive information on this condition can be found on a range of reliable, validated websites. Further information on these resources can be found in our **Medical Information on the Internet** article on page 21.

Support

British Sjögren Syndrome Association

PO Box 10867, Birmingham B16 0ZW   Tel: 0121 455 6532

e-mail: office@bssa.uk.net   Web: http://www.bssa.uk.net

The Association is a National Registered Charity No. 1101571, established in 1990. It offers support , advice and information by telephone, letter and e-mail and a forum for the exchange of views on living with the condition via its regional group network. It publishes a quarterly newsletter and has a variety of information available, details on request. The Association has over 2,500 members.

Group details last updated September 2007.

SMITH-LEMLI-OPITZ SYNDROME

Background

Smith-Lemli-Opitz syndrome (SLOS) is a multiple congenital abnormality syndrome first described in 1964. Thirty years later, SLOS became the first such syndrome to be identified as an 'inborn error of metabolism', in this case due to deficiency of the enzyme called 7-dehydrocholesterol reductase.

What are the symptoms?

Congenital abnormalities that are present in children with SLOS include microcephaly (see entry), cleft palate (see entry, Cleft Lip and/or Palate), abnormalities of the fingers and toes (polydactyly and syndactyly) and abnormalities in development of the heart, kidneys, liver, and lungs (see entries). Not all these organs are affected in each case. Underdevelopment of external genitalia occurs in males.

Some infants are very severely affected and, in the past, the most severe form of the condition was called SLOS type II. Miscarriage, stillbirth or death in the first weeks of life may occur in such severe cases. In surviving infants, slow growth and poor weight gain is the rule and feeding via a gastrostomy may be required.

As the infant gets older, severe learning difficulties usually become evident but it is not uncommon for mildly affected individuals to present with behavioural problems, often with autistic-type behaviours (see entry, Autism Spectrum disorders) and tendency to self-injury. Individuals with SLOS are very rarely able to live independently.

Psychological and behavioural characteristics

The information below has been drawn up by Dr A Kuczynski, Child Clinical Psychologist, South London & Maudsley NHS Trust, London, UK and Dr O Udwin, Consultant Clinical Child Psychologist, West London Mental Health NHS Trust, London, UK. It has also been approved by the Society for the Study of Behavioural Phenotypes.

In addition to the genetic, physiological, and physical features, Smith-Lemli-Opitz syndrome is also associated with psychological and behavioural characteristics.

As noted above, most affected individuals have a learning disability. This can be severe or profound, but intellectually more able people have also been reported. Occasionally, IQ estimates can be around the "borderline" or lower limit of the normal range.

A substantial proportion of those with the syndrome, perhaps even the majority, display repeated self-injurious behaviour, such as head-banging or biting. Many exhibit a distinctive forceful upper body arching and thrusting movement, known as opistokinesis, in which they can throw themselves backwards. Some have other repetitive movements.

Behavioural features may also include heightened sensitivity or hyperreactivity to sensory stimuli, including light, disturbance of the sleep cycle, temperature dysregulation, and difficulties in social communication. The pattern of behavioural impairments is often consistent with diagnosis of an autistic spectrum disorder.

What are the causes?

The enzyme 7-dehydrocholesterol reductase normally drives the conversion of the chemical called 7-dehydrocholesterol to cholesterol. Therefore, deficiency of the enzyme leads to increased 7-dehydrocholesterol level and simultaneously restricts the body's ability to produce cholesterol. Although increased cholesterol in the blood leads to heart disease in adult life, cholesterol is also an essential chemical that governs normal development of the fetus during pregnancy and permits optimal growth and brain development after birth.

How is it treated?

In surviving infants and children, good medical care and nutritional supplements have extended life span. In view of the enzyme deficiency and low level of cholesterol in the blood, treatments with cholesterol supplements are currently being assessed to determine whether these will improve health and lessen the incidence of behavioural problems.

Inheritance patterns and prenatal diagnosis

Inheritance patterns

SLOS is inherited as an autosomal recessive condition.

Prenatal diagnosis

Prenatal testing is available through measurement of 7-dehydrocholesterol levels in tissue obtained from the pregnancy (by chorionic villus sampling or by amniocentesis). This is a specialised test that should be planned in advance. Molecular genetic (DNA) tests are available if the specific gene changes or mutations that cause the disease in an affected individual can be identified. Carriers may be identified by this method. In theory, pre-implantation genetic diagnosis may be possible for some families.

Medical text written July 2003 by Contact a Family. Approved July 2003 by Dr J Tolmie, Consultant Clinical Geneticist, Ferguson-Smith Centre for Clinical Genetics, Glasgow, UK. Psychological and behavioural characteristics last updated February 2004 by Dr A Kuczynski, Child Clinical Psychologist, South London & Maudsley NHS Trust, London, UK and Dr O Udwin, Consultant Clinical Child Psychologist, West London Mental Health NHS Trust, London, UK.

Further online resources

Medical texts in *The Contact a Family Directory* are designed to give a short, clear description of specific conditions and rare disorders. More extensive information on this condition can be found on a range of reliable, validated websites. Further information on these resources can be found in our **Medical Information on the Internet** article on page 21.

Support

While there is no specific support group in the UK for this condition, information is available from Climb (see entry, Metabolic diseases) and support is available from a group of families under the umbrella of Climb.

In 2008 a new carer's strategy for England will be announced by the Department of Health.

SMITH-MAGENIS SYNDROME

Background

Smith-Magenis syndrome (SMS) is a rare condition that is associated with developmental delay, learning difficulties, behavioural difficulties and a disturbed sleep pattern. SMS was first described by Ann Smith and colleagues in 1982. About 1 in 25,000 children are born with this condition, and it is probably under diagnosed.

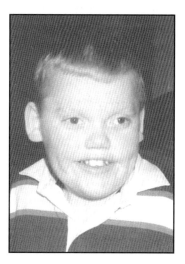

What are the symptoms?

Most children with SMS have developmental delay and moderate to severe learning difficulties. In infancy low muscle tone, feeding difficulties, failure to thrive and frequent ear infections are common. Speech delay tends to be more pronounced than motor delay, and language comprehension is more impaired than expression.

The most distinctive features of SMS are the behavioural problems. These include self-injurious behaviours such as hand biting, self-pinching or scratching, picking at sores, hitting the head or body, and tearing or picking fingernails or the skin around the nails. Some affected patients also demonstrate 'self-hugging' and 'lick and flip' (licking their fingers and rapidly flicking the pages of a book) behaviours. Other behavioural problems include aggression, frequent temper tantrums, hyperactivity, restlessness and distractibility, and severe sleep disturbance, including difficulties falling asleep, shortened sleep cycles, frequent and prolonged night waking and early morning waking. These abnormalities and a phase shift of the circadian rhythm of melatonin are suggestive of an underlying biological clock problem in the syndrome. Autistic-type behaviours such as resistance to change, repetitive questioning, and preoccupations with particular topics are also common.

In many cases the severe behaviour difficulties in children with the syndrome persist into adulthood. Some individuals show improved behaviour with age, but others show a worsening of the aggression and self injury or no change. At the same time, people with SMS are often described as loving and caring, eager to please and with a good sense of humour. They love adult attention and enjoy interacting with adults.

Facial features of SMS are fairly distinctive and include a flat, broad head and prominent forehead, heavy brows, up-slanting eyes, depressed nasal bridge, and a wide mouth with fleshy and inverted central portion of the upper lip. Other features include a relatively hoarse, deep voice, short stature, eye problems (squint and iris abnormalities), hearing loss and scoliosis (spinal curvature). Congenital heart disease, epilepsy and kidney abnormalities are less consistent features. Clinical signs of peripheral neuropathy are found in seventy-five per cent of individuals, and include decreased sensitivity to pain and temperature, gait disturbances and muscle weakness.

What are the causes?

It is caused by a small deletion (microdeletion) on chromosome 17 (17p 11.2), which can be detected cytogenetically and/or by a special diagnostic test called Fluorescent in situ hybridisation (FISH) analysis.

How is it diagnosed?

The characteristic behaviour and sleep disturbance coupled with the distinctive facial features often suggest the diagnosis, which can be confirmed by FISH analysis to look for the 17 p 11.2 microdeletion.

Inheritance patterns and prenatal diagnosis

Inheritance patterns

Most cases of SMS are sporadic in origin. Rarely, the 17p11.2 microdeletion may arise in a child because one of the parents might carry a "balanced" rearrangement involving this region of the short arm of one chromosome 17. Therefore, if the diagnosis of SMS is confirmed in a child the parents' chromosomes should also be checked. If the parental chromosomes are normal then the recurrence risk of SMS is likely to be very small.

Prenatal diagnosis

Parents of children with SMS can be offered prenatal diagnosis in future pregnancies. This involves chorionic villus sampling (CVS) between eleven to thirteen weeks gestation, or amniocentesis between fifteen to sixteen weeks gestation, followed by FISH analysis to look for the 17p11.2 microdeletion.

Medical text written July 2003 by Contact a Family. Approved July 2003 by Dr J Tolmie, Consultant Clinical Geneticist, Duncan Guthrie Institute of Medical Genetics, Glasgow, UK. **Last reviewed January 2004 by Dr M Suri, Consultant Clinical Geneticist, City Hospital, Nottingham, UK. Additional material provided by Dr O Udwin, Consultant Clinical Child Psychologist, West London Mental Health NHS Trust, London, UK.**

Further online resources

Medical texts in *The Contact a Family Directory* are designed to give a short, clear description of specific conditions and rare disorders. More extensive information on this condition can be found on a range of reliable, validated websites. Further information on these resources can be found in our **Medical Information on the Internet** article on page 21.

Support

Smith-Magenis Foundation
24 Brook Road, Dersingham, King's Lynn, Norfolk PE31 6LG Tel: 01328 730782
e-mail: info@smith-magenis.co.uk   Web: http://www.smith-magenis.co.uk
The Foundation is a National Registered Charity No. 1072573, established in 1992. It offers support by letter, email and telephone. It also aims to raise awareness of the condition. It publishes a newsletter and has information available, details on request. The Foundation has over 100 families in membership.
Group details last updated September 2005.

Latest figures show that there are thought to be about 770,000 disabled children under 16 living in the UK.

SOTOS SYNDROME

Sotos syndrome: Cerebral Gigantism in Childhood

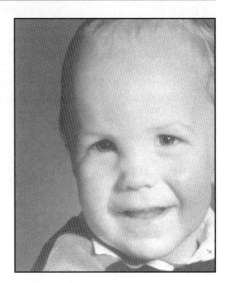

Background
In this rare syndrome babies are generally significantly larger and heavier than average caused by excessive prenatal and early post-natal growth.

What are the symptoms?
Characteristics include macrocephaly (large head) with accelerated bone maturation, delayed development and language problems, widely spaced eyes, prominent jaw, and high arched palate. Intelligence varies from normal to mild learning disability. Children may be clumsy or ataxic (unsteady).

Growth rate usually slows at four to five years. Early adolescent development usually occurs. Adults are usually within normal height parameters. **Weaver syndrome** is a condition characterised by: accelerated growth; mild hypotonia (see entry); loose skin; thin hair; and camptodactyly (permanent immobility of a flexed finger joint).

Psychological and behavioural characteristics
Whereas growth in Sotos syndrome may be seen as accelerated, other aspects of development are often delayed, including achievement of early motor and language milestones. Marked clumsiness, an unsteady gait and poor co-ordination are common, but these difficulties tend to improve with age. Although perhaps half of individuals with Sotos syndrome have mild or borderline learning difficulties, many are of low average or average intellectual ability.

Probably most children with Sotos syndrome are able to attend mainstream schools with appropriate classroom support. Many attain useful skills in reading and writing. Some practical competencies such as understanding of time and money concepts and some daily living skills may represent other areas of strength. That said, some may have specific difficulties with numeracy, and use of language may be repetitive.

Affected individuals are especially prone to anxiety in new situations or when separated from familiar carers and some acquire specific fears or phobias. Some children are also described as having a "difficult" temperament or as irritable, and reports of hyperactivity are common.

Little is known about the long-term psychological and behavioural outcome for adults with Sotos syndrome.

Inheritance patterns and prenatal diagnosis

Inheritance patterns

Most cases are sporadic mutations. Once, established inheritance is autosomal dominant. Weaver syndrome inheritance probably has some pattern of inheritance though this has not been fully determined.

Prenatal diagnosis

Macrocephaly, large hands, long arms and excessive growth are detectable using ultrasound scanning. Genetic counselling is available for affected families.

Medical text written November 1991 by Contact a Family. Approved November 1991 by Professor M Patton, Professor of Medical Genetics, St Georges Hospital Medical School, London, UK and Dr J E Wraith, Consultant Paediatrician, Royal Manchester Children's Hospital, Manchester, UK. Last updated November 1995 by Dr R Stanhope. **Last reviewed July 2006 by Dr R Stanhope, Consultant Paediatric Endocrinologist, Great Ormond Street Hospital, London, UK.**

Further online resources

Medical texts in *The Contact a Family Directory* are designed to give a short, clear description of specific conditions and rare disorders. More extensive information on this condition can be found on a range of reliable, validated websites. Further information on these resources can be found in our **Medical Information on the Internet** article on page 21.

Support

As Sotos syndrome is a growth disorder, information, support and advice is available from the Child Growth Foundation (for contact details see entry, Restricted Growth).

SPEECH AND LANGUAGE IMPAIRMENT

Background
Speech and language impairments can vary greatly in severity. A language difficulty is identified when a child has problems in the acquisition and development of receptive and/or expressive language.

What are the symptoms?
Primary communication difficulties, often called Specific language impairment (SLI) or specific speech and language difficulties (SSLD) occur where the child has developed or is developing within the normal range, and there is no evidence that the difficulty is related to or an outcome of a physical disability (for example, severe or profound hearing loss) or an intellectual impairment. Characteristics in individual cases may vary, and many children do have associated difficulties including mild/moderate hearing impairment, behaviour difficulties, impaired self esteem, and general cognitive ability at the lower end of the normal range.

A **secondary communication difficulty** may be associated with severe or profound hearing or intellectual impairment, and with specific syndromes, chromosome defects, cerebral palsy, accident, injury or disease.

What are the causes?
Causes of language impairment vary greatly.

Inheritance patterns and prenatal diagnosis
Inheritance patterns
Primary problem patterns of inheritance are not known, but there is increasing evidence for genetic predispositions to difficulties with speech and language development.

Secondary problem - will depend upon the cause of the condition but there is good evidence of increased risk of difficulties in acquiring literacy skills, especially reading and spelling, with emerging evidence of increased likelihood of writing difficulties. These children are also at increased risk of behavioural, emotional and social difficulties.
Prenatal diagnosis
This will be possible when the secondary problem is associated with a specific disorder for which prenatal diagnosis has been developed.

Medical text written November 1991 by Contact a Family. Approved November 1991 by Professor M Patton, Professor of Medical Genetics, St Georges Hospital Medical School, London, UK and Dr J E Wraith, Consultant Paediatrician, Royal Manchester Children's Hospital, Manchester, UK. Updated November 2001 by Professor Geoff Lindsay and Professor Julie Dockrell, Institute of Education, London, UK. **Last updated December 2005 by Professor Geoff Lindsay, Professor of Special Educational Needs and Educational Psychology, University of Warwick, Coventry, UK.**

Further online resources

Medical texts in *The Contact a Family Directory* are designed to give a short, clear description of specific conditions and rare disorders. More extensive information on this condition can be found on a range of reliable, validated websites. Further information on these resources can be found in our **Medical Information on the Internet** article on page 21.

Support

Afasic

1st Floor, 20 Bowling Green Lane, London EC1R 0BD
Tel: 0845 355 5577/ 020 7490 9420/21 Helpline   Tel: 020 7490 9410   Fax: 020 7251 2834
e-mail: info@afasic.org.uk   Web: http://www.afasic.org.uk
The organisation is a National Registered Charity No. 1045617, established in 1968. It offers support and information for parents and professional workers together with a nationwide network of self help groups. It publishes a newsletter for members three times a year and has a wide range of information available, details on request.
Group details last updated February 2008.

I CAN Charity

8 Wakley Street, London EC1V 7QE   Tel: 0845 225 4073   Fax: 0845 225 4072
e-mail: info@ican.org.uk   Web: http://www.talkingpoint.org.uk
I CAN is a National Registered Charity No. 210031, established in 1888. I CAN works to support the development of speech, language and communication skills in all children with a special focus on those who find this hard: children with a communication disability. I CAN works to ensure all people who have a responsibility to children, either directly or indirectly, from parents and teachers to policy makers, understand the importance of good communication skills. It does this through information, training, support, raising awareness, campaigning, consultancy and outreach services. They are also involved in direct service provision through two schools for children with severe complex disabilities, and a network of early years provision.
Group details last updated February 2008.

SPINA BIFIDA

Background

Spina bifida is a neural tube defect and is a developmental anomaly which occurs very early in pregnancy. The neural tube develops to form the spinal cord, brain and spine. When Spina Bifida occurs, the tube is split and one or more vertebrae (small bones of the back) fail to form properly, thus leaving a gap.

What are the symptoms?

There are three main types of spina bifida.

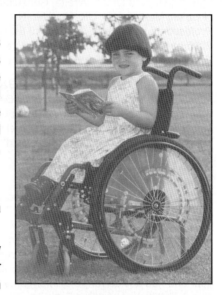

Spina bifida occulta where the only sign of the malformation is a dimple or hair at the site of the defect on the skin of the back. This condition is very mild and is usually symptomless although occasionally there may be continence problems and difficulties with mobility.

In **Spina bifida cystica** a sac or cyst is visible on the back covered by a thin layer of skin. There are two forms: a meningocele and a myelomeningocele. In a **meningocele** the sac contains tissues which cover the spinal cord and cerebro-spinal fluid. The nerves are not normally badly damaged and there is little or no malfunction. This is the least common form of spina bifida. Myelomeningocele is the most common and severest form and is characterised by the inclusion in the sac of nerves and part of the spinal cord as well as tissue and cerebral-spinal fluid. Some degree of paralysis and loss of sensation occur below the site of the defect. The extent of the disability is dependent upon the extent of nerve damage.

Cranium bifida is a failure of development of the bones of the skull. In this form the sac is called an encephalocele. In some cases part of the brain is also enclosed in the sac while in others it contains only tissue and cerebro-spinal fluid. Anencephaly (absent brain) and iniencephaly (badly malformed brain) may also occur and in such cases the child will not survive.

Hydrocephalus is caused by an imbalance between the production and absorption of cerebro-spinal fluid in the brain. About eighty per cent of people with Spina Bifida have Hydrocephalus (see entry).

Inheritance patterns and prenatal diagnosis

Inheritance patterns

Spina bifida has some genetic predisposition. Where a couple have an affected child there is a 1 in 25 chance of an affected pregnancy. For an affected person the risk of an affected child is 1 in 25.

Prenatal diagnosis

A raised alpha-feto protein blood test at sixteen weeks can indicate the presence of a neural tube defect. Amniocentesis at sixteen to eighteen weeks and detailed ultrasound scanning (at over sixteen weeks) can also identify neural tube defects. Unfortunately diagnostic screening for spina bifida is not one hundred per cent accurate. It is now known that taking Folic Acid Supplement of 0.4mg daily prior to conception and for the first three months of pregnancy reduces the risk for all women of having a baby with spina bifida. Women considered to be at risk should take a higher dose (4mg) prescribed by their doctor.

Medical text written November 1991 by Contact a Family. Approved November 1991 by Professor M Patton, Professor of Medical Genetics, St Georges Hospital Medical School, London, UK and Dr J E Wraith, Consultant Paediatrician, Royal Manchester Children's Hospital, Manchester, UK. Last updated May 1997 by Dr C R Birch, Consultant Physician and Medical Director, Grantham and District Hospital, Grantham, UK. **Last reviewed July 2007 by Mr I K Pople, Consultant Neurosurgeon, Frenchay Hospital, Bristol, UK**

Further online resources

Medical texts in *The Contact a Family Directory* are designed to give a short, clear description of specific conditions and rare disorders. More extensive information on this condition can be found on a range of reliable, validated websites. Further information on these resources can be found in our **Medical Information on the Internet** article on page 21.

Support

Association for Spina Bifida and Hydrocephalus (ASBAH)

42 Park Road, Peterborough PE1 2UQ   Tel: 0845 450 7755 Helpline   Tel: 01733 555988 Fax: 01733 555985   e-mail: helpline@asbah.org   Web: http://www.asbah.org

The Association is a National Registered Charity No. 249338, established in 1966. It offers advice and information to individuals with hydrocephalus and/or spina bifida and their families or carers. It has a network of area advisers covering most parts of the country backed up by a team of specialist advisers in medical aspects of the conditions and education matters. It works with around 50 local associations in England, Wales and Northern Ireland. ASBAH publishes 'LINK' Journal quarterly and has a wide range of information available, details on request. The Association has over 8,000 families and individuals on its database.

Group details last updated August 2007.

Scottish Spina Bifida Association

The Dan Young Building, 6 Craighalbert Way, Dullatur, Glasgow G68 0LS
Tel: 08459 11 11 12 (Lo-call Helpline)   Tel: 01236 794516/01236 794500
Fax: 01236 736435   e-mail: familysupport@ssba.org.uk   Web: http://www.ssba.org.uk
The Association is a National Registered Charity No. SCO13328, established in 1965.
It offers a family support service throughout Scotland from a purpose-built family centre,
providing information, support and advice to all users and their families. Home visits can
also be arranged. It publishes a magazine 'talk:BACK' three times per year, which is
provided free to all users. There is also a wide range of information leaflets, publication list
available on request. The Association has over 3,000 users.
Group details last updated August 2007.

Contact a Family has a team of
Volunteer Parent Representatives
based around the UK. They are all
parents of disabled children who
provide information and support to
other parents locally. Call the Contact a
Family Helpline for more information.

SPINAL INJURIES

Background

The spinal cord is an extension of the brain, a thick bundle of nerve fibres from which individual nerves branch off to connect the brain with the muscles, skin and internal organs. Nerves carry messages in both directions: from the brain to individual muscles, telling them to move; and from the skin and other organs to the brain, communicating sense of touch, pain, pressure or heat and cold.

The spinal cord is carried in a hollow channel through the centre of the spinal column, a stack of thirty-three bony rings (the vertebrae). As well as containing the vital cord which controls all movement and perception below the level of the neck, the spinal column is the main component of the body's bone structure, connecting together the head, shoulders, chest and pelvis, which are linked in turn to the arms and legs. The spine has to be immensely strong to support the body weight and anything that is lifted; supple to withstand a lifetime of shocks caused by walking, running and jumping; and flexible to allow the trunk and neck to bend and rotate.

Each vertebra is separated from its neighbour by a flat pad of gristle (a disc). The stack of discs and vertebrae make up a hollow channel called the spinal canal. This channel has a silky lining material (the meninges) and is filled with a colourless liquid (cerebro-spinal fluid or CSF) which provides nutrition and further cushioning for the spinal cord. Up the centre of the canal runs the spinal cord itself, about as thick as a finger, grey in colour and about 20 inches long, starting at the base of the brain, and ending in the small of the back in a bundle of nerve roots called, from its appearance, the cauda equina ('horse's tail').

From the spinal cord thirty-one paired spinal nerves branch out to different parts of the body. From the upper part of the cord, these roots connect to the nerves of the upper torso, arms and hands; from the lower cord they lead to the abdomen, thighs, calves and feet.

There are four major divisions of the spinal column:

Cervical (C) or neck region contains the first seven vertebrae and the first eight spinal nerves.

Thoracic (T) or chest region (also sometimes called Dorsal) contains the next twelve vertebrae and twelve spinal nerves.

Lumbar (L) or lower back region, contains the next five vertebrae and five spinal nerves.

Sacral (S) or tailbone region contains the last nine vertebrae fused together into two sections, the sacrum and the coccyx, and containing six spinal nerves.

What are the symptoms?

Injury to the spinal cord is an extremely severe blow to the body's central nervous system. The body responds by going into 'shock' for a period which can last from a few hours to six weeks. During this period loss of sensation will be almost complete. While the doctors will know, from x-rays and by testing the reflexes, the approximate location and extent of the injury, they won't know for sure how serious the effects will be.

If the spinal injury has been produced by an accident (trauma), affected people will not be allowed to sit up or get out of bed for some weeks after the period of spinal shock is over, in case unhealed bones cause further damage to the spinal cord.

Paralysis

If the spinal cord is damaged, the nerves which join the spinal cord *below* the point of damage may be partially or completely cut off from the brain. Nerves joining *above* the point of damage should be intact and will continue to operate normally. Nerves below the damage point will continue to conduct messages, but the messages won't get through to the brain and messages from the brain will not reach their destination.

Injury to the human spinal cord causes paralysis, the inability to deliberately move or feel particular parts of the body. In general, the higher the level of the injury, the more limbs will be paralysed and the more the disruption to normal bodily functions.

Paraplegia

If the spine is injured below the level of the neck a person is said to be a paraplegic and will be paralysed to some degree in the legs and abdomen. Movement in the trunk and chest will depend on how high the lesion is.

Tetraplegia

If the neck is broken or if there is injury to the spine in the cervical region, the arms also will be partially or fully paralysed. Hence all four limbs are affected, and a person is said to be tetraplegic or quadriplegic. The chest muscles will also be affected, and there may be difficulty with breathing, coughing and clearing the chest.

Autonomic paralysis

As well as the parts of the nervous system that control movement and transmit sensation, the body has another system which controls the involuntary functions of internal organs and glands. This is known as the autonomic nervous system. It is outside of but close to and connected with the spinal cord. Its messages control the bowel and bladder, male (but not female) sexual function, blood circulation and pressure and sweating. Damage to the spinal cord will usually affect the autonomic nervous system also.

Level of lesion

The *level* of the lesion (injury) is the exact point along the spinal cord where the injury occurred, measured by counting the nerves in the four regions of the spinal cord. The level of the lesion determines which of the limbs and functions are affected because the nerves which control the muscles and bodily functions and provide sensation are each connected to the spinal cord at a particular point.

- **Upper motor neurone paralysis** is such that the spinal cord and nerves below the level of lesion, whilst continuing to function normally, cannot get their messages through to the brain. Reflex connections within the grey matter of the spinal cord still work and are often exaggerated because of the loss of the brain's influence. This results in increased reflexes when tested, increased muscle tone (or stiffness) and spasms;

- **Lower motor neurone paralysis** occurs when the nerve roots outside the spinal cord are damaged. This is seen as no reflexes, flaccid or floppy muscles and muscle wasting.

The extent of paralysis and the degree to which specific bodily functions are affected depends on the *completeness* of the lesion. If the spinal cord is only partly damaged, some messages may continue to pass between the brain and the muscles and organs. This explains why some spinal cord injured people retain some leg movement, and a few are able to walk to some degree.

Spinal cord injured people are often described by the level and completeness of their lesion. Someone who broke their neck in a diving accident might be a tetraplegic and a 'C4 complete', meaning that their spinal cord was damaged at the level of the fourth cervical nerve, and that the damage was complete. Someone who broke their back while horse riding might be a 'T12 incomplete', meaning that their cord was injured at the level of the twelth thoracic nerve, but that they retain some function in lower nerves.

There are a number of different types of incomplete spinal cord injury:

Anterior cord syndrome: damage is to the front of the cord, usually leading to partial or complete loss of pain, temperature and touch sensations below the level of lesion, but leaving some pressure and joint sensation. Some people injured in this way will recover movement.

Central cord syndrome: damage is to the centre of the cord, with a lot of swelling there. There is usually complete loss of arm movement, but some sparing of leg function. Bladder and bowel function are often partially spared. There may be recovery, starting gradually from the lower legs and progressing upwards.

Posterior cord syndrome: damage to the back of the cord, which may leave good power and pain and temperature sensation, but leave the injured person with great difficulty co-ordinating movement.

Brown-Séquard syndrome: damage mainly to one side of the cord, often as a result of stab injuries. Power is reduced or absent on the injured side, but pain and temperature sensation are relatively normal. The opposite is true on the non-injured side: power is normal, but pain and temperature sensation are reduced or absent.

Cauda equina lesion: the cauda equina is the mass of nerves which fan out from the base of the spinal cord. Injury here will cause patchy loss of motor power and sensation. If the nerve roots are not completely crushed, they can regrow and functional recovery can occur over a period of twelve to eighteen months.

Other factors

The precise nature and effect of paralysis will vary in each individual, and depend on age and weight, general state of health and life-style before injury, whether other injuries are involved; it also depends on the psychological state of the affected individual and the extent to which they are able to adapt to life with the injury.

What are the causes?
Spinal cord damage

Most spinal cord damage is caused by physical injuries - road traffic accident, fall, diving accident, shot or stab wound, etc., and occasionally by a medical accident during surgery. Broken vertebrae or a foreign body pierce or crush the spinal cord itself. This is called a traumatic lesion of the spine. However, viruses and viral infections (such as transverse myelitis), cysts and tumours on or near the spinal cord, can cause permanent damage leading to progressive paralysis.

Inheritance patterns and prenatal diagnosis
Inheritance patterns
None.
Prenatal diagnosis
None.

Medical text written September 2001 by the Spinal Injuries Association. Approved September 2001 by Dr D Short. **Last reviewed January 2006 by Dr D Short, Consultant in Rehabilitation and Spinal Injuries, Midlands Centre for Spinal Injuries, Oswestry, UK.**

Further online resources

Medical texts in *The Contact a Family Directory* are designed to give a short, clear description of specific conditions and rare disorders. More extensive information on this condition can be found on a range of reliable, validated websites. Further information on these resources can be found in our **Medical Information on the Internet** article on page 21.

Support

Spinal Injuries Association

SIA House, 2 Trueman Place, Oldbrook, Milton Keynes MK6 2HH

Tel: 0800 980 0501 Helpline (Mon-Fri, 9.30am-1pm & 2-4.30pm)

Tel: 0845 678 6633   Fax: 0845 070 6911   e-mail: sia@spinal.co.uk

Web: http://www.spinal.co.uk

The Association is a National Registered Charity No. 1054097, established in 1974. SIA offers information, advice and on-going support to spinal cord injured people on all aspects of living with their disability. SIA's services include a Helpline providing information and advice, a Peer Support scheme to assist those undergoing treatment in Spinal Injuries Centres and a range of expert publications, including a bi-monthly magazine, addressing a wide spectrum of issues of interest and concern to spinal cord injured people. The Association has around 6,000 members including affected individuals and health care professionals.

Group details last confirmed October 2007.

Spinal Injuries Scotland

Festival Business Centre, 150 Brand Street, Glasgow G51 1DH

Tel: 0800 0132 305 Support Helpline Tel: 0141 314 0056

Fax: 0141 427 9258 e-mail: info@sisonline.org Web: http://www.sisonline.org

The organisation is a Scottish Registered Charity No. SCO15405, established in 1960. It is the national voluntary organisation concerned with new and long term spinal cord injured people, their relatives and friends, along with those involved in the management, care and rehabilitation of the injury.

Group details last updated May 2007.

SPINAL MUSCULAR ATROPHY

Background

Spinal Muscular Atrophies (SMA) in children are a group of three inheritable neuro-muscular conditions of varying severity in which there is degeneration of the anterior horn cells of the spinal cord with resultant muscular weakness, usually symmetrical.

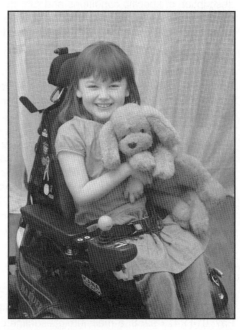

What are the symptoms?

Character-istically, the legs are more severely affected than the arms. Additionally the proximal muscles (those closer to the body) are more severely affected than the distal ones (those closer to the hands and feet). Distinct clinical syndromes can be defined on the basis of the severity of the symptoms displayed. An international classification was agreed in Summer 1990 as follows:

Severe SMA - unable to sit unsupported (also known as Werdnig-Hoffmann disease or Type 1).

Intermediate SMA - able to sit unsupported, unable to stand or walk unaided (also known as Type 2).

Mild SMA - able to stand and walk unaided (also known as Kugelberg-Welander disease or Type 3).

Inheritance patterns and prenatal diagnosis

Inheritance patterns

Autosomal recessive inheritance

Prenatal diagnosis

The gene for all childhood onset Spinal Muscular Atrophies which maps to chromosome 5, has been identified and named the survival motor neurone (SMN) gene. Mutations in the gene are present in almost all cases, particularly Type 1 and 2, and also provide an accurate means of prenatal diagnosis by chorionic villus sampling during early pregnancy.

Medical text written November 1991 by Contact a Family. Approved November 1991 by Professor M Patton, Professor of Medical Genetics, St Georges Hospital Medical School, London, UK and Dr J E Wraith, Consultant Paediatrician, Royal Manchester Children's Hospital, Manchester, UK. **Last updated January 2004 by Professor Francesco Muntoni, Professor of Paediatric Neurology, Imperial College London, London, UK.**

Further online resources

Medical texts in *The Contact a Family Directory* are designed to give a short, clear description of specific conditions and rare disorders. More extensive information on this condition can be found on a range of reliable, validated websites. Further information on these resources can be found in our **Medical Information on the Internet** article on page 21.

Support

Jennifer Trust for Spinal Muscular Atrophy

Elta House, Birmingham Road, Stratford upon Avon CV37 0AQ

Tel: 0800 975 3100 Helpline for families 9am-9pm every day

Tel: 0870 774 3651   Fax: 0870 774 3652

e-mail: jennifer@jtsma.org.uk   Web: http://www.jtsma.org.uk

The Trust is a National Registered Charity No. 1106815, established in 1985. The Trust is the only national charity in the UK dedicated both to supporting people affected by SMA and investing in essential research into causes, treatments and eventually a cure for the disorder. Each year, around 2,000 families, individuals, and healthcare professionals turn to them for information, support, and advice about living with or caring for someone with, all types of SMA.

Group details last updated September 2007.

As spinal muscular atrophy is a neuromuscular disease advice and information about the condition is also available from the Muscular Dystrophy Group (see entry, Muscular Dystrophy and neuromuscular disorders).

STAMMERING

Background

Stammering (or stuttering) is not just a speech problem, it is a problem of communication. It is "characterised by stoppages and disruptions in fluency which interrupt the smooth flow and timing of speech. These stoppages may take the form of repetitions of sounds, syllables or words, or of prolongations of sounds so that words seem to be stretched out, and can involve silent blocking of the airflow of speech when no sound is heard" (Enderby, 1996). Speech may sound forced, tense or jerky. People who stammer may avoid certain words or situations which they know will cause them difficulty.

What are the symptoms?

Stammering usually begins in early childhood when the child is developing his/her speech and language skills. It can, however, also start later in childhood, adolescence and adulthood although these incidences are less common.

As a communication problem, for the child or adult who stammers, confidence and self-esteem can be seriously affected. This means they may experience difficulties in a range of social, educational and employment settings. Sometimes stammering may develop into a "hidden" problem as the person may avoid relationships, situations and opportunities in attempt to hide their stammer. It has been known for parents to believe their child no longer stammers and for partners/spouses to be unaware of this complex disorder of fluency when the person becomes so competent at avoidance behaviours.

How is it treated?

Therapy is available for people of all ages who stammer and a variety of treatment approaches may be offered including individual and/or group therapy.

Research has shown that early intervention by a speech and language therapist, especially in the pre-school years, may prevent the development of persistent stammering. It is recommended, therefore, that parents seek referral to speech and language therapy as soon as their child shows signs of stammering.

Inheritance patterns and prenatal diagnosis

Inheritance patterns

In about sixty per cent of cases of childhood stammering there is a positive family history of stammering or other speech and language difficulties.

Prenatal diagnosis

None

Contact a Family Helpline 0808 808 3555

Medical text written November 1999 by Elaine Christie. BSc. Reg. MRCSLT., Specialist Speech and Language Therapist, British Stammering Association, London, UK. **Last updated October 2004 by Karen E Allen, BSc. Reg MRCSLT., Specialist Speech and Language Therapist, British Stammering Association, London, UK.**

Support

The British Stammering Association

15 Old Ford Road, London E2 9PJ
Tel: 0845 603 2001 Helpline (Mon-Fri, times vary - see website) Tel: 020 8983 1003
Fax: 020 8983 3591 e-mail: info@stammering.org Web: http://www.stammering.org
The Association is a National Registered Charity No. 1089967, established in 1978. It offers a free information and advice service on specialist speech therapy and a lending library of books, audio tapes and videos concerned with stammering. It maintains details of local groups. It publishes a quarterly magazine, 'Speaking Out', has free information packs for people of all ages who stammer and professionals, and a wide range of other information, details on request. The Association has around 1,500 members.
Group details last updated October 2007.

"When I moved house, I didn't know anyone in the new area with my special kind of childcare responsibilities. The local Contact a Family project were very welcoming - I realised I was not alone." Parent.

STARGARDT MACULAR DYSTROPHY

Stargardt Macular Dystrophy: Stargardt Disease

Background

Stargardt Macular Dystrophy is the most common juvenile onset form of inherited macular dystrophy and should not be confused with age related macular degeneration. The condition was first described in 1909 by Dr Karl Stargardt, a German ophthalmologist, and is named after him. The hallmark of Stargardt Macular Dystrophy is loss of central vision in younger people and is usually identified between the ages of six and twenty although affected people might not be aware of the condition until their 30s or even 40s. It is thought that the incidence of Stargardt Macular Dystrophy is between 1 in 1,660 and 1 in 15,000 affecting both males and females.

What are the symptoms?

What was thought to be a separate condition known as Fundus Flavimaculatus, characterised by yellow-white spots scattered in the peripheral retina and minor changes at the macula with only a small degree of loss of central vision, is now thought to be a variant Stargardt Macular Dystrophy.

People affected by Stargardt Macular Dystrophy experience in varying degrees:

- Decreased central vision progressing over a period of years;
- Loss of colour vision;
- Gradual loss of ability to distinguish faces;
- Reduced ability to see clearly.

What are the causes?

The term Macular Dystrophy describes the appearance of the macula (central part of the retina). The cause of Stargardt Macular Dystrophy is progressive loss of cones from this central part of the retina. In the outer areas of the retina the other visual cells, which are called rods, remain unaffected and peripheral (side) vision is, therefore, usually retained. Cones or photoreceptors ensure good central vision, colour perception and the ability to see fine detail. Defects in the ABCR (also called ABCA4) gene on Chromosome 1p21-p13, identified in 1997, are thought to lead to the loss of cones. However, there may be other genes causing Stargardt Macular Dystrophy that are not yet identified.

How is it diagnosed?

A diagnosis of Stargardt Macular Dystrophy is made on the results of a Fluorescein Angiogram and an electroretinogram (ERG). In a Fluorescein Angiogram a dye is injected in the arm and photographs of the retina are taken for an ophthalmologist to interpret. An ERG measures the electrical response of the eye's light-sensitive cones. Electrodes are placed on the cornea and the skin near the eye to measure the electrical currents coming from the cells when a light is flashed.

How is it treated?

There is no cure for Stargardt Macular Dystrophy. Treatment is symptomatic for the features affecting the individual and is aimed at optimising the affected person's vision. There are a number of aids available such as binocular lens, magnifying screens and low vision aids.

Inheritance patterns and prenatal diagnosis

Inheritance patterns

Autosomal recessive.

Prenatal diagnosis

In families already known to be affected, screening to identify carriers of the ABCR gene may lead to the possibility of a prenatal diagnosis.

Medical text written January 2005 by Contact a Family. Approved January 2005 by Mr T ffytch, Consultant Ophthalmic Surgeon, London Clinic, London, UK.

Further online resources

Medical texts in *The Contact a Family Directory* are designed to give a short, clear description of specific conditions and rare disorders. More extensive information on this condition can be found on a range of reliable, validated websites. Further information on these resources can be found in our **Medical Information on the Internet** article on page 21.

Support

Stargardt Support Group

53 Cavendish Road, Manchester M7 4NQ   Tel: 0161 792 7392

e-mail: gillamiriamchait@yahoo.co.uk

The Group is a small, informal network offering a listening ear and linking where possible. Approximately 30 families are in touch. Telephone contact is preferred.

Group details last confirmed July 2007.

Information, support and advice is also available from the Macular Disease Society (see entry, Macular disease.)

STICKLER SYNDROME

Stickler syndrome: Hereditary progressive Arthro-Ophthalmopathy

Background

Stickler syndrome is a genetic progressive condition that affects the body's collagen (connective tissue).

What are the symptoms?

Individuals affected by this condition may present with any number of the following:

- Ocular manifestations of early onset myopia (nearsightedness), usually congenital (born with) and non-progressive. There is a high risk of retinal detachments, which can occur in both eyes. Typically, there are early cataracts, both wedge and comma shaped. Regular checks by an eye specialist are vital to maintain and preserve sight;

- Hypermobility (looseness) of joints assessed objectively using the Beighton scoring system to allow comparison with a matched population. Stiffness and premature osteoarthritis developing typically in the 3rd and 4th decade, prominent joints and the widening of the ends of long bones;

- Any facial clefting (fissures) that occurred in embryonic development, high-arched palate, under-sized jaw (see entry, Pierre Robin syndrome) mid-facial hypoplasia (arrested development) and micrognathia (protruding tongue);

- Sensorineural and/or conductive hearing loss and otitis media (glue ear).

Inheritance patterns and prenatal diagnosis

Inheritance patterns

Inheritance is autosomal dominant. Several genes that control and direct collagen synthesis (the building up of complex substances by the joining and interaction of simpler materials), may cause Stickler syndrome. So far, four types of Stickler syndrome are known to the medical profession with further research taking place:

- Type 1 Stickler syndrome. The gene, COL2A1, which is on the long arm of chromosome 12 is responsible for Stickler syndrome in the majority of people diagnosed with the condition. Most patients will have 'full' Stickler syndrome effecting the eyes (see entry, Vision Disorders in Childhood), joints (see entry, Hypermobility), hearing (see entry, Deafness), and oro-pharynx, but a small but important sub-group have only ocular changes and can easily be missed without careful ophthalmic assessment. It is important that this sub-group is picked up so they can be referred to genetic clinics. Findings also show that those patients with Type 1 Stickler syndrome have an increased incidence of cleft abnormalities;

- Type 2 Stickler syndrome. The gene responsible is COL11A1 and is found on the short arm of chromosome 1. Again this causes 'full' Stickler syndrome, affecting the eyes, joints, hearing, eye and oro-pharynx. Patients with this anomaly have an increased incidence of deafness;
- COL112A causes a 'stickler-like' syndrome, which affects only the joints and hearing with no eye problems. This condition has now been given the name oto-spondylo-megaepiphyseal dysplasia (OSMED);
- A fourth group of individuals, also known to have Stickler syndrome, do not have a fault on any of the known genes, and work is continuing to identify this unknown gene or genes. This group also have 'full' Stickler syndrome affecting the eyes, joints, hearing and oro-pharynx.

Prenatal diagnosis

Ultrasound screening may identify cleft palate.

Medical text written August 2005 by the Stickler Syndrome Support Group. Approved August 2005 by MP Snead, Consultant Vitreoretinal Surgeon, Addenbrookes Hospital, Cambridge, UK.

Further online resources

Medical texts in *The Contact a Family Directory* are designed to give a short, clear description of specific conditions and rare disorders. More extensive information on this condition can be found on a range of reliable, validated websites. Further information on these resources can be found in our **Medical Information on the Internet** article on page 21.

Support

Stickler Syndrome Support Group

PO Box 371, Walton on Thames KT12 2YS Tel: 01932 267635

e-mail: info@stickler.org.uk Web: http://www.stickler.org.uk

The Group is a National Registered Charity No. 1060421, established in 1989. It offers support by telephone, letter and e-mail. It publishes a newsletter and has information booklets on all aspects of the condition, including a booklet for teachers, and a 52-page booklet for medical and healthcare professionals which includes eight medical illustrations. The Group is in touch with about 500 families in the UK and abroad.

Group details last updated March 2007.

STIFF MAN SYNDROME

Background

Stiff Man syndrome (SMS) is a rare, autoimmune, neurological disease which affects approximately 1 in 200,000 individuals - both males and females. The immune system protects the body from disease; whereas the autoimmune system functions to destroy part of the body in conditions such as SMS.

What are the symptoms?

This condition is characterised by progressive stiffness and painful spasms in the back and lower limbs which are often triggered by touch, noise or anxiety. The unpredictable onset and nature of the symptoms associated with SMS may be experienced as frightening. Where the limbs are predominately involved, the condition is also known as Stiff Limb syndrome.

This is a progressive condition, and stiffness may increase to the extent that the individual becomes a wheelchair user. Both the rigidity and the frequency of spasms may be relieved by sleep, general anaesthesia, nerve block and peripheral nerve block. About forty per cent of individuals also have Type 1 diabetes (see entry, Diabetes Mellitus) which is an autoimmune disease.

Three types of Stiff Man syndrome have been described:

- **Classical Stiff Man syndrome** Painful spasms and rigidity occur around the back, stomach and sometimes thighs and neck. As the condition progresses, classical curvature of the lower back can occur. Classical Stiff Man syndrome is commonly associated with Type 1 Diabetes;
- **Stiff Limb syndrome** The legs, including the feet, are affected by painful spasms and occasionally fixed rigidity. More rarely, the hands can be affected;
- **Jerking Stiff Person syndrome** Otherwise known as progressive encephalomyelitis with rigidity, this is the rarest form of SMS. It is a more aggressive form of SMS and can lead to progressive disability over a number of years.

Some individuals with Stiff Man syndrome/Stiff Limb syndrome show an immune response to an enzyme called glutamic acid decarboxylase (GAD). Individuals with classic Type 1 Diabetes show a similar immune response. GAD is an important enzyme in the formation of a chemical messenger in the brain and spinal cord and also in the transmission of insulin. When a patient is developing SMS or Type 1 Diabetes, antibodies to GAD are produced which leads to its destruction, thus interrupting transmission.

How is it diagnosed?

Diagnosis of SMS is often painstakingly slow, simply because it is so rare and the symptoms can baffle doctors. Individuals are often initially mis-diagnosed and labeled psychosomatic. There are two important tests that can be carried out as a means to obtaining a diagnosis. One is to test for antibodies to GAD and the other is to carry out EMG (electromyelogram - muscle testing) studies.

How is it treated?

While treatments do not lead to a cure, they can control symptoms in the majority of individuals. Although there is no known cure for SMS, some individuals are more responsive to certain treatments than others

Research has been conducted into the role of GAD in the development of Type 1 insulin dependent Diabetes and in Stiff Man syndrome. Future research studies may compare the immune response to GAD in individuals with SMS and in Type 1 insulin dependent Diabetes; and in so doing determine whether those individuals with SMS and Diabetes show a different immune response, genetic profile and clinical features from those individuals with SMS without Diabetes. Such research may lead to a therapy to modulate the immune response in both diseases.

Inheritance patterns and prenatal diagnosis

Inheritance patterns

The cause of SMS is not yet known.

Prenatal diagnosis

None available.

Medical text written July 2004 by Contact a Family. Approved July 2004 by Professor P Brown, Professor of Neurology, Institute of Neurology, London, UK.

Further online resources

Medical texts in *The Contact a Family Directory* are designed to give a short, clear description of specific conditions and rare disorders. More extensive information on this condition can be found on a range of reliable, validated websites. Further information on these resources can be found in our **Medical Information on the Internet** article on page 21.

Support

Stiff Man Syndrome Support Group
c/o Contact a Family, 209-211 City Road, London EC1V 1JN   Tel: 01482 868 881
e-mail: lizblows@smssupportgroup.co.uk Web: http://www.smssupportgroup.co.uk
The Group is a National Registered Charity No. 1099206 established in 1998 providing support, information and linking for affected individuals and their families in the UK. It produces a periodic newsletter. The Group also aims to raise awareness and assist with research. They are happy to hear from medical professionals and anyone else with an interest in this condition. The Group has over 90 members.
Group details last updated October 2007.

STILLBIRTHS AND NEONATAL DEATHS

Background

A stillbirth describes when a baby dies before or during birth, after twenty-four weeks of pregnancy. Around ten babies are stillborn every day in the UK, leaving four thousand families bereaved every year.

A neonatal death describes when a baby who was born alive at any gestation dies in the first month of life. Six such babies die every day in the UK.

The death of a baby is a catastrophic event and impacts upon all family members and friends. This can cause great isolation unless there are lines of communication to overcome it. Many difficult and painful feelings are experienced at such a time. Each baby is precious and irreplaceable and will always be part of the lives of those who love them.

What are the causes?

The main known causes of death include prematurity and birth defects. Additionally, multiple pregnancy, smoking, a mother aged over thirty-five, infection and maternal medical problems are known to be risk factors for stillbirth and neonatal death. However, currently at least half of all stillbirths are classified as 'unexplained'; although the evidence shows that around half of these babies have not fulfilled their optimal growth potential.

Inheritance patterns and prenatal diagnosis

Inheritance patterns

These will depend upon the cause of the death.

Prenatal diagnosis

This will depend upon the presence of any underlying anomaly.

Medical text written April 2007 by Pat McGeown, Head of Midwifery, Perinatal Institute, Birmingham, UK. Approved April 2007 Professor Jason Gardosi, Director, Perinatal Institute, Birmingham, UK.

Support

SANDS (Stillbirth and Neonatal Death Society)
28 Portland Place, London W1B 1LY
Tel: 020 7436 5881 Helpline (Mon-Fri, 10am-5.30pm)
Tel: 020 7436 7940 Information Line (Mon-Fri, 10am-5.30pm)   Fax: 020 7436 3715
e-mail: support@uk-sands.org   Web: http://www.uk-sands.org
SANDS is a National Registered Charity No. 299679, established in 1978. It supports parents whose baby has died, and works with health and social care professionals to improve the quality of services provided to bereaved families. SANDS also promotes research into the causes of stillbirths and neonatal deaths and changes in practice that could save more babies' lives.
Group details last updated September 2007.

STROKE

Background

Stroke is defined as a sudden and focal neurological deficit. It is a common disease in the UK affecting around 300 in 100,000 people. Although the risk of stroke is dependent principally on age with the risk increasing with every decade from middle age, the commonest modifiable risk factor is high blood pressure.

What are the symptoms?

Ischaemic stroke (caused by an interruption in the flow of blood to the brain) is the commonest type of stroke and accounts for around eighty per cent of all strokes. The causes are predominantly atherosclerotic related manifesting in arterial cholesterol plaques (abnormal patches of fatty substance

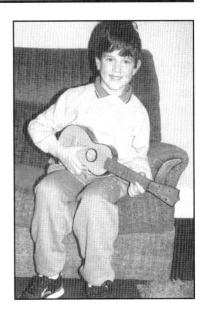

in the arteries), hardening of the arteries and arterial thrombosis (blood clot). Sometimes this type of stroke can also occur in patients from a dislodged blood clot in the heart making its way to the brain. Other risk factors for this type of stroke include blood clotting abnormalities, excess alcohol intake, smoking and obesity.

Transient ischaemic attack (TIA) is a form of ischaemic stroke often called a 'mini-stroke'. The distinguishing feature of this type of stroke is that its neurological effects last less than twenty-four hours. Within that time the patient should fully recover. However, this is an arbitrary distinction based on time and the causes for a TIA are similar to a full stroke. TIA should be regarded as a warning shot-across-the-bow and urgent neurological investigations are warranted to prevent further TIA's or full strokes.

Haemorrhagic strokes result from arterial bleeds rather than occlusions (obstructions). The symptoms however are indistinguishable from ischaemic strokes, although the subsequent management is different in terms of investigations, treatment and future prevention.

Young patients also suffer stroke. Approximately twenty-five per cent of patients are below the age of sixty-five years and a percentage are teenagers and children. There are a few differences in the very young patient. The causes of stroke tend not to be the result of diseased atheromatous (fatty degeneration of the inner coat of the arteries or abnormal fatty deposits in an artery) vessels but rather abnormalities of the vessels themselves. These can be related to trauma or congenital abnormalities developed from birth. It is important to realise that this does not necessarily mean that the condition is inherited or that offspring will be affected. Also any vessel malformation tends to be localised and not generalised. Abnormalities of the clotting system can also manifest themselves as stroke and these would be managed directly.

Recovery in childhood stroke tends to be better than in adult stroke as the child's brain attempts to compensate. Nevertheless stroke occurring in children is often met with surprise and dismay. Clinical investigations should be comprehensively taken in a specialised unit. Counselling should be offered to the patient and their family and this may need to be continued as the child progresses through to teenage years and as a young adult.

Inheritance patterns and prenatal diagnosis
Inheritance patterns
There is little doubt that stroke has an underlying genetic contribution. However, the likely number of genes and their individual effects are small. A few directly inherited genetic conditions do exist such as CADASIL (see entry) and MELAS but these are very rare. Specialised services for these and other familial causes of stroke exist in a number of acute stroke units with a particular interest in genetics of stroke.

Prenatal diagnosis
This may be possible for an individual member of a family with a known mutation leading to a condition such as CADASIL.

Medical text written September 2004 by Dr P Sharma, Consultant Neurologist & Head of Hammersmith Hospital Acute Stroke Unit, Hammersmith Hospitals & Imperial College, London, UK.

Further online resources
Medical texts in *The Contact a Family Directory* are designed to give a short, clear description of specific conditions and rare disorders. More extensive information on this condition can be found on a range of reliable, validated websites. Further information on these resources can be found in our **Medical Information on the Internet** article on page 21.

Support
Different Strokes
9 Canon Harnett Court, Wolverton Mill, Milton Keynes MK12 5NF   Tel: 08451 307172
Fax: 01908 313501   e-mail: info@differentstrokes.co.uk
Web: http://www.differentstrokes.co.uk
The organisation is a National Registered Charity No. 1092168, established in 1996. It offers a telephone helpline staffed by stroke survivors, access to counselling and information on benefits, further and higher education, special training and work opportunities. It publishes a quarterly newsletter and has information available, details on request. The organisation is in touch with over 11,000 stroke affected persons and their families. Group details last confirmed September 2007.

Contact a Family Helpline 0808 808 3555

The Stroke Association
Stroke House, 240 City Road, London EC1V 2PR
Tel: 0845 30 33 100 Stroke Helpline (Mon-Fri, 9am – 5pm)
Tel: 020 7566 0300 Administration (Mon-Fri, 9am – 5.30pm)
Fax: 020 7490 2686   e-mail: info@stroke.org.uk   Web: http://www.stroke.org.uk
The Association is a Registered Charity No. 211015, established in 1899. The Association is the only national charity solely concerned with helping everyone affected by stroke. It provides information and support to stroke people and their families through its helpline and community services. It also provides information about all aspects of stroke from prevention to rehabilitation and can provide details of local support groups and other relevant organisations. A wide range of leaflets and factsheets are produced including a free quarterly magazine. The Association also funds research into stroke, and provide a welfare grants service.
Group details last confirmed August 2007.

Chest, Heart and Stroke Scotland
65 North Castle Street, Edinburgh EH2 3LT
Tel: 0845 077 6000 Advice Line (Mon-Fri, 9.30am-12.30pm & 1.30pm-4pm) Out of hours answer machine. Contact via mopile phone by texting "chss" followed by your message to 07766 404 142 Head Office: 0131 225 6963 Fax: 0131 220 6313
e-mail: admin@chss.org.uk (general) e-mail: adviceline@chss.org.uk (staffed by specialist nurses) Web: http://www.chss.org.uk
The organisation is a Registered Charity No. SCO 18761. It offers a confidential, independent advice line run by trained nurses for affected persons, their families, carers and health professionals. It gives welfare grants and has a network of support groups including some young stroke groups but no children's groups. It also funds medical research. It publishes an annual newsletter 'Update' and has a wide range of information available, details on request.
Group details last updated August 2007.

NICHSA
Northern Ireland Chest Heart & Stroke, 21 Dublin Road, Belfast BT2 7HB
Tel: 08456 011658 Advice Helpline: 08457 697299 Fax: 028 9033 3487
e-mail: mail@nichsa.com   Web: http://www.nichsa.com
The Northern Ireland Chest Heart and Stroke Association (NICHSA) is a Registered Charity No. XN 47338. Its aim is to promote the prevention of and alleviate the suffering resulting from chest, heart and stroke related illnesses. NICHS provides programmes of health promotion, research, rehabilitation, advice and support services.
Group details last updated July 2007.

Direct services for children and adults affected by Stroke are also provided by the National Institute of Conductive Education (see Foundation for Conductive Education, under separate entry, Cerebral Palsy)

STURGE-WEBER SYNDROME

Background

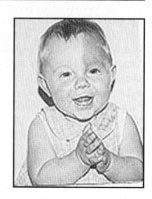

Sturge-Weber syndrome (SWS) is a congenital disorder involving the brain, skin and eyes.

There is a facial birth mark (port wine stain), a layer of blood vessels over the covering of the brain (venous angioma of the leptomeninges) and there may be an angioma (collections of abnormal blood vessels) involving the inner lining of the eye (choroidal angioma). The angioma usually involves one side of the brain and varies in extent. More rarely it may involve both sides of the brain.

What are the symptoms?

The port wine stain involves the skin around the eye, forehead or scalp. In some cases it may involve other areas of the body in addition to the typical facial distribution. In approximately thirteen per cent of cases of SWS the facial port wine stain may be absent.

Other features may include epilepsy (see entry) in seventy-five to ninety per cent of cases, learning disability (see entry), hemiparesis (weakness of one side of the body) which may be evident during infancy or may occur in relation to seizures or in association with migraine-like headache, glaucoma (raised pressure in the eye) (see entry) and episodic migraine-like headache.

There is much variation in the manifestation of the condition between different individuals.

Inheritance patterns and prenatal diagnosis

Inheritance patterns

Sporadic with no evidence of familial involvement.

Prenatal diagnosis

None.

Medical text written March 2003 by Dr S Aylett, Consultant Paediatric Neurologist, Great Ormond Street Hospital, London, UK and the National Centre For Young People With Epilepsy, Surrey, UK.

Further online resources

Medical texts in *The Contact a Family Directory* are designed to give a short, clear description of specific conditions and rare disorders. More extensive information on this condition can be found on a range of reliable, validated websites. Further information on these resources can be found in our **Medical Information on the Internet** article on page 21.

Support

Sturge-Weber Foundation (UK)
Burleigh, 348 Pinhoe Road, Exeter EX4 8AF   Tel: 01392 464675
e-mail: support@sturgeweber.org.uk   Web: http://www.sturgeweber.org.uk
The Foundation is a National Registered Charity No. 1016688, established in 1990. It offers support for families. It aims to raise public awareness and promote medical research. It publishes a bi-annual newsletter and has information available, details on request. The Foundation has over 200 members with affected children and adults.
Group details last updated August 2007.

Parent Partnership services provide independent advice, support and information to parents and carers in England and Wales whose children have special educational needs. Call the Contact a Family Helpline for details of your local service.

SUBACUTE-SCLEROSING PANENCEPHALITIS

Subacute-sclerosing panencephalitis: SSPE

Background

Subacute Sclerosing Panencephalitis is a serious viral encephalitis of children and young adults. It is a late manifestation of measles virus infection, developing between usually six to twelve years after natural measles infection. Cases can also follow immunisation with measles vaccine but at a lesser frequency than after natural measles. The annual incidence is about 1 in 1,000,000. It is believed that measles immunisation significantly reduces the risk of developing SSPE. Males are more commonly affected, as are those living in rural areas. Mortality is very high. Those who survive do so with considerable intellectual and also physical impairment.

What are the symptoms?

The onset of the illness is insidious, the first signs are behavioural disturbances or a decline in school performance. Not infrequently the family are told that the cause for these behavioural or school problems is 'psychological.' Progression of the illness will vary from child to child but evidence that this is a more serious illness usually begins with loss of motor control and co-ordination. This often starts with characteristic jerking movements which may at first appear as clumsiness. These jerking movements are known as myoclonic seizures. Grand mal (also called tonic-clonic) seizures may also occur. As the condition worsens problems with swallowing and speech develop and vision may be impaired.

The duration of the illness can be as short as six weeks or as long as ten years or more. Long-term survival has been reported and up to five per cent may experience spontaneous long-term improvement.

What are the causes?

The precise sequence of events that results in the development of this disease in a tiny proportion of the population is not known. The great majority of children who develop SSPE are known to have had an attack of classical measles, usually many years before. Over fifty per cent of cases have had the disease at the unusually early age of under two years.

How is it treated?

Treatment with Inosiplex (isoprinosine) may be of benefit in slowly progressive cases. Very occasionally, more aggressive treatments may be used, including 'Interferons', although this treatment is not proven to work.

Inheritance patterns and prenatal diagnosis

Inheritance patterns

Not applicable.

Prenatal diagnosis

Not applicable.

Medical text written November 2001 by Dr R Appleton. **Last updated January 2006 by Dr R Appleton, Consultant Paediatric Neurologist, Alder Hey Children's Hospital, Liverpool, UK.**

Further online resources

Medical texts in *The Contact a Family Directory* are designed to give a short, clear description of specific conditions and rare disorders. More extensive information on this condition can be found on a range of reliable, validated websites. Further information on these resources can be found in our **Medical Information on the Internet** article on page 21.

Support

As *Subacute-Sclerosing Panencephalitis is a form of Encephalitis, information, advice and support is provided by the Encephalitis Support Group (see entry, Encephalitis).*

SYDENHAM CHOREA

Background

Sydenham Chorea usually follows infection with the Streptococcus bacterium. It classically follows a bout of tonsillitis and forms part of the spectrum of Rheumatic fever. The true incidence is not known and most cases seen in the UK occur sporadically, but clusters or epidemics can occur. Girls are slightly often more affected in the adolescent age range.

What are the symptoms?

Chorea describes a disorder of constant abrupt movements. These can appear as clumsiness but, if severe, it can lead to 'St Vitus' dance' (prevention of standing or walking). Muscle weakness is present in all affected individuals but, if severe, may result in chorea mollis or paralytic chorea (a motionless state). Difficulties with eye movements and voice control also occur. In the cases where Sydenham Chorea follows an infection, there may be a long delay between the infection and the start of symptoms.

The body's response to infection causes injury to areas of the brain involved in the monitoring of movement, thought and emotion. Swings in mood and other disturbances of feelings have been described. Children may develop features of Obsessive Compulsive Disorder (OCD) or Attention Deficit Hyperactivity Disorder (ADHD), although the full disorder might not develop.

A related condition has been described where there may be prominent changes in behaviour alone (tics, ADHD or OCD) that come and go with documented streptococcal infection. This is known as Paediatric Autoimmune Neuropsychiatric disorder associated with Streptococcus (PANDAS). Tics can occur in children with Sydenham Chorea and can cause diagnostic difficulty. Severe multiple motor and vocal tics in combination may justify a diagnosis of Tourette syndrome (see entry).

How is it diagnosed?

Blood tests and throat swabs may show evidence of the infection. A blood test for Systemic Lupus Erythematosus (see entry, Lupus) may be indicated as, very rarely, this can present in a similar way to Sydenham Chorea. An electrocardiogram (a test to record the electrical activity of the heart) and echocardiogram (a test that uses sound waves to create a moving picture of the heart) will show if there is heart involvement as can occur in Rheumatic fever. Other tests are not usually indicated.

How is it treated?

An antibiotic is given in a high dose for ten days. Low dose antibiotics may be recommended to continue until the age of eighteen years.

The movement disorder may justify drug treatment in some cases, although the clinical response to this is, at best, variable. Awareness of the possible changes in mood and behaviour can be helpful. Symptoms of OCD or ADHD may require treatment in their own right.

Abnormal movements settle over several months but may worsen with illness. Recurrence due to reinfection with Streptococcus is the reason for prescribing low dose antibiotics in the long-term. The long-term impact on behaviour and learning is not fully understood.

Inheritance patterns and prenatal diagnosis

Inheritance patterns
Not applicable.

Prenatal diagnosis
Not applicable.

Medical text written August 2006 by Dr N Cordeiro, Specialist Registrar in Paediatric Neurology, Dr L Dorris, Consultant Neuropsychologist, Dr R McWilliam, Consultant Paediatric Neurologist and Dr M Morton, Consultant Child and Adolescent Psychiatrist, Royal Hospital for Sick Children, Yorkhill, Glasgow, UK.

Further online resources

Medical texts in *The Contact a Family Directory* are designed to give a short, clear description of specific conditions and rare disorders. More extensive information on this condition can be found on a range of reliable, validated websites. Further information on these resources can be found in our **Medical Information on the Internet** article on page 21.

Support

There is no support group for Sydenham Chorea. Cross referrals to other entries in the Contact a Family Directory are intended to provide relevant support for those particular features of the disorder. Organisations identified in those entries do not provide support specifically for Sydenham Chorea. Families can use Contact a Family's Freephone Helpline for advice, information and, where possible, links to other families. Contact a Family's web-based linking service Making Contact.org can be accessed at http://www.makingcontact.org

SYRINGOMYELIA

Background

Syringomyelia refers to a cystic like change (syrinx) within the spinal cord. It can have many different causes such as spinal cord trauma, spinal cord tumours, (see entry), spinal cord tethering and Chiari malformation, or it may have no identifiable cause. Hydrocephalus (see entry) can be an associated condition and treatment of it and some of the other associated problems above may resolve the syringomyelia.

What are the symptoms?

The cyst like change within the spinal cord can extend over a variable length and the symptoms it can cause reflects the level of the change within the spinal cord. Sometimes they can actually be asymptomatic. However, often they can affect sensory perception and ultimately can cause deranged motor function. As the syrinx is usually secondary to another condition the patient most commonly presents with the symptoms attributable to that condition. Therefore in cases of syringomyelia secondary to another condition the treatment is not aimed at the syrinx but at the cause.

Chiari Malformation

Originally referred to as Arnold Chiari malformation it is also known as hindbrain hernia. In essence it is herniation (protrusion) of the bottom of the cerebellum, an area at the back and base of the brain, through the foramen magnum (the hole in the bottom of the skull for the spinal cord to exit). There are two basic types that are most commonly seen. Type one has no other associated cause and type two is associated with spina bifida (see entry). The treatment of type two may involve treatment of the spina bifida. Both types can cause syringomyelia. The treatment can cause resolution of the problem.

Idiopathic, or type one Chiari malformation, can present with headaches particularly at the back of the head, made worse by coughing, sneezing, straining etc. There may also be dizziness, disturbance of vision and abnormal sensations in the arms and legs. Treatment is usually surgical but not in every case. Specialists will consider various approaches. Hydrocephalus may be associated and its treatment may resolve the Chiari malformation.

How is it treated?

The treatment of syringomyelia with no identifiable cause can be controversial as in many cases no treatment may be required and periodical follow up with neurological examination and scanning may be necessary.

Inheritance patterns and prenatal diagnosis

Inheritance patterns

In general, none. However, some conditions causing syringomyelia may be genetic.

Prenatal diagnosis

Where another condition is the cause, ultrasound scanning may be used in diagnosis.

Medical text written December 2002 by Mr N Buxton. **Last updated June 2007 by Mr N Buxton, Consultant Paediatric Neurosurgeon, Alder Hey Children's Hospital, Liverpool, UK.**

Further online resources

Medical texts in *The Contact a Family Directory* are designed to give a short, clear description of specific conditions and rare disorders. More extensive information on this condition can be found on a range of reliable, validated websites. Further information on these resources can be found in our **Medical Information on the Internet** article on page 21.

Support

The Ann Conroy Trust

33 Southam Road, Dunchurch, Rugby CV22 6NL   Tel: 01788 537676   Fax: 01788 569996
e-mail: enquiries@theannconroytrust.org.uk   Web: http://www.theannconroytrust.org.uk
The Trust is a National Registered Charity No. 510582, established in 1980. It offers support for affected individuals and their families together with advice on problems associated with the condition and contact with others in the same situation where possible. It has information available, details on request. Please send SAE. The Trust has around 400 members.
Group details last confirmed October 2007.

TAR SYNDROME

TAR syndrome: Thrombocytopenia and Absent Radius

Background

Thrombocytopenia means low platelets. The thrombocytes are the platelets and 'penia' means 'not very much of.'

In **T**hrombocytopenia and **A**bsent **R**adius there are low platelets and absence of the radius on both sides (bilaterally). The radius and the ulna are the two bones in the forearm. The radius is the bone that is on the side of the forearm where the thumb is and the ulna is on the side of the arm where the little finger is. There may be other bones involved as well but the unique feature of

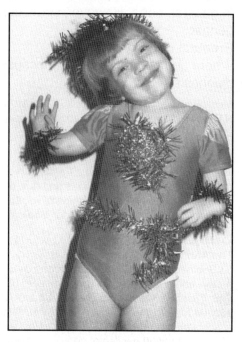

Thrombocytopenia and Absent Radius is that although the radius is absent, the thumb is present. Most other limb anomalies that involve the radius also affect the thumb.

There are a number of other disorders that involve elements of the blood and abnormal structure of bones of the arm and it is important to realise that TAR is a very specific condition. TAR is considered a congenital abnormality since the bone structure is abnormal at birth. TAR has an ongoing problem since during childhood most affected individuals continue to have low platelets. Viral illnesses and other kinds of stress can cause the platelets to become very low and even require platelet transfusions.

What are the symptoms?

All individuals with TAR have low platelets but often as they grow older, it becomes less of a problem and affected individuals can outgrow the risk of bleeding related to low platelets. About ninety per cent of individuals with TAR are symptomatic during the first year of life with easy bruising, bleeding from the GI tract or even bleeding into the brain. The level of platelets will fall and rise throughout low platelet episodes. A normal platelet count is greater than two hundred thousand platelets per millilitres squared of blood. Individuals with TAR may have less than ten thousand platelets per millilitres squared when they are having severe episodes.

In addition to problems with platelets, some individuals with TAR may make too many white cells at times. This is termed a leukaemoid reaction and should not be confused with leukaemia in the sense of being a malignancy. Leukaemoid reaction most often occurs in early infancy along with low platelets in a very sick child.

Occasionally, the bone marrow makes too much of one type of blood cell called the eosinophil. The eosinophil is a white blood cell reddish granules. It is usually associated with allergies and asthma. Many individuals with TAR seem to have an allergy to cow's milk and they will usually be found to have an increase in the eosinophils.

Individuals with TAR often have anaemia (anemia - US) or low red cells. This can be because of bleeding but it is thought that during the first year of life, fewer red cells are made than in the average individual. Affected individuals tend to outgrow anaemia.

The consistent skeletal feature of TAR is absence of the radius but presence of the thumb. The legs may be affected as well. There can be dislocation of the hips so that the head of the femur doesn't sit properly into the hip socket. There can be abnormalities of the knees leading to bending abnormally one way or the other, loose kneecaps, or the bones of the knee slipping on each other. Occasionally the bones of the knee are even fused. Frequently there are abnormalities of toe positioning with 'scrambling' of the toes and occasionally there is some puffiness to the foot.

It would appear the more severely involved the upper limb is, the more likely the lower limbs are to be involved as well. However, if the lower limb is involved, it appears that all five toes and a normal foot is usually seen. At least twenty per cent of affected individuals have significant lower limb involvement.

Minor abnormalities of the ribs, the spine or the jaw can be seen.

Most individuals with TAR are shorter than other family members. No important endocrine abnormalities or growth hormone deficiency have been seen in TAR.

The most frequent other type of anomaly found in individuals with TAR is a hole in the heart. About thirty per cent of affected individuals have some kind of structural abnormality of the heart. This can lead to complications in heart surgery due to the low platelets. However, there are a number of individuals who have had quite complicated heart surgery and, with the aid of platelet transfusions, have done extremely well.

Learning disability can be seen in TAR but this appears to be in individuals who have had a bleed into the brain.

Most affected individuals have bruising at birth. Many develop cow's milk allergy and diarrhoea in infancy. Diarrhoeal illness seems to precipitate low platelets and is of real concern. During the first year of life, there seems to be episodes of low platelets. It is important to avoid cow's milk if it is an irritant. It is also important to avoid viral illnesses particularly gastroenterological ones for the first two years of life.

Inheritance patterns and prenatal diagnosis

Inheritance patterns

Autosomal recessive inheritance.

Prenatal diagnosis

Ultrasound scan at eighteen weeks may show up the absent radii and other limb deformities.

Medical text abridged July 2001 by Contact a Family from a paper by Professor J Hall.
Last updated December 2005 by Professor J Hall, Professor Emerita of Pediatrics and Medical Genetics, Department of Pediatrics, British Columbia Children's Hospital, Vancouver, Canada.

Further online resources

Medical texts in *The Contact a Family Directory* are designed to give a short, clear description of specific conditions and rare disorders. More extensive information on this condition can be found on a range of reliable, validated websites. Further information on these resources can be found in our **Medical Information on the Internet** article on page 21.

Support

TAR Syndrome Support Group
Little Wings, Whatfield Road, Elmsett, Ipswich IP7 6LS   Tel: 01473 657535 (8-9pm)
e-mail: tarsupportgroup@telia.com   Web: http://www.ivh.se/TAR
The Group is a Self Help Group which was started in 1986. It offers support and information about the syndrome and care issues. The Group has a link list for families. It publishes occasional newsletters and leaflets, and holds a family day every two years. The Group has over 50 families in membership worldwide.
Group details last confirmed September 2007.

TAY SACHS DISEASE

Background

Tay Sachs is a life-threatening, progressive, genetic, lysosomal storage disease. Like all metabolic diseases there is a block because a catalyst or enzyme, necessary to perform essential chemical reactions in the body, is absent or malfunctioning. This defect results in the build up of chemicals on one side of the metabolic blockage and a deficiency of vital chemicals on the other. In this case the enzyme concerned is hexosaminidase A (hex-A). In its absence a lipid GM(2) ganglioside builds up abnormally in the body. The nerve cells in the brain are particularly affected.

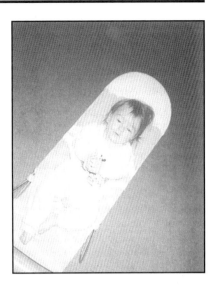

What are the symptoms?

This process begins in the fetus during pregnancy. However the baby usually develops normally until about six months of age. The nervous system is progressively affected and the disease is usually fatal by the age of three to five years.

Late-Onset Tay Sachs Disease (LOTS) is much less common than the classic infant form of the disease. Individuals diagnosed with LOTS have a much smaller amount of the enzyme rather than a complete absence.

Onset of LOTS is usually between adolescence and the mid-thirties and individuals vary in the way it affects them, with much variation among affected persons. The first symptoms may only be recognised in retrospect as they may not be obvious; these include:

- Clumsiness;
- Mood changes.

As the features of LOTS develop, they can include:

- Speech difficulties;
- Difficulty in comprehension;
- Memory impairment;
- Muscle twitching, wasting and weakness;
- Movement problems such as dystonia (see entry);
- Behaviour changes, short attention span and personality changes;
- Depression and psychotic episodes in a number of affected individuals.

Inheritance patterns and prenatal diagnosis

Inheritance patterns

Autosomal recessive inheritance. 1 in 25 Ashkenazi Jews and 1 in 250 of the general population are carriers of this disease. Carrier detection is available through genetic clinics.

Prenatal diagnosis

Chorionic villus sampling at ten to twelve weeks.

Medical text written November 1991 by Contact a Family. Approved November 1991 by Professor M Patton, Professor of Medical Genetics, St Georges Hospital Medical School, London, UK and Dr J E Wraith. **Last updated December 2005 by Contact a Family. Approved December 2005 by Dr J E Wraith, Consultant Paediatrician, Royal Manchester Children's Hospital, Manchester, UK.**

Further online resources

Medical texts in *The Contact a Family Directory* are designed to give a short, clear description of specific conditions and rare disorders. More extensive information on this condition can be found on a range of reliable, validated websites. Further information on these resources can be found in our **Medical Information on the Internet** article on page 21.

Support

While there is no specific support group in the UK for this condition, information is available from Climb (see entry, Metabolic diseases) and support is available from a group of families under the umbrella of Climb.

THALASSAEMIA MAJOR
(ß Thalassaemia)

Thalassaemia Major: Thalassemia Major - US; ß Thalassaemia; Thalassaemia; Mediterranean anaemia; Cooley's anaemia; Homozygous ß thalassaemia

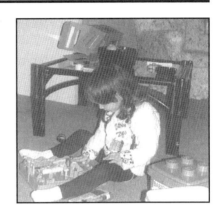

Background
ß Thalassaemia major is a life threatening, genetically inherited, progressive anaemia common in the Mediterranean, Asian, South East Asian and Middle Eastern countries.

What are the symptoms?
Children with ß Thalassaemia major are healthy at birth but become pale within the first few months of life, they fail to thrive, are prone to infections and often have an enlarged spleen and liver. ß Thalassaemia is treatable with two to three weekly red cell transfusions throughout life and the removal of excess iron which is the result of these frequent blood transfusions. The drug currently used for this iron removal is Desferal which is administered by injections. Desferal may cause local skin irritations at the injection site. It may also interfere with spinal growth and can cause hearing problems and interfere with eye sight. Those who are sensitive to this drug or are unable to comply to the injections can now be treated with Ferriprox tablets. Ferriprox is less effective in removing iron from the body than Desferal and may cause a low blood count which may result in severe infections. Those patients who can consistently comply to the prescribed medications can live normal lives, those whose compliance is erratic will experience many endocrinological complications caused by iron overload (growth disturbance, failure of pubertal development, thyroid and parathyroid dysfunction and diabetes) and eventually early death from heart problems.

What are the causes?
The condition is caused by defective production of the beta chain of haemoglobin with resultant abnormal haemoglobin function.

How is it treated?
Treatment is by bone marrow transplantation from a Human Leukocyte Antigen (HLA) identical donor, a brother, sister or rarely from a mother or father.

Inheritance patterns and prenatal diagnosis
Inheritance patterns
Autosomal recessive. Persons with the carrier, or trait, state are generally healthy. They need a simple blood test to detect thalassaemia carrier state.

Prenatal diagnosis
Chorionic villus sampling from ten weeks of gestation and fetal blood sampling from sixteen to twenty weeks of gestation.

Medical text written December 2001 by Dr B Wonke, Consultant Haematologist, Whittington Hospital, London, UK. **Last reviewed October 2006 by Dr Paul Telfer, Senior Lecturer, Centre for Haematology, Barts and The London, Queen Mary's School of Medicine and Dentistry, London. UK.**

Further online resources
Medical texts in *The Contact a Family Directory* are designed to give a short, clear description of specific conditions and rare disorders. More extensive information on this condition can be found on a range of reliable, validated websites. Further information on these resources can be found in our **Medical Information on the Internet** article on page 21.

Support
UK Thalassaemia Society
19 The Broadway, Southgate, London N14 6PH   Tel: 020 8882 0011   Fax: 020 8882 8618
e-mail: office@ukts.org.uk   Web: http://www.ukts.org
*The Society is a National Registered Charity No. 275107, established in 1976. The group covers **thalassaemia major** and **thalassaemia trait**. There are several other forms of thalassaemia. It offers advice and support for affected families together with counselling for carriers, affected individuals and families. It publishes a quarterly newsletter and has a wide range of information available, details on request. The Society has around 680 members.*
Group details last confirmed March 2007.

THROMBOTIC THROMBOCYTOPENIC PURPURA

Background

Thrombotic Thrombocytopenic Purpura (TTP) is a rare condition which is identified by five key features:

- a low platelet count;
- microangiopathic haemolytic anaemia (fragmentation and destruction of the red blood cells as they flow through partially obstructed blood vessels);
- fluctuating neurological features (which may include headaches, unusual behaviour, fits, sensory abnormalities and reduced consciousness);
- impairment of kidney function;
- and fever.

What are the symptoms?

In TTP, thrombi (clots) form in the small blood vessels primarily supplying the brain and kidneys. These clots are composed of platelets that stick together and impede the flow of blood through the vessels. This process causes red blood cells to fragment and break up, leading to anaemia. Formation of the clots is initiated by the presence of a protein (ULVWF) which normally does not circulate in the bloodstream in this form due to the action of an enzyme (ADAMTS13). ULVWF causes the platelets to stick together. In patients with TTP the activity of ADAMTS13 has been found to be very low, usually less than five per cent of the normal value. Without this enzyme platelets stick together and clots form. This blocks the blood flow supplying the kidneys and brain and causes the symptoms associated with TTP.

The idiopathic acquired form of TTP usually occurs in adulthood (or older children) with a very low platelet count. Again the activity of ADAMTS13 is usually very low but this time this is due to an antibody produced by the patient that inhibits the enzyme.

What are the causes?

There are a number of sub-types of TTP. These have different causes and require different treatments:

- An inherited (otherwise known as congenital) form of TTP;
- TTP caused by drugs such as quinine, ticlodipine, cyclosporin;
- TTP caused by infection such as HIV;
- TTP following bone marrow transplantation;
- TTP as a feature of pregnancy, cancers, systemic lupus erythematous (SLE);
- Idiopathic TTP in which no cause has been identified.

How is it diagnosed?

Diagnosis is not always straightforward and is sometimes made when only a low platelet count and haemolytic anaemia (hemolytic anemia - US) are present in the absence of any other identifiable cause. TTP is a serious and life threatening condition, especially if it is not treated quickly.

The inherited or congenital form of TTP is very rare but once the diagnosis has been made it is treatable. This form of TTP usually comes to light during infancy or early childhood with recurrent episodes of low platelets and haemolytic anaemia. In mild cases the disease may not be apparent until later in life. The five key features described above are usually present and are often precipitated by a viral illness. TTP then recurs at regular intervals of about three weeks. Once a diagnosis of the congenital form of TTP has been made, the aim of treatment is to prevent the patient from having recurrent episodes of TTP. This is achieved through transfusion. Although transfusion is very safe there is always a very small risk of transmission of an infection so all patients should be immunised against hepatitis B and C.

How is it treated?

The treatment is plasma exchange which needs to be started as soon as possible, (within twenty-four hours) as any delays in treatment result in complications and decrease the survival rate. Although remission is achieved in the majority of patients, about one third will relapse at some point within a ten year period. It is not yet possible to identify those patients at risk of relapse. Urgent self-referral is advised if a patient develops symptoms suggestive of a relapse so that plasma exchange can be started as soon as possible.

TTP remains a rare condition. Research continues to understand more about the biology of the condition and develop better treatments.

Inheritance patterns and prenatal diagnosis

Inheritance patterns

The inherited form of TTP is autosomal recessive caused by a defect in the ADAMTS13 gene.

Prenatal diagnosis

Not applicable. Parents may be unaware that they carry an abnormality of the ADAMTS13 gene. Not all children are severely affected and relapses can be prevented by transfusion.

Medical text written November 2003 by Dr R Auer, LRF Clinician Scientist, Barts & The London Queen Mary School of Medicine, London, UK.

Further online resources

Medical texts in *The Contact a Family Directory* are designed to give a short, clear description of specific conditions and rare disorders. More extensive information on this condition can be found on a range of reliable, validated websites. Further information on these resources can be found in our **Medical Information on the Internet** article on page 21.

Contact a Family Helpline 0808 808 3555

Support

TTP Network

c/o Contact a Family, 209-211 City Road, London EC1V 1JN   Tel: 0808 808 3555 Helpline
Fax: 020 7608 8701   e-mail: jo@ttpnetwork.org.uk   Web: http://www.ttpnetwork.org.uk
*This is a small informal network started in 1996. Those in touch include affected
individuals, their families and professionals working in the field. It offers information via the
website and information exchange and mutual support through the message board.*
Group details last updated March 2007.

Did you know that genetic counselling
is available on the NHS for all families
expecting a child with a genetic
condition. Call the Contact a Family
Helpline for more information and a
copy of the guide, 'About Diagnosis'.

THYROID DISORDERS

Thyroid underactivity (Hypothyroidism)

Underactivity of the thyroid gland (hypothyroidism) can arise for a number of reasons. Hypothyroidism can occur in newborn infants (Congenital Hypothyroidism, CHT) as well as later on in childhood (acquired Hypothyroidism, AHT.) Affected newborns look, and usually act, normal for the first few days and the national screening programme for CHT, by blood spot collection, ensures that affected infants are identified and treated as early as possible. The commonest cause of CHT is a poorly developed or absent thyroid gland; the underlying basis to this abnormality is not understood. CHT can also occur if there is a defect in thyroxine production within the gland. These defects may be permanent or transient. Although every child with CHT should be started on thyroxine promptly, they should be evaluated at some time later to exclude a transient problem.

The commonest causes of acquired hypothyroidism include an immune reaction against the thyroid gland by the body itself (Autoimmune Hypothyroidism, Hashimoto's disease) or damage to the thyroid gland or the part of the brain which controls the thyroid.

Symptoms and signs of hypothyroidism vary depending on a number of factors such as the cause of hypothyroidism, age of onset and the duration of the interval leading to treatment. In untreated or inadequately treated cases, features may include dry skin with a yellowish tinge, coarse brittle hair, puffy eyelids, thick broad tongue, hoarse voice, slow heart rate, constipation, short stature, delayed pubertal development and learning disabilities.

Congenital Hypothyroidism in women

It is most important that women with Congenital Hypothyroidism who are pregnant ensure that they have regular thyroxine treatment in the periconceptual period (around the time of conception) and in the first three months of pregnancy. This is important as there is evidence that minor degrees of hypothyroidism can affect the baby. An endocrinologist and obstetrician needs to be involved from an early stage.

Inheritance patterns and prenatal diganosis (Hypothyroidism)

Inheritance patterns

Some defects of thyroxine synthesis are inherited in an autosomal recessive pattern. It is very rare to have more than one affected individual in any one family with abnormal development of the thyroid gland.

Prenatal diagnosis

This may be available if the genetic abnormality is already known. As affected newborns do very well if thyroxine therapy is started following early postnatal diagnosis, there is no clinical need at the present for prenatal diagnosis.

Thyroid Overactivity (Hyperthyroidism, thyrotoxicosis)

Hyperthyroidism can occur if children with hypothyroidism are on an inappropriately high dose of thyroxine or because of overactivity of the thyroid gland, which occurs most commonly in late childhood. In most cases the overactivity is due to the action of antibodies produced by one's own body which stimulate the thyroid gland (Graves' disease.) This condition is opposite to hypothyroidism caused during Hashimoto's thyroiditis. Sometimes the latter may be preceded by the former in the same individual. Hyperthyroidism accelerates a number of biochemical processes in the body and the affected child may grow faster, become more anxious, restless with disturbed sleep and develop increased appetite (but weight loss), excessive sweating and diarrhoea. The gland, situated in the front of the neck, may become enlarged and the eyes may become prominent. Rarely, Thyroid Overactivity may occur in the newborn. This is often a temporary phenomenon and is due to the transfer of antibodies across the placenta of a mother with Graves' disease. The hyperthyroidism subsides as the antibody levels reduce over the first couple of months of life.

Thyroid overactivity is treated by drug management, radioiodine treatment or surgery. However, surgery is not commonly performed in children.

Inheritance patterns and prenatal diagnosis (Hyperthyroidism)

Inheritance patterns

Other family members have a higher likelihood of both disorders; no simple genetic tests are available, yet.

Prenatal diagnosis

None

Medical text written June 1999 by Dr S Faisal Ahmed and Dr P Hindmarsh. **Last reviewed January 2004 by Dr S Faisal Ahmed, Consultant Paediatric Endocrinologist & Hon. Senior Lecturer, Royal Hospital for Sick Children, Glasgow, UK and Dr P Hindmarsh, Consultant Paediatric Endocrinologist and Reader in Paediatric Endocrinology, University College London Medical School, London, UK.**

Further online resources

Medical texts in *The Contact a Family Directory* are designed to give a short, clear description of specific conditions and rare disorders. More extensive information on this condition can be found on a range of reliable, validated websites. Further information on these resources can be found in our **Medical Information on the Internet** article on page 21.

Support

British Thyroid Foundation
PO Box 97, Clifford, Wetherby LS23 6XD   Tel: 01423 709707 / 709448
e-mail: b.m.nevens@btf-thyroid.org   Web: http://www.btf-thyroid.org
The Foundation is a National Registered Charity No. 1006391, established in 1991. It offers support for affected adults and support for families of children with thyroid disorders and thyroid cancer. It publishes a quarterly newsletter with occasional paediatric articles and has a wide range of information available, details on request. Please send SAE. The Foundation has over 7,000 members including the families of over 50 children.
Group details last confirmed October 2007.

Support is also available from a group of families of children with Hypothyroidism under the umbrella of Climb (see entry, Metabolic diseases).

---

162 new condition entries have been added to the Contact a Family Directory over the last seven editions.

THYROID EYE DISEASE

Thyroid Eye disease: Thyroid Ophthalmopathy; Thyroid Associated Ophthalmopathy; Graves' Eye disease; Graves' Ophthalmopathy

Background

Thyroid Eye disease is an autoimmune condition in which damage to the eye muscles and fatty tissue behind the eye is caused by the body's own white blood cells and antibodies.

What are the symptoms?

Swelling of the damaged tissues behind the eyes can cause the eyes to become red and swelling to occur above and below the eyes. It may also cause the eyes to be pushed forward ('starey eyes', 'proptosis'). In more severe cases, the damage at the back of the eye causes swelling and stiffness of the muscles that move the eye, causing double vision. This occurs especially when looking from side to side as the muscles cannot keep the eyes exactly in line with each other. Occasionally, the swelling behind the eyes is severe enough to press on the nerve from the eyes to the brain affecting vision.

Other features that may occur include mild soreness and grittiness of the eyes usually only affecting one eye, increased watering of the eye, a dislike of bright lights and a feeling of discomfort behind the eyes especially when looking up or side to side. Puffiness of the upper eyelid or around the eyes giving the impression of baggy eyes is also common and is worse first thing in the morning. The eyes often appear 'starey' and drying of the eyes or too many tears can cause blurry vision which comes and goes.

What are the causes?

Ninety per cent of people with Thyroid Eye disease also have an overactive thyroid gland (thyrotoxicosis). Graves' disease is a type of thyrotoxicosis which is autoimmune in aetiology. A feature of both Graves' disease and Thyroid Eye disease is thought to be the common molecule, the thyrotrophin stimulating hormone (TSH) receptor to which stimulating antibodies develop. Thyroid Eye disease and an overactive thyroid gland do not always develop at the same time and the treatment for one does not affect the treatment of the other, with the exception of radioactive iodine treatment. A small number of people with Thyroid Eye disease may have an underactive thyroid with some having no thyroid disturbance at all.

How is it treated?

Treatment for Thyroid Eye disease depends on the severity and ranges from simple eye drops to immunosuppressive therapy and decompressive surgery. The most important aspect of treatment is the preservation of eyesight.

Inheritance patterns and prenatal diagnosis
Inheritance patterns
None.
Prenatal diagnosis
None.

Medical text written April 2002 by Contact a Family. **Last reviewed June 2007 by Dr R Stanhope, Consultant Paediatric Endocrinologist, Institute of Child Health, London, UK.**

Further online resources
Medical texts in *The Contact a Family Directory* are designed to give a short, clear description of specific conditions and rare disorders. More extensive information on this condition can be found on a range of reliable, validated websites. Further information on these resources can be found in our **Medical Information on the Internet** article on page 21.

Support
Thyroid Eye Disease Charitable Trust
PO Box 2954, Calne SN11 8WR   Tel: 0844 800 8133   e-mail: ted@tedct.co.uk
Web: http://www.tedct.co.uk
The Trust (formerly the Thyroid Eye Disease Association) is a National Registered Charity No. 1095967, established in 1995. It offers information, care and support for affected people. It also supports research. It publishes a newsletter and has information available, details on request. The Association has over 800 members.
Group details last updated January 2007.

TINNITUS

Background

Tinnitus is the name given to a symptom described by an individual who experiences perceptions of noises in the head or ears, these noises being generated internally.

What are symptoms?

Tinnitus can a very distressing condition although many people are not troubled by their noises. An individual distressed by tinnitus may often experience difficulty coping and some depression may result. Sleep and concentration may be affected.

Children are sometimes affected by tinnitus, but it is rare for this to become a persistent problem in childhood.

What are the causes?

The condition has many causes among which are natural ageing processes, microscopic damage to the auditory system, damage to the system due to external sources of noise (including industrial, personal stereos and explosions or gunfire). Tinnitus may also be part of a specific condition, for example Menières disease in which it is associated with an increase in pressure of the fluid in the inner ear, vertigo, nausea and vomiting. It should be noted however that in many people with tinnitus no underlying pathology can be found.

How is it treated?

There is no cure for tinnitus but a variety of effective therapies are available. Affected individuals should seek guidance from their GP and may refer for specialist advice.

Inheritance patterns and prenatal diagnosis

Inheritance patterns

Current research does not indicate any hereditary link.

Prenatal diagnosis

None.

Medical text written August 2001 by David Baguley. **Last reviewed December 2005 by David Baguley, Audiological Scientist, Addenbrooke's Hospital, Cambridge, UK and Vice-Chairman of the British Tinnitus Association Professional Advisers Committee.**

Further online resources

Medical texts in *The Contact a Family Directory* are designed to give a short, clear description of specific conditions and rare disorders. More extensive information on this condition can be found on a range of reliable, validated websites. Further information on these resources can be found in our **Medical Information on the Internet** article on page 21.

Support

British Tinnitus Association
Ground Floor, Unit 5, Acorn Business Park, Woodseats Close, Sheffield S8 0TB
Tel: 0800 018 0527 Freephone   Tel: 0114 250 9933   Fax: 0114 258 2279
e-mail: info@tinnitus.org.uk   Web: http://www.tinnitus.org.uk
The Association is a National Registered Charity No. 1011145, established in 1992. It offers information and advice about healthy living and relaxation techniques together with support and contact with others through local groups. It publishes a quarterly journal 'Quiet' and has information available, details on request.
Group details last confirmed September 2007.

RNID Tinnitus Helpline
RNID, 19-23 Featherstone Street,   London EC1Y 8SL
Tel: 0808 808 6666 Freephone Helpline   Tel: 0808 808 0007 Free Textphone
Fax: 020 7296 8199   e-mail: tinnitushelpline@rnid.org.uk   Web: http://www.rnid.org.uk
The RNID Tinnitus Helpline provides support and deals with enquiries about the nature and causes, treatment and management of tinnitus. It offers a wide range of factsheets, leaflets and other publications and produces "Tinnitus Focus" magazine. Factsheets may also be downloaded from RNID's website.
Group details last confirmed September 2006.

"The best part of the day was meeting others who were experiencing similar problems, dilemmas and emotion; being able to talk so freely and not feeling so alone." A grandparent at a workshop for grandparents of disabled children organised by Contact a Family North East. It was the first time any of them had met others in similar situations to themselves.

TOURETTE SYNDROME

Tourette syndrome: Gilles de la Tourette syndrome

Background

This is a condition characterised by multiple tics. Tics are involuntary twitch-like movements involving groups of muscles. In this syndrome, tics characteristically involve the facial area (e.g. blinking, grimacing, nodding) as well as phonic (vocal) tics, although any area can be involved. The tics range from very simple to more complex, purposeful movements. Vocal tics can be as simple as throat clearing or coughing. Tics can be suppressed for a short time and so, for example, the condition may appear different at school compared to home.

What are the symptoms?

The onset of the symptoms is usually between the ages of five to eleven with a maximum starting age of eighteen. There is a very wide range of severity so that many people with the condition may never need to seek medical attention whilst others have a socially disabling condition.

Common associations of the syndrome are Obsessive Compulsive Disorder or Behaviour (OCD/OCB) (see entry, Obsessive Compulsive Disorder) and Attention Deficit Hyperactivity Disorder (ADHD) (see entry). In some cases echolalia (the repetition of phrases, or mimicking of gestures) may be present. A relatively rare feature in more severe cases is coprolalia (the involuntary use of obscene or offensive words) or copropraxia (the involuntary making of obscene gestures.)

Symptoms may occur and disappear, increase or decrease in severity, or new symptoms may arise. In some cases remissions occur. It is thought that Tourette syndrome often decreases in severity around or after adolescence although it can be a lifelong condition. The incidence of the syndrome is three to four times greater in males than females.

Inheritance patterns and prenatal diagnosis

Inheritance patterns

It is thought that in about ninety per cent of cases the condition runs in the family, although other family members may have a mild, barely noticeable disorder. The wide range of features has made it difficult to definitively define the genetic inheritance although the autosomal dominant with incomplete penetrance model has been used. That is, each pregnancy has a 1 in 2 chance of an affected gene with many such cases not manifesting the condition. It is thought that many different genes may be causative in different individuals.

Environmental factors may also play a part with possible interactions with a perinatal insult - for example, a birth trauma such as anoxia (lack of oxygen). In recent years a link with throat infections caused by a bacteria called streptococcus has been proposed. There is probably no single cause of Tourette syndrome, and multiple factors may be involved

Mild cases may not need to be treated. There is no cure but many of the symptoms such as OCD and ADHD can be helped with medication.

Prenatal diagnosis

None. So far only one possible causative gene has been identified, and more may be expected in future. The genetic causes will need to be far better understood before prenatal diagnosis is possible. However, in general the children of someone with Tourette syndrome are not likely to inherit a severe form of the disease, although that possibility cannot be completely ruled out.

Medical text written March 2001 by Dr J Stern. **Last updated January 2006 by Dr J Stern, Consultant Neurologist, St. George's Hospital, London.**

Further online resources

Medical texts in *The Contact a Family Directory* are designed to give a short, clear description of specific conditions and rare disorders. More extensive information on this condition can be found on a range of reliable, validated websites. Further information on these resources can be found in our **Medical Information on the Internet** article on page 21.

Support

Tourette Syndrome (UK) Association

Southbank House, Black Prince Road, London SE1 7SJ   Tel: 0845 458 1252 Helpline Tel: 020 7793 2356 Admin   e-mail: help@tsa.org.uk   Web: http://www.tsa.org.uk

The Association is a National Registered Charity No. 1003317, established in 1980. It offers support for affected individuals and their families. It promotes research and maintains a register of physicians familiar with the condition. It publishes a quarterly newsletter and has information available, details on request.

Group details last updated February 2008.

Tourette Scotland

Algo Business Centre, Glenearn Road, Perth PH2 0NJ   Tel: 01738 450 411 e-mail: info@tourettescotland.org   Web: http://www.tourettescotland.org

The organisation is a Scottish Registered Charity No. SCO21851, established in 1993. It provides advice and support for affected persons and their families, brings together individuals affected by TS and associated disorders, and raises awareness amongst public and professionals. It publishes a newsletter and has information available, details on request. The organisation is in touch with over 300 individuals, families and professionals.

Group details last updated February 2007.

TOWNES-BROCKS SYNDROME

Background

Townes-Brocks syndrome (TBS) is a rare genetic condition present at birth. The main features include ear anomalies leading to hearing loss and characteristic anal and thumb anomalies. The range and severity of these features vary from person to person. TBS affects males and females equally. Since 1972, when the condition was first described by Dr Townes and Dr Brocks, approximately one hundred individuals worldwide have been reported with the syndrome. It is difficult to estimate the true incidence of TBS because there is a possibility that TBS is currently under-diagnosed. On this basis, more individuals than reported may be affected with TBS.

What are the symptoms?

Anal anomalies associated with TBS may include absence of a normal opening (imperforate anus) with a passage connecting the rectum to the vagina (rectovaginal fistula), abnormal placement of the anus and narrowing of the anal passage (anal stenosis). Typically, the ears of individuals with TBS may be large, or small, abnormally developed (dysplastic) ears, lop ear (over-folded ear helix) or have preauricular tags or pits (a rudimentary tag of ear tissue typically located just in front of the ear). Individuals may experience hearing loss (see entry, Deafness) due to structural anomalies in the inner ear (sensorineural deafness) or because of anomalies in the external or middle ear (conductive deafness). The thumbs may be underdeveloped (hypoplastic) or have the appearance more of a finger than a thumb. Webbed fingers (syndactyly) may occur, as well as fusion of the bones in the wrist.

A number of other features may also be associated TBS. These involve other systems in the body. The bones in the feet of some children may be fused with overlapping toes leading to mobility difficulties (see entry, Lower Limb Abnormalities). TBS may affect the kidney, and underdeveloped (hypoplastic) kidneys, multicystic kidneys, abnormal (dysplastic) kidneys and kidney failure have been reported (see entry, Kidney disease). Abnormalities associated with the heart may include tetralogy of fallot and ventricular septal defects (see entry, Heart Defects). Whilst severe heart and kidney problems may be life-threatening, many individuals with TBS have a normal life-span.

Learning difficulties have been reported in some children with TBS. For others, intelligence is within the normal range.

Inheritance patterns and prenatal diagnosis

Inheritance patterns

TBS is inherited as an autosomal dominant trait. Changes in a gene located on chromosome 16 are associated with the characteristic features.

Prenatal diagnosis

It may sometimes be possible to perform prenatal diagnosis by chorionic villus sampling (CVS) or amniocentesis during pregnancy. Genetic counselling may be helpful for individuals and families affected by this condition.

Medical text written September 2003 by Contact a Family. Approved September 2003 by Dr M Whiteford, Consultant Clinical Geneticist, Ferguson-Smith Centre for Clinical Genetics, Glasgow, UK.

Further online resources

Medical texts in *The Contact a Family Directory* are designed to give a short, clear description of specific conditions and rare disorders. More extensive information on this condition can be found on a range of reliable, validated websites. Further information on these resources can be found in our **Medical Information on the Internet** article on page 21.

Support

There is no support group for Townes-Brocks syndrome. Cross referrals to other entries in The Contact a Family Directory are intended to provide relevant support for these particular features of the disorder. Organisations identified in these entries do not provide support specifically for Townes-Brocks syndrome. Families can use Contact a Family's Freephone Helpline for advice, information and, where possible, links to other families. Contact a Family's web-based linking service Making Contact.org can be accessed at http://www.makingcontact.org

TOXOCARIASIS

Background

Human toxocariasis is an infection with the larval stage of the dog roundworm, Toxocara canis, a parasitic worm. The extent of involvement in human disease of the cat roundworm, Toxocara cati, is unknown. The disease is caught by swallowing the microscopic Toxocara egg which is spread in infected dog or cat faeces.

Up to 2 per cent of the 'normal' population may be seropositive for Toxocara antibodies. The ocular form of the disease occurs mainly in children between the ages of six and twelve. It is rare in the UK. Visceral larval migrans usually self-resolves, but is treatable with anthelminthic drugs.

What are the symptoms?

The systemic form results in non-specific ill health and is probably frequently undiagnosed. Signs and symptoms may include fever, wheezy chest, abdominal pain, the source of which is unrecognised, or may be more severe, with hepatomegaly (enlargement of the liver), when toxocariasis may be diagnosed. Subclinical (not detectable by the usual clinical tests) toxocariasis is termed covert toxocariasis.

What are the causes?

Toxocariasis more commonly affects children than adults and characteristically presents as eye disease: ocular toxocariasis, but may also cause systemic disease: visceral larval migrans. Both conditions are caused by the larvae, which hatch in the intestine, immediately burrowing through the gut wall and migrating through the body, unable to complete their life cycle in humans. The migration can continue for months or years. With the ocular form, a larva becomes trapped in the eye causing a granuloma in the retina and visual impairment, possible blindness. Eye damage is usually unilateral, but affects both eyes in up to three per cent of patients.

How is it diagnosed?

Diagnosis is by means of a blood test for toxocaral antibodies, carried out in a specialist laboratory. The test does not distinguish between active and inactive disease.

Inheritance patterns and prenatal diagnosis

Inheritance patterns

Not applicable.

Prenatal diagnosis

None.

T

Medical text written May 1996 by Community Hygiene Concern. Approved May 1996 by Dr P Chiodini. **Last updated August 2006 by Professor P Chiodini, Hospital for Tropical diseases, London, UK.**

Support

Community Hygiene Concern

Manor Gardens Centre, 6-9 Manor Gardens, London N7 6LA   Tel: 020 7686 4321
e-mail: bugbusters2k@yahoo.co.uk   Web: http://www.chc.org
The Organisation is a National Registered Charity No. 801371, established in 1988. It offers counselling and linking affected families where possible. It publishes a periodic journal, 'Shared Wisdom' and has information available, details on request.
Group details last confirmed June 2007.

Contact a Family continuously updates and expands a Group Action Pack which gives developmental advice to new and established support groups.

TOXOPLASMOSIS

Background

Toxoplasmosis is an infection which is caused by the parasite Toxoplasma gondii which affects all warm blooded animals including humans. Infection is caught by eating anything infected or contaminated with the parasite such as raw or under cooked meat, food contaminated with infected cat faeces or the soil where cats mess, and unpasteurised goat's milk.

What are the symptoms?

In healthy adults and children infection may be without symptoms, a mild flu-like illness and occasionally symptoms similar to glandular fever. The infection can cause serious health problems for anyone with suppressed or damaged immunity, for example people on immune suppressing drugs or people with AIDS.

Toxoplasmosis is one of a small group of infections which can transmit to the fetus if caught for the first time during pregnancy. The risk of transmission and the degree of damage done depend on when in pregnancy the woman catches the infection. In the first trimester, the damage may be very severe as the fetus is so vulnerable, however it is less likely that infection is transmitted at this stage of pregnancy. Later on in pregnancy the damage is less severe, but the infection is more likely to transmit and cause congenital infection.

Severe damage includes hydrocephalus (excess fluid on the brain), calcifications of the brain tissue that can lead to developmental delay and epilepsy, and damage to the retina of one or both eyes called retinochoroiditis. The majority of people with congenital toxoplasmosis have impaired sight in one or both eyes. The more severe damage to the brain is rare.

Damage in a severely affected infant will be apparent soon after birth, but in most cases the congenital infection will only show in childhood, the teens or even later, and this will be as retinochoroiditis.

How is it diagnosed?

In most cases congenital infection will only be detected after birth when there are eye problems and the patient presents with retinochoroiditis. These patients need to be carefully investigated by Reference Laboratories, and treatment for congenital infection may be up to one year.

Inheritance patterns and prenatal diagnosis

Inheritance patterns

Not applicable

Prenatal diagnosis

This requires a specific blood test on the pregnant woman. This is not done routinely in the UK, although in other European countries there are national screening programmes. If a woman feels she has been at risk through something she ate, or if she has symptoms which could indicate toxoplasma infection, she can request a blood test. All positive tests should be sent to the Toxoplasma Reference Laboratory for confirmation and in the case of current infection, for tests which estimate the onset of infection. If the onset of infection is considered to be recent, the fetus can be tested, using amniocentesis or cordocentesis: but as these tests carry a risk of miscarriage, they are only offered where the risk of infection to the fetus is high and must be performed by a specialist in this field. Ultrasound scans can show up severe damage, but not the minor forms and only a blood test could confirm toxoplasmosis as the cause. Specific antibiotic treatment can help limit the risk of the infection crossing to the fetus where an infection is diagnosed during pregnancy. If the fetus is found to be infected, stronger antiparasitic drugs may be given to help limit the damage, and this treatment would also be given to all infants born with congenital infection.

Medical text written May 1996 by Contact a Family. Approved May 1996 by Dr T Brand, Toxoplasmosis Trust, London UK. **Last updated February 2004 by Dr D Ho-Yen, Director, Scottish Toxoplasma Reference Laboratory, Raigmore Hospital, Inverness, UK.**

Further online resources

Medical texts in *The Contact a Family Directory* are designed to give a short, clear description of specific conditions and rare disorders. More extensive information on this condition can be found on a range of reliable, validated websites. Further information on these resources can be found in our **Medical Information on the Internet** article on page 21.

Support

Tommy's, the baby charity
Nicholas House, 3 Laurence Pountney Hill, London EC4R 0BB
Tel: 0870 777 3060 Pregnancy Information Line   Tel: 08707 70 70 70
Fax: 08707 70 70 75   e-mail: info@tommys.org   Web: http://www.tommys.org
Tommy's is a National Registered Charity No. 1060508. It funds a national programme of medical research and information. It provides information for parents, parents-to-be, health professionals and the general public, to help maximise the chance of having a healthy pregnancy, through a telephone pregnancy information line, e-mail and web access to health professionals, plus a range of free publications.
Group details last updated January 2006.

TRACHEO-OESOPHAGEAL FISTULA and/ or OESOPHAGEAL ATRESIA

Background

Oesophageal Atresia (OA) and Tracheo-Oesophageal Fistula (TOF) are rare congenital conditions of the oesophagus (food pipe) and/or trachea (airway) that affect newborn babies.

What are the symptoms?

With OA, the oesophagus forms a closed off pouch that prevents food from reaching the stomach. Prior to corrective surgery, this pouch can fill up with food and saliva, which can eventually overflow into the baby's trachea (windpipe), entering the lungs and causing choking.

With TOF, the oesophagus is connected to the windpipe. Without surgical intervention, this allows air to pass from the windpipe to the food pipe and stomach. It can also allow stomach acid to pass into the lungs.

Approximately 1 in 3,500 babies is born with a TOF/OA related condition, most with both TOF and OA.

VACTERL Association

Babies with TOF/OA may also have other health problems, particularly heart defects, imperforate anus and kidney, spinal or limb anomalies. There is a recognised association between a particular group of abnormalities, which has been called the VACTERL Association (see entry).

How is it diagnosed?

The main diagnostic criteria include frothing at the mouth, laboured breathing and/or blueness of the lips and fingertips. If oesophageal atresia is suspected, the passage of a rigid tube down the oesophagus from the mouth will confirm the diagnosis (if it is held up in the blind upper pouch) or exclude it (if the tube reaches the stomach).

How is it treated?

Babies with TOF/OA require intensive neo-natal care prior to corrective surgery, usually within days of being born. Some children have to undergo additional surgical interventions later on in life.

Inheritance patterns and prenatal diagnosis

Inheritance patterns

None in the majority of cases.

Prenatal diagnosis

Maternal polyhydramnios (excessive quantity of amniotic fluid) may indicate the presence of oesophageal atresia especially if accompanied by a small or absent stomach in the developing fetus.

Medical text written December 2005 by Mr Bruce Jaffray, Consultant Paediatric Surgeon, Royal Victoria Infirmary, Newcastle upon Tyne, UK.

Support

TOFS (Tracheo-Oesophageal Fistula Support)
St George's Centre, 91 Victoria Road, Netherfield, Nottingham NG4 2NN
Tel: 0115 961 3092   Fax: 0115 961 3097   e-mail: office@tofs.org.uk
Web: http://www.tofs.org.uk
TOFS is a National Registered Charity No. 327735, established in 1982. It provides support and information to families of children with TOF/OA and VACTERL Association. TOFS enables mutual support through telephone, letters and visits. It can put members in touch with each other and also offers contact through local meetings and social events in some areas. TOFS publishes a quarterly newsletter "Chew", a book, "The TOF Child" and a range of leaflets on practical and medical topics. Its website provides access to many of these leaflets and also to online discussion forums. The charity has over 1,000 members, including medical specialists and health professionals.
Group details last confirmed March 2007.

TRACHEOSTOMY

Background

A tracheostomy is an artificial opening into the trachea (windpipe) usually between the second and fourth tracheal rings. It is held open by a tracheostomy tube. A tracheotomy refers to the actual surgical 'cutting' into the trachea and a tracheostomy refers to the actual hole and the tube that sits into it.

Usually the decision to perform a tracheostomy is reached as a result of many investigations and tests. However, on some occasions, the need to perform a tracheostomy is the result of an acute upper airway emergency.

Indications for tracheostomy in the paediatric population differ somewhat from the adult population. A tracheostomy will ensure a patent (open) airway when the child's condition results in an obstruction causing a narrowed upper airway. Some children may require long or short term mechanical support from a ventilator, and some may require it to protect the lower airways from aspiration.

A child with a tracheostomy requires constant close observation and careful suctioning to keep the tube clear and to minimise undesirable effects.

There are different types of tracheostomy tubes available and the child should be given the tube that best suits its needs. The frequency of these tube changes will depend on the type of tube the child has and may possibly alter during the winter or summer months. Practitioners should refer to specialist practitioners and/or the manufacturers for advice.

Tracheostomies may be permanent or temporary. A temporary tracheostomy will be indicated until the child's medical condition stabilises or has been surgically corrected. Once it has been established that the tracheostomy is likely to be in place for a period of time, plans for community care will be started. A home care programme will be discussed with the child and family so that carers are sufficiently trained in all aspects of tracheostomy care before discharge from hospital.

Inheritance patterns and prenatal diagnosis

Inheritance patterns
Not applicable.

Prenatal diagnosis
None.

Medical text last updated November 2002 by J Cooke, Tracheostomy Nurse Specialist, Great Ormond Street Hospital, London, UK. **Last reviewed February 2008 by Mr B Hartley, Consultant ENT Surgeon, Great Ormond Street Hospital, London, UK.**

Support
ACT

Lammas Cottage, Stathe, Bridgwater TA7 0JL   Tel: 01823 698398
e-mail: support@actfortrachykids.com   Web: http://www.actfortrachykids.com
The Group is a National Registered Charity No. 326511, established in 1983. It offers
support and encouragement to families together with contact with others where possible.
It publishes a quarterly newsletter and has information available, details on request. The
Group has over 700 members including professionals (over 500 affected children).
Group details last confirmed March 2007.

If you look after a disabled child and caring has a major impact in your life then a carer's assessment could help you. Call the Contact a Family Helpline for more information and a copy of a guide to disabled children's services.

TRANSVERSE MYELITIS

Background

Transverse Myelitis (TM) is a rare neurological disorder of the central nervous system caused by inflammation across the spinal cord. TM can affect adults and children of both sexes and all ethnic groups. It is thought to have an incidence of between 1 and 5 in 1,000,000.

Onset of TM is usually sudden over a day or two but in some people it can develop over a longer period. Swelling, caused by inflammation, blocks messages to the brain relating to touch, pain and temperature, resulting in numbness or altered feeling. Messages from the brain also cannot get down the cord causing weakness or paralysis in the limbs, usually the legs. Control of bladder and bowel can also be affected by the inflammation in the cord. Although the effects disappear as the swelling reduces, damage can be more long term.

What are the symptoms?

The features of TM vary in individuals and will depend on which nerve fibres in the spinal cord are affected by inflammation. Changed function is experienced below the level of the inflammation but remains normal above. The severity of the symptoms is related to the intensity of the inflammation. Features can include:

- Leg weakness;
- Altered sensation including pins and needles;
- Back pain;
- Numbness;
- Inability to distinguish temperature of objects and liquids;
- Loss of control of the bowel or bladder;
- Loss of sexual function.

The area of spinal cord inflammation will determine the nature of some of the features of TM.

What are the causes?

The cause of TM is not known but viral infections, spinal cord injury, immune reactions and an insufficient blood flow through spinal cord blood vessels have been suggested as causes. In some cases, TM can be the initial presentation of Multiple Sclerosis (see entry) and can also occur as part of Multiple Sclerosis.

How is it diagnosed?

A diagnosis of TM will be based on the observation of characteristic clinical features. Before a diagnosis can be made, other causes of pressure or inflammation of the spinal cord must be eliminated; this will usually involve carrying out a magnetic resonance imaging scan (MRI) and blood tests. Some patients require a lumbar puncture (spinal tap).

How is it treated?

Treatment of TM is symptomatic and supportive. It may include drug therapy, physiotherapy and, for some, the insertion of a catheter into the bladder. Pain relief may also be indicated in individuals affected by muscle strain or pressure on nerves. Most people improve but recovery can vary from complete recovery (which may take some time), to little improvement with significant motor, sensory or bowel deficits or even to no recovery. Rehabilitation can be aided by physiotherapy and rest when indicated but keeping active is also important. Mechanical aids including walking frames and wheel chairs will be helpful during recovery. Usually TM only occurs once but occasionally there may be a recurrence, possibly due to an underlying condition such as Multiple Sclerosis.

Inheritance patterns and prenatal diagnosis

Inheritance patterns

None.

Prenatal diagnosis

Not applicable.

Medical text written May 2006 by Contact a Family. Approved June 2006 by Professor R A C Hughes, Professor of Neurology, King's College London School of Medicine, London, UK.

Further online resources

Medical texts in *The Contact a Family Directory* are designed to give a short, clear description of specific conditions and rare disorders. More extensive information on this condition can be found on a range of reliable, validated websites. Further information on these resources can be found in our **Medical Information on the Internet** article on page 21.

Support

Transverse Myelitis Society
c/o Contact a Family, 209-211 City Road, London EC1V 1JN   Tel: 01539 434677
e-mail: Geoff.Treglown@btinternet.com   Web: http://www.myelitis.org.uk
The Transverse Myelitis Society is a National Registered Charity No. 1108179, established in 2004. It offers support to affected people and families by telephone and e-mail.
The Society has a number of local support groups offering meetings. It has a range of information, details on the website. Over 400 members are in touch with about ten per cent being the families of children or young people.
Group details last confirmed June 2007.

TREACHER COLLINS SYNDROME

Treacher Collins syndrome: Mandibulo Dysostosis; Franceschetti-Klein

Background

It is a genetic condition characterised by malformed cheek bones, chin, nose, and jaw.

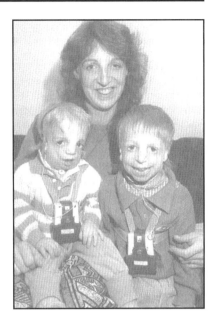

Three similar conditions are: **Nager** which is a syndrome with similar mandibular dysostosis anomalies to Treacher Collins but with additional arm and digital anomalies: **Aural atresia** of the ears (congenital imperforation of the normal channel or pathological closure of the channel in the ears): **First and second arch** syndromes which are inclusive titles for developmental errors of the facial bones and which include Treacher Collins syndrome.

What are the symptoms?

Features include: drooping eyelids which may be associated with a nick in the lower lid; variable degrees of malformed or absent ears, the middle ear may also be malformed or missing causing conductive deafness; receding chin at birth; hairline and palate may also be unusual (cleft palate or choanal atresia may occur in severe cases). Associated problems may include dental, breathing and eye infections.

Inheritance patterns and prenatal diagnosis

Inheritance patterns

In Treacher-Collins inheritance is autosomal dominant with variable expression. Over half of cases are sporadic mutations.

Prenatal diagnosis

Prenatal diagnosis can sometimes be performed by molecular testing.

Medical text written November 1991 by Contact a Family. Approved November 1991 by Professor M Patton, Professor of Medical Genetics, St Georges Hospital Medical School, London, UK and Dr J E Wraith, Consultant Paediatrician, Royal Manchester Children's Hospital, Manchester, UK. Last updated May 2001 by Professor M Dixon. **Last reviewed October 2005 by Professor M Dixon, Professor of Dental Genetics, University of Manchester, Manchester, UK.**

Further online resources

Medical texts in *The Contact a Family Directory* are designed to give a short, clear description of specific conditions and rare disorders. More extensive information on this condition can be found on a range of reliable, validated websites. Further information on these resources can be found in our **Medical Information on the Internet** article on page 21.

Support

Treacher Collins Family Support Group

114 Vincent Road, Thorpe Hamlet, Norwich NR1 4HH   Tel: 01603 433736
e-mail: info@treachercollins.net   Web: http://www.treachercollins.net
The Group is a National Registered Charity No. 1006300, established in 1987. The group also covers First and Second Arch syndromes, Atresia of the Ear, and any other condition combining conductive deafness with facial/head malformation. It offers support and friendship for affected families. It publishes a regular newsletter and has information available, details on request. The Group holds an annual Family Conference and has over 250 members in touch.
Group details last confirmed June 2007.

TRIGEMINAL NEURALGIA

Trigeminal Neuralgia: Tic Douloureux

Background

Trigeminal Neuralgia (TN) is an extremely severe facial pain that tends to come and go unpredictably in sudden shock-like attacks. The pain is often described as stabbing, shooting, excruciating, burning, extremely strong. The pain usually lasts for a few seconds, but there can be many bursts of pain in quick succession. It is a chronic disorder of the trigeminal nerve (or fifth cranial nerve) and affects about 8 people in 100,000.

The Trigeminal Nerve has three branches (or divisions):

- The upper branch (Ophthalmic) which runs above the eye, forehead and front of the head;
- The middle branch (Maxillary) which runs through the cheek, upper jaw, teeth and gums, side of the nose;
- The lower branch (Mandibular) which runs through the lower jaw, teeth and gums.

TN can involve one or more branches. Most frequently, the middle and lower branches are affected. It usually affects people over 50 years old, but many cases have been reported in young adults, and very rarely among children.

It affects women more than men, and it is more often on the right side of the face. It is not hereditary.

What are the symptoms?

- Spasms of sharp, stabbing pain, often described as like a jolt of lightning;
- The pain is confined in the area served by the branches of the TN nerve: lower jaw, upper jaw, cheek, eye, and forehead. The pain may include one, two or all three branches of the TN nerve;
- Pain is almost always on one side of the face, most commonly the right-hand side;
- The pain is usually provoked by a light touch on the face, movements of the face (and therefore mouth), washing the face, a light breeze. Trigger points are usually around the nose and lip;
- The pain might disappear by itself for weeks, even months, and return.

What are the causes?

The cause of TN is still an area for debate among medical professionals. Most believe that the deterioration of the myelin (protective coating of the nerve) allows the transmission of abnormal messages of pain. The damage of the myelin sheath may be caused by pressure from blood vessels or arteries, tumours, Multiple Sclerosis, injury to the nerve, consequences of shingles, or just the ageing process.

How is it diagnosed?

Diagnosis of idiopathic trigeminal neuralgia is made entirely on history but tests for tumours pressing on the nerve or Multiple Sclerosis may be required to be eliminate symptomatic trigeminal neuralgia. Magnetic imaging resonance (MRI) of the brain is done to determine if a blood vessel is pressing on the nerve.

How is it treated?

If, after several visits to a dentist, a GP or an oral surgeon, TN is suspected, the patient is sent to a neurologist. He will perform some neurological tests to rule out or discover other diseases. He will also ask for a precise description of the pain. Most doctors will recommend a MRI scan in order to see if there is any obvious cause.

A number of drugs, mainly anti-epileptic, are used to treat TN singly or in combination. As these drugs have a number of side effects such as drowsiness or a feeling of inability to concentrate, the specific drugs for an individual are dictated by efficacy and affect. If a drug regime fails to alleviate pain or leads to unacceptable side effects, surgery may be considered. There are a wide variety of surgical procedures available, all with their own risks but they give much longer pain relief periods. Due to the rarity of the condition and its severity, sufferers can feel isolated and fearful. Contact with a trigeminal neuralgia support group may be very helpful.

Inheritance patterns and prenatal diagnosis

Inheritance patterns

None.

Prenatal diagnosis

None.

Medical text written November 2007 by Professor Joanna Zakrzewska, Professor of Pain in Relation to Oral Medicine and Honorary Consultant in Oral Medicine, Institute of Dentistry, Barts and the London NHS Trust, London, UK.

Further online resources

Medical texts in *The Contact a Family Directory* are designed to give a short, clear description of specific conditions and rare disorders. More extensive information on this condition can be found on a range of reliable, validated websites. Further information on these resources can be found in our **Medical Information on the Internet** article on page 21.

Support

Trigeminal Neuralgia Association UK
PO Box 234, Oxted RH8 8BE   Tel: 01883 370 214 e-mail: help@tna.org.uk
Web: http://www.tna.org.uk
The Association is a National Registered Charity No. 1093022, established in 1999.
It provides information and support to members, and raises awareness of Trigeminal
Neuralgia amongst medical professionals and the public. Members receive access to
the helpline, a quarterly newsletter and invitation to attend the Association's AGM and
conferences.
Group details last updated November 2007.

"I have received more information
about the condition from Contact a
Family in the past week than I have
from anyone else in the last 15 years."
Parent.

TRIPLE-X SYNDROME

Background

Triple-X is a chromosomal condition which occurs only in females. A chromosome is a rod-like structure present in the nucleus of all body cells, with the exception of the red blood cells, which stores genetic information. Normally humans have twenty-three pairs of chromosomes, forty-six chromosomes in total. The twenty-third pair, otherwise referred to as the sex chromosomes, stores genetic information which determines our sex. A male has a XY pair and a female has a XX pair of chromosomes.

A female affected by triple-X syndrome has an XX pair of chromosomes, as well as additional X chromosome, resulting in the formation of XXX. A mosaic form also occurs where only a percentage of body cells contain XXX while the remainder carry XX. The extent to which an individual is affected by the condition will depend upon the proportion of XXX to XX throughout.

What are the symptoms?

The effect of having an extra X chromosome can be very varied. Some females with triple-X syndrome show no, or very few, symptoms and are entirely 'normal', whilst others have learning difficulties, developmental delay and/or behavioural problems. Individuals may show some or all features and furthermore may be differently affected by the severity of their symptoms. It is not possible to offer a precise prediction of the symptoms either before or even immediately after the birth of each triple-X girl.

At birth, girls with triple-X are usually normally developed, although babies may be floppy (hypotonic) and weight may be slightly lower than average. Many girls have a 'growth spurt' up until the age of eight years and women tend to be a little taller than average. In the 'full blown' condition, girls with triple-X are at risk of delays in neuromotor development, learning ability and/ or impaired psychosocial adaptation. This leads to co-ordination problems including both gross motor skills and/or fine motor skills.

Delays in speech and language development are frequent but individuals respond well to speech therapy. Behavioural problems including tantrums, shyness and emotional immaturity are rather more frequent than in girls with XX chromosomes.

Sexual development is normal and triple-X women are fertile though there is a slight increased risk of sex chromosome changes in their children and an amniocentesis test is available to confirm this. Some women have been reported to have an early menopause, however further follow-up studies are required to confirm how likely this is for the majority of triple-X women. Individuals with triple-X have no increased risk of any diseases during childhood or in adult life.

How is it treated?

Females with triple-X are at risk of becoming socially isolated, particularly in the face of environmental stressors. A supportive and encouraging environment providing psychological, social and motor stimulation is, therefore, beneficial.

Inheritance patterns and prenatal diagnosis

Inheritance patterns

Triple-X occurs sporadically and is not usually passed on from a triple-X mother to her daughters. However, there is an increased risk in the children of older mothers.

Prenatal diagnosis

Chorionic villus sampling at ten to twelve weeks or amniocentesis at about sixteen weeks is available to all mothers with Triple X syndrome, and routinely to older mothers, to confirm or exclude Triple X syndrome.

Medical text written August 2002 by Contact a Family. **Last reviewed February 2008 by Dr R Stanhope, Consultant Paediatric Endocrinologist, Institute of Child Health, London, UK.**

Further online resources

Medical texts in *The Contact a Family Directory* are designed to give a short, clear description of specific conditions and rare disorders. More extensive information on this condition can be found on a range of reliable, validated websites. Further information on these resources can be found in our **Medical Information on the Internet** article on page 21.

Support

Triple-X Family Network Support Group
32 Francemary Road, London SE4 1JS   Tel: 020 8690 9445
e-mail: helenclements@hotmail.com
This is a small support network started in 1997 offering support to families of affected children. It publishes a biannual newsletter and has information available, details on request. There are 230 families in the UK and abroad in touch with the network.
Group details last updated July 2004.

TUBERCULOSIS

Background

Tuberculosis (or 'TB') is an infection caught from other people, as with a cold or 'flu. It most often occurs in the lungs and lymph glands but can affect any part of the body.

What are the symptoms?

The commonest symptom of TB is a cough sometimes accompanied by phlegm which can be bloodstained. There may also be chest pain, loss of appetite and weight, a fever with sweating particularly at night, and swollen lymph glands in the neck.

How is it treated?

TB is now readily curable if it is correctly diagnosed and the right drugs are used. The emergence of multi drug resistant TB, in which the bug is resistant to one or two drugs means that it is important that it is detected quickly and correct treatment initiated. Treatment is with a combination of tablets which must be taken every single day for six to nine months. Treatment may be longer in cases of multi drug resistance.

In the UK, the BCG vaccination programme delivered through schools will be replaced with a programme of targeted vaccination for those individuals who are at greatest risk. This programme will vaccinate babies and older people who are most likely to catch the disease, especially those living in areas with a high rate of TB or whose parents or grandparents were born in a country with high TB prevalence.

Current information on vaccination is available from the Department of Health, Web: http://www.immunisation.org.uk. BCG vaccination does not give complete protection against TB, but does help the body's defences to fight it off.

Inheritance patterns and prenatal diagnosis

Inheritance patterns

Not applicable.

Prenatal diagnosis

Not applicable.

Medical text written November 1995 by Dr Robert Winter, Consultant Respiratory Physician, Barnet Hospital, London, UK. **Last updated July 2005 by Dr Adam Jaffe, Consultant and Honorary Senior Lecturer in Respiratory Research, Great Ormond Street Hospital for Children and Institute of Child Health, London, UK.**

Support

Support for Tuberculosis can be obtained from Breath Easy, the support network of the British Lung Foundation (see entry, Lung diseases).

TUBEROUS SCLEROSIS

Background

Tuberous Sclerosis (TSC) is a complex and heterogeneous genetic disorder which may affect many of the body systems.

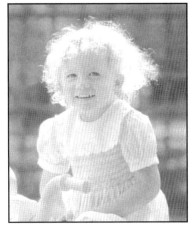

Tuberous Sclerosis, which literally means a swelling or enlargement and hardening of tissue, has typical manifestations which occur in the brain, skin, and kidneys. Manifestations may also affect the eye, heart, lungs and rarely other organs.

What are the symptoms?

Characteristic features include:

- in the brain, calcified nodules and non-calcified swellings which show on a CAT or MRI scan;
- on the skin, hypomelanic (white) patches;
- on the face, a rash termed angiofibromatosis (previously called adenoma sebaceum);
- on the forehead, fibrous plaque;
- on the lumbar area, a shagreen patch (thickened and discoloured skin);
- in the kidney, angiomyolipomas (benign fatty growths) or cysts;
- in the heart, rhabdomyomas (benign growth of heart muscle).

Epileptic seizures occur in at least seventy-five per cent of cases and often start in the first year of life with characteristic infantile spasms. Some degree of learning difficulty (see entry, Learning Disability) occurs in about forty per cent of cases. Additionally, behaviour problems and autistic tendencies (see entry, Autism Spectrum disorders including Asperger syndrome) are very common features of the condition. However the severity and diversity of the presenting manifestations is very variable in individual cases. It is possible to have the condition but have very few symptoms or signs; or to be severely affected, for example with no speech, limited mobility and severe epilepsy, or anywhere in between.

Psychological and behavioural characteristics

The information below has been drawn up by Dr Orlee Udwin of the Society for the Study of Behavioural Phenotypes.

Intellectual abilities range from profound learning difficulties to above average abilities, with normal intelligence in fifty per cent of children. There can be specific language difficulties in those with normal intelligence and these problems increase as learning disability becomes more severe. A significant number of individuals have no speech. Children affected by Tuberous Sclerosis can show overactivity, and attention deficits as well as autism (social communication difficulties, ritualistic behaviours and resistance to change.) These conditions lead to behaviour problems (destructiveness, aggression, screaming episodes) which often decrease with age. Severe sleep disturbance is also a feature of the condition, with settling and night waking difficulties, and this is related to underlying epilepsy.

Inheritance patterns and prenatal diagnosis

Inheritance patterns

Autosomal dominant inheritance with very variable expression but essentially complete penetrance. Sporadic mutations account for over fifty per cent of new cases. A severely affected child may have a very mildly affected parent and great care must be taken when trying to establish the status of relatives in genetic counselling.

Prenatal diagnosis

The diagnosis of Tuberous Sclerosis is usually made according to accepted clinical diagnostic criteria. Two Tuberous Sclerosis associated genes have been identified TSC2 (encoding tuberin) and TSC1 (encoding hamartin). Molecular genetic diagnosis of TSC by analysis of a blood sample is now available but the genes are unusually large and complex. Mutations can be identified in about eighty per cent of cases. Identification of the family-specific mutation enables early pre-natal diagnosis by chorion villus biopsy for couples who wish to take this step. A small proportion of patients with Tuberous Sclerosis also have Polycystic Kidney disease. This is because the PKD1 gene that is associated with polycystic kidneys lies next to the TSC2 gene on chromosome 16. Extra tests are needed to identify the mutation in these unusual cases.

Situations in which molecular genetic testing is appropriate in persons/families with, or at risk of, Tuberous Sclerosis include:

- Genetic counselling - Detection of a mutation in one of the two TSC genes in the affected member of a family means that relatives at risk can have their genetic status determined by an unequivocal blood test. This is a more simple approach than by conventional clinical and radiographic tests.
- Prenatal diagnosis – Where a prospective parent has TSC, the identification of a causative mutation allows very reliable DNA-based prenatal diagnosis. The same is true for clinically unaffected couples who have an affected child, if they are concerned about the small recurrence risk posed by gonadal mosaicism (about one or two per cent). In families where the mutation cannot yet be identified, an ultrasound scan can be done at eighteen to twenty weeks to diagnose

heart tumours with a further scan at twenty-two to twenty-three weeks to confirm the diagnosis.

- Clinical diagnostic uncertainty - Detection of a mutation in one of the two TSC genes in a person presenting with one or more features suggestive of Tuberous Sclerosis, but which do not fulfil the accepted clinical diagnostic criteria for the disorder, can clarify the person's status. However, a negative gene test result doesn't help much and so this approach requires careful consideration.

Medical text written November 1991 by Contact a Family. Approved November 1991 by Professor R Mueller, Consultant in Clinical Genetics, St James University Hospital, Leeds, UK. **Last updated September 2006 by Professor J Sampson, Consultant in Clinical Genetics, Institute of Medical Genetics, Cardiff, UK.**

Further online resources

Medical texts in *The Contact a Family Directory* are designed to give a short, clear description of specific conditions and rare disorders. More extensive information on this condition can be found on a range of reliable, validated websites. Further information on these resources can be found in our **Medical Information on the Internet** article on page 21.

Support

Tuberous Sclerosis Association
PO Box 12979, Barnt Green, Birmingham B45 5AN   Tel/Fax: 0121 445 6970
e-mail: support@tuberous-sclerosis.org   Web: http://www.tuberous-sclerosis.org
The Association is a National Registered Charity No. 1039549, established in 1977. It provides advice, information and training and offers practical and emotional support. The Association employs TS Specialist Advisers to support and advocate for families. It publishes a newsletter 3 times a year and has a wide range of information available, details on request. Please send SAE. The Association has over 1,600 families and 450 professional workers in membership.
Group details last confirmed June 2007.

TURCOT SYNDROME

Turcot syndrome: Association of multiple polyps of the colon and a primary tumour of the Central Nervous System

Background

Turcot syndrome was first described by Drs Turcot, Despré and St. Pierre in 1959. Turcot syndrome is a very rare inherited disorder of tumours of the brain and colon. The syndrome affects people of both sexes and all ethnic groups and presents in childhood and adolescence. Approximately one hundred and fifty cases are known to medical literature.

What are the symptoms?

Features of Turcot syndrome include:

- **Brain tumours.** There have been two types of primary brain tumour (see entry) described in Turcot syndrome: malignant gliomas (such as anaplastic astrocytoma or glioblastoma); and medulloblastoma (a malignant tumour of the central nervous system);
- **Colon.** Polyps (growths that develop on the inside wall of a tubular body part), which undergo malignant transformation into a cancer of the colon.

What are the causes?

There are two major inheritable syndromes leading to multiple polyps in the colon; familial adenomatous polyposis (FAP) and hereditary nonpolyposis colorectal cancer (HNPCC). The genetics of these syndromes is now well described with FAP arising in the majority of cases from a defect in the APC gene (chromosome 5) and HNPCC arising from defects in genes involved in DNA repair (chromosomes 3 and 7).

Very rarely a patient with either of these two syndromes will develop a primary brain tumour and it is thought that the underlying genetic abnormality may predispose that patient to central nervous system tumours.

How is it diagnosed?

Turcot syndrome is diagnosed clinically in a patient with known multiple colonic polyps who develops a primary brain tumour with a relevant family history.

How is it treated?

Treatment of Turcot syndrome includes:

- Appropriate management of the underlying colonic polyps by a gastroenterologist experienced in FAP or HNPCC;
- Appropriate management of the primary brain tumour by a neuro-oncology team;
- Clinical genetic counselling.

Inheritance patterns and prenatal diagnosis

Inheritance patterns

This has been controversial as some authors have reported an autosomal dominant pattern (as in FAP & HNPCC) and others an autosomal recessive inheritance. Genetic counselling should be sought to discuss testing in families known to be at risk.

Prenatal diagnosis

In families where a gene mutation has been identified, this is possible by amniocentesis at sixteen to eighteen weeks or Chorionic Villus Sampling (CVS) at ten to twelve weeks. However, prenatal testing for adult onset conditions is not common.

Medical text written August 2005 by Contact a Family. Approved August 2005 by Dr D Hargrave, Consultant Paediatric Oncologist, Royal Marsden Hospital, Sutton, UK.

Further online resources

Medical texts in *The Contact a Family Directory* are designed to give a short, clear description of specific conditions and rare disorders. More extensive information on this condition can be found on a range of reliable, validated websites. Further information on these resources can be found in our **Medical Information on the Internet** article on page 21.

Support

There is no support group for Turcot syndrome but reference can be made to the Cancer entry. Cross referrals to other entries in the Contact a Family Directory are intended to provide relevant support for these particular features of the disorder. Organisations identified in these entries do not provide support specifically for Turcot syndrome. Families can use Contact a Family's Freephone Helpline for advice, information and, where possible, links to other families. Contact a Family's web-based linking service Making Contact.org can be accessed at http://www.makingcontact.org

TURNER SYNDROME

Turner syndrome: Bonnevie-Ullrich; Gonadal Dysgenesis (XO); MonosomyX; Turner-Ullrich; XO syndrome

Background

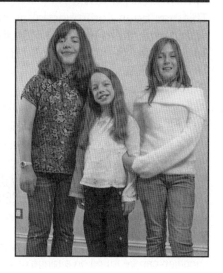

Although the features of the syndrome in girls were described earlier, the syndrome is named after Dr Henry Turner who reported a number of girls with the features of the syndrome in a paper of 1938. Turner syndrome is a chromosomal condition affecting 1 in 2,500 girls where the second X chromosome is absent or abnormal. It is one of the most common chromosomal disorders. The diagnosis is confirmed by examination of chromosomes from the blood cells (Karyotype). Sometimes the second X chromosome is missing from, or abnormal in, only some cells in the body, but not all. This is referred to as Turner mosaicism.

What are the symptoms?

Turner syndrome is generally characterised by short stature and non functioning ovaries, usually leading to the absence of pubertal development and infertility. Though growth hormone secretion is nearly always normal the treatment with growth hormone has demonstrated an increase in growth rate. At an appropriate age girls are given oestrogen for the development of secondary sexual characteristics and the introduction of regular uterine withdrawal bleeds, which is important to keep the uterus healthy.

Physical features associated with Turner syndrome may include Coarctation of the aorta, webbing of the neck, wide spaced nipples and puffy hands and feet. Sleeping and feeding difficulties may occur in early childhood and though intelligence spans the normal range there can be learning and behavioural difficulties, which benefit from appropriate support and the diligence of the girls themselves.

Psychological and behavioural characteristics

Girls with Turner syndrome usually attain overall IQ scores in the normal range. However, they have consistently been found to have significantly better verbal than visuospatial abilities. For example, nonverbal reasoning and memory skills tend to be weaker than verbal reasoning and memory. Visuomotor co-ordination may also be an area of weakness. Correspondingly, reading may be relatively good but mathematics is often an area of academic weakness. Visuospatial deficits may also contribute to difficulties in processing some socially important information, such as recognising faces and facial expressions.

Many affected girls experience difficulties in their peer relationships. They may seem immature, have poor social skills and be unassertive, shy and socially anxious. They may also have difficulties related to poor concentration, distractibility, and overactivity. There is a risk of low self-esteem, and social withdrawal and depression in adulthood. In a small but significant minority of girls, autistic features may be recognised. Interestingly, girls who inherited their single X chromosome from their mother tend to have more difficulties in this respect than those who inherited the chromosome from their father.

That said, many adult women attain high goals in their personal, academic, and occupational lives.

How is it diagnosed?
The diagnosis is confirmed by examination of chromosomes from the blood cells (Karyotype). Sometimes the second X chromosome is missing from, or abnormal in, only some cells in the body, but not all. This is referred to as Turner mosaicism.

Inheritance patterns and prenatal diagnosis
Inheritance patterns
This is a sporadic event.
Prenatal diagnosis
Chorionic villus sampling at nine to twelve weeks and amniocentesis at sixteen weeks.

Medical written November 1995 by Dr Richard Stanhope. **Last updated September 2005 by Dr Richard Stanhope, Consultant Paediatric Endocrinologist, Great Ormond Street Hospital, London, UK. Psychological and behavioural characteristics last updated February 2004 by Dr O Udwin, Consultant Clinical Child Psychologist, West London Mental Health NHS Trust, London, UK and Dr A Kuczynski, Child Clinical Psychologist, South London & Maudsley NHS Trust, London, UK.**

Further online resources
Medical texts in *The Contact a Family Directory* are designed to give a short, clear description of specific conditions and rare disorders. More extensive information on this condition can be found on a range of reliable, validated websites. Further information on these resources can be found in our **Medical Information on the Internet** article on page 21.

Support

Turner Syndrome Support Society

13 Simpson Court, 11 South Avenue, Clydebank Business Park, Clydebank G81 2NR
Tel: 0845 230 7520 Helpline   Tel: 0141 952 8006   Fax: 0141 952 8025
e-mail: Turner.syndrome@tss.org.uk   Web: http://www.tss.org.uk
*The Society is a National Registered Charity 1080507, established in 1999. It offers
support and information to girls and women who have Turner syndrome, their families and
friends. The Society works with medical specialists to raise awareness about the condition
and to encourage research into all aspects of Turner syndrome. It publishes a quarterly
newsletter and hosts Society Open Days and an Annual Conference. It encourages
enquiries from Health, Educational and Social Services professionals. It can provide further
information and details of membership on request. The Society has over 700 members.*
Group details last updated October 2006.

*Support and information on Turner syndrome can also be obtained from the Child Growth
Foundation (for contact details see entry, Restricted Growth).*

Contact a Family deals with 18,000
enquiries each year.

TWINS WITH SPECIAL NEEDS/ MULTIPLE BIRTHS

Background

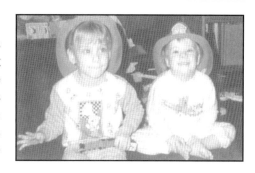

Over ten thousand multiple births occur in the UK each year. A significant percentage of multiple births are premature (before thirty-seven weeks gestation) and this can be a factor in the predisposition to some forms of disability. Twins, triplets or more present special problems of care. However, where one child in a pair of twins has a disability the problems are multiplied and stress is immeasurably increased.

What are the symptoms?

Disabilities in one twin can encompass any condition and include conditions such as cerebral palsy (see entry). Where a condition is genetic, monozygotic (identical) twins will both be affected, but may manifest the same condition in different ways. Binovular or dizygotic (non-identical) twins may have one affected and one non-affected child.

Children of multiple births may die in infancy more commonly than single infants: therefore neonatal death (see entry, Stillbirths) may also be an associated problem of multiple births. The death of one or more children in a multiple birth is particularly stressful for the parents.

Inheritance patterns and prenatal diagnosis

Inheritance patterns

Not applicable.

Prenatal diagnosis

Not applicable.

Medical text written November 1991 by Contact a Family. Approved November 1991 by Professor Michael Patton, Professor of Medical Genetics, St George's Hospital Medical School, London, UK and Dr J E Wraith, Consultant Paediatrician, Royal Manchester Children's Hospital, Manchester, UK. **Last updated February 2005 by the Twins and Multiple Births Association (TAMBA).**

Further online resources

Medical texts in *The Contact a Family Directory* are designed to give a short, clear description of specific conditions and rare disorders. More extensive information on this condition can be found on a range of reliable, validated websites. Further information on these resources can be found in our **Medical Information on the Internet** article on page 21.

T

Support

Multiple Births Foundation

Hammersmith House, Level 4, Queen Charlotte and Chelsea Hospital, Du Cane Road, London W12 0HS   Tel: 020 8383 3519   Fax: 020 8383 3041   e-mail: mbf@hhnt.nhs.uk
Web: http://www.multiplebirths.org.uk
The Foundation is a National Registered Charity No. 1094546, established in 1988. It offers a support service and has information available, details on request.
Group details last confirmed June 2007.

TAMBA Special Needs Group

2 The Willows, Gardner Road, Guildford GU1 4PG   Tel: 0870 770 3305
Tel: 0800 138 0509 Helpline (Mon-Fri, 10am-1pm & 7-10pm)
Fax: 0870 770 3303   e-mail: enquiries@tamba.org.uk   Web: http://www.tamba.org.uk
TAMBA Special Needs group is part of TAMBA, (Twins and Multiple Births Association) a National Registered Charity No. 1076478, started in 1978. The Special Needs Group offers support and information to families where one or all of their multiple birth have special needs. As well as receiving the 'Twins, Triplets and More' magazines quarterly, members also receive a newsletter twice a year from the group co-ordinator. Also there is a special section on their message board where members of the group can post to each other. To be able post on the message board you have to have a valid Tamba membership.
Group details last updated October 2007.

UNDIAGNOSED CHILDREN

Background

There is a continuing increase in knowledge about the causes of complex illness or disability in children. Doctors may recognise a pattern in the medical problems, or there may be clues in the child's appearance.

How is it diagnosed?

In many cases a firm diagnosis can now be reached. There remain, however, children for whom the diagnosis at present is unclear. With the growth of knowledge resulting from human genome mapping data, more tests to identify rare, hitherto unidentified, disorders may become available. Contact with others who have been in a similar position may be very helpful.

Even without a firm diagnosis much can usually be done to support the child and the family. Medical and nursing treatment or therapy may be offered. Appropriate educational help, social services support and benefits should be available depending on the child's needs, not on a medical label.

Inheritance patterns and prenatal diagnosis

Inheritance patterns

Without a specific diagnosis this may be unclear, although specialists can sometimes advise, based on general genetic principles.

Prenatal diagnosis

This may depend on the actual medical features, some of which might be picked up on ultrasound scanning.

Medical text written March 2000 by Dr P Corry. **Last updated August 2005 by Dr P Corry, Consultant Community Paediatrician, Child Development Centre, St Luke's Hospital, Bradford, UK.**

Support

SWAN (Syndromes Without A Name)
6 Acorn Close, Great Wyrley, Walsall WS6 6HP   Tel/Fax: 01922 701234
e-mail: info@undiagnosed.org.uk   Web: http://www.undiagnosed.org.uk
Swan is a National Registered Charity 1074829, established in 1996. It offers support for families by phone, letter and e-mail. It publishes a newsletter and has information available, details on request. Swan has over 1,100 members and links with similar groups in several other countries.
Group details last confirmed October 2007.

UPPER LIMB ABNORMALITIES

Background

Traumatic

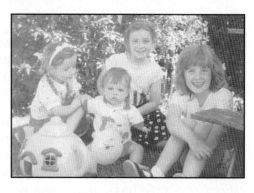

These may include birth trauma such as injuries to the nerve plexus of the arm (brachial plexus palsy), in which the baby is often big, and may present shoulder first causing a traction injury to the nerves to the arm. Typically patterns of injury are recognised (Erb's palsy or Klumpke's palsy). Most babies recover within three months, but some may develop a weak arm that is small. In such cases, where surgery to the brachial plexus may be warranted, expert advice is necessary

Congenital

Whole limb

- The whole limb may fail to grow. The cause for this may be multifactorial as in congenital amputation, or may be due to a specific environmental factor such as in many cases of Phocomelia (caused by maternal ingestion of Thalidomide). Treatment includes prostheses from a young age, and very occasionally surgery. Many individuals function well even without a prosthesis.

Elbow

- The outer bone in the forearm (thumb side) is the radius. At the elbow the radial head forms a joint with the humerus bone of the upper arm. Radial head dislocation causes mild loss of forearm rotation and a cosmetic bulge over the outer elbow. It is sometimes associated with other skeletal anomalies such as Nail-Patella syndrome, Hereditary Multiple Exostoses or Ollier disease and may be secondary to a short ulna. Surgical treatment is reserved for the painful or dysfunctional elbow.

- A bony bridge between the two bones of the forearm (Radioulnar synostosis) is usually a pain-free condition, but results in a stiff forearm. Surgery is indicated if both arms are affected to improve the functional position of the forearm.

Hand

Congenital hand abnormalities occur in about 1 in 1,000 live births and the following are the commonest manifestations:

- **Failure of the fingers to separate from each other** (Syndactyly) in the womb. Twenty per cent are inherited. Severity ranges from mild skin webbing to complete bony fusion of the fingers. Surgery is most successful in the milder forms, but is necessary early in severe cases to avoid progressive deformity.

- **Polydactyly** (extra fingers) may sometimes be inherited. Surgery is performed to remove extra digits at an early age.
- **Camptodactyly** (bent finger towards the palm) commonly affects the little finger at the proximal joint. This condition is often inherited. Treatment is rarely necessary, but if progressive may respond to splinting, or surgery.
- **Clinodactyly** (bent finger in the plane of the palm) is common, and surgery is only warranted if there is an underlying bony abnormality with progressive severe deformity. Again there is likely to be a strong family history.
- **Failure of formation of the radius bone** (radial club hand) occurs in 1 in 30,000 live births, and has many possible causes. Sometimes other body systems are involved (cardiac, haematological, spine, gastro-intestinal, renal) in various named syndromes (see Holt-Oram syndrome, VACTERL Association or TAR syndrome entries). Treatment depends on functional needs, and may include early splinting, surgery to centralise the wrist on the forearm and prevention of radial drift of the hand. Secondary thumb reconstructive surgery may also be necessary.

There are also further specific syndromes which include arm defects amongst their characteristic features:
- Poland syndrome (see entry);
- Hanhart syndrome (Hypoglassia-Hypo-Dactylia);
- Cornelia de Lange syndrome (see entry);
- Femur/Fibula/Ulna syndrome;
- Focal Dermal Hypoplasia (see entry).

Inheritance patterns and prenatal diagnosis
Inheritance patterns
Most arm and hand deficiencies are sporadic events. Inheritance in VATER Association is sporadic. In TAR syndrome inheritance is autosomal recessive.
Prenatal diagnosis
Prenatal ultrasound scanning may pick up anomalies of limb development.

Medical text written September 2002 by Mr D E Porter, Senior Lecturer & Hon. Consultant in Orthopaedic Surgery, University of Edinburgh, Edinburgh, UK. **Last updated July 2007 by Mr A C Watts, Specialist Registrar in Orthopaedics, Royal Infirmary of Edinburgh, Edinburgh, UK.**

Support

Reach

PO Box 54, Helston TR13 8WD   Tel: 0845 130 6225   Fax: 0845 130 0262
e-mail: reach@reach.org.uk   Web: http://www.reach.org.uk
Reach is a National Registered Charity No. 278679, established in 1979. It offers a network of local branches promoting contact between families. It provides insurance cover for the 'good arm' of children over 2 years of age (UK only) as an automatic benefit of membership. It publishes a quarterly magazine 'Within Reach' and has a wide range of information available, details on request. Reach has approximately 1,200 families and professional workers in membership.
Group details last confirmed May 2007.

"I felt ready to face the challenges my child gives me every day and how I could react to him decisively." Parent at a workshop on challenging behaviour organised jointly by Contact a Family West Midlands and Autism West Midlands.

UREA CYCLE DISORDERS

Background
The urea cycle is the metabolic pathway by which waste nitrogen is converted to urea, which is then excreted in the urine.

What are the causes?
The cycle has several steps, each catalysed by a different enzyme. Urea cycle defects result when there is a deficiency of one of these enzymes:
- N-acetyl glutamate synthase (NAGS) deficiency;
- Carbamyl phosphate synthase (CPS) deficiency;
- Ornithine transcarbamylase (OTC) deficiency;
- Citrullinaemia (Argininosuccinate synthase deficiency);
- Argininosuccinic aciduria (Argininosuccinate lyase deficiency);
- Hyperargininaemia (Arginase deficiency).

The most common of the urea cycle disorders is OTC deficiency. Disturbance of the urea cycle results in a rise in ammonia concentrations in the blood and brain with associated irritability, vomiting, drowsiness and coma. The disorders commonly present in the first month of life but symptoms may start at almost any age. Arginase deficiency mostly presents with a neurological disorder (spastic diplegia) and developmental delay.

How is it treated?
Management aims to control ammonia concentrations and prevent episodes of decompensation, as these are potentially serious. General measures include a protein restricted diet, arginine supplementation (as this becomes an essential amino acid in these disorders with the exception of hyperargininaemia), and the use of alternate pathway medicines which help rid the body of excess nitrogen bypassing the urea cycle. During periods of infection, protein intake is stopped, and glucose is given either by mouth or intravenously.

Inheritance patterns and prenatal diagnosis
Inheritance patterns
The mode of inheritance of all these disorders is autosomal recessive, except OTC deficiency which is an X-linked disorder. Female carriers of OTC deficiency may be at risk of developing symptoms themselves.
Prenatal diagnosis
Prenatal diagnosis is available for all the conditions.

Medical text written October 2001 by Dr M Champion. **Last updated January 2006 by Dr M Champion, Consultant in Paediatric Metabolic Medicine, Evelina Children's Hospital, London, UK.**

Further online resources

Medical texts in *The Contact a Family Directory* are designed to give a short, clear description of specific conditions and rare disorders. More extensive information on this condition can be found on a range of reliable, validated websites. Further information on these resources can be found in our **Medical Information on the Internet** article on page 21.

Support

As Urea Cycle Disorders are metabolic diseases, support and advice are also available from Climb (see entry, Metabolic diseases).

"I take my son everywhere, but I long to see other disabled children there too. I often wonder where they are and what they are doing." Parent quoted in a joint report by Contact a Family West Midlands and Action for Leisure entitled "Come on In: Developing inclusive play and leisure services."

USHER SYNDROME

Background

Usher syndrome is a genetic condition characterised by sensory neural hearing loss with Retinitis Pigmentosa (see entry). The hearing loss is usually congenital and may be total or partial. Retinitis pigmentosa, a progressive deterioration of the retina which causes night blindness, tunnel vision and finally severely reduced central vision, may not occur until late childhood or early adulthood. In some forms, poor balance is an associated problem.

What are the symptoms?

There are three types of the syndrome. Type I is characterised by profound congenital hearing loss, poor balance and retinitis pigmentosa before the age of 10. Type II presents moderate to severe hearing loss, normal balance and retinitis pigmentosa develops in the late teens or early 20's. Type III is characterised by progressive hearing loss and Retinitis Pigmentosa progressing at a variable rate, generally with onset around the second or third decade of life.

How is it diagnosed?

Diagnosis of Usher syndrome may occur while the child has no visual problems, by means of electrical tests of retinal function (electroretinogram or ERG). More often, diagnosis may be delayed until the visual problems have become significant because peripheral and night vision are not routinely tested in school children, and because the optimal age for such screening testing is unknown.

Inheritance patterns and prenatal diagnosis

Inheritance patterns

Autosomal recessive

Prenatal diagnosis

Several genes have been identified which may, in theory, allow prenatal diagnosis. However genetic testing, and therefore prenatal diagnosis, are difficult due to the number and size of the genes which have to be screened. Methods for this are improving all the time.

Medical text written November 1991 by Contact a Family. Approved November 1991 by Professor M Patton, Professor of Medical Genetics, St Georges Hospital Medical School, London, UK and Dr J E Wraith, Consultant Paediatrician, Royal Manchester Children's Hospital, Manchester, UK. **Last updated June 2006 by Dr. Maria Bitner-Glindzicz, Academic Head of the Clinical and Molecular Genetics Unit, Institute of Child Health, London, UK.**

Further online resources

Medical texts in *The Contact a Family Directory* are designed to give a short, clear description of specific conditions and rare disorders. More extensive information on this condition can be found on a range of reliable, validated websites. Further information on these resources can be found in our **Medical Information on the Internet** article on page 21.

Support

Usher Services, National Acquired Deafblind Team Sense
Sense South East, Newplan House, 41 East Street, Epsom, Surrey KT17 1BL
Tel: 01372 840326 Text (Direct line) Tel: 0845 127 0076 (Referrals Officer)
Tel: 0845 127 0078 Textphone Fax: 0845 127 0077
e-mail: usher@sense.org.uk Web: http://www.sense.org.uk
Usher Services belongs to the National Acquired Deafblind Team, which is part of Sense, a National Registered Charity No. 289268. They are in contact with people with Usher syndrome, their family, friends and interested professionals. They work directly with Usher people and their families and liaise with schools, social services and hospitals as appropriate, via Sense Regional staff as required. They run training courses about Usher syndrome for the staff of schools, social services, hospitals and other organisations, and also for firms and organisations which have Usher employees. They have around 800 Usher contacts. The Hearing and Sight Impaired UK (HSI UK) group, a branch of Sense, is a social and support group for hearing aid users with Usher or similar types of acquired deafblindness. Usher Services produces a wide range of information on Usher. Details about all information and services are available on request or via the website. Professionals should send a SAE or e-mail requests for information.
Group details last updated February 2008.

UVEITIS

Background

Uveitis is the term given to a number of rare eye conditions and is now used to describe any inflammation which occurs inside the eye (as opposed to outside the eye, for example conjunctivitis). This has lead to the term 'intraocular inflammation' being used as an alternative name. Strictly speaking uveitis denotes inflammation of the uvea, one of a number of 'layers' within the eye which are shown shaded in the diagram.

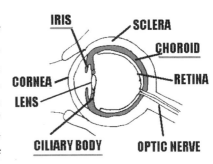

What are the symptoms?

There are many types of uveitis and even several different types of cause.

Uveitis may be divided into two main types, based on the part of the eye affected:

Anterior uveitis. This affects the front of the eye. This condition is often referred to as iritis. Typical symptoms include pain, sensitivity to light and possible blurring of vision. Anterior uveitis may be acute, lasting for a short time or chronic, lasting for more than three months although it may wax and wane.

Posterior uveitis. This describes inflammation at the back of the eye. This is usually a painless but potentially a more sight-threatening condition.

This is a very simple way of categorising uveitis. It must be stressed that there are many sub types and patients may suffer both anterior and posterior (panuveitis). Uveitis may also be one feature of a wider medical condition such as sarcoidosis, toxoplasmosis or juvenile idiopathic arthritis (see entry, Arthritis (Juvenile Idiopathic)).

There is a lack of good data concerning vision loss in uveitis. This can be explained by firstly, there are many, quite different types of uveitis, and, secondly, there are different ways in which the vision may be affected by uveitis. It must be said that many people, especially those with acute anterior uveitis, will not lose any vision. However uveitis, particularly posterior uveitis, may cause significant vision loss. Uveitis typically affects people of working age and may also affect very young children.

Apart from vision loss resulting directly from the effects of the inflammation, the most likely means of losing vision are through the more indirect complications of uveitis, including: cataract, raised intraocular pressure (leading to glaucoma), macula oedema and vitritis.

What are the causes?

There are known associations with certain infections, for example toxoplasmosis (see entry) and with certain medical conditions, for example sarcoidosis. Many cases are examples of autoimmune disease in which the body reacts against itself. The trigger for this is unknown but might be infection in susceptible individuals.

How is it treated?

The aim of treatment is to completely control the inflammation on the lowest possible dosage of drugs, and to monitor and to treat any sight threatening complications such as raised intraocular pressure and macula oedema.

Treatment varies depending upon the severity of uveitis. For sight-threatening disease treatment it includes drugs taken orally, normally steroids, and sometimes with certain immunosuppressant drugs. Less severe uveitis may be controlled by steroid eye drops.

Inheritance patterns and prenatal diagnosis

Inheritance patterns

Uveitis is not an hereditary condition that runs in families as there is no identifiable gene that causes the disease. However, certain people will have an increased susceptibility due to the genes they have. Certain types of uveitis have an association with gene types such as HLA B27, HLA B51 and HLA A29.

Prenatal diagnosis

None.

Medical text written October 2001 by Professor A D Dick. **Last updated December 2005 by Professor A D Dick, Professor and Head of the Division of Ophthalmology, University of Bristol, UK.**

Support

Uveitis Information Group
South House, Sweening, Vidlin, Shetland ZE2 9QE   Tel: 01806 577310
e-mail: info@uveitis.net   Web: http://www.uveitis.net
The Group is Scottish charity no.SC028439, established in 1998. It offers support by telephone, post or e-mail. It publishes a newsletter and has extensive information on uveitis, and specifically on uveitis in children, both on its web site and by post, details on request. Public meetings are help annually in London, Scotland and Bristol. The Group has around 350 members in the UK and an international e-mail list.
Group details last confirmed February 2008.

VACTERL ASSOCIATION

Background

'VACTERL' is the name for a group of developmental defects that often occur as a group (or 'association') in newborn babies.

What are the symptoms?

Babies with health problems in three or more of the seven following areas are identified as having VACTERL:

V   **Vertebral** (spine/back bone). Anomalies in the vertebral bones that form the spine may result in scoliosis (see entry) or kyphosis (abnormal spinal shapes). There may also be abnormalities in the associated muscles and nerves.

A   **Anal** (back passage). Anal problems can vary from a low imperforate anus (an intact bowel with a blind end) to abnormal connections between the bowel and the bladder or vagina. The complexity of surgery required will depend on the severity of the problem.

C   **Cardiac** (heart). The most common type of cardiac abnormality is a Ventricular Septal Defect (VSD) in which there is a hole in the wall that separates the two large chambers of the heart, preventing the heart from functioning efficiently. The impact on the child's health depends on the size of the hole, with surgery being required in more serious cases. Other heart defects may occur in isolation or with a VSD.

T   **Tracheal** (windpipe).

E   **Esophageal** (food pipe – US spelling of oesophageal used as the term VACTERL originates from the US). Tracheo-Oesophageal Fistula/ Oesophageal Atresia (TOF/OA) (see entry) is a feature of VACTERL. With OA, the oesophagus (food pipe) forms a closed off pouch that prevents food from reaching the stomach. This can fill up with food and saliva, which can eventually overflow into the trachea (windpipe), entering the lungs and causing choking. With TOF, the oesophagus is connected to the windpipe. This allows air to pass from the windpipe to the food pipe and stomach. It can also allow stomach acid to pass into the lungs. Surgery soon after birth is required, with possible medical interventions later on.

R   **Renal** (kidney). Renal problems can be due to the total failure of one or both kidneys to form. Absence of both kidneys can have serious health implications. There is a range of other renal problems that vary in their impact on a child's health. (see entry, Kidney disease).

L   **Limb** (arms/legs). Partial or total failure of the radius (one of the arm bones), and the muscles which attach to it, to develop is common in children with VACTERL. Splints or surgery may be required. There may also be abnormalities with the feet or legs (see entries, Upper Limb abnormalities and Lower Limb abnormalities).

Whilst the term 'VACTERL' is not in itself a 'diagnosis', the list of anomalies that occur together helps medical professionals to know what to look for. The severity of the defects can vary considerably from one individual to another.

As well as the problems listed above, there may be associated endocrinopathies.

Inheritance patterns and prenatal diagnosis
Inheritance patterns
VACTERL Association occurs sporadically.

Prenatal diagnosis
Ultrasound scanning can reveal the radial anomaly and oesophageal atresia.

Medical text written December 2005 by Mr Bruce Jaffray, Consultant Paediatric Surgeon, Royal Victoria Infirmary, Newcastle upon Tyne, UK.

Further online resources
Medical texts in *The Contact a Family Directory* are designed to give a short, clear description of specific conditions and rare disorders. More extensive information on this condition can be found on a range of reliable, validated websites. Further information on these resources can be found in our **Medical Information on the Internet** article on page 21.

Support
VACTERL Association Support Group
76 Foxwood Gardens, Plymstock, Plymouth PL9 9HX   Tel: 01752 482568
e-mail: support@vacterl-association.org.uk   Web: http://www.vacterl-association.org.uk
The Association is a small parent support group, established in 2003. It offers support by phone and e-mail. The Association hosts an online forum on its website.
Group details last confirmed March 2007.

Support and information on VATER and VACTERL Association is also available from TOFS (see entry, Tracheo-Oesophageal Fistula and/or Oesophageal Atresia).

VASCULAR BIRTHMARKS

Background

There are many different types of vascular birthmarks which present at birth or within a few weeks after birth. The most common are:

- Telangiectasia (stork marks or spider naevi);
- Port wine stains;
- Haemangiomas (Hemangiomas - US).

Telangiectasia

- **Stork marks.** These can present on the forehead, upper eyelids and on the back of the neck. They tend to be pale pink in colour. Stork marks, especially those on the upper eyelids, fade within two years. Those on the forehead may take up to four years to fade. The ones on the back of the neck usually persist.
- **Spider Naevi.** Individual marks which are superficial blood vessels, often have the appearance of a spider with a central darker red punctate with radiating blood vessels like thread veins, Others can be slightly raised from the surface of the skin as a red spot or diffused with a flat mark known as a matt telangiectasia.

Port wine stains

A port wine stain is a type of blood vessel birthmark which presents at birth as a uniform flat red, purple or pink mark on the skin, often on one side of the body, usually the face. Occasionally port wine stains can occur on both sides of the body. Sometimes this type of mark is referred as a naevus flammus.

Port wine stains are due to an abnormal development of blood vessels in that area of the skin. They are permanent stains and never go away. They are not inherited and therefore not passed from one generation to the next. They are not related to anything that the parents may have done during pregnancy.

The incidence of port wine stain is 3 in 1,000 children. They are twice as common in girls than boys. They may darken with age, thicken with raised bumps (papules) or ridges and increase in size proportionally to the child's growth.

Until two decades ago, the help that could be given was to cover the port wine stain with camouflage make-up. In recent years, the pulsed dye lasers have revolutionized the treatment of port wine stain with excellent results and minimal side effects. Following completion of laser therapy (two to four years later) 1 in 10 children may have a recurrence of their port wine stain. The child should have further treatment and usually the response is very good especially with the newer lasers that are now available which allow delivery of higher laser strength using the dynamic cooling device. This reduces the risk of skin change or superficial scarring.

Sometimes complications may occur with this type of birthmark. These may present as Glaucoma (see entry) if the port wine stain is around the eye or Sturge-Weber syndrome (see entry) if the mark extends onto the forehead or scalp. Occasionally the tissue around a port wine stain may enlarge causing soft tissue hypertrophy (on a lip, for example) or may be associated with extra growth of that limb called Klippel Trenaunay syndrome (see entry). For these associated conditions different specialists need to get involved so that the child can be treated appropriately.

Haemangiomas

The word haemangioma comes from the Latin words 'haem' meaning blood and "angioma" meaning growth of cells. A haemangioma is a collection of small blood vessels that produces a lump in the skin. Haemangiomas can be superficial (capillary) or deep (cavernous). They are sometimes called strawberry marks. Approximately 1 in 10 babies have haemangioma, and they tend to be more common in girls, twins, triplets and premature babies or in mothers who presented with bleeding in pregnancy. They are usually not present at birth but develop a few days to weeks later. Initially there may be a small area of pale skin followed by a red spot. They grow rapidly in the first three months increasing in size and may intensify in colour. It is unusual for a haemangioma to grow after ten months. After this the haemangioma tends to have a rest period and will gradually improve with time. By the age of three years there are obvious signs of' reduction in size and most small haemangiomas will disappear leaving little or no mark on the skin by the age of five years. Large haemangiomas may continue to reduce in size up to seven to nine years of age.

Deep (cavernous) haemangiomas may appear bluish in colour because the abnormal blood vessels are deeper in the skin. Some haemangiomas may distort or stretch the skin around the lesion when it has completely disappeared. Sometimes there may be 'left over' fatty tissue following the regression of the haemangioma. In these situations, plastic surgery may be necessary.

Haemangiomas can appear anywhere on the body; rarely they can also be present in the internal organs. If this is the case, ultra sound scanning, magnetic resonance imaging (MRI), or rarely CT scan, may be indicated. Sometimes there can be more then one haemangioma in the same patient.

Most haemangiomas do not require any treatment, but some may need to be treated soon after birth if they interfere with feeding, breathing or other body functions. If the haemangioma presents on the child's eyelid, it may need urgent treatment in the first few weeks of life, as it may interfere with the development of the child's vision.

Some children with haemangiomas may require treatments with a pulsed dye laser, steroids or surgery. Those that have ulcerated or become sore may need to be admitted to hospital for treatment with antibiotics, dressings and regular nursing care.

Inheritance patterns and prenatal diagnosis

Inheritance patterns

None.

Prenatal diagnosis

A huge congenital haemangioma may be identified on ultrascan towards the end of pregnancy. This can only be confirmed at birth. In this case the haemangioma is probably atypical and of the rare type, for example: NICH (Non Involuting Capillary Haemangioma); RICH (Rapidly Involuting Capillary Haemangioma); KHE with KMP (Kaposiform Haemangio-endothelioma with Kasabach Merritt Phenomena); or a Tufted Angioma. This group of haemangiomas need urgent review by a paediatrician or specialists working in the vascular birthmark units, for further management.

Medical text written August 2001 by Dr S B Syed. **Last updated January 2006 by Dr S B Syed, Associate Specialist in Paediatric Dermatology, Great Ormond Street Hospital, London, UK.**

Support

Angioma Alliance UK

2 St Helens Road, Dorset, Dorchester DT1 1SD
(Telephone number available for those without internet access, please call Contact a Family for details on Tel: 0800 808 3555)
e-mail: info@angiomaalliance.org.uk
Web: http://www.angiomaalliance.org.uk
The Alliance is a National Registered Charity No.1114145 established in 2004. The group offers information and support. The group has close links with the American group, Angioma Alliance. Angioma Alliance UK (with financial assistance from Awards for All, funded by the National Lottery) held a medical conference in London in 2007. The Alliance hope the conference will be an annual Forum.
Group details last updated September 2007.

Birthmark Support Group

BM, London WC1N 3XX   Tel: 0845 045 4700
e-mail: info@birthmarksupportgroup.org.uk
Web: http://www.birthmarksupportgroup.org.uk
The Group is a National Registered Charity No. 1090952, established in 1998. It offers information, medical advice, coping strategies and an effective support network available to all family members. It runs four free family fun days a year which are spread all over the country and supported by medical and cosmetic professionals who give free advice and support. The group also has a group for adults (face it together) and one for teenagers (teentalk). They have approximately 800 members.
Group details last updated January 2007.

VEIN OF GALEN MALFORMATION

Background

Vein of Galen malformation (VGM) is an uncommon blood vessel disorder usually identified in childhood. It is estimated that around ten children with this condition are born in the UK each year.

Arteriovenous shunting has several potential effects. As blood usually flows faster in arteries than in veins, arteriovenous shunting means that the rate of flow in the veins is increased. This increased flow puts a strain on other organs of the body, especially the heart in young babies. Arteriovenous shunting also means that it is difficult for the veins to do their job of soaking up and circulating water from the brain. This may mean that the brain is deprived of nutrients and energy. Finally, there is a risk of bleeding from the abnormal vessels, although this is relatively low.

What are the symptoms?

The manifestations of Vein of Galen malformation will vary between individuals; however, some patterns are recognised:

- Antenatal diagnosis: sometimes VGM is identified on an ultrasound done before the baby is born. The mother may be transferred closer to a centre with experience of VGM prior to delivery so that the baby can be assessed soon after birth;
- Neonatal presentation: Some babies present in the early days of life with heart failure secondary to the increased flow though the VGM;
- Infants may present with difficulties in achieving developmental milestones or with a large head size (due to increased water in the brain);
- Older children may present with seizures, developmental difficulties or a large head size.

What are the causes?

The malformation is the result of persistence of a vein (blood vessel) which is normally present early on during pregnancy (during embryonic development) but which usually disappears before the baby's birth. If this blood vessel persists, it results in an abnormal communication between the arteries and veins of the brain. Arteries are blood vessels which take blood to the brain and veins take blood away; they are usually separated by a network of finer vessels called capillaries. In VGM, there is direct communication between arteries and veins, bypassing capillaries, a process called arteriovenous shunting. There can be single or multiple communications.

How is it treated?

Treatment of children with VGM consists of treatment of the abnormal blood vessels and treatment of secondary complications, such as cardiac failure. Treatment of the vascular problem is undertaken in a procedure known as embolisation. This is a technique used to block the abnormal communication(s) between arteries and veins, commonly using glue. More than one session of treatment may be required.

Inheritance patterns and prenatal diagnosis

Inheritance patterns

Not applicable.

Prenatal diagnosis

It is possible that in some cases of VGM can be identified on Ultrascan.

Medical text written June 2005 by Dr V Ganesan, Senior Lecturer and Hon. Consultant Paediatric Neurologist, Institute of Child Health, London, UK.

Further online resources

Medical texts in *The Contact a Family Directory* are designed to give a short, clear description of specific conditions and rare disorders. More extensive information on this condition can be found on a range of reliable, validated websites. Further information on these resources can be found in our **Medical Information on the Internet** article on page 21.

Support

Vein of Galen Support Group
28 Southgate Drive, Wincanton BA9 9ET   Tel: 01963 34393
e-mail: support@veinofgalen.co.uk   Web: http://www.veinofgalen.co.uk
This is a parent support group, established in the UK in 1999 by parents of affected children. It offers support by telephone, letter and e-mail, information on the condition and linking families where possible. There is a forum for families available on the group's website. The group aims to increase awareness of Vein of Galen malformation within the medical profession and provide information for families who have children with this rare condition. Via the website, the group is in contact with parents worldwide.
Group details last confirmed November 2007.

VISION DISORDERS IN CHILDHOOD

Background

When eyesight is tested, a great deal of emphasis is placed upon the ability to see letters on a chart several metres away and the ability to read from a book. Clearness of vision or 'Visual acuity' is then expressed as the smallest size of letter identified on the chart. It is often not comfortable to read at this threshold of vision for long periods.

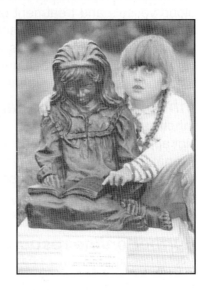

Vision in the real world is not that simple. More than 40% of the brain is devoted to visual function. To have normal vision is to have the ability to perform a number of visual 'tasks'. A child often will have difficulties in more than one of these 'tasks'. The extent of difficulties they have will vary with the eye problem they have and with the child.

To understand the tasks that the eye must perform it helps to think of the eye like a camera.

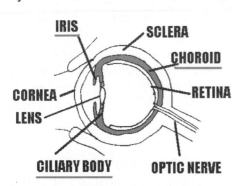

The clear **cornea** at the front and the **lens** inside the eye focus like camera lenses.

The **retina** (light sensitive film) inside the eye is the film that turns the picture into an electrical signal.

The **optic nerve** brings the signals to the brain much like a cable connecting a camera to a computer.

Normal vision is the ability to carry out the following 'tasks':

Focus

Focussed vision is being able to have clear vision (good acuity) both far away and close to you. The **cornea** of the eye works as the main lens focussing an image onto the **retina**, but needs the help of the **eye lens** which changes shape to bring things at different distances into focus. The image is blurred if the cornea is the wrong shape, the eye is too long or too short or if the lens does not **accommodate** (change shape properly).

"My eyesight is blurry without glasses"

It is common for children to need glasses to see clearly. In some parts of the world glasses for short sight are so commonly needed, for school aged children to see clearly, that children without glasses are in the minority. Glasses help the eye to focus. A child's eye is still growing so the strength of glasses changes with age.

When glasses are worn, vision is normal in most cases. Failing to realise that a child needs glasses can disadvantage them especially at school. In some cases failing to wear glasses needed to see clearly can stop the vision part of the brain developing correctly and lead to **amblyopia** (lazy eye) and to the eyes not working together (**strabismus**, 'squint' or 'turn').

Problems with focus of the eye include:

Myopia (short sight)

If you are short sighted you can see small things clearly if you hold them very close to your eyes, but you cannot read the whiteboard at school until you put you glasses on. People with myopia usually have long eyeballs and they grow with age so glasses often need to be stronger whilst you are still growing.

Hypermetropia (long sight)

Many young people with long sight can see clearly both far away and near, but may develop a headache looking at small things close up. This becomes more of a problem with age and reading glasses may be needed. With higher hypermetropia vision is blurred at all distances especially for near. Glasses are then needed all the time. Hypermetropic individuals may develop a **strabismus** (squint) with one eye turning inwards. Glasses reduce the focussing effort and the squint. Most longsighted eyes are short eyes or have a weak focussing system. As the eye grows the glasses needed may be thinner and may only be needed for reading.

Astigmatism (oval front of eye)

Often astigmatism is combined with short or long sight. If you have astigmatism small things both far away and near are distorted so you cannot see what they are clearly. This is because the **cornea** (clear front of your eye) is shaped like an egg or rugby ball rather than a spherical football shape.

Accommodation (poor change of focus)

As we age the lens in our eye becomes less elastic and cannot change shape to focus on close objects. It is like a spongy ball gradually turning into a hard ball. At the same time the **ciliary muscle** (muscle inside the eye) that changes the shape of the lens weakens. Reading glasses help overcome this problem. It is very unusual for a child's lens to become more rigid but some children appear to have weak ciliary muscles or a poor nerve signal from the brain to trigger focussing.

Children with more complex visual disorders rarely have one single problem with their eyes. They may need glasses to best use the vision they have, but even strong glasses would not make their vision normal. This is because part of their eye, the optic nerve (the connection of their eye to their brain) or the visual pathways in the brain did not develop normally or are damaged.

Contrast

Contrast vision is the ability to see an object separate from it's background. Acuity is usually tested using high contrast black pictures or letters on a white, often lit up, background. This test is used because it is not usually affected by background lighting of the room. To test contrast vision, charts with letters in varying shades of grey are used, and the background lighting is kept constant.

> **"I cannot see if teacher writes on the whiteboard with a yellow pen or a black pen that is running out of ink."**

> **"I can see a bright star in the sky, but I don't always see a cyclist when I cross the road on a rainy day."**

With normal eye sight it is harder to see letters on a chart if they are grey rather than black, or if there is shine on the chart. With impaired contrast vision the difficulty is greatly magnified if the chart is poorly lit or the letters grey. There is difficulty in seeing objects that are poorly contrasting from their background such as grey print on a page or yellow pen on a white board.

Problems with contrast vision:

A child with a disorder such as **optic atrophy** (a damaged optic nerve) may, in good lighting, see half of the high contrast normal eye chart, but will not see even the largest letter if the chart is dull and the letters grey.

Colour

Colour vision is the ability to distinguish between different colours. Anomalies of colour vision are very common in males and the commonest form of "colour blindness" and in most cases it does not affect everyday life. Some individuals may even be unaware that they perceive colours differently to most of us. Most people with colour vision deficiency do see colours they just see them differently to people with normal colour vision.

> **"I can see the grass is green and that the sky is blue, but my friends sometimes tease me when I cannot tell if their shirt is pink or green"**

> **"When I look at a coloured map my friends see more different colours than I do. Some colours look just the same as each other to me"**

Problems with colour vision:

In one rare form of "colour blindness" the colour red appears dim so a red light such as a traffic light may not always be noticed. Teachers need to be aware of common red/green confusions and avoid the need to distinguish between these colours in educational materials. Black print may totally disappear on a red or green page for these children. Individuals with the common colour vision anomalies have normal acuity (detail vision) and visual field. Children with the common colour vision problems have them from birth and their ability to see colours does not change.

Other problems with colour vision, that develop due to an abnormality in the eye are more commonly associated with poor acuity and contrast sensitivity and it is these factors that have greater impact on vision.

Visual Field

The visual field describes the entire range that a person can see even if a person is looking straight ahead they can also see some of the environment on either side of them.

> **"Some people think I am rude or clumsy because when I am walking I sometimes bump into them or trip on steps."**

> **"When I look at my Mum's face I cannot see the toy she is holding out to me."**

Problems with Visual Field:

If the visual field is abnormally narrow, it is like looking through a tunnel. A normal excited toddler focused on a person or object ahead of them may trip on a toy. An older child with a narrow field of vision may remain clumsy and trip on steps or objects beneath their feet if they are looking ahead. Children with tunnel vision may appear clumsy or even rude as they bump into people. If the field of vision is severely restricted a person may be registered as blind despite being able to see and read the finest print, as it is difficult to move around safely in unfamiliar surroundings without the skilled use of a touch cane. If the field of vision is reduced to one side (**homonymous hemianopia**) there may be difficulty finding the start of a new line. It may help to move a ruler down the page or a piece of black card with a letterbox opening to view the line. Children with **hemianopia** may appear to be not 'paying attention' when they are, as they often compensate by turning their head to one side to centralise their useful field of vision. Generally the causes of problems in the visual field are irreversible.

Stereovision and depth perception

Stereoacuity is the ability to see close objects in depth (3D). This ability is used by those performing fine manipulations at a close distance, such as using scissors, working through a microscope, or threading a needle. Many with poor stereovision but otherwise normal eyesight have no practical difficulties in everyday life. Perception of the depth of more distant targets such as steps is a different function. Distance depth perception is gauged by multiple clues such as interpretation of size differences and of overlapping edges.

'Vision for action' and 'spatial skills'

Parts of the brain called the Posterior Parietal Lobes control 'Vision for Action' and 'Spatial Skills', these are both important in various vision related tasks:

- To be aware of various parts of a scene at the same time;
- To find a particular object in a crowded area;
- To move eyes towards an interesting object;
- To break off looking at an object;
- To accurately grasp an object or to post a letter into a letterbox;
- To step onto a moving escalator.

"**I can find my toy car on the carpet, but it is hard if there are other small toys there too**"

"**There is too much on this page. It is better if the sentences are spaced out**"

Reading a letter from a line of letters, a word from a sentence, finding a person in a crowd, finding a toy from a mass of toys is important for normal vision. A person with problems performing these tasks may have the '**crowding phenomenon**'. These children may appear not to see a picture on a page if there are too many pictures, but then surprise their parents by noting very small detail in a single picture on a page. The same child may appear not to see print unless it is enlarged but will see small print if only a single line of print is on a page rather than a full page of print.

Visual acuity is not only a measure of a child's ability to see detail, but of their ability to pick out an object from several other objects. This ability is measured by the ability to name a letter or pictures from amongst a line of letters or shapes. This is a harder task than identifying single letters or pictures one at a time. Most children can perform a simple matching test of letters, or name single pictures by three years of age and match letters from a line by four years of age.

Motion vision

In walking or running, the environment appears to stay still as the brain compensates for the movement. In some rare disorders when higher processing of vision in the brain's pathways is affected, a moving object will appear to 'disappear' whilst the stationary environment is seen clearly.

There are also rare individuals who appear blind on conventional testing who retain some motion detection. These individuals may 'see' if they are moving relative to objects; for example if they are rocking in a chair or a passenger in a car.

Other problems with vision

Visual Tracking

Eyes have the ability to see and track an object, providing it is not moving too quickly. Most specific reading problems are due to processing problems within the brain, and not to problems with eye movement, although the two can occur together. Children with **nystagmus** (regular rapid eye movements such as occurs in individuals with albinism) are often excellent readers as long as they can hold the page close, but they may find prolonged reading causes fatigue.

Saccadic (rapid eye movement) is important for choosing to look in a new direction such as looking towards a parent who has just entered or a toy that is being held towards a child. When this doesn't work, compensating strategies will often be adopted. These include the child shaking their head to bring their eyes towards the interesting object or blinking to move their gaze. There may however still be difficulties, especially with reading, as it may be hard to locate the beginning of a new line of print. Individuals with abnormal **saccades** also often have additional processing problems in the visual pathways and difficulty with global brain processing.

'Visual library'

The temporal lobes located in the right side of the brain are responsible for our Visual library and help us to read maps and remember faces.

> **"I have difficulty in remembering people's faces, even my own family. I also find it difficult to name different animals"**

> **"I cannot remember which drawer my socks are in. I could not find my bedroom by myself until my door was painted a different colour to the others"**

For the brain to find one letter from several others and identify it as a remembered shape is called processing. A child may have the optical system to see small detail but have problems with reading due to problems with processing. It is rare that glasses or any optical 'training' will be of benefit in these cases whereas educational strategies are more helpful.

The complicated task of reading from a line of letters requires good focussing and healthy eye structures, especially normal function of the light sensitive retina which forms the image. Information the eye sees or 'receives' is then passed to an area of the brain, which maps the image and passes the information to other parts of the brain for processing. If a child has a problem with processing then they will have difficulty with standard vision tests. Processing of vision is complex and standard eye tests do not explore different difficulties in these areas.

Reflex subconscious vision

We may react to something in our vision before we have 'seen' it. This is our primitive vision system reflexes working to 'protect' us from the 'threat' of the sudden movement in our visual field. Children with very severe vision handicap may still have primitive vision reflexes.

Medical text written September 2002 by Miss Isabelle Russell-Eggitt FRCS FRCOphth.
Last updated December 2007 by Miss Isabelle Russell-Eggitt FRCS FRCOphth, Consultant Ophthalmic Surgeon, Great Ormond Street Hospital, London, UK.

Support

Support Groups for children and families:
Vision Aid
106 Junction Road, Deane, Bolton BL3 4NE   Tel: 01204 64265   Fax: 01204 855937
e-mail: visionaiduk@aol.com
Vision Aid is a National Registered Charity No. 518641, established in 1984. It aims to offer practical help and advice to the families of vision impaired children throughout the UK. Children with additional needs are also welcome. The range of free services include: resource centre; guidance on education and benefits; a range of publications; library service for toys and books; weekly drop-in sessions; parent-to-parent contact; visual stimulation programmes; and equipment loan. The organisation also offers advice to professionals working with vision impaired children. The Group is in contact with 5,000 families nationwide.
Group details last updated June 2007.

LOOK
c/o Queen Alexandra College, 49 Court Oak Road, Birmingham B17 9TG
Tel: 0121 428 5038   Fax: 0121 427 9800   e-mail: office@look-uk.org
Web: http://www.look-uk.org
LOOK is a National Registered Charity No. 1007282, established in 1991. It is an umbrella organisation for groups concerned with visual impairment in children. It offers the opportunity for parents and parent support groups to co-operate in order to enhance the education, welfare and leisure opportunities for visually impaired children. It publishes a quarterly newsletter.
Group details last confirmed August 2007.

Victa Children Ltd
PO Box 5791, Milton Keynes MK10 1BE
Tel: 01908 240831 Information and grants   Tel: 01908 691338 Fundraising
e-mail: admin@victa.org.uk   Web: http://www.victa.org.uk
Visually Impaired Children Taking Action (VICTA) is a National Registered Charity No. 1065029, established in 1987. It will consider grant applications for individual children for equipment/services that will aid their education or social skills. VICTA will also consider grant applications from groups and charities supporting visually impaired children. Please contact VICTA for more information.
Group details last updated October 2007.

Contact a Family Helpline 0808 808 3555

National Blind Children's Society
2nd Floor, Shawton House, 792 Hagley Road West, Oldbury B68 0PJ
Tel: 0800 781 1444 Helpline   Tel: 01278 764770   Fax: 01278 764790
e-mail: enquiries@nbcs.org.uk
The Society is a National Registered Charity No. 1051607, established in 1996. It
offers services for children and young people with a visual impairment, from birth to the
completion of full time education. NBCS provides family support, educational advocacy,
IT advice and support, and CustomEyes large print children's books. NBCS can provide
grants for computers, speech and magnification software, educational toys etc.
Group details last updated January 2007.

Support Groups for adults and children:
RNIB (Royal National Institute of the Blind)
105 Judd Street, London WC1H 9NE   Tel: 0845 766 9999 Helpline (UK only)
Tel: 020 7388 1266 Switchboard/Overseas callers   Fax: 020 7388 2034
e-mail: helpline@rnib.org.uk   Web: http://www.rnib.org.uk
The Institute is a National Registered Charity No. 226227, established in 1868. It offers
information about school choices and contact with advisory teachers in their Local
Education Authority. It has information about parent support groups, practical advice for
employers and employees, and a Talking Book Service. It runs schools for various ages
and abilities, some catering for children with additional needs. It also runs Colleges for
Further Education and vocational courses. It also has rehabilitation centres, resource and
education centres and has a holiday service. Products, aids and publications are available
from the Customer Services Department. It publishes 'Visability' and 'Eye Contact'
magazines for parents and teachers and has a wide range of information available, details
on request. The Institute is a membership organisation.
Group details last confirmed January 2007.

Henshaw's Society for Blind People
John Derby House, 88-92 Talbot Road, Old Trafford, Manchester M16 0GS
Tel: 0161 872 1234   Fax: 0161 848 9889   e-mail: info@hsbp.co.uk
Web: http://www.hsbp.co.uk
The Society is a National Registered Charity No. 221888, established in 1837. Henshaw
children and family services offers support to families with a visual impairment within
the North of England. It provides domiciliary visits within Greater Manchester and has a
Resource Centre in Manchester incorporating a Specialist Toy Library, Soft Play area and
Sensory Stimulation room. It also runs a College of Further Education providing vocational
education and training opportunities for young people who are visually impaired, many with
additional physical and learning disabilities. It publishes a newsletter three times a year
and has information available, details on request. Please send SAE.
Group details last updated June 2007.

The Partially Sighted Society
7/9 Bennetthorpe, Doncaster DN2 6AA   Tel: 0844 477 4966   Fax: 0844 477 4969
e-mail: info@partsight.org.uk   e-mail: doncaster@partsight.org.uk
The Society is a National Registered Charity No. 254052, established in 1973. It offers
advice and information for people with vision impairment or their carers, to help them make
the best use of their remaining vision. It publishes a quarterly magazine, 'The Oculus',
and offers a free brochure/catalogue on request. The Society has approximately 2,000
members ond over 30,000 contacts.
Group details last updated May 2007.

Action for Blind People

14-16 Verney Road, London SE16 3DZ   Tel: 0800 915 4666 (Helpline)

Fax: 020 7635 4900   e-mail: info@actionforblindpeople.org.uk

Web: http://www.actionforblindpeople.org.uk

Action for Blind People is a National Registered Charity No. 205913, established in 1857.
It provides direct services for visually impaired people through regional teams in four
key areas: support, (including a wide range of information and specialist welfare advice),
employment advice and development for blind and partially sighted jobseekers and those
in work who are losing their sight, independent living and specialist housing advice, holiday
break opportunities in purpose built and specially adapted hotels and a network of activities
clubs for visually impaired children.

Group details last confirmed January 2007.

"It's great to know you are there to turn to in a troubling situation. It has been reassuring to have someone else looking and finding out things for us."
Parent.

VITILIGO

Background

In Vitiligo there is an absence of melanocytes within the epidermis.

The clinical hallmark of Vitiligo is patches of absent pigmentation giving rise to areas of very white skin, the hair may also be affected. The patches often present in a strikingly symmetrical pattern on both sides of the body, they may spread over time and are highly vulnerable to sunburn.

How is it treated?

Treatment of Vitiligo is often difficult and, except for a very small depigmented patches, is usually lengthy. In addition, none appears to alter the course of the underlying disease and, although pigmentation may be satisfactory at the end of treatment, a risk of relapse persists indefinitely.

Inheritance patterns and prenatal diagnosis

Inheritance patterns

Although the cause(s) of Vitiligo is unknown, there is undoubtedly a genetic aspect as Vitiligo quite often runs in families with a history of so called 'autoimmune' diseases such as diabetes, thyroid disease and pernicious anaemia (anemia - US). A study of twins showed that both identical twins are more likely to develop the disease than both non-identical twins.

Prenatal diagnosis

None

Medical text written August 2000 by Dr D J Gawkrodger. **Last reviewed September 2005 by Professor D J Gawkrodger, Consultant Dermatologist, Royal Hallamshire Hospital, Sheffield, UK.**

Further online resources

Medical texts in *The Contact a Family Directory* are designed to give a short, clear description of specific conditions and rare disorders. More extensive information on this condition can be found on a range of reliable, validated websites. Further information on these resources can be found in our **Medical Information on the Internet** article on page 21.

Support

The Vitiligo Society
125 Kennington Road, London SE11 6SF   Tel: 0800 018 2631 Helpline
Tel: 020 7840 0844   Fax: 020 7840 0866   e-mail: ken125@vitiligosociety.org.uk
Web: http://www.vitiligosociety.org.uk
The Society is a National Registered Charity No. 1069607, established in 1985. It offers support and understanding to affected people. It publishes a regular newsletter and has a wide range of information available, details on request. The Society has approximately 2,000 members.
Group details last confirmed February 2008.

VON HIPPEL-LINDAU SYNDROME

Background

Von Hippel-Lindau (VHL) syndrome is an uncommon genetic disorder in which tumours and cysts occur in a variety of organs. Most frequently these are the cerebellum (hind part of the brain), the spinal cord, the kidneys, the pancreas and the retina of the eye. Angiomas (enlarged blood vessels) can occur on the retina, while haemangioblastomas (benign cysts or tumours) may occur in the cerebellum or spinal cord. Kidney tumours and cysts are common and early detection of kidney tumours is important. Phaeochromocytomas occur in about ten per cent of patients, pancreatic tumours in up to ten per cent and endolymphatic sac tumours (causing deafness) occur in up to fifteen per cent. Pancreatic and epididymal cysts are common but rarely cause clinical problems.

What are the symptoms?

The presenting symptoms vary greatly in individual cases. This means that in different generations, or among siblings, affected individuals will not have the same organ affected: for example, one individual may have an affected kidney whilst in another individual the eyes are affected.

Early childhood onset is infrequent and but can occur and so surveillance should be started in the first few years of life. Most people with VHL develop clinical complications between the age of fifteen to thirty years but, in some cases, no effects are noted until after the age of 50. Hence it is important that all individuals at risk are offered screening for subclinical involvement. Detailed information and advice on screening and follow-up is available from local Genetics Centres.

What are the causes?

The gene responsible for the disorder is on chromosome 3 and was identified in 1993.

How is it diagnosed?

Pre-symptomatic diagnosis is available to most families by direct mutation analysis.

Inheritance patterns and prenatal diagnosis

Inheritance patterns

Autosomal dominant, new mutations may also occur.

Prenatal diagnosis

Not usually requested but possible in many cases by DNA testing.

Contact a Family Helpline 0808 808 3555

Medical text written November 1991 by Contact a Family. Approved November 1991 by Professor M Patton, Professor of Medical Genetics, St Georges Hospital Medical School, London, UK and Dr J E Wraith, Consultant Paediatrician, Royal Manchester Children's Hospital, UK. **Last updated August 2004 by Professor E R Maher , Professor of Medical Genetics, Department of Paediatrics and Child Health, University of Birmingham Medical School, Birmingham, UK.**

Further online resources

Medical texts in *The Contact a Family Directory* are designed to give a short, clear description of specific conditions and rare disorders. More extensive information on this condition can be found on a range of reliable, validated websites. Further information on these resources can be found in our **Medical Information on the Internet** article on page 21.

Support

Von Hippel-Lindau Contact Group
c/o Contact a Family, 209-211 City Road, London EC1V 1JN   Tel: 01204 886112
e-mail: maryweetman@waitrose.com   Web: http://www.vhlcg.com
The Group is a support network, established in 1990. It offers a listening ear to affected individuals, their families and carers. An information pack can be requested by telephone or e-mail. The Group is in touch with over 50 families.
Group details last confirmed February 2008.

WAARDENBURG SYNDROME

Background

Waardenburg syndrome (WS) is an inherited condition which may be associated with a range of features. The main characteristics of WS include hearing impairment (see Deafness), pigmentation changes of iris, hair, and skin, and a characteristic facial appearance.

What are the symptoms?

Individuals with WS may show some or all of these features and, in addition, may be differently affected by the severity of their symptoms. For example, some individuals with WS may have profound deafness and no pigmental changes, whilst others may have a white forelock, slightly widely spaced eyes and mild hearing impairment. Hearing impairment due to defects of the inner ear (sensorineural), may affect one ear or both ears. Individuals may have different coloured eyes, usually one eye is blue and the other brown. However, sometimes one eye may be two different colours. An individual may also have a white lock of hair growing above the forehead and premature greying or whitening of the hair may appear by as early as twelve years. Some individuals may have a wide space between the eyes (dystopia canthorum), connecting eyebrows and/or a low frontal hairline. Infrequently, WS may be associated with other conditions such as the gastrointestinal problems of Hirschsprung's disease (see entry, Gut Motility Disorders) or features including upper limb abnormalities (see entry) and cleft lip and/or palate (see entry). Individuals with WS have a normal lifespan.

How is it diagnosed?

Researchers have described four main types of WS. A diagnosis of the particular type of WS depends upon detecting the fault in the causative gene. The different types of WS vary in the physical characteristics present. The most common types of WS are Type 1 and Type 2, which are distinguished on the basis of widely spaced eyes. This feature is present in Type 1 and absent in Type 2. However, hearing impairments are more common in Type 2. Type 3 (Klein-Waardenburg syndrome) is rare and is associated with widely spaced eyes and upper limb abnormalities. Type 4 (Waardenburg-Hirschsprung's disease), which is also uncommon, is associated with colon problems originating from the time of birth.

Inheritance patterns and prenatal diagnosis

Inheritance patterns

WS Types 1 and 2 are inherited as autosomal dominant traits; Types 3 and 4 may be dominant or recessive in different families. A number of different genes have been associated with WS, but only Type 1 is a well-defined single genetic condition. Type 3 is caused by the same gene as Type 1, but is more severe. Type 2 is genetically heterogeneous (involvement of several genes); so far only one causative gene has been clearly identified and this is responsible for only a small proportion of cases. Mutations in three different genes have been seen in different cases of Type 4.

Prenatal diagnosis

This may be possible but those wishing to pursue this should ask to see a specialist in medical genetics to discuss whether or not this applies in their particular circumstances.

Medical text written September 2001 by Contact a Family. Approved September 2001 by Professor Valerie Newton, Professor in Audiological Medicine, University of Manchester, Manchester, UK. **Last updated March 2006 by Professor Valerie Newton, Professor Emerita in Audiological Medicine.**

Further online resources

Medical texts in *The Contact a Family Directory* are designed to give a short, clear description of specific conditions and rare disorders. More extensive information on this condition can be found on a range of reliable, validated websites. Further information on these resources can be found in our **Medical Information on the Internet** article on page 21.

On-going research

Deafness Research UK

330-332 Grays Inn Road, London WC1X 8EE

Tel: 0808 808 2222 Freephone Information Service (Mon-Fri, 9.30am-5.30pm)

Tel: 020 7915 1412 Textphone   Tel: 020 7833 1733   Fax: 020 7278 0404

e-mail: info@deafnessresearch.org.uk   Web: http://www.deafnessresearch.org.uk

Research Registry for Hereditary Hearing Loss, Omaha, USA

e-mail: deafgene.registry@boystown.org

Support

A support group for Waardenburg syndrome has not yet been established. However, a one-to-one linking system between parents who have children with Waardenburg syndrome is offered within Contact a Family. This service has been formulated and adapted to provide a confidential and sensitive service aimed to meet individual needs.

A number of organisations provide information and support services about conditions which may be associated with Waardenburg syndrome (for example, hearing impairment, hypopigmentation, eye abnormalities etc).

WEST SYNDROME

West syndrome; Infantile spasms

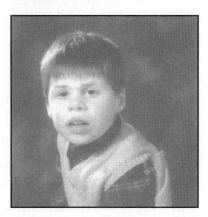

Background

West syndrome is the term used to describe a type of epilepsy (see entry) which most typically starts in the first year of life, between four and eight months of age. It may, however, start younger than this.

What are the symptoms?

The hallmark of West syndrome is the occurrence of a particular type of epileptic seizure called a spasm. Spasms typically produce a sudden jerk of the body followed by stiffening of the limbs. Different types of spasms may occur but most typically a child will suddenly bend forward with elevation of the arms or legs. These attacks usually occur in runs or clusters when one spasm occurs after another for a period of several minutes. These episodes may occur several times per day. Very commonly, when a child starts to have spasms there is change in their behaviour and they appear to switch off and lose interest in their surroundings.

What are the causes?

West syndrome is not one condition but is a symptom of many different brain disorders. A cause can be found in most children but in a small proportion no obvious cause can be identified. Sometimes West syndrome occurs in children with severe abnormalities of the brain such as congenital infections, severe brain injury due to birth asphyxia or severe malformations of the brain. Sometimes very rare genetic or metabolic diseases cause West syndrome. One of the commonest causes of West syndrome is tuberous sclerosis (see entry). Chromosome abnormalities may also cause West syndrome. It is therefore very important when a diagnosis of West syndrome is made that an extensive search is carried out to find the underlying cause.

How is it diagnosed?

The diagnosis of West syndrome is based on the occurrence of infantile spasms and the presence of a very abnormal EEG (brain wave recording). The most typical EEG abnormality is called hypsarrhythmia but other abnormal patterns may occur.

How is it treated?

The most common treatments for West syndrome are Vigabatrin (an anti-epileptic drug) or steroids (Prednisolone, Hydrocortisone or ACTH). In many children the spasms will stop with appropriate treatment, however after a period of time they will often relapse and require a change of treatment.

The prognosis for West syndrome depends in part upon the underlying cause. However, overall it is one of the more severe forms of epilepsy and most children with West syndrome will have long-term problems which may include developmental delay, learning disability (see entry), epilepsy or any combination of these three. Around twelve to fifteen per cent of children with West syndrome will stop having spasms and will develop normally.

Inheritance patterns and prenatal diagnosis

Inheritance patterns

This depends on the underlying cause and genetic advice should be sought.

Prenatal diagnosis

None.

Medical text written November 2002 by Dr J Livingston, Consultant Paediatric Neurologist, Leeds General Infirmary, Leeds, UK.

Further online resources

Medical texts in *The Contact a Family Directory* are designed to give a short, clear description of specific conditions and rare disorders. More extensive information on this condition can be found on a range of reliable, validated websites. Further information on these resources can be found in our **Medical Information on the Internet** article on page 21.

Support

West Syndrome Support Group
c/o Contact a Family, 209-211 City Road, London EC1V 1JN   Tel: 01252 654057
e-mail: info@cafamily.org.uk
The current West Syndrome Support Group was re-established in 2002, having been originally, established in 1994. It is run by parents and can offer support and a sympathetic ear to families of affected children.
Group details last updated May 2007.

WILLIAMS SYNDROME

Infantile Hypercalcaemia: Williams-Beuren syndrome

Background

Williams syndrome is a sporadic congenital syndrome due to a microdeletion of chromosome 7 (7q11, 23) at the elastin gene focus. There is a typical facies and global developmental delay. There may be abnormalities of calcium metabolism and problems may occur in any of the major systems.

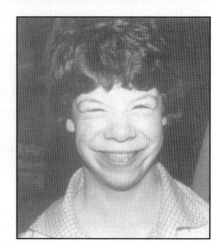

What are the symptoms?

Features include facial similarities (prominent cheeks, upturned nose, wide mouth, irregular teeth). Children may have a heart problem, typically supravalvular aortic stenosis, peripheral pulmonary artery stenosis, or both. These heart murmurs are often present at birth. Some children develop hypercalcaemia, usually within the first two years of life. This may cause failure to thrive, feeding problems, irritability, vomiting, constipation and kidney problems.

Behaviour problems, hyperactivity, short attention span and obsessional behaviour occur. Peculiar to the syndrome is an increased verbal ability in comparison to other cognitive skills. Hypersensitivity to loud noises (hyperacusis) is reported in ninety per cent of children.

Psychological and behavioural characteristics

Children with Williams syndrome are developmentally delayed, with moderate or severe learning difficulties, though a few come within the borderline to low average range of abilities. Most will need to attend a special needs school. They may be slow to develop language in the pre-school years, but by school-age their verbal abilities are in most cases markedly superior to their perceptual abilities and to their gross and fine motor skills. Their spoken language tends to be grammatically correct, complex and fluent at a superficial level, with a well developed and precocious vocabulary, but with poor turn-taking and topic maintenance skills. The children tend to be very chatty, and their auditory memory, mimicry skills and social use of language are particularly well developed. In contrast, they are often clumsy and have difficulties in the integration of visual- spatial information and in sequencing and constructional tasks.

Most children with Williams syndrome are outgoing and socially disinhibited towards adults, including strangers, but they tend to have poor relationships with peers. Typical behaviour difficulties include overactivity, poor concentration and distractibility, excessive anxiety, attention seeking behaviours, and high rates of preoccupations and obsessions with particular activities or objects. In some cases depression, anxiety and/or preoccupations and obsessions worsen in adulthood. Many of the children are hypersensitive to particular sounds, including electrical noises like vacuum cleaners and drills, and sudden loud noises like thunder. The basis for this hyperacusis is not clear, and it often becomes less of a problem in adulthood.

Despite their relatively good verbal and social skills, most adults with Williams syndrome are unable to live independently and require ongoing support and supervision in everyday activities. This is most likely due to their characteristic over-friendliness and social disinhibition, their limited social awareness, distractibility, and high levels of anxiety and fearfulness.

Inheritance patterns and prenatal diagnosis

Inheritance patterns

Most cases are sporadic and presumed to be new mutations. Affected individuals would be expected to display autosomal dominant inheritance.

Prenatal diagnosis

None available.

Medical text written November 1991 by Contact a Family. Approved November 1991 by Professor M Patton, Professor of Medical Genetics, St Georges Hospital Medical School, London, UK and Dr J E Wraith, Consultant Paediatrician, Royal Manchester Children's Hospital,UK. **Last updated June 2004 by Dr Mike Wolfman, General Practitioner and Secretary to the Professional Panel, Williams Syndrome Foundation, Tonbridge, UK. Psychological and behavioural characteristics last reviewed January 2004 by Dr Orlee Udwin, Consultant Clinical Child Psychologist, West London Mental Health NHS Trust, London, UK.**

Further online resources

Medical texts in *The Contact a Family Directory* are designed to give a short, clear description of specific conditions and rare disorders. More extensive information on this condition can be found on a range of reliable, validated websites. Further information on these resources can be found in our **Medical Information on the Internet** article on page 21.

W

Support

Williams Syndrome Foundation Ltd
161 High Street, Tonbridge TN9 1BX   Tel: 01732 365152   Fax: 01732 360178
e-mail: john.nelson-wsfoundation@btinternet.com
Web: http://www.williams-syndrome.org.uk
The Foundation is a National Registered Charity No.281014, established in 1980. It offers parent contact and support through a network of regional groups with financial help to attend meetings if necessary. It publishes a newsletter twice a year and has information available, details on request. The Foundation represents the families of over 900 affected children and adults.
Group details last confirmed July 2007.

As Williams syndrome is a metabolic disease, support and advice are also available from Climb (see entry, Metabolic diseases).

The Royal College of Physicians has estimated that 2-3 per cent of births in the UK result in babies with either congenital or genetically-determined abnormalities, that's over 13,000 babies and their families affected in a year.

WOLF-HIRSCHHORN SYNDROME

Wolf Hirschhorn syndrome, 4p-, Pitt-Rogers-Danks syndrome (occasional)

Background

Wolf-Hirschhorn syndrome is a rare chromosome disorder affecting approximately 1 in 90,000 births.

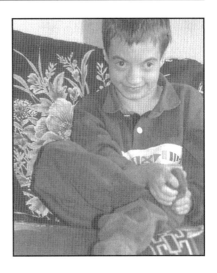

What are the symptoms?

There is a wide variation in the degree of problems seen in this condition. Children with Wolf-Hirschhorn have a low birth weight and will usually have slow weight gain and difficulty with feeding. They have a small head size for their age (see entry, microcephaly) and most will have epilepsy (see entry). Individuals with Wolf-Hirschhorn tend to have similar facial features. These may include a broad bridge to the nose, wider spaced eyes than average and a small chin. Learning difficulties (see entry, Learning Disability) are variable and can be moderate to severe. In the past, children whose deletion was too small to be seen with a light microscope, were described as having Pitt-Rogers-Danks syndrome. These children are now felt to represent the mild end of the Wolf-Hirschhorn syndrome spectrum.

Children with Wolf-Hirschhorn syndrome may be born with some other congenital problems. The most commonly recognised include: cleft lip and/or palate (see entry), congenital heart disease (see entry, Heart defects), kidney problems (see entry, Kidney disease), eye anomalies, undescended testes and hypospadias (see entry).

What are the causes?

It is caused by a missing section (deletion) of genetic information from the tip of the short arm of chromosome 4. Chromosomes are rod like structures which store genetic information in the centre of most of our body cells.

Inheritance patterns and prenatal diagnosis

Inheritance patterns

Once a child has been diagnosed, the chromosomes of the parents should be checked. In the majority of cases these will be normal indicating that the deletion or rearrangement was present in the egg or sperm cell. In this situation, a couple's chance of having another affected child is low (under one per cent).

In the remaining cases there may be a more complex chromosome rearrangement or translocation which one parent may carry in a balanced form. If this is the case, then the chance of having a second affected child is assessed on an individual basis and in addition, blood tests may be arranged for other family members.

Genetic counselling is available.

Prenatal diagnosis

Chorionic villous sampling at eleven to twelve weeks gestation and amniocentesis from sixteen weeks gestation are available.

Medical text written February 2004 by Dr O Quarrell, Consultant in Clinical Genetics, Centre for Human Genetics, Sheffield, UK and Dr N Shannon, Consultant in Clinical Genetics, Clinical Genetics Centre, Nottingham, UK.

Support

Wolf-Hirschhorn Syndrome Support Group

Bungalow 2, Pettycur Bay Caravan Park, Kinghorn, Fife KY3 9YE

Tel: 0845 603 5338 e-mail: enquiries@whs4pminus.co.uk

Web: http://www.whs4pmins.co.uk

The Group is a National Registered Charity No. 1038219, established in 1987. It offers contact with other parents of affected children where possible. It publishes a newsletter each April, August and December. Information is available on request, please send SAE. The Group has two medical advisers and has over 160 families in membership.

Group details last updated January 2008.

WORSTER-DROUGHT SYNDROME

Worster-Drought syndrome: Congenital Suprabulbar Paresis

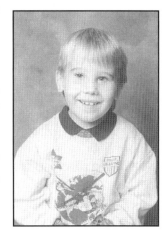

Background

This condition is a form of cerebral palsy. The main problems occur with the mouth, tongue and swallowing muscles as a result of the bulbar muscles being affected. There are usually no obvious causes in the pregnancy or birth but some varieties are genetically determined. Because of the range of problems the diagnosis is often made quite late.

What are the symptoms?

The signs and symptoms of Worster-Drought syndrome include difficulties with voluntary lip, tongue and palate movements with a brisk jaw jerk. Sometimes there is an abnormal shape to the jaw and tooth alignment and, therefore, dental care is important. The arms and legs may show signs of mild spasticity and incoordination. Minor congenital abnormalities including contractures of the feet are sometimes seen.

The first indication of the condition is usually when the baby has difficulties with feeding. Attempts at feeding may cause choking and inhalation which may lead to chest infections. In the severest cases sucking difficulties may necessitate tube feeding for several months.

In less severe cases the major problems occur when solid foods are introduced. These include difficulties with lip closure and tongue mobility, so that food is not moved to the back of the mouth or cleared efficiently from the mouth cavity or hard palate. Chewing and swallowing are often impaired which may lead to inhalation of food into the respiratory tract. These problems may gradually improve over the first two to three years or persist for many years. The second major clinical problem is usually a severe speech delay which may even prevent all early speech (see entry, Speech and Language Impairment.)

Persistent dribbling is very common but may show steady improvement during childhood. In some cases speech therapy, medication and occasionally surgical intervention are sometimes required. As a result of the swallowing problems there is an increased incidence of middle ear infection and conductive hearing loss.

A mild delay in walking and running with clumsiness of the hands is common. Many children have mild learning and behaviour difficulties which may include hyperactivity.

In a minority of cases Epilepsy (see entry) can occur which is treated with medication in the usual way.

The management of Worster-Drought syndrome is dependent on the degree of feeding and speech problems. The condition is non-progressive.

Although separately described as a syndrome of quite severe epilepsy, Bilateral Perisylvian syndrome (see entry, Congenital Bilateral Perisylvian syndrome) overlaps almost totally with Worster-Drought syndrome. In this latter condition, magnetic resonance imaging shows the characteristic abnormality called perisylvian polymicrogyria. All of the clinical problems are similar to those of the Worster-Drought syndrome with the exception that the rate of epilepsy is higher. There are families with one child with this MRI abnormality and another child with typical Worster-Drought findings and a normal MRI scan. There are some genetic clues now to perisylvian polymicrogyria which are being actively explored.

Inheritance patterns and prenatal diagnosis
Inheritance patterns
Most cases are sporadic but there have been families with more than one affected member for which the inheritance is still unclear.
Prenatal diagnosis
None

Medical text written April 1999 by Professor B Neville. **Last updated February 2004 by Professor B Neville, Professor of Childhood Epilepsy, Institute of Child Health, London, UK.**

Further online resources
Medical texts in *The Contact a Family Directory* are designed to give a short, clear description of specific conditions and rare disorders. More extensive information on this condition can be found on a range of reliable, validated websites. Further information on these resources can be found in our **Medical Information on the Internet** article on page 21.

Support
Worster-Drought Syndrome Support Group
10 St Vincent Chase, Braintree, Essex CM7 8UJ Tel: 01376 348 948
e-mail: national.contact@wdssg.org.uk Web: http://www.wdssg.org.uk
The Group is a National Registered Charity No. 1095290, established in 1994. It offers support by telephone and letter and linking of families where possible. It publishes a newsletter three time a year and has information available, details on request. The Group has over 100 members.
Group details last confirmed July 2007.

X-LINKED HYPOPHOSPHATEMIA

X-Linked Hypophosphatemia: X-Linked Hypophosphataemia - UK; Vitamin D Resistant Rickets; Familial Hypophosphatemic Rickets

Background

X-Linked Hypophosphatemia is a relatively rare syndrome that affects about 1 in 20,000 people. In the past, the syndrome has been referred to as Vitamin D Resistant Rickets.

What are the symptoms?

It is characterised by low phosphorus in the blood (hypophosphatemia) associated with high phosphate excretion in the urine (hyperphosphaturia), and symptoms of rickets (bowed or knock-kneed legs). Dental problems, particularly unexplained abscesses in primary teeth, are also a common sign of the disease.

How is it diagnosed?

Typically, if there is no apparent family history, parents become concerned when a toddler's legs appear bowed. Diagnosis can be difficult; usually blood tests show an elevated alkaline phosphatase and a profoundly low phosphorus level.

How is it treated?

Treatment is usually directed toward stabilising the blood phosphorus levels, by means of oral phosphate medications and the active Vitamin D hormone, 1,25 D3 (calcitriol) or 1-alpha D3. Although in some cases osteotomies are required to correct pronounced lower leg deformities, in other cases a dramatic response to the medication is achieved, and the lower legs straighten over several years of growth. Complications can include an associated increase in renal calcium (nephrocalcinosis) and elevated parathyroid hormone (PTH) levels. Regular monitoring of these blood tests, and ultrasound examination of the kidneys, are part of the standard care associated with this condition.

Inheritance patterns and prenatal diagnosis

Inheritance patterns

X-linked dominant. Fathers only pass the disorder to their daughters. The XLH syndrome can appear when there has been no family history of bone problems. Sometimes, in these so-called sporadic cases, tests for blood phosphorus will indicate that one parent has hypophosphatemia without any associated bone disease; alternatively there may be no apparent family history of any phosphate handling problems.

Prenatal diagnosis

This is possible, if there is a family history, although in practise it may be difficult to find a molecular biology laboratory that would provide such a service. The gene affected in this syndrome is called PHEX, and it codes for an endopeptidase associated with bone and parathyroid cells, which is believed to act on a phosphate-handling hormone.

Medical text written October 2000 by Contact a Family. Approved October 2000 by Dr A Morris. **Last reviewed August 2005 by Dr A Morris, Consultant Paediatrician with Special Interest in Metabolic disease, Willink Biochemical Genetics Unit, Royal Manchester Children's Hospital, Manchester, UK.**

Further online resources

Medical texts in *The Contact a Family Directory* are designed to give a short, clear description of specific conditions and rare disorders. More extensive information on this condition can be found on a range of reliable, validated websites. Further information on these resources can be found in our **Medical Information on the Internet** article on page 21.

Support

XLH Network

Elpha Green Cottage, Sparty Lea, Allendale, Hexham NE47 9UT   Tel: 01434 685047
e-mail: info@xlhnetwork.org   Web: http://www.xlhnetwork.org
The Network was established in 1996 as an Internet based worldwide support group. It also supports individuals and families with Autosomal Dominant Hypophosphatemic Rickets (ADHR). It offers support by telephone and letter to individuals and families who are not online and links families where possible. It has a wide range of information available, mainly on the website. The XLH Network has over 500 members worldwide, representing 41 countries, and from a continuing poll of the members, is confident that its contact base is approaching 1,000 people directly affected by XLH. The XLH Network Inc.is incorporated in the USA as a nonprofit organisation and is actively involved in understanding the basis of the bone and mineralisation disorder that links its members. Group details last updated August 2007.

XERODERMA PIGMENTOSUM

Background

Xeroderma pigmentosum (XP) is a group of rare inherited conditions that is characterised by defective repair of DNA damaged by ultraviolet light, particularly from the sun. There are at least eight different subtypes recognised, which are referred to as complementation groups A to G and XP variant. Each subtype has a different genetic abnormality and capacity to repair DNA. The subtypes show different degrees of severity.

What are the symptoms?

The condition leads to variable degrees of pigmentary change such as freckling, skin dryness, premature skin ageing and early skin cancers. The eyes can also be affected with photophobia, conjunctivitis and damage to the cornea and conjunctiva. Neurological abnormalities occur in some patients with learning disabilities, spasticity, poor co-ordination and deafness. XP patients may be of small stature and show developmental delay.

How is it treated?

The treatment for XP should include genetic counselling and rigorous protection against UV light with sunscreens, wearing of UV blocking clothing and eyewear and modification of lifestyle to minimize UV exposure. Pre-malignant skin lesions should be treated and neoplasms should be removed early. In some patients, oral Isotreteioin has been showed to delay the risk of skin cancer.

Inheritance pattterns and prenatal diagnosis

Inheritance patterns

It is inherited in an autosomal recessive pattern.

Prenatal diagnosis

This can be performed by amniocentesis. For some families earlier and more reliable results can be achieved with molecular genetic methods by performing chorionic villus sampling.

Medical text written December 1999 by Dr J Reed, Specialist Registrar, Department of Dermatology, Amersham Hospital, Amersham UK. **Last updated July 2004 by Dr. Sheru George, Consultant Dermatologist, Amersham Hospital, Amersham ,UK.**

Further online resources

Medical texts in *The Contact a Family Directory* are designed to give a short, clear description of specific conditions and rare disorders. More extensive information on this condition can be found on a range of reliable, validated websites. Further information on these resources can be found in our **Medical Information on the Internet** article on page 21.

Support

XP Support Group

2 Strawberry Close, Prestwood, Great Missenden HP16 0SG   Tel: 01494 890981
Fax: 01494 864439   e-mail: info@xpsupportgroup.org.uk
Web: http://www.xpsupportgroup.org.uk
The Group is a National Registered Charity No. 1075302, established in 1998. The group also supports those with other Ultra-Violet related disorders. It offers support by telephone and letter and links with other families and affected individuals where possible. It publishes a newsletter three times a year and has information available, details on request. There is an annual night-time camp for families to meet other families and experts in a safe environment. The Group has over 400 members.
Group details last updated August 2007.

Contact a Family produce a bi-monthly newsletter specifically aimed at parent support groups, professional workers and anybody interested in policy issues concerning rare disorders.

XYY SYNDROME

Background

XYY syndrome is a chromosomal condition which occurs only in males and is found with a frequency of 1 in 1,000. A chromosome is a rod-like structure present in the nucleus of all body cells, with the exception of the red blood cells. Chromosomes store genetic information. Normally humans have twenty-three pairs of chromosomes, forty-six chromosomes in total. The twenty-third pair, otherwise referred to as the sex chromosomes, store genetic information which determine our sex. A female has a XX pair and a male has a XY pair of chromosomes.

A male affected by XYY syndrome has an additional Y chromosome as well as the usual XY pair of chromosomes resulting in the formation of XYY. Sometimes the additional Y chromosome is present in only some of the cells of the body, but not all. This is referred to as a mosaic form of XYY syndrome. The extent to which such an individual is affected by XYY syndrome depends upon the proportion of XYY cells to XY cells throughout the body.

What are the symptoms?

The effect of having an extra Y chromosome in some or all cells varies between individuals. Some males with XYY syndrome show very few symptoms. The majority are never diagnosed whilst others may be more severely affected. Additionally, individuals may be differently affected by the severity of their features. It is not possible, therefore, to offer a precise prediction of the symptoms before or even immediately after the birth of each XYY boy.

XYY boys grow taller than average, they have a 'growth spurt' during childhood which results in an average height of 6'2". In early childhood, XYY boys are very active, with good eating and sleeping patterns. During adolescence they may experience severe acne.

In some cases, XYY males show learning difficulties, with slightly lowered intelligence scores for the group compared with XY males. They may have delayed speech development and have difficulties in communication. Boys with an extra Y chromosome seem to be at higher risk of having problems at school. However, regular assessment of educational achievement allows early intervention and helps to prevent secondary behavioural problems. Some XYY boys have obtained degrees at University.

Behavioural problems involve difficult and defiant behaviour which usually starts in childhood. Temper tantrums are common. It has been suggested that XYY males are predisposed to commit criminal acts more frequently than expected. Long-term follow-up studies are currently underway to shed more light on this issue and, to date, show that the frequency of conviction does not differ from that found in XY boys of the same level of intelligence. Sexual development is normal including development of sex organs and of secondary sex characteristics. Fertility is not affected.

Inheritance patterns and prenatal diagnosis

Inheritance patterns

XYY occurs sporadically and is not usually passed on from a XYY father to his sons.

Prenatal diagnosis

Chorionic villus sampling at ten to twelve weeks or amniocentesis at about sixteen weeks is available during pregnancy but is usually carried out only in mothers who are thirty-five or older; there is no increase in the frequency of having a boy with XYY over age 35, hence many will not be recognised.

Medical text written July 2002 by Contact a Family. **Last reviewed June 2007 by Dr S Ratcliffe, Consultant Paediatrician (Retired), Kent, UK.**

Support

Support for XYY syndrome is provided by Unique, the Rare Chromosome Support Group (see entry, Chromosome Disorders).

INDEX

The purpose of this Index is to list in alphabetical order all the conditions featured in *The Contact a Family Directory* cross-referenced to their more commonly used alternative names. All conditions shown in **Bold** have an entry in the alphabetical sections of *The Contact a Family Directory*.

Acute Idiopathic Polyneuritis see **Guillain-Barré syndrome**

Acute Inflammatory Polyneuropathy see **Guillain-Barré syndrome**

Acute Intermittent Porphyria see **Porphyria**

Acute Leukaemia see **Leukaemia and other allied blood disorders**

Acute Lymphoblastic Leukaemia see **Leukaemia and other allied blood disorders**

Acute Myeloid Leukaemia see **Leukaemia and other allied blood disorders**

Acute Pancreatitis see **Pancreatitis**

Acute Viral encephalitis see **Encephalitis**

Adams-Oliver syndrome

Addison disease

Adenine Phosphoribosyltransferase deficiency see **Purine & Pyrimidine Metabolic diseases**

Adenosine Deaminase deficiency see **Primary Immunodeficiencies**

Adenylosuccinase deficiency see **Purine & Pyrimidine Metabolic diseases**

Adipogenital Retinitis Pigmentosa-Polydactyly see **Bardet-Biedl syndrome**

Adrenal Hyperplasia see **Congenital Adrenal Hyperplasia** Adrenal Hypoplasia see **Addison disease**

Adrenoleukodystrophy

Adrenomyeloneuropathy see **Adrenoleukodystrophy**

Aganglionosis see **Hirschsprung's disease**

Agenesis of the Corpus Callosum

Agyria see **Cortical Malformations**

Aicardi syndrome

Aicardi-Goutières syndrome

Alagille's syndrome see **Liver disease**

Albinism

Albright Hereditary Osteodystrophy

Albright syndrome see **McCune-Albright syndrome**

Alexander disease

Alexander Leukodystrophy see **Alexander disease**

Alkaptonuria

Allergies

Alobar HPE see **Holoprosencephaly**

Alopecia

Alopecia Areata see **Alopecia**

Alopecia Totalis see **Alopecia**

Alopecia Universalis see **Alopecia**

Alpers disease see **Metabolic diseases** and see **Mitochondrial Cytopathies and related disorders**

Alpha One Antitrypsin deficiency see **Liver disease**

Alpha Thalassaemia/Mental Retardation on the X Chromosome

Alports syndrome see **Metabolic diseases**

Alström syndrome

Alternating Hemiplegia

Alymphocytosis see **Primary Immunodeficiencies**

Alzheimer's disease

Amblyopia see **Vision Disorders in Childhood**

Amsterdam dwarfism see **Cornelia de Lange syndrome**

Amyloidosis see **Metabolic diseases**

Amyoplasia Congenita see **Arthrogryposis**

Amyotrophic Lateral Sclerosis see **Motor Neurone disease**

Anaphylaxis

Andersen disease see **Glycogen Storage diseases**

Anderson-Fabry disease see **Fabry disease**

Androgen Insensitivity syndrome

Androgen Resistance syndrome see **Androgen Insensitivity syndrome**

Androgenetic Alopecia see **Alopecia**

Anencephaly

Angelman syndrome

Angiokeratoma Corporis Diffusum see **Fabry disease**

Aniridia

Ankylosing Spondylitis

Ano-cerebral-digital syndrome see **Pallister Hall syndrome**

Anomalous Pulmonary Venous Drainage see **Heart Defects**

Anophthalmia

Anorchia see **Congenital Absence of the Testes**

Anorchidism see **Congenital Absence of the Testes**

Anorexia Nervosa see **Eating Disorders**

Anterior Chamber Cleavage syndrome see **Peters anomaly/Peters Plus syndrome**

Anterior Uveitis see **Uveitis**

Antley Bixler syndrome see **Craniofacial**

Contact a Family Helpline 0808 808 3555

Conditions

Anxiety Disorders

Aortic Stenosis see **Heart Defects**

Apert syndrome see **Craniofacial Conditions**

Aphasia

Aplastic Anaemia (Acquired) see **Acquired Aplastic Anaemia**

Aplastic Anaemia (Congenital) see **Fanconi Anaemia**

Apoliprotein B deficiency see **Neuroacanthocytosis disorders**

Arachidonic Acid, Absence of see **Metabolic diseases**

Arboviral Encephalitides

Arginase deficiency see **Urea Cycle Disorders**

Argininosuccinate Lyase deficiency see **Urea Cycle Disorders**

Argininosuccinate Synthase deficiency see **Urea Cycle Disorders**

Argininosuccinic Aciduria see **Urea Cycle Disorders**

Arm or Hand Deficiencies see **Upper Limb Abnormalities**

Arnold Chiari Malformation see **Syringomyelia**

Aromatic Amino Acid Decarboxylase deficiency see **Metabolic diseases**

Arterial Calcification of Infancy

Arteriovenous malformations

Arteriovenous malformations of the brain see **Arteriovenous malformations**

Arthritis see **Arthritis (Adult)** or see **Arthritis (Juvenile Idiopathic)**

Arthritis (Adult)

Arthritis (Juvenile Idiopathic)

Arthrochalasia Type Ehlers-Danlos syndrome see **Ehlers-Danlos syndrome**

Arthrochalasis-Multiplex Congenita see **Ehlers-Danlos syndrome**

Arthrogryposis

Arylsulphatase A deficiency see **Metabolic diseases**

Aspartylglycosaminuria see **Mucopolysaccharide diseases and associated diseases**

Asperger syndrome see **Autism Spectrum disorders including Asperger syndrome**

Aspergillosis see **Lung diseases**

Asthma

Asymmetry Dwarfism see **Silver-Russell syndrome**

Ataxia-Telangiectasia

Athetosis see **Cerebral Palsy**

Atrial Septal Defect see **Heart Defects**

Atrioventricular Septal Defect see **Heart Defects**

Attention Deficit Disorder see **Attention Deficit Hyperactivity Disorder**

Attention Deficit Hyperactivity Disorder

Auditory Processing disorder

Aural Atresia see **Treacher Collins syndrome**

Auriculovertebral Dysplasia see **Goldenhar syndrome**

Autistic Spectrum disorders see **Autism Spectrum disorders including Asperger syndrome**

Autism see **Autism Spectrum disorders including Asperger syndrome**

Autism Spectrum disorders including Asperger syndrome

Autoimmune and inflammatory neuropathies see **Peripheral Neuropathy**

Autoimmune encephalitis see **Encephalitis**

Autoimmune Hepatitis see **Liver disease**

Autoimmune Hypothyroidism see **Thyroid Disorders**

Autoimmune neutropenia see **Neutropenia (Severe Chronic)**

Autosomal Dominant Kidney disease see **Polycystic Kidney disease**

Autosomal Recessive Kidney disease see **Polycystic Kidney disease**

BBS see **Bardet-Biedl syndrome**

BPD see **Broncho Pulmonary Dysplasia**

BRRS see **Bannayan-Riley-Ruvalcaba syndrome**

Bannayan-Riley-Ruvalcaba syndrome

Bannayan-Zonana syndrome see **Bannayan-Riley-Ruvalcaba syndrome**

Bardet-Biedl syndrome

Barth syndrome

Bartters syndrome see **Metabolic diseases**

Basal Cell Naevus syndrome see **Gorlin syndrome**

Bassen-Kornzweig syndrome see

Neuroacanthocytosis disorders

Batten disease

Becker MD see **Becker Muscular Dystrophy**

Becker Muscular Dystrophy

Beckwith-Wiedemann syndrome

Benign Intracranial Hypertension

Benign Joint Hypermobility syndrome see **Hypermobility**

Berardinelli Lipodystrophy syndrome see **Metabolic diseases**

Best disease see **Macular disease**

Beta Ketothiolase deficiency see **Metabolic diseases**

Beta-Methylcrotonylglycinuria see **Organic Acidaemias**

Bilateral Frontal Polymicrogyria see **Congenital Bilateral Perisylvian syndrome**

Bilateral Parasagittal Parietooccipital Polymicrogyria see **Congenital Bilateral Perisylvian syndrome**

Bilateral Perisylvian Polymicrogyria see **Congenital Bilateral Perisylvian syndrome**

Biliary Atresia see **Liver disease**

Biliary Hypoplasia see **Liver disease**

Biotin deficiency see **Metabolic diseases**

Bipolar Affective disorder see **Bipolar disorder**

Bipolar disorder

Birthmarks see **Vascular Birthmarks**

Blackfan Diamond syndrome see **Diamond Blackfan syndrome**

Bladder Exstrophy

Blepharospasm see **Dystonia**

Blindness see **Vision Disorders in Childhood**

Bloch-Sulzberger syndrome see **Incontinentia Pigmenti**

Bonnevie-Ullrich syndrome see **Turner syndrome**

Bloom syndrome

Brachial Plexus Paralysis see **Erb's Palsy**

Brachio-Oto-Renal syndrome see **Deafness**

Brachmann de Lange syndrome see **Cornelia De Lange syndrome**

Brain Injuries

Brain Tumours

Brainstem encephalitis see **Encephalitis**

Breughel syndrome see **Dystonia**

Brissaud II see **Tourette syndrome**

Brittle Asthma see **Asthma**

Brittle Bone diseases (Osteogenesis Imperfecta)

Broad Thumb-Great Toe syndrome see **Rubinstein Taybi syndrome**

Bronchiectasis see **Lung diseases**

Broncho Pulmonary Dysplasia

Brown-Séquard syndrome see **Spinal Injuries**

Bruton's disease see **Primary Immunodeficiencies**

Budd Chiari syndrome see **Liver disease**

Bulbar Poliomyelitis see **Poliomyelitis**

Bulimia nervosa see **Eating Disorders**

Bullous Ichthyosiform Erythroderma see **Ichthyosis**

Bulls Eye Dystrophy see **Macular disease**

Buphthalmia see **Glaucoma**

Butterfly-shaped Dystrophy see **Retinitis Pigmentosa**

C1 Esterase Inhibitor deficiency

C1 Inhibitor deficiency see **C1 Esterase Inhibitor deficiency**

CADASIL

CAH see **Congenital Adrenal Hyperplasia**

CAIS see **Androgen Insensitivity syndrome**

CATCH 22 see **22q11 Deletion syndromes**

CAVE see **Pallister Hall syndrome**

CBD see **Corticobasal Degeneration**

CBPS see **Congenital Bilateral Perisylvian syndrome**

CD40 Ligand deficiency see **Primary Immunodeficiencies**

CDH see **Congenital Dislocation and Developmental Dysplasia of the Hip**

CFC syndrome see **Cardiofaciocutaneous syndrome**

CFIDS see **Chronic Fatigue Syndrome / Myalgic Encephalmimyelitis**

CFS/ME see **Chronic Fatigue Syndrome / Myalgic Encephalmimyelitis**

CGD see **Chronic Granulomatous Disorder**

ChAc see **Neuroacanthocytosis disorders**

CHARGE association see **CHARGE syndrome**

CHARGE syndrome

Contact a Family Helpline 0808 808 3555

CHT see **Thyroid Disorders**

CIDP see **Guillain-Barré syndrome**

CINCA see **Chronic infantile neurologic cutaneous and articular syndrome**

CJD see **Creutzfeldt-Jakob disease**

CLL see **Leukaemia and other allied blood disorders**

CML see **Leukaemia and other allied blood disorders**

CMN see **Congenital Melanocytic Naevi**

CMT see **Charcot-Marie-Tooth disease**

CMV see **Cytomegalovirus**

COFS see **Cockayne syndrome**

COPD see **Lung diseases**

COX see **Metabolic diseases** and see **Mitochondrial Cytopathies and related disorders**

CPD-choline phosphotrasferase deficiency see **Purine & Pyrimidine Metabolic diseases**

CPS deficiency see **Urea Cycle Disorders**

CPT I see **Fatty Acid Oxidation Disorders**

CPT II see **Fatty Acid Oxidation Disorders**

CVID see **Primary Immunodeficiencies**

California encephalitis see **Encephalitis**

Calve-Perthes disease see **Perthes disease**

Canavan disease

Cancer

Carbamyl Phosphate Synthase see **Urea Cycle Disorders**

Carbohydrate Deficient Glycoprotein syndrome see **Congenital Disorders of Glycosylation**

Cardiofaciocutaneous syndrome

Cardiomyopathies

Carnitine Acylcarnitine Translocase deficiency see **Fatty Acid Oxidation Disorders**

Carnitine Palmitoyl-Transferase I (CPT I) deficiency see **Fatty Acid Oxidation Disorders**

Carnitine Palmitoyl-Transferase II (CPT II) deficiency see **Fatty Acid Oxidation Disorders**

Carpenter syndrome see **Craniofacial Conditions**

Cataplexy see **Narcolepsy**

Cataract-oligophrenia see **Marinesco-Sjögren syndrome**

Cataracts

Cauda Equina Lesion see **Spinal Injuries**

Cavernous Haemangioma see **Vascular Birthmarks**

Central Areolar Choroidal Dystrophy see **Retinitis Pigmentosa**

Central Core disease see **Muscular Dystrophy and neuromuscular disorders**

Central Hypoventilation syndrome see **Congenital Central Hypoventilation syndrome**

Centronuclear Myopathy see **Myotubular Myopathy**

Cerebellar Ataxia

Cerebellar Atrophy see **Friedreich's Ataxia**

Cerebellitis see **Encephalitis**

Cerebral Autosomal Dominant Arteriopathy with Subcortical Infarcts and Leucoencephalopathy see **CADASIL**

Cerebral Palsy

Cerebro-Acro-Visceral Early Lethality Multiplex syndrome see **Pallister Hall syndrome**

Cerebro-Oculo-Facio-Skeletal see **Cockayne syndrome**

Cerebro-Oculo-Muscular Dystrophy see **Cortical Malformations**

Cerebroside Lipidosis see **Gauchers disease**

Cerebrotendinous Xanthomatosis see **Metabolic diseases**

Cerebrovascular Accident see **Stroke**

Cervical Dystonia see **Dystonia**

Charcot-Marie-Tooth disease

Chediak-Higashi syndrome see **Albinism**

Chiari Malformation see **Syringomyelia**

Choledochal Cyst see **Liver disease**

Chondroectodermal Dysplasia see **Ellis-Van Creveld syndrome**

Chorea-acanthocytosis see **Neuroacanthocytosis disorders**

Choreoancanthocytosis see **Neuroacanthocytosis disorders**

Choroideraemia see **Retinitis Pigmentosa**

Christmas disease see **Haemophilia, von Willebrand disease and other coagulation defects**

Chromosome 4p- syndrome see **Wolf-Hirschhorn syndrome**

Chromosome 5 short arm deletion see **Cri du Chat syndrome**

Chromosome 5p- syndrome see **Cri du**

Chat syndrome

Chromosome 11 q- syndrome see **Jacobsen syndrome**

Chromosome 13 + syndrome see **Patau syndrome**

Chromosome 18 + syndrome see **Edwards' syndrome**

Chromosome Disorders

Chronic Bronchitis see **Lung diseases**

Chronic Degenerative Chorea see **Huntington's disease**

Chronic Fatigue and Immune Dysfunction syndrome see **Chronic Fatigue syndrome / Myalgic Encephalmimyelitis**

Chronic Fatigue syndrome / Myalgic Encephalmimyelitis

Chronic Glomerulonephritis see **Kidney disease**

Chronic Granulomatous Disorder

Chronic Idiopathic Demyelinating Polyradiculoneuropathy see **Guillain-Barré syndrome**

Chronic Idiopathic Polyneuritis see **Guillain-Barré syndrome**

Chronic infantile neurologic cutaneous and articular syndrome

Chronic Inflammatory Demylenating Polyneuropathy see **Guillain-Barré syndrome**

Chronic Iridocyclitis see **Arthritis (Juvenile Idiopathic)**

Chronic Leukaemia see **Leukaemia and other allied blood disorders**

Chronic Lymphocytic Leukaemia see **Leukaemia and other allied blood disorders**

Chronic Mucocutaneous Candidiasis see **Primary Immunodeficiencies**

Chronic Myeloid Leukaemia see **Leukaemia and other allied blood disorders**

Chronic Obstructive Pulmonary disease see **Lung diseases**

Chronic Pancreatitis see **Pancreatitis**

Ciliary Dyskinesia see **Primary Ciliary Dyskinesia**

Citrullinaemia see **Urea Cycle Disorders**

Classical Lissencephaly see **Cortical Malformations**

Classical Type Ehlers-Danlos syndrome see **Ehlers-Danlos syndrome**

Cleft Lip and/or Palate

Cleidocranial Dysostosis

Cloacal Exstrophy see **Bladder Exstrophy**

Cloverleaf Skull see **Craniofacial Conditions**

Clubfoot see **Congenital Talipes Equinovarus**

Clumsy Child syndrome see **Dyspraxia**

Coagulation Defects see **Haemophilia, von Willebrand disease and other coagulation defects**

Coarctation of the Aorta see **Heart Defects**

Coats disease

Coats' retinitis see **Coats disease**

Cobalamin C/G deficiency see **Metabolic diseases**

Cobblestone Lissencephaly see **Cortical Malformations**

Cockayne syndrome

Coeliac disease

Coffin-Lowry syndrome

Cogan's Apraxia see **Congenital Ocular Motor Apraxia**

Cohen syndrome

Coloboma

Colorado tick fever see **Encephalitis**

Common Variable Immunodeficiency see **Primary Immunodeficiencies**

Communication Disorder see **Speech and Language Impairment**

Complete Androgen Insensitivity syndrome see **Androgen Insensitivity syndrome**

Complex Regional Pain syndrome see **Reflex Sympathetic Dystrophy**

Conduct disorder **see Conduct Disorder and Oppositional Defiant disorder**

Conduct disorder and Oppositional Defiant disorder

Cone disorders see **Vision Disorders in Childhood**

Cone Dystrophy see **Macular disease**

Congenital abnormality of the iris see **Aniridia**

Congenital Absence of the Testes

Congenital Adrenal Hyperplasia

Congenital Aplastic Anaemia see **Fanconi Anaemia**

Congenital Aregenerative Anaemia see **Diamond Blackfan syndrome**

Congenital Asplenia see **Primary Immunodeficiencies**

Congenital Bilateral Perisylvian

Contact a Family Helpline 0808 808 3555

syndrome

Congenital Cataracts see **Cataracts**

Congenital Central Hypoventilation syndrome

Congenital Diaphragmatic Hernia see **Diaphragmatic Hernia**

Congenital Dislocation and Developmental Dysplasia of the Hip

Congenital Disorders of Glycosylation

Congenital Fibre Type Disproportion see **Muscular Dystrophy and neuromuscular disorders**

Congenital Heart Abnormality see **Heart Defects**

Congenital Hyperinsulinism

Congenital Hypothyroidism see **Thyroid Disorders**

Congenital Insensitivity/Indifference to Pain

Congenital Melanocytic Naevi

Congenital Microcephaly see **Microcephaly**

Congenital Mitochondrial Myopathy see **Mitochondrial Cytopathies and related disorders** and see **Muscular Dystrophy and neuromuscular disorders**

Congenital Muscular Dystrophy

Congenital Myasthenia see **Myasthenia Gravis and other Myasthenic syndromes**

Congenital Myopathies see **Muscular Dystrophy and neuromuscular disorders**

Congenital Nephrotic syndrome see **Nephrotic syndrome**

Congenital neutropenia see **Neutropenia (Severe Chronic)**

Congenital Ocular Motor Apraxia

Congenital Pancreatic Insufficiency with neutropenia and Growth Failure see **Shwachman syndrome**

Congenital porphyria see **Porphyria**

Congenital Pseudarthrosis of the Tibia see **Lower Limb abnormalities**

Congenital Short Femur see **Lower Limb abnormalities**

Congenital Suprabulbar Paresis see **Worster-Drought syndrome**

Congenital Talipes Equinovarus

Congenital Telangiectatic Erythema see **Bloom syndrome**

Congenital Tibia Recurvatum see **Lower Limb abnormalities**

Conradi-Hunermann syndrome

Cooley's Anaemia see **Thalassaemia Major (ß Thalassaemia)**

Coprolalia Generalised Tic see **Tourette syndrome**

Cori disease see **Glycogen Storage diseases**

Corneal Dystrophies see **Vision Disorders in Childhood**

Cortical Blindness see **Vision Disorders in Childhood**

Cortical Malformations

Cornelia De Lange syndrome

Corticobasal Degeneration

Costello syndrome

Cot Death

Cowden disease

Cowden syndrome see **Cowden disease**

Coxa Plana see **Perthes disease**

Cranial Dystonia see **Dystonia**

Craniocarpotarsal Dystrophy see **Freeman Sheldon syndrome**

Craniofacial Conditions

Craniopharyngioma see **Pituitary Disorders**

Craniostenosis see **Craniofacial Conditions**

Craniosynostosis see **Craniofacial Conditions**

Cranium Bifida see **Spina Bifida**

Cree encephalitis see **Aicardi-Goutières syndrome**

Crescentic Glomerulonephritis see **Glomerulonephritis**

Creutzfeldt-Jakob disease

Cri du Chat syndrome

Crigler-Najjar syndrome see **Liver disease**

Crohn's disease and Ulcerative Colitis

Crouzon disease

Cushing syndrome/disease

Cutaneous Porphyrias see **Porphyria**

Cutaneous Mastocytosis see **Mastocytosis**

Cutis Hyperelastica see **Ehlers-Danlos syndrome**

Cutis Laxa

Cutis Marmorata Telangiectasia Congenita syndrome see **M-CMTC syndrome**

Cyclical neutropenia see **Neutropenia (Severe Chronic)**

Cyclical Vomiting

Cystic Dysplasia see **Kidney disease**

Cystic Encephalomalacia see **Porencephaly**

Cystic Fibrosis

Cystic Hygroma

Cystinosis see **Metabolic diseases**

Cystinuria see **Metabolic diseases**

Cytochrome C Oxydase deficiency see **Metabolic diseases** and see **Mitochondrial Cytopathies and related disorders**

Cytomegalovirus

D+HUS see **Haemolytic Uraemic syndrome**

DAF syndrome see **Niemann-Pick disease**

DAMP see **Attention Deficit Hyperactivity Disorder**

DDH see **Congenital Dislocation and Developmental Dysplasia of the Hip**

DGS see **22q11 Deletion syndromes**

DHPA see **Purine & Pyrimidine Metabolic diseases**

DHPD see **Purine & Pyrimidine Metabolic diseases**

DM see **Dermatomyositis and Polymyositis**

DRS see **Duane Retraction syndrome**

Dancing Eye syndrome

Darier disease

De Lange 1 syndrome see **Cornelia de Lange syndrome**

De Morsiers syndrome see **Septo-Optic Dysplasia**

Deafblindness

Deafness

Deficiency of HLA Expression see **Primary Immunodeficiencies**

Degos disease

Dejerine-Sottas disease see **Muscular Dystrophy and neuromuscular disorders**

Dementia, Hereditary Multi-infarct Type see **CADASIL**

Dementia in Children

Dementia with Lewy bodies see **Dementias**

Dementias

Depression in children and young people

Dermatitis Herpetiformis see **Coeliac disease**

Dermatomyositis and Polymyositis

Dermatosparaxis Type Ehlers-Danlos syndrome see **Ehlers-Danlos syndrome**

Developmental Delay see **Global Developmental Delay**

Developmental Dysplasia of the Hip see **Congenital Dislocation and Developmental Dysplasia of the Hip**

Diabetes Insipidus see **Pituitary Disorders**

Diabetes - Maturity Onset Diabetes of the Young

Diabetes Mellitus

Diabetic neuropathy see **Peripheral Neuropathy**

Diamond Blackfan syndrome

Diaphragmatic Hernia

Diaphyseal Aclasis see **Hereditary Multiple Exostoses**

Diastrophic Dwarfism see **Diastrophic Dysplasia**

Diastrophic Dysplasia

DiGeorge syndrome see **22q11 Deletion syndromes**

Dihyropyrimidine dehydrogenase deficiency see **Purine & Pyrimidine Metabolic diseases**

Dihyropyrimidinase deficiency see **Purine & Pyrimidine Metabolic diseases**

Dilated Cardiomyopathy see **Cardiomyopathies**

Distal Muscular Dystrophy see **Muscular Dystrophy and neuromuscular disorders**

Donohue syndrome see **Metabolic diseases**

Double Inlet Ventricular see **Heart Defects**

Down syndrome

Down syndrome with Heart Defect

Duane Retraction syndrome

Duane syndrome see **Duane Retraction syndrome**

Dubowitz syndrome

Duchenne Muscular Dystrophy

Duncan's syndrome see **Primary Immunodeficiencies**

Durands syndrome see **Mucopolysaccharide diseases and associated diseases**

Dyscalculia

Dyskeratosis Congenita

Dyslexia

Dysmyelination see **Metabolic diseases**

Contact a Family Helpline 0808 808 3555

Dysphasia see **Aphasia**
Dyspraxia
Dystonia
Dystrophia Myotonica see **Myotonic Dystrophy/Congenital Myotonic Dystrophy**
Dystrophic Epidermolysis Bullosa see **Epidermolysis Bullosa**

E.Coli 0157 infection see **Haemolytic Uraemic syndrome**
EB Simplex see **Epidermolysis Bullosa**
EDS see **Ehlers-Danlos syndrome**
EMG syndrome see **Beckwith-Wiedemann syndrome**
Eagle-Barrett syndrome see **Prune Belly syndrome**
Early Infantile Epileptic Encephalopathy see **Ohtahara syndrome**
Eastern equine encephalitis see **Encephalitis**
Eating Disorders
Ectodermal Dysplasia
Eczema
Edwards' syndrome
Ehlers-Danlos syndrome
Ellis-Van Creveld syndrome
Emery-Dreifuss disease see **Muscular Dystrophy and neuromuscular disorders**
Emphysema see **Lung diseases**
Encephalitis
Encephalofacial Angiomatosis see **Sturge-Weber syndrome**
Enchondromatosis see **Ollier disease**
Endocardial Fibroelastosis see **Metabolic diseases**
Enthesitis-related Arthritis see **Arthritis (Juvenile Idiopathic)**
Eosinophilic granuloma see **Histiocytosis**
Epidemic Neuromyasthenia see **Chronic Fatigue Syndrome / Myalgic Encephalmimyelitis**
Epidermal Naevus syndrome see **Hemimegalencephaly**
Epidermolysis Bullosa
Epilepsy
Epilepsy syndromes in Childhood
Epispadias see **Bladder Exstrophy**
Epispadias Complex see **Bladder Exstrophy**
Erb's Palsy

Erythrogenesis imperfecta see **Diamond Blackfan syndrome**
Erythromelalgia see **Raynaud's Phenomenon**
Erythropoietic Protoporphyria see **Porphyria**
Ethylmalonic Aciduria see **Metabolic diseases**
Ethylmalonic Adipic Aciduria see **Metabolic diseases**
Eulenberg's disease see **Muscular Dystrophy and neuromuscular disorders**
Exomphalos see **Abdominal Exstrophies**
Exomphalos-Macroglossia-Gigantism see **Beckwith-Wiedemann syndrome**
Exostoses see **Hereditary Multiple Exostoses**
Exstropy/Epispadias Complex see **Bladder Exstrophy**
Extended Oligoarthritis see **Arthritis (Juvenile Idiopathic)**
Exudative retinitis see **Coats disease**
Exudative retinopathy see **Coats disease**
Eye Defects see **Vision Disorders in Childhood**

FAS see **Fetal Alcohol Spectrum disorder**
FCMD see **Cortical Malformations**
FCS syndrome see **Costello syndrome**
FG syndrome see **Opitz-Kaveggia syndrome/FG syndrome**
FJHN see **Purine & Pyrimidine Metabolic diseases**
FOP see **Fibrodysplasia Ossificans Progressiva**
FSHD see **Facioscapulohumeral Muscular Dystrophy**
FTLD see **Frontotemporal Lobar degeneration including Frontotemporal Dementia**
Fabry-Anderson disease see **Fabry disease**
Fabry disease
Facial Difference
Facial Disfigurement see **Facial Difference**
Facioauriculovertebral Spectrum see **Goldenhar syndrome**
Faciocutaneoskeletal syndrome see **Costello syndrome**
Facioscapulohumeral Muscular

Contact a Family Helpline 0808 808 3555

Dystrophy

Facioscapuloperoneal Muscular Dystrophy
see **Facioscapulohumeral Muscular
Dystrophy**

Factor V Leiden see **Hereditary
Thrombophilia**

Familial Combined Hyperlipidaemia see
Familial Hyperlipidaemias

Familial Dysautonomia

Familial Haemorrhagic Telangiectasia
see **Hereditary Haemorrhagic
Telangiectasia**

Familial Hypercholesterolaemia see
Familial Hyperlipidaemias

Familial Hyperlipidaemias

Familial Hypertriglyceridaemia see **Familial
Hyperlipidaemias**

Familial Juvenile Hyperuricaemia
Nephropathy see **Purine & Pyrimidine
Metabolic diseases**

Familial Rectal Pain see **Paroxysmal
extreme pain disorder**

Familial Spastic Paraplegia

Familial Splenic Anaemia see **Gauchers
disease**

Fanconi anaemia

Fanconi's anaemia see **Fanconi anaemia**

Fatty Acid Oxidation Disorders

Female Androgenetic Alopecia see
Alopecia

Female pattern hair loss see **Alopecia**

Feminising Testes syndrome see
Androgen Insensitivity syndrome

Femoral Torsion see **Lower Limb
abnormalities**

Fetal Abnormality

Fetal Alcohol Spectrum disorder

Fetal Alcohol Syndrome see **Fetal Alcohol
Spectrum disorder**

Fetal Anti-Convulsant syndrome

Fibrodysplasia Ossificans Progressiva

Fibrosing Alveolitis see **Lung diseases**

Fibrous Dysplasia see **Brittle Bone
diseases (Osteogenesis Imperfecta)**

Fibular Hemimelia see **Hemimelia**

Fingerprint Body Myopathy see **Muscular
Dystrophy and neuromuscular
disorders**

First Arch syndrome see **Treacher Collins
syndrome**

Fisher syndrome see **Guillain-Barré
syndrome**

Fish Odour syndrome see **Metabolic
diseases**

Fits and Faints see **Reflex Anoxic
Seizures**

Floating-Harbor syndrome

Focal and Segmental Glomeruloschlerosis
see **Glomerulonephritis**

**Focal Dermal Hypoplasia (Goltz
syndrome)**

Foetal Abnormality see **Fetal Abnormality**

Foetal Alcohol syndrome see **Fetal Alcohol
syndrome**

Foetal Anti-Convulsant syndrome see **Fetal
Anti-Convulsant syndrome**

Fong's disease see **Nail-Patella syndrome**

Forbes disease see **Glycogen Storage
diseases**

Fragile X syndrome

Franceschetti-Klein see **Treacher Collins
syndrome**

Freeman Sheldon syndrome

Friedreich's Ataxia

Frontal Lobe Degeneration see
**Frontotemporal Lobar degeneration
including Frontotemporal Dementia**

Frontotemporal Dementia **see
Frontotemporal Lobar degeneration
including Frontotemporal Dementia**

**Frontotemporal Lobar degeneration
including Frontotemporal Dementia**

Fructose Intolerance, Hereditary see
Metabolic diseases

Fructose 1/6 Dyphosphatase deficiency
see **Metabolic diseases**

Fucosidosis see **Mucopolysaccharide
diseases and associated diseases**

Fukuyama Congenital Muscular Dystrophy
see **Cortical Malformations**

G syndrome see **Opitz G/BBB syndrome**

GDD see **Global Developmental Delay**

GOSHS see **Goldberg-Shprinzten
syndrome**

Galactokinase deficiency see **Metabolic
diseases**

Galactosaemia

Gangliosidosis GM1 see **Metabolic
diseases**

Gangliosidosis GM2 see **Metabolic
diseases**

Gastro-oesophageal reflux see **Gut
Motility Disorders**

Contact a Family Helpline 0808 808 3555

Gastroschisis see **Abdominal Exstrophies**
Gauchers disease
Gender Identity disorder
Genital Herpes Simplex see **Herpes Virus Infection**
Genetic Haemochromatosis see **Haemochromatosis**
Gilbert-Dreyfus syndrome see **Androgen Insensitivity syndrome**
Gilberts disease see **Metabolic diseases**
Gilles de la Tourette syndrome see **Tourette syndrome**
Gitelman's disease see **Metabolic diseases**
Glanzmann's Thrombasthenia
Glaucoma
Gliomas see **Brain Tumours**
Global Developmental Delay
Global Disaccharide Intolerance see **Metabolic diseases**
Glomerulonephritis
Glucose-6-Phosphate Dehydrogenase deficiency see **Metabolic diseases**
Glucose Galactose Malabsorption deficiency see **Metabolic diseases**
Glutaric Aciduria Type I see **Organic Acidaemias**
Glutaric Aciduria Type II see **Metabolic diseases**
Glutathion Synthetase deficiency see **Metabolic diseases**
Glycerol Kinase deficiency see **Metabolic diseases**
Glycogen Storage diseases
Goldberg-Maxwell syndrome see **Androgen Insensitivity syndrome**
Goldberg-Shprinzten syndrome
Goldberg-Shprinzten megacolon syndrome see **Goldberg-Shprinzten syndrome**
Goldenhar syndrome
Goltz syndrome see **Focal Dermal Hypoplasia (Goltz syndrome)**
Gonadal Dysgenesis (XO) see **Turner syndrome**
Gorlin-Goltz syndrome see **Gorlin syndrome**
Gorlin syndrome
Gout see **Arthritis (Adult)**
Granulomatous disease see **Chronic Granulomatous Disorder**
Graves' disease see **Thyroid Disorders**
Graves' Eye disease see **Thyroid Eye disease**
Graves' Ophthalmopathy see **Thyroid Eye disease**
Group B Streptococcus
Growth Hormone deficiency
Guanidinoacetic Acid Methyltransferase deficiency see **Metabolic diseases**
Guillain-Barré syndrome
Guinon's Myospasia Impulsiva see **Tourette syndrome**
Gut Motility Disorders

HAE see **C1 Esterase Inhibitor deficiency**
HCH See **Hypochondroplasia**
HCM see **Cardiomyopathies**
HGG see **Primary Immunodeficiencies**
HGPRT deficiency see **Lesch Nyhan syndrome**
HH see **Hypothalmic Hamartoma**
HHH see **Metabolic diseases**
HHT see **Hereditary Haemorrhagic Telangiectasia**
HIV Infection and AIDS
HLH see **Histiocytosis**
HLHS see **Hypoplastic Left Heart syndrome**
HME see **Hemimegalencephaly**
HMG CoA Lyase deficiency see **Organic Acidaemias**
HMS see **Hypermobility**
HOCM see **Cardiomyopathies**
HOOD see **Nail-Patella syndrome**
HPE see **Holoprosencephaly**
HPRT see **Lesch Nyhan syndrome**
HSAN see **Congenital Insensitivity/ Indifference to Pain**
HSAN Type I see **Congenital Insensitivity/ Indifference to Pain**
HSAN Type II see **Congenital Insensitivity/Indifference to Pain**
HSAN Type III see **Congenital Insensitivity/Indifference to Pain**
HSAN Type IV see **Congenital Insensitivity/Indifference to Pain**
HSCR cleft palate-mental retardation see **Goldberg-Shprinzten syndrome**
HSP see **Henoch Schonlein Purpura**
Haemangiomas see **Vascular Birthmarks**
Haemochromatosis
Haemolytic Uraemic syndrome
Haemophagocytic Lymphohistiocytosis see **Histiocytosis**

Haemophilia, von Willebrand disease and other coagulation defects

Haemorrhagic nodular glycolipid lipidosis see **Fabry disease**

Hallervorden-Spatz syndrome see **Neuroacanthocytosis disorders**

Hand Schuller Christian syndrome see **Histiocytosis**

Harlequin Ichthyosis see **Ichthyosis**

Hartnup disease see **Metabolic diseases**

Hashimoto's disease see **Thyroid Disorders**

Hashimoto's Encephalitis

Head Injuries see **Brain Injuries**

Heart and Heart/Lung Transplant

Heart Defects

Hemifacial Microsomia see **Goldenhar syndrome**

Hemimegalencephaly

Hemimelia

Hemiplegia

Henoch Schonlein Purpura

Hepatitis A see **Liver disease**

Hepatitis B see **Liver disease**

Hepatitis C see **Liver disease**

Hepatoblastoma see **Liver disease**

Hereditary oligophrenic cerebellolental degeneration see **Marinesco-Sjögren syndrome**

Hereditary and Sensory Autonomic Neuropathy see **Congenital Insensitivity/ Indifference to Pain**

Herediary Angiodema see **C1 Esterase Inhibitor deficiency**

Hereditary Coproporphyria see **Porphyria**

Hereditary Haemorrhagic Telangiectasia

Hereditary Motor and Sensory Neuropathy see **Charcot-Marie-Tooth disease**

Hereditary Multiple Exostoses

Hereditary Orotic Aciduria see **Purine & Pyrimidine Metabolic diseases**

Hereditary-Osteo-Onycho-Dysplasia see **Nail-Patella syndrome**

Hereditary Progressive Arthro-Ophthalmopathy see **Stickler syndrome**

Hereditary Renal Hypouricaemia see **Purine & Pyrimidine Metabolic diseases**

Hereditary Spastic Paraplegia see **Familial Spastic Paraplegia**

Hereditary Thrombophilia

Hermansky-Pudlak syndrome see **Albinism**

Herpes Simplex encephalitis see **Encephalitis**

Herpes Simplex Virus Infection see **Herpes Virus Infection**

Herpes Virus Infection

Hers disease see **Glycogen Storage diseases**

Hexosaminidase A deficiency see **Metabolic diseases**

Hind Brain Malformation see **Syringomyelia**

Hirschsprung Disease-Microcephaly-Mental Retardation syndrome see **Mowat-Wilson syndrome**

Hirschsprung's disease

Histiocytosis

Histiocytosis X see **Histiocytosis**

Hodgkin's disease see **Lymphoma**

Holocarboxylase deficiency see **Organic Acidaemias**

Holoprosencephaly

Holt-Oram syndrome

Homocystinuria see **Metabolic diseases**

Homozygous Beta Thalassaemia see **Thalassaemia Major (ß Thalassaemia)**

Horner syndrome see **Erb's Palsy**

Hunter syndrome see **Mucopolysaccharide diseases and associated diseases**

Huntington's Chorea see **Huntington's disease**

Huntington's disease

Hurler Scheie see **Mucopolysaccharide diseases and associated diseases**

Hurler syndrome see **Mucopolysaccharide diseases and associated diseases**

Hydranencephaly

Hydrocephalus

Hydrophthalmia see **Glaucoma**

Hydroxicarboxylic Aciduria see **Metabolic diseases**

Hyobetalipoproteinaemia see **Neuroacanthocytosis disorders**

Hyobetalipoproteinemia see **Neuroacanthocytosis disorders**

Hyperactivity see **Attention Deficit Hyperactivity Disorder**

Hyperammonaemia see **Metabolic diseases**

Contact a Family Helpline 0808 808 3555

Hyperargininaemia see **Urea Cycle Disorders**

Hypercalcaemia Hypocalcinuria see **Metabolic diseases**

Hypercalcinuria see **Metabolic diseases**

Hypercarotinaemia see **Metabolic diseases**

Hypercholesterolaemia see **Metabolic diseases**

Hyperchylomicronaemia see **Metabolic diseases**

Hyperekplexia

Hyperexplexia see **Hyperekplexia**

Hyperglycinaemia see **Metabolic diseases**

Hyper IgE syndrome see **Primary Immunodeficiencies**

Hyper IgM syndrome see **Primary Immunodeficiencies**

Hyperinsulinism see **Metabolic diseases**

Hyperkinetic disorder see **Attention Deficit Hyperactivity Disorder**

Hyperlipidaemia see **Metabolic diseases**

Hyperlipoproteinaemia see **Metabolic diseases**

Hypermobility

Hypermobility Type Ehlers-Danlos syndrome see **Ehlers-Danlos syndrome**

Hyperornithinaemia see **Metabolic diseases**

Hyperornithinaemia-Hyperammonaemia-Homocitrullinaemia see **Metabolic diseases**

Hyperoxaluria (Type 1) see **Metabolic diseases**

Hyperprolinaemia see **Metabolic diseases**

Hypertelorism see **Craniofacial Conditions**

Hypertelorism-hypospadias syndrome see **Opitz G/BBB syndrome**

Hyperthyroidism see **Thyroid Disorders**

Hypertriglyceridaemia see **Metabolic diseases**

Hypertrophic Cardiomyopathy see **Cardiomyopathies**

Hypertrophic Obstructive Cardiomyopathy see **Cardiomyopathies**

Hypobetalipoprotinaemia see **Metabolic diseases**

Hypochondrodysplasia see **Hypochondroplasia**

Hypochondroplasia

Hypogammaglobulinaemia see **Primary Immunodeficiencies**

Hypoglycaemia see **Metabolic diseases**

Hypolipoproteinaemia see **Metabolic diseases**

Hypomania see **Bipolar disorder**

Hypomelanosis of Ito

Hypomelanosis (Pigmentary Mosaicism) see **Hypomelanosis of Ito**

Hypoparathyroidism see **Metabolic diseases**

Hypophosphatasia see **Metabolic diseases**

Hypophosphatemic Rickets see **X-Linked Hypophosphatemia**

Hypoplastic Congenital Anaemia see **Diamond Blackfan syndrome**

Hypoplastic Left Heart syndrome

Hypoprothrombinaemia see **Metabolic diseases**

Hypospadias

Hypothalmic Hamartoblastoma syndrome see **Pallister Hall syndrome**

Hypothalmic Hamartoma

Hypothyroidism see **Thyroid Disorders**

Hypotonia

Hypoxanthine Guanine Phosphoribosyl Transferase deficiency see **Lesch Nyhan syndrome**

Hypoxanthine Phosphoribosyltransferase see **Purine & Pyrimidine Metabolic diseases**

I Cell disease see **Mucopolysaccharide diseases and associated diseases**

IHSS see **Cardiomyopathies**

ILS see **Cortical Malformations**

ITD see **Dystonia**

ITP see **Immune (Idiopathic) Thrombocytopenic Purpura**

Ichthyosis

Ichthyosis Vulgaris see **Ichthyosis**

idic (15) see **Isodicentric 15**

Idiopathic Erythroblastopenia see **Diamond Blackfan syndrome**

Idiopathic Hypertrophic Sub-Aortic Stenosis see **Cardiomyopathies**

Idiopathic Intracranial Hypertension see **Benign Intracranial Hypertension**

Idiopathic Juvenile Osteoporosis see **Osteoporosis (Juvenile)**

Idiopathic Leukoderma see **Vitiligo**

Contact a Family Helpline 0808 808 3555

Idiopathic Neonatal Hepatitis see **Liver disease**

Idiopathic neutropenia see **Neutropenia (Severe Chronic)**

Idiopathic Torsion Dystonia see **Dystonia**

IgA Nephropathy see **Glomerulonephritis**

Immotile Cilia syndrome see **Primary Ciliary Dyskinesia**

Immunoglobulin Light Chain deficiency see **Primary Immunodeficiencies**

Immune (Idiopathic) Thrombocytopenic Purpura

Incomplete Androgen Insensitivity see **Androgen Insensitivity syndrome**

Incontinentia Pigmenti

Incontinentia Pigmenti Acromians see **Hypomelanosis of Ito**

Infantile Neuroaxonal Dystrophy see **Metabolic diseases**

Infantile Paralysis see **Poliomyelitis**

Infantile Spasms see **West syndrome**

Infectious encephalitis see **Encephalitis**

Infective Myositis see **Muscular Dystrophy and neuromuscular disorders**

Inherited Disciform Macular Degeneration see **Retinitis Pigmentosa**

Inosine triphosphate pyrophosphohydrolase deficiency see **Purine & Pyrimidine Metabolic diseases**

Insulin Dependence see **Diabetes Mellitus**

Intellectual disability see **Learning disability**

Interleukin deficiency see **Primary Immunodeficiencies**

Intoeing see **Lower Limb Abnormalities**

Intraocular Inflamation see **Uveitis**

Inverted Duplication 15 see **Isodicentric 15**

Iritis see **Uveitis**

Irritable Bowel syndrome

Isodicentric 15

Isolated Lissencephaly Sequence see **Cortical Malformations**

Isolated Premature Thelarche see **Premature Sexual Maturation**

Isovaleric Acidaemia see **Organic Acidaemia**

Ito syndrome see **Hypomelanosis of Ito**

Ivemark syndrome

JDM see **Dermatomyositis and Polymyositis**

JPM see **Dermatomyositis and Polymyositis**

Jackknife Convulsions see **West syndrome**

Jacobsen syndrome

Jansky-Bielschowsky disease (late infantile Type) see **Batten disease**

Japanese Encephalitis see **Arboviral Encephalitides**

Jerking Stiff Person syndrome see **Stiff Man syndrome**

Jervell-Lange-Nielson syndrome see **Long QT syndrome**

Job's syndrome see **Primary Immunodeficiencies**

Joubert syndrome

Junctional EB see **Epidermolysis Bullosa**

Juvenile Dermatomyositis see **Dermatomyositis and Polymyositis**

Juvenile Dystonic Lipidosis see **Niemann-Pick disease**

Juvenile Idiopathic Arthritis see **Arthritis (Juvenile Idiopathic)**

Juvenile Nephronopthisis see **Kidney disease**

Juvenile Osteoporosis see **Osteoporosis (Juvenile)**

Juvenile Polymyositis see **Dermatomyositis and Polymyositis**

KID syndrome see **Ichthyosis**

Kabuki Make-Up syndrome see **Kabuki syndrome**

Kabuki syndrome

Kallman syndrome see **Pituitary Disorders**

Kartagener syndrome see **Primary Ciliary Dyskinesia**

Kawasaki disease

Kawasaki syndrome see **Kawasaki disease**

Kearns-Sayre disease see **Metabolic diseases** and see **Mitochondrial Cytopathies and related disorders**

Keller syndrome see **Opitz-Kaveggia/ FG Syndrome**

Keratoconus

Kidney disease

Kinsbourne syndrome see **Dancing Eye syndrome**

Kleeblattschäedel syndrome see **Craniofacial Conditions**

Klein-Waardenburg syndrome see **Waardenburg syndrome**

Contact a Family Helpline 0808 808 3555

Klinefelter syndrome
Klippel-Feil syndrome
Klippel-Trenaunay syndrome
Klumpke's Paralysis see **Erb's Palsy**
Kohlers disease see **Perthes disease**
Kohlmeier-Degos disease see **Degos disease**
Krabbe disease
Krabbe Leukodystrophy see **Krabbe disease**
Krause-Kivlin syndrome see **Peters anomaly/Peters Plus syndrome**
Kufs disease (adult type) see **Batten disease**
Kugelberg-Welander disease see **Spinal Muscular Atrophy**
Kyphoscoliosis Type Ehlers-Danlos syndrome see **Ehlers-Danlos syndrome**

LCA see **Leber's Congenital Amaurosis**
LCAD see **Fatty Acid Oxidation Disorders**
LCH see **Histiocytosis**
LCHAD see **Fatty Acid Oxidation Disorders**
LEMS see **Myasthenia Gravis and other Myasthenic syndromes**
LFL see **Li-Fraumeni syndrome**
LFS see **Li-Fraumeni syndrome**
LIMD see **Mitochondrial Cytopathies and related disorders**
LOTS see **Tay Sachs disease**
Lactic Acidosis see **Metabolic diseases** and see **Mitochondrial Cytopathies and related disorders**
Lafora Body disease see **Metabolic diseases**
Lambert-Eaton Myasthenia syndrome see **Myasthenia Gravis and other Myasthenic syndromes**
Lamellar Ichthyosis see **Ichthyosis**
Landau-Kleffner syndrome
Landouzy-Dejerine see **Facioscapulohumeral Muscular Dystrophy**
Landry's Ascending Paralysis see **Guillain-Barré syndrome**
Langer-Giedion syndrome
Langerhans Cell Histiocytosis see **Histiocytosis**
Language Disorder see **Speech and**

Language Impairment
Larsen syndrome
Laryngeal Dystonia see **Dystonia**
Late Onset Tay Sachs disease see **Tay Sachs disease**
Laurence-Moon-Bardet-Biedl syndrome see **Bardet-Biedl syndrome**
Laurence-Moon-Biedl see **Bardet-Biedl syndrome**
Learning Disability
Learning Problem see **Dyslexia**
Leber's Amaurosis see **Leber's Congenital Amaurosis**
Leber's Congenital Amaurosis
Leber's Hereditary Optic Neuropathy
Leber's Optic Atrophy see **Leber's Hereditary Optic Neuropathy**
Leber's Optic Neuropathy see **Leber's Hereditary Optic Neuropathy**
Leg length discrepancy see **Lower Limb abnormalities**
Legg-Calve-Perthes disease see **Perthes disease**
Leigh's disease see **Leigh syndrome**
Leigh's Encephalopathy see **Leigh syndrome**
Leigh syndrome
Lejeune syndrome see **Cri du Chat syndrome**
Lennox-Gastaut syndrome
Leprechaunism see **Metabolic diseases**
Leroy syndrome (ML II) see **Mucopolysaccharide diseases and associated diseases**
Lesch Nyhan syndrome
Lethal Infantile Mitochondrial disease see **Mitochondrial Cytopathies and related disorders**
Letterer Siwe disease see **Histiocytosis**
Leukaemia and other allied blood disorders
Leukocyte Adhesion Defect Type II see **Congenital Disorders of Glycosylation**
Leukodystrophy see **Metabolic diseases**
Levine-Critchley syndrome see **Neuroacanthocytosis**uscular
Li-Fraumeni syndr~~ ~~omuscular
Limb Girdle Defects see **Lower Limb**
D~~

Contact a Family Helpline 0808 808 3555

Abnormalities

Limbic encephalitis see **Encephalitis**

Linear Naevus Sebaceous syndrome see
Hemimegalencephaly

Lipodystrophy see **Metabolic diseases**

Lissencephaly see **Cortical Malformation**

Liver disease

Lobar HPE see **Holoprosencephaly**

Localised Nodular Myosotis see **Muscular
Dystrophy and neuromuscular
disorders**

Long Chain Acyl deficiency see **Fatty Acid
Oxidation Disorders**

Long Chain Hydroxyacyl-CoA
Dehydrogenase (LCHAD) deficiency
see **Fatty Acid Oxidation Disorders**

Long QT syndrome

Louping ill Virus see **Arboviral
Encephalitides**

Lowe syndrome

Lower Limb abnormalities

Lower Limb deficiency see **Lower Limb
abnormalities**

Lower limb reduction defects see **Lower
Limb abnormalities**

Lub's syndrome see **Androgen
Insensitivity syndrome**

Luft disease see **Mitochondrial
Cytopathies and related disorders**

Lung diseases

Lung Transplant see **Heart and Heart/
Lung Transplant**

Lupus

Lymphocytic Interstitial Pneumonitis see
HIV Infection and AIDS

Lymphoedema

Lymphoedema-Distichiasis syndrome see
Lymphoedema

Lymphoma

MAD see **Fatty Acid Oxidation Disorders**

MCAD see **Fatty Acid Oxidation
Disorders**

M-CMTC syndrome

MDA see **Purine & Pyrimidine Metabolic
Diseases**

MDC1C s... Dy... Congenital Muscular
Dystroph...

MDS see Cortical... ital Muscular

ME see Chronic F...

...ns

Myalgic Encephalopathy

MEB see **Congenital Muscular Dystrophy**
and **Cortical Malformations**

MED see **Perthes disease**

MELAS see **Metabolic diseases** and
see **Mitochondrial Cytopathies and
related disorders**

MEN I see **Multiple Endocrine Neoplasia
Type I**

MEN II see **Multiple Endocrine Neoplasia
Type II**

MEN IIA see **Multiple Endocrine
Neoplasia Type II**

MEN IIB see **Multiple Endocrine
Neoplasia Type II**

MERRF see **Mitochondrial Cytopathies
and related disorders**

MG see **Myasthenia Gravis and other
Myasthenic syndromes**

MH see **Malignant Hyperthermia**

MICS see **Aicardi-Goutières syndrome**

ML I see **Mucopolysaccharide diseases
and associated diseases**

ML II see **Mucopolysaccharide diseases
and associated diseases**

ML III see **Mucopolysaccharide diseases
and associated diseases**

ML IV see **Mucopolysaccharide diseases
and associated diseases**

MMD see **Moya Moya disease**

MNGIE see **Mitochondrial Cytopathies
and related disorders**

MODY see **Diabetes - Maturity Onset
Diabetes of the Young**

MOP see **Fibrodysplasia Ossificans
Progressiva**

MOPD II see **Majewski Osteodysplastic
Primordial Dwarfism Type II**

MPHD see **Growth Hormone deficiency**

MPS I see **Mucopolysaccharide diseases
and associated diseases**

MPS II see **Mucopolysaccharide
diseases and associated diseases**

MPS III see **Mucopolysaccharide
diseases and associated diseases**

MPS IV see **Mucopolysaccharide
diseases and associated diseases**

MPS VI see **Mucopolysaccharide
diseases and associated diseases**

MPS VII see **Mucopolysaccharide
diseases and associated diseases**

MS see **Multiple Sclerosis**

Contact a Family Helpline 0808 808 3555

MSA see **Multiple System Atrophy**

MTAP see **Purine & Pyrimidine Metabolic diseases**

MURCS see **Klippel-Feil syndrome**

Macrocephaly – Cutis Marmorata Telangiectasia Congenita syndrome see **M-CMTC syndrome**

Macrocephaly, Multiple Lipomas and Haemangioma see **Bannayan-Riley-Ruvalcaba syndrome**

Macular degeneration see **Macular disease**

Macular disease

Macular Dystrophy see **Macular disease**

Majewski Osteodysplastic Primordial Dwarfism Type II

Male balding see **Alopecia**

Male pattern hair loss see **Alopecia**

Male Pseudo-Hermaphroditism see **Androgen Insensitivity syndrome**

Malignant Atrophic Papulosis see **Degos disease**

Malignant Histiocytosis see **Histiocytosis**

Malignant Hyperpyrexia see **Malignant Hyperthermia**

Malignant Hyperthermia

Mandibulo Dysostosis see **Treacher Collins syndrome**

Manic depression see **Bipolar disorder**

Mannosidosis see **Mucopolysaccharide diseases and associated diseases**

Maple Syrup Urine disease see **Organic Acidaemias**

Marfan syndrome

Marinesco-Garland syndrome see **Marinesco-Sjögren syndrome**

Marinesco-Sjögren syndrome

Marinesco-Sjögren-Garland syndrome see **Marinesco-Sjögren syndrome**

Maroteaux Lamy see **Mucopolysaccharide diseases and associated diseases**

Mastocytosis

McArdle disease see **Glycogen Storage diseases**

McCune-Albright syndrome

McLeod Neuroacanthocytosis syndrome see **Neuroacanthocytosis disorders**

McLeod syndrome see **Neuroacanthocytosis disorders**

Mediterranean Anaemia see **Thalassaemia Major (ß Thalassaemia)**

Medium-chain acyl-CoA dehydrogenase (MCAD) deficiency see **Fatty Acid Oxidation Disorders**

Medulloblastomas see **Brain Tumours**

Meige syndrome see **Dystonia**

Melorheostosis

Melnick-Needles syndrome

Membranous Nephropathy see **Glomerulonephritis** and **Nephrotic syndrome**

Ménière's disease

Meniere's disease see **Ménière's disease**

Meningitis

Meningoencephalitis see **Encephalitis**

Menkes see **Metabolic diseases**

Mental Health

Mental Handicap see **Learning Disability**

Metachromatic Leukodystrophy see **Metabolic diseases**

Metabolic diseases

Metatarsus Adductus see **Lower Limb abnormalities**

Methionine Adenosyl Transferase see **Metabolic diseases**

Methionine Synthetase deficiency see **Metabolic diseases**

Methylenetetrahydrofolate Reductase deficiency see **Metabolic diseases**

Methylmalonic Aciduria see **Organic Acidaemias**

Methylthioadenosine Phosphorylase Deficiency see **Purine & Pyrimidine Metabolic diseases**

Microcephaly

Microcephaly-intracranial calcification syndrome see **Aicardi-Goutières syndrome**

Microlissencephaly see **Cortical Malformations**

Microphthalmia see **Anophthalmia**

Microphthalmus see **Coloboma**

Migraine

Miller-Dieker syndrome see **Cortical Malformations**

Miller-Fisher syndrome see **Guillain-Barré syndrome**

Milroy disease see **Lymphoedema**

Minimal Change disease see **Nephrotic syndrome**

Mitochondrial Complex I see **Metabolic diseases**

Mitochondrial Complex 2/3 see **Metabolic**

diseases and see **Mitochondrial Cytopathies and related disorders**

Mitochondrial Cytopathies and related disorders

Mitochondrial DNA Mutations see **Mitochondrial Cytopathies and related disorders**

Mitochondrial deficiency see **Metabolic diseases**

Mitochondrial diseases see **Mitochondrial Cytopathies and related disorders**

Mitochondrial Encephalomyopathy see **Metabolic diseases** and see **Mitochondrial Cytopathies and related disorders**

Mitochondrial Fatty Oxidase Disorders see **Mitochondrial Cytopathies and related disorders**

Mitochondrial mi (maternal inheritance) DNA see **Metabolic diseases** and see **Mitochondrial Cytopathies and related disorders**

Mitochondrial Myopathy see **Mitochondrial Cytopathies and related disorders** and see **Muscular Dystrophy and neuromuscular disorders**

Mitochondrial Myopathy, Encephalopathy, Lactic Acidosis and Mitoketothiolase deficiency see **Metabolic diseases**

Möbius syndrome see **Moebius syndrome**

Moebius syndrome

Molybdenum co-factor deficiency see **Metabolic diseases**

Molybdenum co-factor deficiency - Combined XOD/sulphate oxidase deficiency see **Purine & Pyrimidine Metabolic diseases**

Mononeuritis Multiplex see **Peripheral Neuropathy**

Mononeuropathy see **Peripheral Neuropathy**

Monosomy X see **Turner syndrome**

Morbus Coats' see **Coats disease**

Morquio see **Mucopolysaccharide diseases and associated diseases**

Morris's syndrome see **Androgen Insensitivity syndrome**

Motor Impairment see **Cerebral Palsy**

Motor Neurone disease

Mowat-Wilson syndrome

Moya Moya disease

Moyamoya disease see **Moya Moya disease**

Mucocutaneous Lymph Node syndrome see **Kawasaki disease**

Mucolipidosis see **Mucopolysaccharide diseases and associated diseases**

Mucopolysaccharide diseases and associated diseases

Mucosal Neuroma syndrome see **Multiple Endocrine Neoplasia Type II**

Muenke syndrome see **Craniofacial Conditions**

Multi-Infarct Dementia see **Dementias**

Multicystic Encephalomalacia see **Hydranencephaly**

Multiple Acyl-CoA Dehydrogenase (MAD) deficiency (= Glutaric aciduria type II, GA II) see **Fatty Acid Oxidation Disorders**

Multiple Births see **Twins with Special Needs/Multiple Births**

Multiple Carboxylase deficiency see **Metabolic diseases**

Multiple Endocrine Neoplasia Type I

Multiple Endocrine Neoplasia Type II

Multiple Epiphyseal dysplasia

Multiple Hamartoma syndrome see **Cowden disease**

Multiple Myeloma see **Leukaemia and other allied blood disorders**

Multiple Osteochondromatosis see **Hereditary Multiple Exostoses**

Multiple Pituitary Hormone deficiency see **Growth Hormone deficiency**

Multiple Sclerosis

Multiple Sulphatase deficiency see **Mucopolysaccharide diseases and associated diseases**

Multiple System Atrophy

Muscle-Eye-Brain disease see **Cortical Malformations**

Muscular Dystrophy and neuromuscular disorders

Muscular Sub-Aortic Stenosis see **Cardiomyopathies**

Myalgic Encephalomyelitis see **Chronic Fatigue syndrome / Myalgic Encephalopathy**

Myasthenia Gravis and other Myasthenic syndromes

Myasthenic-Myopathic syndrome see **Myasthenia Gravis and other Myasthenic syndromes**

Contact a Family Helpline 0808 808 3555

Mycoplasma encephalitis see **Encephalitis**

Myoadenylate Deaminase see **Purine & Pyrimidine Metabolic diseases**

Myoclonic Encephalopathy see **Dancing Eye syndrome**

Myoclonic Epilepsy and Ragged-Red Fibre's see **Mitochondrial Cytopathies and related disorders**

Myoneurogastrointestinal Disorder and Encephalopathy see **Mitochondrial Cytopathies and related disorders**

Myopia see **Vision Disorders in Childhood**

Myositis see **Dermatomyositis and Polymyositis**

Myositis Ossificans Progressiva see **Fibrodysplasia Ossificans Progressiva**

Myotonia Congenita see **Muscular Dystrophy and neuromuscular disorders**

Myotonic Dystrophy/Congenital Myotonic Dystrophy

Myotubular Myopathy

NAGS deficiency see **Urea Cycle Disorders**

NARP see **Mitochondrial Cytopathies and related disorders**

NBCCS see **Gorlin syndrome**

NOMID see **Chronic infantile neurologic cutaneous and articular syndrome**

NPS see **Nail-Patella syndrome**

N-acetyl glutamate synthase see **Urea Cycle Disorders**

Naevus Flammus see **Vascular Birthmarks**

Nager syndrome

Nail-Patella syndrome

Narcolepsy

Necrotising Fasciitis

Nemaline Myopathy see **Muscular Dystrophy and neuromuscular disorders**

Neonatal Death see **Stillbirths and Neonatal Deaths**

Neonatal Haemochromatosis see **Liver disease**

Neonatal Hepatitis see **Liver disease**

Neonatal Hypoglycemia-Visceromegaly-Macroglossia-Microcephaly see **Beckwith-Wiedemann syndrome**

Neonatal Onset Multisystem Inflammatory Disease see **Chronic infantile neurologic cutaneous and articular syndrome**

Nephrogenic Diabetes Insipidus see **Pituitary Disorders**

Nephronopthisis see **Kidney disease**

Nephrotic syndrome

Nesidioblastosis see **Congenital Hyperinsulinism**

Netherton disease see **Netherton syndrome**

Netherton syndrome

Neural Tube Defect see **Spina Bifida**

Neuroacanthocytosis see **Neuroacanthocytosis disorders**

Neuroacanthocytosis disorders

Neuroblastoma

Neurodevelopmental Regression in Children see **Dementia in Children**

Neurofibromatosis

Neuronal Ceroid Lipofuscinosis Type 1 (infantile) see **Batten disease**

Neuronal Ceroid Lipofuscinosis Type 2 (late infantile) see **Batten disease**

Neuronal Ceroid Lipofuscinosis Type 3 (juvenile) see **Batten disease**

Neuropathy, Ataxia and Retinitis Pigmentosa see **Mitochondrial Cytopathies and related disorders**

Neurovisceral Storage disease see **Niemann-Pick disease**

Neutral Lipid Storage disease see **Ichthyosis**

Neutropenia (Severe Chronic)

Nevilles disease see **Niemann-Pick disease**

Nevoid basal cell carcinoma syndrome see **Gorlin syndrome**

Niemann-Pick disease

Non-Bullous Ichthyosiform Erythroderma see **Ichthyosis**

Non-Epileptic Seizures see **Reflex Anoxic Seizures**

Non-Hodgkin's Lymphoma see **Lymphoma**

Noonan syndrome

Normal Pressure Hydrocephalus

Norman-Roberts syndrome see **Cortical Malformations**

Norrie disease

Nuclear DNA Mutations see **Mitochondrial Cytopathies and related disorders**

Nystagmus

OCD see **Obsessive Compulsive disorder**

OMIM 609460 see **Goldberg-Shprinzten syndrome**

OSMED see **Stickler syndrome**

OTC deficiency see **Urea Cycle Disorders**

Obsessive Compulsive disorder

Obstetric Brachial Plexus Palsy see **Erb's Palsy**

Occlusive Infantile Arteriopathy see **Metabolic diseases**

Occupational Lung diseases see **Lung diseases**

Ocular Albinism see **Albinism**

Ocular Muscular Dystrophy see **Muscular Dystrophy and neuromuscular disorders**

Ocular Myasthenia see **Myasthenia Gravis and other Myasthenic syndromes**

Oculopharyngeal Muscular Dystrophy see **Muscular Dystrophy and neuromuscular disorders**

Oculoauriculovertebral Dysplasia see **Goldenhar syndrome**

Oculo-Cerebro-Renal syndrome see **Lowe syndrome**

Oculo-cutaneous Albinism see **Albinism**

Oesophageal Atresia see **Tracheo-Oesophageal Fistula and/or Oesophageal Atresia**

Ohdo Blepharophimosis syndrome see **Ohdo syndrome**

Ohdo syndrome

Ohtahara syndrome

Oligoarthritis see **Arthritis (Juvenile Idiopathic)**

Olivopontocerebellar Atrophy see **Metabolic diseases**

Ollier disease

Omenn's syndrome see **Primary Immunodeficiencies**

Ondine's see **Congenital Central Hypoventilation syndrome**

Ondine's Curse see **Congenital Central Hypoventilation syndrome**

Opitz FG syndrome see **Optiz-Kaveggia/ FG syndrome**

Opitz G/BBB syndrome

Opitz-Frias syndrome see **Opitz G/BBB syndrome**

Opitz-Kaveggia / FG syndrome

Oppositional Defiant disorder see **Conduct Disorder disorder and Oppositional Defiant disorder**

Opsoclonus-Myoclonus see **Dancing Eye syndrome**

Optic Nerve hypoplasia

Organic Acidaemias

Ornithinaemia see **Metabolic diseases**

Ornithine Transcarbamylase see **Urea Cycle Disorders**

Oromandibular Dystonia see **Dystonia**

Osgood Schlatter disease see **Perthes disease**

Osler-Rendu-Weber see **Hereditary Haemorrhagic Telangiectasia**

Osteoarthritis see **Arthritis (Adult)**

Osteochondritis of the Upper Femoral Epiphysis see **Perthes disease**

Osteodysplasia see **Melnick-Needles syndrome**

Osteodysplasty see **Melnick-Needles syndrome**

Osteogenesis Imperfecta see **Brittle Bone diseases (Osteogenesis Imperfecta)**

Osteopetrosis

Osteoporosis see **Osteoporosis (Adult)** and see **Osteoporosis (Juvenile)**

Osteoporosis (Adult)

Osteoporosis (Juvenile)

Oto-Spondylo-Megaepiphyseal Dysplasia see **Stickler syndrome**

Oxygen Dependency see **Broncho Pulmonary Dysplasia**

PAIS see **Androgen Insensitivity syndrome**

PANDAS see **Sydenham Chorea**

PAVMs see **Hereditary Haemorrhagic Telangiectasia**

PBP see **Motor Neurone disease**

PCOS see **Polycystic Ovary syndrome**

PCT see **Porphyria**

PDA see **Pathalogical Demand Avoidance syndrome**

PDA see **Heart Defects**

PDH see **Metabolic diseases** and see **Mitochondrial Cytopathies and related disorders**

PEHO syndrome

PEO see **Mitochondrial Cytopathies and related disorders**

Contact a Family Helpline 0808 808 3555

PEPCK see **Mitochondrial Cytopathies and related disorders**

PFFD see **Lower Limb abnormalities**

PFIC see **Liver disease**

PHHI see **Congenital Hyperinsulinism**

PHP see **Albright Hereditary Osteodystrophy**

PID see **Primary Immunodeficiencies**

PKAN see **Neuroacanthocytosis disorders**

PKD see **Polycystic Kidney disease**

PKU see **Phenylketonuria**

PLS see **Motor Neurone disease**

PM see **Dermatomyositis and Polymyositis**

PMA see Motor Neurone disease

PMG see **Cortical Malformations**

PNFA see **Frontotemporal Lobar degeneration including Frontotemporal Dementia**

PNP see **Purine & Pyrimidine Metabolic diseases**

PPH see **Primary Pulmonary Hypertension**

PR PS see **Purine & Pyrimidine Metabolic diseases**

PSP see **Progressive Supranuclear Palsy**

PVFS see **Chronic Fatigue Syndrome / Myalgic Encephalmimyelitis**

PVNH see **Cortical Malformations**

PXE see **Pseudoxanthoma Elasticum**

Pachygyria see **Lissencepahly**

Paediatric Autoimmune Neuropsychiatric disorder associated with Streptococcus see **Sydenham Chorea**

Paediatric HIV Infection see **HIV Infection and AIDS**

Paget Disease

Paget's Disease of Bone see **Paget Disease**

Pallid Infantile Syncope see **Reflex Anoxic Seizures**

Pallister Hall syndrome

Pallister-Killian syndrome

Pancreatitis

Panic Attack see **Anxiety Disorders**

Pantothenate Kinase-associated Neurodegeneration see **Neuroacanthocytosis disorders**

Panuveitis see **Uveitis**

Paramyotonia Congenita see **Muscular Dystrophy and neuromuscular disorders**

Paraneoplastic encephalitis see **Encephalitis**

Paraneoplastic Pemphigus see **Pemphigus Vulgaris**

Paraplegia see **Spinal Injuries**

Parkinson's disease

Paroxysmal extreme pain disorder

Partial Androgen Insensitivity syndrome see **Androgen Insensitivity syndrome**

Patau syndrome

Pathalogical Demand Avoidance syndrome

Pearson syndrome see **Mitochondrial Cytopathies and related disorders**

Pelizaeus-Merzbacher disease

Pemphigus Foliaceus see **Pemphigus Vulgaris**

Pemphigus Vulgaris

Pendred syndrome

Perceptuo-Motor Dysfunction see **Dyspraxia**

Peripheral Neuropathy

Periventricular Nodular Heterotopia see **Cortical Malformations**

Peroneal Muscular Atrophy see **Charcot-Marie-Tooth disease**

Peroxisomal Defects see **Metabolic diseases**

Persistent Ductus Arteriosus see **Heart Defects**

Persistent Hyperinsulinaemic Hypoglycaemia of Infancy see **Congenital Hyperinsulinism**

Persistent Oligoarthritis see **Arthritis (Juvenile Idiopathic)**

Perthes disease

Peters anomaly/Peters Plus syndrome

Peters Plus syndrome see **Peters anomaly/Peters Plus syndrome**

Petit Mal see **Epilepsy**

Pfeiffer syndrome see **Craniofacial Conditions**

Phenosulphotransferase P deficiency see **Metabolic diseases**

Phenylketonuria

Phobia see **Anxiety Disorders**

Phosphoenolpyruvate Carboxykinase deficiency see **Mitochondrial Cytopathies and related disorders**

Phosphoribosylpyrophospate Synthetase

Superactivity see **Purine & Pyrimidine Metabolic diseases**

Phosphorylation diseases see **Mitochondrial Cytopathies and related disorders**

Pick's disease see **Frontotemporal Lobar degeneration including Frontotemporal Dementia**

Pierre Robin sequence see **Pierre Robin syndrome**

Pierre Robin syndrome

Pigmentary Mosaicism see **Hypomelanosis of Ito**

Pitt-Rogers-Danks syndrome see **Wolf-Hirschhorn syndrome**

Pituitary Disorders

Pneumocystic Carinii Pneumonia see **HIV Infection and AIDS**

Pneumocystis Pneumonia see **HIV Infection and AIDS**

Poland syndrome

Poliomyelitis

Polyarthritis see **Arthritis (Juvenile Idiopathic)**

Polyarticular Arthritis see **Arthritis (Juvenile Idiopathic)**

Polycystic Kidney disease

Polycystic Ovarian disease see **Polycystic Ovary syndrome**

Polycystic Ovary syndrome

Polymalgia Rheumatica see **Arthritis (Adult)**

Polymicrogyria see **Cortical Malformations**

Polymyositis see **Dermatomyositis and Polymyositis**

Polyneuropathy see **Peripheral Neuropathy**

Pompe disease

Porencephaly

Porphyria

Porphyria - Protoporphyria Proto see **Porphyria**

Porphyria Cutanea Tarda see **Porphyria**

Port Wine Stains see **Vascular Birthmarks**

Post-infectious encephalitis see **Encephalitis**

Post infectious Radiculoneuropathy see **Guillain-Barré syndrome**

Post-Polio syndrome see **Poliomyelitis**

Post Viral Fatigue syndrome see **Chronic Fatigue Syndrome / Myalgic**

Encephalmimyelitis

Posterior Uveitis see **Uveitis**

Potassium channel antibody encephalitis see **Encephalitis**

Potter Syndrome

Powassan virus see **Arboviral Encephalitides**

Prader-Willi syndrome

Precocious Puberty see **Premature Sexual Maturation**

Pre-eclampsia

Pre-eclamptic Toxaemia see **Pre-eclampsia**

Premature Adrenarch see **Premature Sexual Maturation**

Premature Babies see **Prematurity and sick newborn**

Premature Sexual Maturation

Prematurity and sick newborn

Primary Ciliary Dyskinesia

Primary Focal Dystonia see **Dystonia**

Primary Gout see **Purine & Pyrimidine Metabolic diseases**

Primary Haemophagocytic Lymphohistiocytosis see **Histiocytosis**

Primary Immunodeficiencies

Primary Lateral Sclerosis see **Motor Neurone disease**

Primary Progressive Aphasia see **Frontotemporal Lobar degeneration including Frontotemporal Dementia**

Primary Pulmonary Hypertension

Primary Red Cell Anaemia see **Diamond Blackfan syndrome**

Primary (systemic) Carnitine deficiency see **Fatty Acid Oxidation Disorders**

Progeria see **Metabolic diseases**

Progressive Bulbar Palsy see **Motor Neurone disease**

Progressive External Opthalmoplegia see **Mitochondrial Cytopathies and related disorders**

Progressive Familial Intrahepatic Cholestasis see **Liver disease**

Progressive Hypertrophic Interstitial Polyneuropathy see **Muscular Dystrophy and neuromuscular disorders**

Progressive Muscular Atrophy see **Motor Neurone disease**

Progressive Non-Fluent Aphasia see **Frontotemporal Lobar degeneration**

Contact a Family Helpline 0808 808 3555

including **Frontotemporal Dementia**
Progressive Supranuclear Palsy
Prolactinoma see **Pituitary Disorders**
Properdin deficiency see **Primary Immunodeficiencies**
Propionic Acidaemia see **Organic Acidaemias**
Proteus syndrome
Prothrombin Gene Mutation see **Hereditary Thrombophilia**
Proximal Focal Femoral deficiency see **Lower Limb abnormalities**
Prune Belly syndrome
Pseudo TORCH syndrome see **Aicardi-Goutières syndrome**
Pseudo Achondroplasia see **Restricted Growth**
Pseudo Hurler Polydystrophy see **Mucopolysaccharide diseases and associated diseases**
Pseudo Tumour Cerebri see **Benign Intracranial Hypertension**
Pseudoachondroplasia see **Restricted Growth**
Pseudocholinesterase deficiency see **Metabolic diseases**
Pseudohypoaldosteronism see **Metabolic diseases**
Pseudohypoparathyroidism Type 1a see **Albright Hereditary Osteodystrophy**
Pseudohypoparathyroidism Types 1b & 2 see **Metabolic Diseases**
Pseudopseudo Hypoparathyroidism see **Metabolic diseases**
Pseudoxanthoma Elasticum
Psoriasis
Psoriatic Arthritis see **Arthritis (Juvenile Idiopathic)**
Psoriatic Arthropathy
Psoriatic Spondylitis see **Psoriatic Arthropathy**
Pulmonary Arteriovenous malformations see **Arteriovenous malformations**
Pulmonary Fibrosis see **Lung diseases**
Pulmonary Hypertension of the newborn
Pulmonary Stenosis see **Heart Defects**
Purine & Pyrimidine Metabolic diseases
Purine Metabolism see **Purine & Pyrimidine Metabolic diseases**
Purine Nucleoside Phosphorylase deficiency see **Purine & Pyrimidine Metabolic diseases**

Pyrimidine 5' - nucleotidase deficiency see **Purine & Pyrimidine Metabolic diseases**
Purtillo's syndrome see **Primary Immunodeficiencies**
Pyridoxine Dependent Vitamin B deficiency see **Metabolic diseases**
Pyroglutamic Aciduria see **Metabolic diseases**
Pyruvate Dehydrogenase Complex deficiency see **Metabolic diseases** and see **Mitochondrial Cytopathies and related disorders**
Pyruvate Dehydrogenase deficiency see **Metabolic diseases** and see **Mitochondrial Cytopathies and related disorders**
Pyruvate Kinase deficiency see **Metabolic diseases**

RE see **Rasmussen's Encephalitis**
RSMD1 see **Congenital Muscular Dystrophy**
RSV see **Lung diseases**
Radial Hemimelia see **Hemimelia**
Rasmussen's encephalitis
Raynaud's Phenomenon
Reading Disorders see **Dyslexia**
Recessive Spino-cerebellar Degeneration see **Friedreich's Ataxia**
Reflex Anoxic Seizures
Reflex Sympathetic Dystrophy
Refsum's disease see **Ichthyosis**
Reifenstein syndrome see **Androgen Insensitivity syndrome**
Relapsing Polychondritis
Renal Failure see **Kidney disease**
Rendu-Osler-Weber see **Hereditary Haemorrhagic Telangiectasia**
Respiratory Chain Disorders see **Mitochondrial Cytopathies and related disorders**
Respiratory Syncytial Virus see **Lung diseases**
Restricted Growth
Reticular Dysgenesis see **Primary Immunodeficiencies**
Retinal Dystrophy see **Vision Disorders in Childhood**
Retinitis Pigmentosa
Retinoblastoma
Retinopathy see **Vision Disorders in**

Childhood

Rett syndrome

Reye syndrome

Rheumatoid Arthritis see **Arthritis (Adult)**
or see **Arthritis (Juvenile Idiopathic)**

Rhinitis see **Allergies**

Rhizomelic Chondrodysplasia Punctata see **Restricted Growth**

Right Atrial Isomerism see **Ivemark syndrome**

Riley-Day syndrome see **Metabolic diseases**

Riley-Smith syndrome see **Bannayan-Riley-Ruvalcaba syndrome**

Robin Anomalad see **Pierre Robin syndrome**

Rod Disorders see **Vision Disorders in Childhood**

Rod with Cone Disorders see **Vision Disorders in Childhood**

Romano-Ward syndrome see **Long QT syndrome**

Rosai-Dorfman disease see **Histiocytosis**

Rubella

Rubella Panencephalitis see **Encephalitis**

Rubinstein Taybi syndrome

Russell-Silver syndrome see **Silver-Russell syndrome**

Russian spring-summer encephalitis see **Arboviral Encephalitides**

Ruvalcaba-Myhre-Smith syndrome see **Bannayan-Riley-Ruvalcaba syndrome**

SCAD see **Fatty Acid Oxidation Disorders**

SCH see **Cortical Malformations**

SCID see **Primary Immunodeficiencies**

SD see **Frontotemporal Lobar degeneration including Frontotemporal Dementia**

SED see **Restricted Growth**

SIDS see **Cot Death**

SLE see **Lupus**

SLOS see **Smith-Lemli-Opitz syndrome**

SMA see **Spinal Muscular Atrophy**

SMS see **Stiff Man syndrome**

SOD see **Septo-Optic Dysplasia**

SSPE see **Subacute-Sclerosing Panencephalitis**

S-adenosylhomocysteine hydolase deficiency see **Purine & Pyrimidine**

Metabolic diseases

Saccade Initiation Failure see **Congenital Ocular Motor Apraxia**

Sacral Agenesis

Saethre-Chotzen see **Craniofacial Conditions**

Sagital Craniosynostosis see **Craniofacial Conditions**

Salaam attacks see **West syndrome**

Sandhoff's disease see **Metabolic diseases**

Sanfilippo see **Mucopolysaccharide diseases and associated diseases**

Santavuori disease see **Batten disease**

Santavuori-Haltia disease (infantile) see **Batten disease**

Sarcoidosis

Scapulohumeral Dystrophy see **Muscular Dystrophy and neuromuscular disorders**

Scapuloperoneal Dystrophy see **Muscular Dystrophy and neuromuscular disorders**

Schilder's disease see **Adrenoleukodystrophy**

Scheie see **Mucopolysaccharide diseases and associated diseases**

Scheurmanns disease see **Perthes disease**

Schilder's disease see **Metabolic diseases**

Schizencephaly see **Cortical Malformations**

Schizophrenia

Scleroderma

Scoliosis

Second Arch syndrome see **Treacher Collins syndrome**

Secondary Arthritis see **Arthritis (Adult)**

Secondary Haemophagocytic Lymphohistiocytosis see **Histiocytosis**

Segawa's syndrome see **Dystonia**

Seizures (epileptic) see **Epilepsy**

Seizures (anoxic) see **Reflex Anoxic Seizures**

Selective IgA deficiency see **Primary Immunodeficiencies**

Selective Mutism

Semantic Dementia see **Frontotemporal Lobar degeneration including Frontotemporal Dementia**

Semilobar HPE see **Holoprosencephaly**

Septo-Optic Dysplasia

Contact a Family Helpline 0808 808 3555

Serum Cholinesterase deficiency see **Metabolic diseases**

Severe Combined Immune deficiency see **Primary Immunodeficiencies**

Severs disease see **Perthes disease**

Short-Chain Acyl-CoA Dehydrogenase (SCAD) deficiency see **Fatty Acid Oxidation Disorders**

Short Stature see **Restricted Growth**

Shprintzen syndrome see **22q11 Deletion syndromes**

Shwachman-Diamond syndrome

Shwachman syndrome see **Shwachman-Diamond syndrome**

Shy Drager syndrome see **Multiple System Atrophy**

Sialic Acid Storage disease see **Mucopolysaccharide diseases and associated diseases**

Sialidosis see **Mucopolysaccharide diseases and associated diseases**

Sickle Cell Anaemia see **Sickle Cell disorders**

Sickle Cell disorders

Sick New Born Babies see **Prematurity and sick newborn**

Silver-Russell syndrome

Silver's syndrome see **Silver-Russell syndrome**

Sinus-Histiocytosis with Massive Lymphadenopathy see **Histiocytosis**

Sipple syndrome see **Multiple Endocrine Neoplasia Type I**

Sjögren-Larsson syndrome see **Ichthyosis**

Sjogren-Larsson syndrome see **Ichthyosis**

Sjögren syndrome

Sjogren syndrome see **Sjögren syndrome**

Sly see **Mucopolysaccharide diseases and associated diseases**

Small Eye see **Coloboma**

Smith-Lemli-Opitz syndrome

Smith Magenis syndrome

Sotos syndrome

Spasmodic Torticollis see **Dystonia**

Spasticity see **Cerebral Palsy**

Speech and Language Impairment

Sphingomyelin Lipidosis see **Niemann-Pick disease**

Spina Bifida

Spina Bifida Cystica see **Spina Bifida**

Spina Bifida Occulta see **Spina Bifida**

Spinal Cord Injury see **Spinal Injuries**

Spinal Injuries

Spinal Muscular Atrophy

Spondylo Epiphyseal Dysplasia see **Restricted Growth**

Spongiform Leukodystrophy see **Metabolic diseases**

Squint see **Vision Disorders in Childhood**

St Louis encephalitis, see **Encephalitis**

Stammering

Stargardt disease see **Stargardt Macular Dystrophy**

Stargardt Macular Dystrophy

Startle disease see **Hyperekplexia**

Steele Richardson Olszewski syndrome see **Progressive Supranuclear Palsy**

Stein-Leventhal syndrome see **Polycystic Ovary syndrome**

Steinert's disease see **Myotonic Dystrophy/Congenital Myotonic Dystrophy**

Steroid Sulphatase deficiency with Icthiosis and Microcephaly with Global Delay see **Metabolic diseases**

Stickler syndrome

Stiff Limb syndrome see **Stiff Man syndrome**

Stiff Man syndrome

Stillbirths and Neonatal Deaths

Stills disease see **Arthritis (Juvenile Idiopathic)**

Stork Marks see **Vascular Birthmarks**

Strawberry Birthmark see **Vascular Birthmarks**

Strep B see **Group B Streptococcus**

Streptococcus Agalactiae see **Group B Streptococcus**

Streptococcus (Group B) see **Group B Streptococcus**

Stroke

Stroke-like Episodes see **Metabolic diseases** and see **Mitochondrial Cytopathies and related disorders**

Strumpell disease see **Familial Spastic Paraplegia**

Sturge-Weber syndrome

Subacute-Sclerosing Panencephalitis

Sucrose Isomaltose Enzyme deficiency see **Metabolic diseases**

Sudanophilic Leukodystrophy see **Adrenoleukodystrophy**

Sudden Infant Death syndrome see **Cot Death**

Supranuclear Opthalmoplegic Lipidosis see **Niemann-Pick disease**

Sydenham Chorea

Syringomyelia

Systemic Arthritis see **Arthritis (Juvenile Idiopathic)**

Systemic Lupus Erythematosus see **Lupus**

systemic Mastocytosis see **Mastocytosis**

Systemic Sclerosis see **Scleroderma**

TAR syndrome

TB see **Tuberculosis**

TBS see **Townes-Brocks syndrome**

TPMT see **Purine & Pyrimidine Metabolic diseases**

TSC see **Tuberous Sclerosis**

TTP see **Thrombotic Thrombocytopenic Purpura**

Talipes see **Congenital Talipes Equinovarus**

Tangier disease see **Metabolic diseases**

Tauri disease see **Glycogen Storage diseases**

Tay Sachs disease

T-cell Activation deficiency see **Primary Immunodeficiencies**

T-cell Receptor deficiency see **Primary Immunodeficiencies**

Telangiectasia see **Vascular Birthmarks**

Termination of Pregnancy see **Fetal Abnormality**

Testicular Feminisation see **Androgen Insensitivity syndrome**

Tetrahydrobiopterin deficiency see **Metabolic diseases**

Tetralogy of Fallot see **Heart Defects**

Tetraplegia see **Spinal Injuries**

Thalassaemia Major (ß Thalassaemia)

Thiopurine Methyltransferase deficiency/ superactivity see **Purine & Pyrimidine Metabolic diseases**

Thomsen disease see **Muscular Dystrophy and neuromuscular disorders**

Thrombocytopenia with Absent Radii see **TAR syndrome**

Thrombotic Thrombocytopenic Purpura

Thymic Aplasia see **Primary Immunodeficiencies**

Thymoma with Hypogammaglobulinaemia see **Primary Immunodeficiencies**

Thyroid Associated Ophthalmopathy see **Thyroid Eye disease**

Thyroid Disorders

Thyroid Eye disease

Thyroid Ophthalmopathy see **Thyroid Eye disease**

Thyrotoxicosis see **Thyroid Disorders**

Tibial Hemimelia see **Hemimelia**

Tibial Torsion see **Lower Limb abnormalities**

Tic Douloureux see **Trigeminal Neuralgia**

Tick-Borne Encephalitis see **Arboviral Encephalitides**

Tinnitus

Torsten Sjögren see **Marinesco-Sjögren syndrome**

Torticollis see **Dystonia**

Tourette syndrome

Townes-Brocks syndrome

Toxic and drug induced neuropathies see **Peripheral Neuropathy**

Toxocariasis

Toxoplasmosis

Tracheo-Oesophageal Fistula and/or Oesophageal Atresia

Tracheostomy

Transcobalamin II deficiency see **Primary Immunodeficiencies**

Transient Hypogammaglobulinaemia of Infancy see **Primary Immunodeficiencies**

Transient Ischaemic Attack see **Stroke**

Transposition of Great Arteries see **Heart Defects**

Traumatic Mutism see **Selective Mutism**

Treacher Collins syndrome

Trichorhinophalangeal syndrome Type II see **Langer-Giedion syndrome**

Tricuspid Atresia see **Heart Defects**

Trifunctional Protein deficiency see **Fatty Acid Oxidation Disorders**

Trigeminal Neuralgia

Trigonocephaly see **Craniofacial Conditions**

Trimethylamineuria see **Metabolic diseases**

Triosephosphate Isomerase deficiency see **Metabolic diseases**

Triple-X syndrome

Trisomy 13 see **Patau syndrome**

Trisomy 18 see **Edwards' syndrome**

Trisomy 21 see **Down syndrome**

Contact a Family Helpline 0808 808 3555

Trisomy 21 with Heart Defect see **Down syndrome with Heart Defect**

Tryptophan Malabsorption see **Metabolic diseases**

Tuberculosis

Tuberous Sclerosis

Turcot syndrome

Turner syndrome

Turner-Kieser syndrome see **Nail-Patella syndrome**

Turner-Ullrich syndrome see **Turner syndrome**

Twins with Special Needs/Multiple Births

Tyrosinaemia Type 1 see **Liver disease**

UMP Hydrolase deficiency see **Purine & Pyrimidine Metabolic diseases**

Ulcerative Colitis see **Crohn's disease and Ulcerative Colitis**

Ullrich Congenital Muscular Dystrophy see **Congenital Muscular Dystrophy**

Ulna Hemimelia see **Hemimelia**

Undiagnosed Children

Unilateral Multilobar Polymicrogyria see **Congenital Bilateral Perisylvian syndrome**

Unilateral Perisylvian Polymicrogyria see **Congenital Bilateral Perisylvian syndrome**

Upper Limb Abnormalities

Urea Cycle Disorders

Usher syndrome

Uveitis

VACTERL Association

VATER Association see **VACTERL Association**

VCFS see **22q11 Deletion syndromes**

vCJD see **Creutzfeldt-Jakob disease**

VLCAD see **Fatty Acid Oxidation Disorders**

VSD see **Heart Defects**

VTEC 0157 infection see **Haemolytic Uraemic syndrome**

VWD see **Haemophilia, von Willebrand disease and other coagulation defects**

Variegate Porphyria see **Porphyria**

Variant Lissencephaly see **Cortical Malformations**

Vascular Birthmarks

Vein of Galen malformation

Velo-Cardio-Facial syndrome see **22q11 Deletion syndromes**

Very-Long-Chain Acyl-CoA Dehydrogenase (VLCAD) deficiency see **Fatty Acid Oxidation Disorders**

Vestibular Schwannoma see **Acoustic Neuroma**

Viral Encephalitis see **Encephalitis**

Viral Fatigue syndrome see **Chronic Fatigue Syndrome / Myalgic Encephalmimyelitis**

Vision Disorders in Childhood

Visual Impairment see **Vision Disorders in Childhood**

Vitiligo

Vitamin D Resistant Rickets see **X-Linked Hypophosphatemia**

Vitamin deficiency derived neuropathies see **Peripheral Neuropathy**

Vogt-Spielmeyer disease see **Batten disease**

Von Gierke disease see **Glycogen Storage diseases**

Von Hippel-Lindau syndrome

Von Recklinghausen's disease see **Neurofibromatosis**

Von Willebrand syndrome see **Haemophilia, von Willebrand disease and other coagulation defects**

WAGR syndrome see Aniridia

WWS see **Cortical Malformations**

Waardenburg-Hirschsprung disease see **Waardenburg syndrome**

Waardenburg syndrome

Walker-Warburg syndrome see **Congenital Muscular Dystrophy** and **Cortical Malformations**

Weil's disease see **Meningitis**

Werdnig-Hoffman disease see **Spinal Muscular Atrophy**

Wermer syndrome see **Multiple Endocrine Neoplasia Type I**

West Nile Encephalitis see **Arboviral Encephalitides**

West syndrome

Western equine encephalitis, see **Encephalitis**

Whistling Face Syndome see **Freeman Sheldon syndrome**

White Breath Holding see **Reflex Anoxic Seizures**

Wiedemann-Rautenstrauch syndrome see
Metabolic diseases
Wildervanck syndrome see **Klippel-Feil
syndrome**
Williams-Beuren syndrome see **Williams
syndrome**
Williams syndrome
Wilson's disease see **Liver disease**
Winchester syndrome see
**Mucopolysaccharide diseases and
associated diseases**
Wiskott-Aldrich syndrome see **Primary
Immunodeficiencies**
Wolf-Hirschhorn syndrome
Wolman's disease see **Metabolic diseases**
Worster-Drought syndrome
Writer's Cramp see **Dystonia**

XLA see **Primary Immunodeficiencies**
XLP see **Primary Immunodeficiencies**
XO syndrome see **Turner syndrome**
XOD see **Purine & Pyrimidine Metabolic
diseases**
XP see **Xeroderma Pigmentosum**
XXX see **Triple-X syndrome**
XXY see **Klinefelter syndrome**
XXXY see **Klinefelter syndrome**
XXXXY see **Klinefelter syndrome**
XYY syndrome
X-Linked Agammaglobulinaemia see
Primary Immunodeficiencies
X-Linked Hypophosphatemia
X-Linked Ichthyosis see **Ichthyosis**
X-Linked Lymphoproliferative syndrome
see **Primary Immunodeficiencies**
Xanthine Oxidase/Sulphite Oxidase
deficiency see **Metabolic diseases**
Xanthinuria deficiency see **Purine &
Pyrimidine Metabolic diseases**
Xeroderma Pigmentosum

Young-Simpson syndrome see **OHDO
syndrome**

Zellweger syndrome see **Metabolic
diseases**

NOTES

HOW YOU CAN HELP
Contact a Family

If you would like to learn more about how you can help Contact a Family please tick the appropriate boxes, complete the address information below and send the form to: Dept FR, Contact a Family, Freepost LON8801, London EC1B 1EE.

☐ Please send me details about the work of Contact a Family

☐ Please send me details about giving through my payroll

☐ Please send me details about making a will

☐ Please send me details about participating in sponsored events for Contact a Family

☐ Please send me details about how I can involve my employers in fundraising for Contact a Family

☐ I would like to make a donation of £.......... towards the work of Contact a Family

☐ I would like Contact a Family to reclaim tax on this donation (Contact a Family can reclaim tax at the rate of 28p in the £ on your donation provided you have paid an amount of income tax or capital gains tax at least equal to the tax the charity reclaims in this tax year)

Please then complete the following information in full.

Name (Mr/Mrs/Ms/Dr) ....

Address ....

....

Postcode .... Tel. No ....

Signature .... Date ....

☐ I am happy for Contact a Family to send me further information about the work of the charity and associated activities